RESPIRATORY CARE
PHARMACOLOGY

RESPIRATORY CARE PHARMACOLOGY

Joseph L. Rau, Jr. *PhD, RRT*

Professor and Chair
Cardiopulmonary Care Sciences
College of Health and Human Sciences
Georgia State University
Atlanta, Georgia

SIXTH EDITION

with 230 illustrations

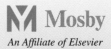
Mosby

An Affiliate of Elsevier

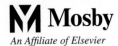

An Affiliate of Elsevier

Acquisitions Editor: **Karen Fabiano**
Developmental Editor: **Mindy Copeland**
Project Manager: **John Rogers**
Project Specialist: **Beth Hayes**
Designer: **Kathi Gosche**
Cover Illustrator: **Christine Oleksyk Perchal**

SIXTH EDITION

NOTICE

Pharmacology is an ever-changing field. Standard safety precautions must be followed, but as new research and clinical experience broaden our knowledge, changes in treatment and drug therapy may become necessary or appropriate. Readers are advised to check the most current product information provided by the manufacturer of each drug to be administered to verify the recommended dose, the method and duration of administration, and contraindications. It is the responsibility of the treating physician, relying on experience and knowledge of the patient, to determine dosages and the best treatment for each individual patient. Neither the publisher nor the editor assumes any liability for any injury and/or damage to persons or property arising from this publication.

Permissions may be sought directly from Elsevier's Health Sciences Rights Department in Philadelphia, PA, USA: phone: (+1) 215 239 3804, fax: (+1) 215 239 3805, e-mail: healthpermissions@elsevier.com. You may also complete your request on-line via the Elsevier homepage (http://www.elsevier.com), by selecting 'Customer Support' and then 'Obtaining Permissions'.

Mosby
11830 Westline Industrial Drive
St. Louis, MO 63146

Printed in the United States of America

Library of Congress Cataloging in Publication Data

Rau, Joseph L.
    Respiratory care pharmacology / Joseph L. Rau, Jr.—6th ed.
      p. ; cm.
    Includes bibliographical references and index.
    ISBN-13: 978-0-323-01696-4   ISBN-10: 0-323-01696-0
    1. Respiratory agents. 2. Respiratory therapy. I. Title.
    [DNLM: 1. Respiratory Therapy. 2. Bronchodilator Agents—administration & dosage.
    3. Bronchodilator Agents—pharmacology. WB 342 R239r 2002]
    RM388 .R383 2002
    616.2'00461—dc21   2001052104
    ISBN-13: 978-0-323-01696-4
    ISBN-10: 0-323-01696-0
    06 07 08 09 CRW 9 8 7 6 5

IN MEMORIAM

Dedicated to the memory of
Agnes S. Rau
(March 3, 1904 – March 3, 2001)

CONTRIBUTORS

HENRY COHEN, BS, MS, PharmD, BCPP
Associate Professor of Pharmacy Practice
Arnold & Marie Schwartz College of Pharmacy
  and Health Sciences
Long Island University
Director of Pharmacotherapy Education, Research,
  and Residency Programs
Department of Pharmacy and Medicine
Kingsbrook Jewish Medical Center
Brooklyn, New York

CHARLES G. DURBIN, JR., MD, FCCM
Professor of Anesthesiology and Surgery
Medical Director, Respiratory Care
University of Virginia Health System
Charlottesville, Virginia

MAMTA FULORIA, MD
Assistant Professor
Department of Pediatrics
School of Medicine
Wake Forest University
Winston-Salem, North Carolina

ERKAN HASSAN, PharmD, FCCM
Director of Pharmacotherapy Services
VISICU
Baltimore, Maryland

JUDITH JACOBI, PharmD, FCCM, FCCP, BCPS
Critical Care Pharmacist
Pharmacy Department
Methodist Hospital/Clarian Health
Indianapolis, Indiana

MANJUNATH P. PAI, PharmD
Assistant Professor
College of Pharmacy
University of New Mexico
Albuquerque, New Mexico

BRAD D. PEARCE, PhD
Assistant Professor of Psychiatry and Behavioral
  Sciences
Program in Pharmacology and Neuropathogenesis
School of Medicine
Emory University
Atlanta, Georgia

SUSAN L. PENDLAND, MS, PharmD
Assistant Professor
Department of Pharmacy Practice
College of Pharmacy
University of Illinois at Chicago
Chicago, Illinois

LIZ RAMOS, BS, PharmD
Critical Care Pharmacy Practice Resident
Kingsbrook Jewish Medical Center
Brooklyn, New York

RUBEN D. RESTREPO, MD, RRT
Assistant Professor
Cardiopulmonary Care Sciences
Georgia State University
Atlanta, Georgia

BRUCE K. RUBIN, Mengr, MD, FRCP(C)
Professor and Vice-Chair
Department of Pediatrics
Professor of Medicine, Physiology, and Pharmacology
Wake Forest University School of Medicine
Winston-Salem, North Carolina

MAHA SADEK, BS, PharmD
Geriatric Pharmacy Practice Resident
Kingsbrook Jewish Medical Center
David Minkin Rehabilitation Center
Clinical Assistant Professor of Pharmacy Practice
Arnold & Marie Schwartz College of Pharmacy
  and Health Sciences
Long Island University
Brooklyn, New York

CHRISTOPHER A. SCHRIEVER, MS, PharmD
Infectious Diseases Fellow
Department of Pharmacy Practice
College of Pharmacy
University of Illinois at Chicago
Chicago, Illinois

ROBERT D. WARHURST, PharmD
Cardiovascular Surgery Pharmacist
Methodist Hospital/Clarian Health
Indianapolis, Indiana

REVIEWERS

REGINA CLARK, MEd, RRT
Program Director
Respiratory Therapy
Northwest Mississippi Community College
Southaven, Mississippi

STANLEY M. PEARSON, MSEd, RRT, CPFT
Program Representative
Respiratory Therapy
Southern Illinois University
Carbondale, Illinois

GARY RUSHWORTH, BSRT, RRT, REMT-B
Clinical Specialist—Emergency Room
Medstar/Franklin Square
Baltimore, Maryland

STEPHEN F. WEHRMAN, RRT, RPFT
Professor
Program Director, Respiratory Care
Kapi'olani Community College
University of Hawaii
Honolulu, Hawaii

PREFACE

The goal of the sixth edition remains the same as that of the previous five editions: to offer an organized and clear compendium of current respiratory care drug information helpful for those in respiratory care. The target audience includes those who wish to understand the topics, mechanisms, and principles of action for drug groups relevant to respiratory care. Primary among this target audience is the respiratory care student. Features intended to facilitate the understanding of this area of pharmacology include a chapter summary of key terms, self-assessment questions, clinical case examples and questions, and a glossary of useful terms. Emphasis is also placed on assessing respiratory care drug therapy, in keeping with the expanded role of respiratory therapists in protocol-driven medical care.

The continuing developments in respiratory drugs, as well as related critical care drug groups, challenge practitioners, students, and authors with increasing complexity and scope of material. In this edition, contributing authors have been sought for their expertise in cardiovascular agents, neuromuscular blocking agents, antiinfective drug groups, and drugs affecting the central nervous system.

Every effort has been made to ensure the accuracy of information on drugs in this text. However, practitioners are urged to review the manufacturer's detailed literature when administering a drug and to keep informed of new information on drug therapy.

ACKNOWLEDGMENTS

The sixth edition of *Respiratory Care Pharmacology* brings with it a greater debt of acknowledgment than any previous edition. Unlike the previous editions, this edition benefits greatly from the generous contribution of individuals who are each expert in various areas of pharmacology. Their names and affiliations, too numerous to list here, are found in the list of Contributors and in the chapters they have authored. They have willingly, and at times under duress, provided invaluable material for a new revision of the text. In particular, I am grateful to Erkan Hassan, Pharm.D., for his help in identifying colleagues in pharmacology as contributors.

I am also indebted to my friend and colleague, Douglas J. Pearce, M.D., Director, Advanced Heart Failure Program, St. Thomas Heart Institute, and Clinical Assistant Professor of Medicine, Vanderbilt University, for case material found in Chapters 19 and 21. Robert Aranson, M.D., pulmonologist, former Medical Director of the Respiratory Care Program at Georgia State University and now in private practice in Maine, provided the case for Chapter 22. I am also grateful to Robert Harwood, M.S.A., R.R.T., former teaching colleague at Georgia State and now with American Biosystems, Inc., for the case material in Chapters 10 and 17.

Mindy Copeland and Karen Fabiano provided welcome editorial and personal support during the usual frustrations attendant with a new edition. I am indebted to Meryl Sheard for assistance with new illustrations in this edition. I also wish to thank unnamed reviewers for their valuable suggestions for improvement. As always, it must be said that any shortcomings of this edition are entirely my own responsibility.

As with every previous edition, the final acknowledgment must go to the students of respiratory care, whose need for knowledge has always been the primary motivation for the book.

"If I have seen further, it is by standing on the shoulders of giants."

(Isaac Newton, letter to Robert Hooke, February 5, 1675)

Joseph L. Rau, Jr., Ph.D., RRT

CONTENTS

BASIC CONCEPTS AND PRINCIPLES IN PHARMACOLOGY

CHAPTER 1

Introduction to Respiratory Care Pharmacology

Joseph L. Rau

Respiratory care pharmacology represents the application of pharmacology to the treatment of pulmonary disorders and, more broadly, critical care. Chapter 1 introduces and defines basic concepts and selected background information useful in the pharmacological treatment of respiratory disease and critical care patients.

PHARMACOLOGY AND THE STUDY OF DRUGS

The many complex functions of the human organism are regulated by chemical agents such as hormones, kinins, and catecholamines. Chemicals interact with an organism to alter its function, thus illuminating the life process and at times providing methods of diagnosis, treatment, or prevention of disease. Such chemicals are termed *drugs.* A drug is any chemical that alters the organism's functions or processes. Examples include oxygen, alcohol, lysergic acid diethylamide (LSD), heparin, epinephrine, and vitamins. The study of drugs is the subject of pharmacology, which may be defined as follows:

Pharmacology: The study of drugs (chemicals), including their origin, properties, and interactions with living organisms

Respiratory care pharmacology, broadly defined, represents the application of pharmacology to the treatment of cardiopulmonary disease and critical care. Pharmacology can be subdivided into the following more specialized topics:

Pharmacy: The preparation and dispensing of drugs
Pharmacognosy: The identification of sources of drugs, from plants and animals
Pharmacogenetics: The study of the interrelationship of genetic differences and drug effects
Therapeutics: The art of treating disease with drugs
Toxicology: The study of toxic substances and their pharmacological actions, including antidotes and poison control

The principles of drug action from dose administration to effect and clearance from the body are the subject of *drug administration, pharmacokinetics,* and *pharmacodynamics.* These topics are defined and presented in detail in Chapter 2. A summary of key developments in the regulation of drugs in the United States is given in Box 1-1.

NAMING DRUGS

Because a drug is a chemical, is officially regulated in the United States and is sold as a competitive

Box 1-1	**Legislation Affecting Drugs**

1906 The first Food and Drugs Act is passed by Congress; the United States Pharmacopeia (USP) and the National Formulary (NF) were given official status.

1914 The Harrison Narcotic Act is passed to control the importation, sale, and distribution of opium and its derivatives, as well as other narcotic analgesics.

1938 The Food, Drug, and Cosmetic Act becomes law. This is the current Federal Food, Drug, and Cosmetic Act to protect the public health and protect physicians from irresponsible drug manufacturers. This act is enforced by the Food and Drug Administration (FDA).

1952 The Durham-Humphrey Amendment defines the drugs that may be sold by the pharmacist only on prescription.

1962 The Kefauver-Harris Law is passed as an amendment to the Food, Drug, and Cosmetic Act of 1938. This act requires proof of safety and efficacy of all drugs introduced since 1938. Drugs in use before that time have not been reviewed but are under study.

1971 The Controlled Substances Act becomes effective; this act lists requirements for the control, sale, and dispensation of narcotics and dangerous drugs. Five schedules of controlled substances have been defined. Schedule I to Schedule V generally define drugs of decreasing potential for abuse, increasing medical use, and decreasing physical dependence. Examples of each schedule are as follows:

Schedule I: All nonresearch use is illegal; examples: heroin, marijuana, LSD, peyote, and mescaline

Schedule II: No telephone prescriptions, no refills; examples: opium, morphine, certain barbiturates, amphetamines

Schedule III: Prescription must be rewritten after 6 months, or five refills; examples: certain opioid doses, glutethimide (Doriden), and some other barbiturates

Schedule IV: Prescription must be rewritten after 6 months or five refills; penalties for illegal possession differ from those for Schedule III drugs; examples: phenobarbital, barbital, chloral hydrate, meprobamate (Equanil, Miltown), and zolpidem (Ambien)

Schedule V: As for any nonopioid prescription drug; examples: narcotics containing nonnarcotics in mixture form, such as cough preparations or Lomotil (diphenoxylate, narcotic with 2.5 mg and atropine sulfate, nonnarcotic).

product by various manufacturers, a drug has a variety of labels rather than a single name. A drug that becomes officially approved for general clinical use in the United States will have accumulated at least five different names: a chemical name, code name, official name, generic name, and brand (or trade) name.

Chemical name: The name indicating the drug's chemical structure.

Code name: A name assigned by a manufacturer to an experimental chemical that shows potential as a drug. An example is aerosol SCH 1000, which was the code name for ipratropium bromide, a parasympatholytic bronchodilator (see Chapter 7).

Generic name: The name assigned to a chemical by the United States Adopted Name (USAN) Council when the chemical appears to have therapeutic use and the manufacturer wishes to market the drug. Instead of a numerical or alphanumerical code, as in the code name, this name often is loosely based on the drug's chemical structure. For example, isoproterenol has an isopropyl group attached to the terminal nitrogen on the amino side chain, whereas metaproterenol is the same chemical structure as isoproterenol except that a dihydroxy attachment on the catechol nucleus is now in the so-called meta position (carbon-3,5 instead of carbon-3,4). The generic name is also known as the *nonproprietary* name, in contrast to the brand name.

Official name: In the event that an experimental drug becomes fully approved for general use and is admitted to the *United States Pharmacopeia–National Formulary* (USP-NF), the generic name becomes the official name. Because an officially approved drug may be marketed by many manufacturers under different names, it is recommended that clinicians use the official name, which is nonproprietary, and not brand names.

Trade name: This is the brand, or proprietary name, given by a particular manufacturer. For example, the generic drug named albuterol is currently marketed by Schering-Plough as Proventil and by Glaxo-Wellcome as Ventolin.

The following is an example of the different names for the drug zafirlukast, an agent intended to control asthma:

> *Code name:* ICI 204,219
> *Chemical name:* 4-(5-cyclopentyloxy-carbony-lamino-1-methyl-indol-3-ylmethyl)- 3-methoxy-*N*-O-tolylsulfonylbenzamide
> *Official name:* Zafirlukast
> *Generic name:* Zafirlukast
> *Trade name:* Accolate (Zeneca Pharmaceuticals)

SOURCES OF DRUG INFORMATION

The official volume giving drug standards in the United States is the *United States Pharmacopeia–National Formulary* (USP-NF). This text was originally produced as two separate works.

The United States Pharmacopeia (USP) was first published in 1820 as a private medical effort. It was given official status in 1906 with the first congressional Food and Drugs Act. The Pharmacopeia specifies standards for drugs such as oxygen, indicated by the USP label. The Pharmacopeia undergoes revision every 5 years.

The National Formulary (NF) was first published in 1888, with the same legal status as the USP. It is published by the United States Pharmacopeial Convention. In 1980, which was the date for revision of the USP, the USP and NF were combined into a single volume. Supplements to the USP-NF are issued periodically during the years between revisions.

Another source of drug information is the *Physician's Desk Reference* (PDR). Although prepared by manufacturers of drugs, and therefore potentially lacking the objectivity of the preceding sources, this annual volume provides useful information, including descriptive color charts for drug identification, names of manufacturers, and general drug actions.

A comprehensive and in-depth discussion of general pharmacological principles and drug classes can be found in several texts. Examples of two of these are the following, with a complete listing in the references:

- *Goodman and Gilman's The Pharmacological Basis of Therapeutics*, edition 9[1]
- *Basic & Clinical Pharmacology*, edition 7[2]

Excellent sources of information on drug products and new releases are provided by Mosby's DRUG*Consult*™ updated yearly, and the monthly subscription service *Drug Facts and Comparisons*.[3,4]

SOURCES OF DRUGS

Although the source of drugs is not a crucial area of expertise for the respiratory care clinician, it can be extremely interesting. Recognition of naturally occurring drugs dates back to Egyptian papyrus records, to the ancient Chinese, to the Central American civilizations and is still seen in remote regions of modern America, such as Appalachia.

For example, the prototype of cromolyn sodium was khellin, found in the Eastern Mediterranean plant *Ammi visnaga*, and the plant was used in ancient times as a muscle relaxant. Today its synthetic derivative is used as an antiasthmatic agent. Another example is curare, derived from large vines and used by South American Indians to coat their arrow tips for lethal effect. Digitalis is obtained from the foxglove plant *(Digitalis purpurea)*, was reputedly used by the Mayans for relief of angina, and was referred to by thirteenth-century Welsh physicians. The notorious poppy seed is the source of the opium alkaloids, immortalized in *Confessions of an English Opium Eater*. Today, the most common source of drugs is chemical synthesis, but plants, minerals, and animals have often contributed the prototype of the active ingredient. Examples of each source include the following:

Animal: Thyroid hormone, insulin, pancreatic dornase

Plant: Khellin *(Ammi visnaga)*, atropine (belladonna alkaloid), digitalis (foxglove), reserpine *(Rauwolfia serpentine)*, volatile oils of eucalyptus, pine, anise

Mineral: Copper sulfate, magnesium sulfate (epsom salts), mineral oil (liquid hydrocarbons)

PROCESS OF DRUG APPROVAL IN THE UNITED STATES

The process by which a chemical moves from the status of a promising potential drug to one fully approved by the FDA for general clinical use is, on the average, long, costly, and complex. Cost estimates vary, but in the 1980s it took an average of 13 to 15 years from chemical synthesis to marketing approval by the FDA, with a cost of $350 million in the United States.[5] The figure of $500 million is also given if failures are included in the cost analysis, because only one of thousands of potential drugs reach general approval. Cost analysis is heavily dependent on premises and what is included or excluded, and these figures are debated.[6] The cost of clinical trials for FDA approval has been given as $25 million, and if adjusted for failures, this figure reaches $56 million.[6]

The major steps in the drug approval process are reviewed by Flieger[7] and Hassall and Fredd.[8] Box 1-2 outlines major steps in the process.

CHEMICAL IDENTIFICATION

Because a drug is a chemical, the first step in drug development is to identify a chemical with the potential for useful physiological effects. This was exemplified by the plant product paclitaxel, which was derived from the needles and bark of the western yew tree. Paclitaxel demonstrated antitumor activity, making it attractive for investigation as an anticancer drug. It was subsequently developed and marketed as paclitaxel (Taxol). The exact structure and physical and chemical characteristics of an active ingredient are established during this step of the process.

ANIMAL STUDIES

Once an active chemical is isolated and identified, a series of animal studies examines its general ef-

fect on the organism and effects on specific organs such as the liver or kidneys. Toxicology studies to examine mutagenicity, teratogenicity, effect on reproductive fertility, and carcinogenicity are also performed.

INVESTIGATIONAL NEW DRUG APPROVAL

At this point an Investigational New Drug (IND) application is filed with the FDA for the chemical being examined. This application includes all of the information previously gathered, as well as plans for human studies. These studies proceed in three phases and usually require around three years to complete.

Phase 1: The drug is investigated in a small group of healthy volunteers to establish its activity. This is the pharmacokinetic description of the drug (rates of absorption, distribution, metabolism, and elimination).
Phase 2: The drug is next investigated as a treatment for a small number of individuals with the disease the drug is intended to treat.
Phase 3: The drug is investigated in large, multicenter studies to establish safety and efficacy.

NEW DRUG APPLICATION

After a successful IND process, a New Drug Application (NDA) is filed with the FDA, and, upon approval, the drug is released for general clinical use. A detailed reporting system is in place for the first 6 months to track any problems that arise with the drug's use. The drug is no longer experimental (investigational) and can be prescribed for treatment of the general population by physicians.

Because of the involved, lengthy, and expensive process of obtaining approval through the FDA to market a new drug in the United States, there is often criticism of the process. The potential for harm from an insufficiently tested drug should not be ignored, however, and is well illustrated by the thalidomide story summarized in Box 1-3.

FOOD AND DRUG ADMINISTRATION NEW DRUG CLASSIFICATION SYSTEM

Because some drugs are simply released in new forms, or are similar to previously approved agents, the Food and Drug Administration has a classification system to help identify the significance of new products.[9] An alphanumeric code is given to provide this information.

Box 1-2　Major Steps in the Process of Marketing a Drug in the United States

Isolation and Identification of the Chemical
Animal studies
General effects
Special effects on organ systems
Toxicology studies

Investigational New Drug (IND) Approval
Phase 1 studies: Small number, healthy subjects
Phase 2 studies: Small number, subjects with disease
Phase 3 studies: Large, multicenter studies

New Drug Application (NDA)
Reporting system for first 6 months

Box 1-3	The Thalidomide Story

In the 1950s a drug named thalidomide was released outside the United States as a hypnotic agent (sleeping aid). The fact that the drug caused severe birth deformities such as phocomelia (limb truncation) in the developing fetus was not known until, tragically, the babies of mothers who had taken the drug were delivered. This drug disaster has reinforced the need for careful testing of potential drugs before their release and has served to point out the possibility of drug interference with fetal development during pregnancy. Of interest, thalidomide is currently used worldwide for the treatment of leprosy. The drug is also under investiga-tion to reverse the weight loss seen in tuberculosis and acquired immunodeficiency syndrome (AIDS) and as an agent that can slow viral replication, including that of the human immunodeficiency virus (HIV). The exact mechanism of action of thalidomide is still not fully understood, although this is under investigation. Thalidomide is an immunomodulatory agent that, among other effects, reduces production of the cytokine tumor necrosis factor–alpha (TNF-α). Overproduction of TNF-α by immune cells can cause tissue wasting, fevers, and night sweats.

Table 1-1

Examples of orphan drugs of interest to respiratory care clinicians showing either a proposed use or an approved use* by the Food and Drug Administration

DRUG	PROPOSED USE
Acetylcysteine	IV for moderate to severe acetaminophen overdose
α_1-Proteinase inhibitor (Prolastin)*	Replacement therapy in the α_1-proteinase inhibitor congenital defect
Beractant (Survanta)*	Prevention or treatment of RDS in the newborn
Colfosceril palmitate (Exosurf Neonatal)*	Prevention or treatment of RDS in the newborn
Cystic fibrosis transmembrane conductance regulator	Treatment of cystic fibrosis
Dornase alfa (Pulmozyme)*	Reduce mucus viscosity and increase airway secretion clearance in cystic fibrosis
Nitric oxide (INOmax)*	Treatment of persistent pulmonary hypertension of the newborn, or acute respiratory distress in adults
Tobramycin by inhalation (TOBI)*	Treatment of *Pseudomonas aeruginosa* in cystic fibrosis or bronchiectasis

*From *Drug Facts and Comparisons,* St Louis, 2000, Facts and Comparisons.
IV, Intravenous; *RDS,* respiratory distress syndrome.

Chemical/pharmaceutical standing

1 = New chemical entity	4 = New combination
2 = New salt form	5 = Generic drug
3 = New dosage form	6 = New indication

Therapeutic potential

A = Important (significant) therapeutic gain over other drugs
AA = Important therapeutic gain, indicated for a patient with acquired immunodeficiency syndrome (AIDS); fast-track
B = Modest therapeutic gain
C = Important options; little or no therapeutic gain

ORPHAN DRUGS

An orphan drug is a drug or biological product for the diagnosis or treatment of a rare disease. *Rare* is de-fined as a disease that affects fewer than 200,000 persons. Alternatively, a drug may be designated as an orphan if used for a disease that affects more than 200,000 persons but there is no reasonable expectation of recovering the cost of drug development. Table 1-1 lists several orphan drugs of interest for respiratory care clinicians.

THE PRESCRIPTION

The prescription is the written order for a drug, along with any specific instructions for compounding, dispensing, and taking the drug. This order may be written by a physician, osteopath, dentist, veterinarian,

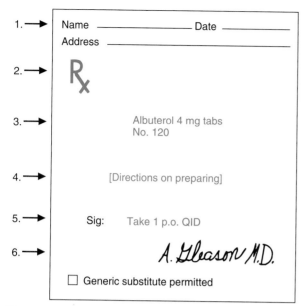

Figure 1-1 Parts of a prescription (see text for identification of elements).

3. The *inscription* lists the name and quantity of the drug being prescribed.
4. When applicable, this is the *subscription,* which is directions to the pharmacist on preparing the medication. As an example, a direction to make an ointment would be "ft ungt," which might be appropriate for certain medications. In many cases, with precompounded drugs, counting out the correct number is the only requirement.
5. *Sig (signa)* means "write." The *transcription* or *signature* is the information the pharmacist writes on the label of the medication as instructions to the patient.
6. *Name of the prescriber.* Note that although the physician signs the prescription, the term *signature,* as described above in 5, denotes the directions to the patient, not the physician's name.

A list of the most common abbreviations seen with prescriptions is provided in Table 1-2.

OVER-THE-COUNTER DRUGS

Many drugs are available to the general population without a prescription; these are referred to as *over-the-counter* (OTC) products. Although the strength and amount per dose may be less than with a prescription formulation, OTC drugs can be hazardous in normal amounts if their effects are not understood and can be taken in large quantities, thereby increasing the risk.

EXAMPLE

The potent sympathomimetic amine, epinephrine, is available OTC as an inhalant solution for asthma. Some of its trade names are AsthmaHaler Mist, Medihaler-Epi, and Primatene Mist. The first two products deliver the equivalent of 0.16 mg of epinephrine per spray, and Primatene Mist delivers 0.2 mg per spray. Epinephrine can provoke cardiac arrhythmias or hypertension and, in particular, can exacerbate these conditions if they preexist in a patient. In addition, someone may self-treat during an asthma episode and avoid seeking medical help until serious or even fatal airway obstruction occurs.

GENERIC SUBSTITUTION IN PRESCRIPTIONS

A physician can indicate to the pharmacist that generic substitution is permitted in the filling of the prescription. In such a case the pharmacist may provide any manufacturer's version of the prescribed drug, and not a specific brand. This is intended to save money, because the manufacturer of the generic substitute has not invested the considerable time and money in developing the original drug product, and presumably the generic substitute will be less expensive to the consumer than the original proprietary brand.

and others, but not chiropractors or opticians. The detailed parts of a prescription are shown in Figure 1-1. It should be noted that both Latin and English, as well as metric and apothecary measures, have been used for drug orders.

The directions (*4* in Figure 1-1) to the pharmacist for mixing or compounding drugs have become less necessary with the advent of the large pharmaceutical firms and their prepared drug products. However, the importance of these directions is in no way diminished, because misinterpretation is potentially lethal when dealing with drugs.

Since passage of the Controlled Substances Act of 1971, physicians must include their registration number provided by the Drug Enforcement Administration (DEA) (usually termed a DEA Registration Number) when prescribing narcotics or controlled substances. Any licensed physician may apply for a DEA Registration Number.

The following parts of the prescription are indicated in Figure 1-1:

1. Patient's name, address, and date.
2. R℞ (meaning "recipe" or "take thou") directs the pharmacist to take the drug listed and prepare the medication. This is referred to as the *superscription.*

Table 1-2

Abbreviations and symbols used in prescriptions

ABBREVIATION	MEANING	ABBREVIATION	MEANING
$\overline{aa}$	of each	OS	left eye
ac	before a meal	OU	both eyes
ad lib	as much as desired	$\overline{p}$	after
alt hor	every other hour	part aeq	equal parts
aq dest	distilled water	pc	after meals
bid	twice daily	pil	pill
C, cong	gallon	placebo	I please (inert substitute)
$\overline{c}$	with	po	by mouth
cap	capsule	prn	as needed
cc	cubic centimeter	pr	rectally
dil	dilute	pulv	powder
dtd	give such doses	q	every
elix	elixir	qh	every hour
emuls	emulsion	qid	four times daily
et	and	qod	every other day
ex aq	in water	qd	every day
ext	extract	q2h	every 2 hours
fld	fluid	q3h	every 3 hours
f t	make	q4h	every 4 hours
gel	a gel, jelly	qs	as much as required (quantity sufficient)
g	gram		
gr	grain	qt	quart
gtt	a drop	Rx, ℞	take
hs	at bedtime	$\overline{s}$	without
IM	intramuscular	sig	write
IV	intravenous	sol	solution
L	liter	solv	dissolve
lin	a liniment	sos	if needed (for one time)
liq	liquid, solution	spt	spirit
lot	lotion	sp frumenti	whiskey
M	mix	$\overline{ss}$	half
mist, mixt	mixture	stat	immediately
ml	milliliter	syr	syrup
nebul	a spray	tab	tablet or tablets
non rep	not to be repeated	tid	three times daily
npo	nothing by mouth	tr, tinct	tincture
o, $\overline{o}$	pint	ung	ointment
OD	right eye	ut dict	as directed
ol	oil	vin	wine

RESPIRATORY CARE PHARMACOLOGY: AN OVERVIEW

Care of the person with pulmonary disease such as cystic fibrosis (CF) or pulmonary derangement such as acute respiratory distress syndrome (ARDS) defines a spectrum of pharmacological care from maintenance support of a stable person through intervention for a critically ill person. The respiratory system can-

not be dissociated from the cardiac and vascular systems, given the interlinked function of these systems. As a result, respiratory care pharmacology involves a relatively broad area of drug classes.

AEROSOLIZED AGENTS GIVEN BY INHALATION

A central group of drugs in respiratory care is the group given by inhaled aerosol for direct treatment of

Table 1-3

Aerosolized agents

DRUG GROUP	THERAPEUTIC PURPOSE	AGENTS
Adrenergic agents	β-*adrenergic:* Relaxation of bronchial smooth muscle and bronchodilation, to reduce R_{aw} and improve ventilatory flow rates in airway obstruction such as COPD, asthma, CF, acute bronchitis. α-*Adrenergic:* E.g., epinephrine: topical vasoconstriction and decongestion.	Epinephrine Isoproterenol Isoetharine Terbutaline Metaproterenol Albuterol Pirbuterol Bitolterol Levalbuterol Salmeterol Formoterol
Anticholinergic agents	Relaxation of cholinergic-induced bronchoconstriction to improve ventilatory flow rates in COPD and asthma.	Ipratropium bromide
Mucoactive agents	Modification of the properties of respiratory tract mucus; current agents lower viscosity and promote clearance of secretions.	Acetylcysteine Dornase alfa
Corticosteroids	Reduce and control the inflammatory response in the airway usually associated with asthma (lower respiratory tract) or with seasonal or chronic rhinitis (upper respiratory tract).	Dexamethasone Beclomethasone dipropionate Triamcinolone acetonide Flunisolide Fluticasone propionate Budesonide
Antiasthmatic agents	Prevention of the onset and development of the asthmatic response, through inhibition of chemical mediators of inflammation.	Cromolyn sodium Nedocromil sodium Zafirlukast Zileuton Montelukast
Antiinfective agents	Inhibition of or eradication of specific infective agents, such as *Pneumocystis carinii* (pentamidine), respiratory syncytial virus (ribavirin), *Pseudomonas aeruginosa* in CF or influenza A and B.	Pentamidine Ribavirin Tobramycin Zanamivir
Exogenous surfactants	Approved clinical use is by direct intratracheal instillation, for the purpose of restoring a more normal lung compliance in respiratory distress syndrome of the newborn.	Colfosceril palmitate Beractant Calfactant Poractant alfa

CF, Cystic fibrosis; *COPD,* chronic obstructive pulmonary disease; R_{aw}, airway resistance.

the upper and lower airway in pulmonary disease. Drugs delivered by oral inhalation or nasal inhalation are intended to provide a local topical treatment of the respiratory tract. The following are advantages of this method and route of delivery:

1. Aerosol doses are smaller than those used for the same purpose and given systemically.
2. Side effects are usually fewer and less severe with aerosol delivery than with oral or parenteral delivery.
3. The onset of action is rapid.
4. Drug delivery is targeted to the respiratory system, with lower systemic bioavailability.
5. The inhalation of aerosol drugs is painless, relatively safe, and may be convenient depending on the specific delivery device used.

The classes of aerosolized agents (including surfactants, that are directly instilled into the trachea), their uses, and individual agents are summarized in Table 1-3.

RELATED DRUG GROUPS IN RESPIRATORY CARE

Additional groups of drugs important in critical care are the following:

- *Antiinfective agents,* such as antibiotics or antituberculous drugs
- *Neuromuscular blocking agents,* such as curariform agents and others
- *Central nervous system agents,* such as analgesics and sedatives/hypnotics
- *Antiarrhythmic agents,* such as cardiac glycosides and lidocaine
- *Antihypertensive and antianginal agents,* such as β-blocking agents or nitroglycerin
- *Anticoagulant and thrombolytic agents,* such as heparin or streptokinase
- *Diuretics,* such as the thiazides or furosemide

SUMMARY KEY TERMS AND CONCEPTS

- Key terms in the study of pharmacology are introduced, including *drug* and *pharmacology.* The study of *respiratory care pharmacology* is broadly defined as the application of pharmacology to cardiopulmonary disease and critical care.
- Each drug has five different names: *chemical, code, official, generic,* and *brand. Sources of drug information* include references such as the *Physician's Desk Reference (PDR),* the *United States Pharmacopeia-National Formulary* (USP-NF), and texts such as *Goodman and Gilman's The Pharmacological Basis of Therapeutics,* as well as subscription services such as *Drug Facts and Comparisons.*
- The *process of drug approval* in the United States is lengthy and expensive, involving multiple phases.
- Certain drugs used for rare diseases, which may not return the cost of their development, are termed *orphan drugs.*
- The selling of many drugs requires a physician's order, known as the *prescription,* and involves Latin terms and abbreviations.
- An *over-the-counter* (OTC) drug does not require a prescription for purchase.
- Central to the respiratory care of pulmonary disease is the group of *aerosolized agents,* which includes adrenergic, anticholinergic, mucoactive, corticosteroid, antiasthmatic, antiinfective agents, as well as surfactants directly instilled into the trachea. *Other drug groups* important in respiratory care include cardiovascular, antiinfective, neuromuscular blocking and diuretic agents.

SELF-ASSESSMENT QUESTIONS

1. What is the definition of the term *drug?*
2. What is the difference between the generic and the trade name of a drug?
3. What part of a prescription contains the name and amount of the drug being prescribed?
4. A physician's order reads as follows: "gtts iv of racemic epinephrine, c̄ 3 cc of normal saline, q4h, while awake." What has been ordered?
5. The drug salmeterol was released for general clinical use in the United States in 1994. Where would you look to find information on this drug, such as the available dosage forms, doses, properties, side effects, and action?

Answers to Self-Assessment Questions are found in Appendix A.

CLINICAL SCENARIO

A 24-year-old male played golf on a newly mown course. He had exhibited allergies in the past few years and was diagnosed as having asthma. He did not have a regular physician or medical treatment site, nor was he on any medications to control his asthma and allergies. He began to experience difficulty breathing later in the day, with wheezing and some shortness of breath (SOB) on mild exertion. He visited his local drugstore and purchased Primatene Mist. Upon use, he obtained immediate relief for his breathing but his heart rate increased from 66 beats/min to 84 beats/min and he felt shaky. By midnight, his wheezing had returned. He continued using the Primatene Mist through the next morning. The relief he experienced with the drug diminished during the afternoon, and a friend found him later that evening with audible wheezing, gasping for air, and in severe respiratory distress. He was rushed to a local emergency room, where he went into respiratory arrest approximately 5 minutes after arrival.

Where could you find information on the drug, Primatene Mist, that he was taking?

In general, what is the fundamental error this person displayed?

Answers to Clinical Scenario Questions are found in Appendix A.

REFERENCES

1. Harman JG, Limbird LE, eds: *Goodman and Gilman's the pharmacological basis of therapeutics,* ed 9, New York, 1996, Pergamon Press.
2. Katzung BG, ed: *Basic & clinical pharmacology,* ed 7, New York, 1998, Lange Medical Books/McGraw-Hill.
3. *Drug Facts and Comparisons,* St Louis, 2000, Facts and Comparisons, Wolters Kluwer.
4. 2002 Mosby's Drug Consult, St. Louis, 2002, Mosby.
5. Gale EAM, Clark A: A drug on the market? *Lancet* 355:61, 2000.
6. Love J: Who pays what in drug development, *Nature* 397:202, 1999.
7. Flieger K: How experimental drugs are tested in humans, *Pediatr Infect Dis J* 8:160, 1989.
8. Hassall TH, Fredd SB: A physician's guide to information available about new drug approvals, *Am J Gastroenterol* 84:1222, 1989.
9. Covington TR: The ABCs of new drugs, *Facts and Comparisons Newsletter* 10:73, 1991.

CHAPTER 2

Principles of Drug Action

Joseph L. Rau • *Brad D. Pearce*

*T*he entire course of a drug's action, from *dose* to *effect*, can be understood in three phases of action: the *drug administration* phase, the *pharmacokinetic* phase, and the *pharmacodynamic* phase. This useful conceptual framework, based on the principles offered by Ariëns and Simonis,[1] organizes the steps of a drug's action from drug administration through effect and ultimate elimination from the body. This framework is illustrated in Figure 2-1, and provides an overview of the interrelationship of the three phases of drug action, each of which is discussed.

THE DRUG ADMINISTRATION PHASE

Definition: The drug administration phase describes the method by which a drug dose is made available to the body.

DRUG DOSAGE FORMS

The drug administration phase entails the interrelated concepts of drug formulation (e.g., compounding a tablet for particular dissolution properties) and drug delivery (e.g., designing an inhaler to deliver a unit dose). Two key topics of this phase are the drug dosage form and the route of administration. The drug *dosage form* is the physical state of the drug in association with nondrug components such as the vehicle. Tablets, capsules, and injectable solutions are common examples of drug dosage forms. The *route of administration* is the portal of entry for the drug into the body, such as oral (enteral), injection, or inhalation. The form in which a drug is available must be compatible with the route of administration desired. For example, the injectable route, such as intravenously, requires a liquid solution of a drug, whereas the oral route is possible with capsules, tablets, or liquid solutions. Some common drug formulations are listed in Box 2-1 for each of the common routes of drug administration.

DRUG FORMULATIONS AND ADDITIVES

A drug is the active ingredient in a dose formulation, but it is usually not the only ingredient in the total formulation. For example, in a capsule of an antibiotic, the capsule itself is a gelatinous material that allows the drug to be swallowed. The capsule material then disintegrates in the stomach, and the active drug ingredient is released for absorption. The rate at which active drug is liberated from a capsule or tablet can be controlled during the formulation process, for example, by altering drug particle size or using a specialized coating or formulation matrix. Aerosolized agents for inhalation and treatment of the respiratory tract also contain ingredients other than the active drug. These include preservatives, propellants for metered dose inhaler formulations (MDIs), dispersants (surfactants), and carrier agents with dry powder inhalers (DPIs). An example of three formulations with differing ingredients for the adrenergic bronchodilator albuterol is given in Table 2-1. In the nebulizer solution, the benzalkonium chloride is a preservative and sulfuric acid adjusts the pH of the solution. In the MDI, the chlorofluorocarbons are propellants and oleic acid is a dispersing agent. Similarly, in the DPI formulation, the lactose acts as a bulking agent to improve uniform dispersion of the drug powder.

ROUTES OF ADMINISTRATION

Advances in drug formulation and delivery systems have yielded a wide range of routes by a which a drug can be administered. In the discussion below, routes of administration have been divided into five broad categories: *enteral, parenteral, inhalation, transdermal,* and *topical.*

ENTERAL

The term *enteral* refers literally to the small intestine, but the enteral route of administration is more broadly applicable to administration of drugs intended for absorption anywhere along the gastrointestinal tract. The most common enteral route is by mouth (oral) because it is convenient, is painless, and offers flexibility in possible dose forms of the drug, as seen Table 2-1. The oral route requires the patient to be able to swallow, and airway protective reflexes should be intact. If the drug is not destroyed or inactivated in the stomach and can be absorbed into the bloodstream, distribution throughout the body and a

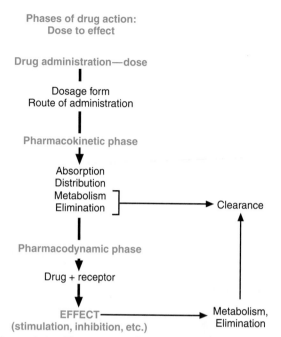

Figure 2-1   The conceptual scheme illustrating the major phases of drug action in sequence, from dose administration to effect in the body. (Modified from Ariëns EJ, Simonis AM: Drug action: target tissue, dose-response relationships, and receptors. In Teorell T, Dedrick RL, Condliffe PG, eds: *Pharmacology and pharmacokinetics,* New York, 1974, Plenum Press.)

Box 2-1   Common Drug Formulations for Different Routes of Administration

Enteral	Parenteral	Inhalation	Transdermal	Topical
Tablet	Solution	Gas	Patch	Powder
Capsule	Suspension	Aerosol	Paste	Lotion
Suppository	Depot			Ointment
Elixir				Solution
Suspension				

Table 2-1

Three different dosage forms for the bronchodilator drug albuterol indicating ingredients other than active drug

DOSAGE FORM	ACTIVE DRUG	INGREDIENTS
Nebulizer solution	Albuterol sulfate	Benzalkonium chloride, sulfuric acid
Metered dose inhaler	Albuterol	Trichloromonofluoromethane, dichlorodifluoromethane, oleic acid
Dry powder inhaler	Albuterol	Lactose

systemic effect can be achieved. Other enteral routes of administration include suppositories inserted in the rectum, tablets placed under the tongue (sublingual), and drug solutions introduced though an indwelling gastric tube.

PARENTERAL (INJECTABLE)

Technically, the term *parenteral* means "besides the intestine," which implies any route of administration other than enteral. However, the parenteral route is commonly taken to mean injection of a drug. Various options are available for injection of a drug, the most common of which are the following:

Intravenous (IV): Injected directly into the vein, allowing nearly instantaneous access to the systemic circulation. Drugs can be given as a bolus, in which case the entire dose is given rapidly, leading to a sharp rise in the plasma concentration, or a steady infusion can be used to avoid this precipitous rise.

Intramuscular (IM): Injected deep into a skeletal muscle. Because the drug must be absorbed from the muscle into the systemic circulation, the drug effects occur more gradually than with intravenous injection, although typically more rapidly than by the oral route.

Subcutaneous (SC): Injected into the subcutaneous tissue beneath the epidermis and dermis.

TRANSDERMAL

An increasing number of drugs are being formulated for application to the skin to produce a systemic effect. The advantage of this route is that it can supply long-term continuous delivery to the systemic circulation. The drug is absorbed percutaneously, obviating the need for a hypodermic needle and decreasing the fluctuations in plasma drug levels that can occur with repeated oral administration.

INHALATION

Drugs can be given by inhalation for either a systemic effect or a local effect in the lung. Two of the most common drug formulations given by this route are gases, which usually are given by inhalation for anesthesia (a systemic effect), and aerosolized agents intended to target the lung or respiratory tract in the treatment of respiratory disease (local effect). The technology and science of aerosol drug delivery to the respiratory tract continues to develop and is described in detail in Chapter 3. A summary of devices commonly used for inhaled aerosol drug delivery is given in Box 2-2. The general rationale for

---

Box 2-2	**Devices for Inhaled Administration of Drugs**

Vaporizer (anesthetic gases)
Atomizer
Nebulizer, small or large
Metered dose inhaler (MDI), with/without spacer
Dry powder inhaler (DPI)
Ultrasonic nebulizer (USN)

---

aerosolized drug delivery to the airways for treating respiratory disease is the local delivery of the drug to the target organ, with reduced or minimal body exposure to the drug and hopefully reduced prevalence or severity of possible side effects.

TOPICAL

Drugs can be applied directly to the skin or mucous membranes to produce a local effect. Such drugs are often formulated to minimize systemic absorption. Examples of topical administration include the application of corticosteroid cream to an area of contact dermatitis (e.g., poison ivy), administration of an eye drop containing a β-adrenergic antagonist to control glaucoma, and instillation of nasal drops containing an α-adrenergic agonist to relieve congestion.

THE PHARMACOKINETIC PHASE

Definition: The pharmacokinetic phase of drug action describes the time course and disposition of a drug in the body, based on its absorption, distribution, metabolism and elimination.

Once presented to the body, as described in the drug administration phase, a drug crosses local anatomical barriers to varying extents depending on its chemical properties and the physiological milieu of the body compartment it occupies. For a systemic effect it is desirable for the drug to get into the bloodstream for distribution to the body; for a local effect this is not desirable and can lead to unwanted side effects throughout the body. The four topics of absorption, distribution, metabolism, and elimination describe the factors influencing and determining the course of a drug after it is introduced to the body. In essence, *pharmacokinetics* describes what the body does to a drug and *pharmacodynamics* describes what the drug does to the body.

ABSORPTION

When given orally for a systemic effect, a pill must first dissolve to liberate the active ingredient. The free drug must then reach the epithelial lining of the stomach or intestine and traverse the lipid membrane barriers of the gastric and vascular cells before reaching the bloodstream for distribution into the body. The lining of the lower respiratory tract also presents barriers to drug absorption. This mucosal barrier consists of the following five identifiable elements:

1. Airway surface liquid
2. Epithelial cells
3. Basement membrane
4. Interstitium
5. Capillary vascular network

After traversing these layers a drug can reach the smooth muscle or glands of the airway. The mechanisms by which drugs move across membrane barriers are briefly outlined and include aqueous diffusion, lipid diffusion, active or facilitated diffusion, and pinocytosis. In general a drug must be sufficiently water-soluble to reach a lipid (cell) membrane and sufficiently lipid-soluble to diffuse across the cell barrier. Figure 2-2 illustrates these basic mechanisms, which will be briefly discussed.

AQUEOUS DIFFUSION

This method of absorption occurs in the aqueous compartments of the body, such as interstitial spaces or within a cell. Transport across epithelial linings is restricted because of small pore size; capillaries have larger pores allowing passage of most drug molecules. Diffusion is by a concentration gradient.

LIPID DIFFUSION

Lipid diffusion is an important mechanism for drug absorption because of the many epithelial membranes that must be crossed if a drug is to distribute in the body and reach its target organ. Epithelial cells have lipid membranes, and a drug must be lipid-soluble to diffuse across such a membrane. Lipid-insoluble drugs tend to be ionized, or have positive and negative charges separated on the molecule (polar).

Lipid insoluble: Ionized, polar, water-soluble drug
Lipid soluble: Nonionized, nonpolar drug

Many drugs are weak acids or weak bases, and the degree of ionization of these molecules is dependent on the pKa (the pH at which the drug is 50% ionized and 50% nonionized), the ambient pH, and whether the

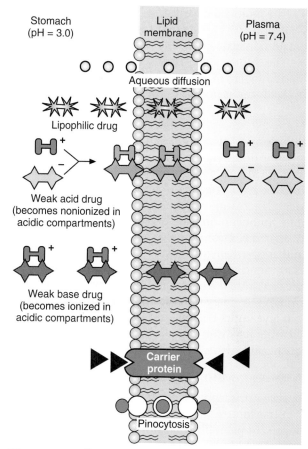

Figure 2-2 Illustration of pathways by which drugs can traverse lipid membranes and enter the circulation. A membrane separating an acidic (stomach) and a neutral compartment (plasma) is shown to illustrate that only the nonionized form of weak acids or weak bases substantially cross these lipophilic barriers.

drug is a weak acid or base. The direction of increasing ionization is opposite for weak acids and weak bases, as ambient pH changes.

Weak acid: Because an acid contributes protons (H^+ ions), the protonated form is neutral, or nonionized.

Drug		Drug$^-$	+	H^+
neutral	$\Longleftrightarrow$	anion		proton
(protonated)				

Weak base: Because a base accepts protons (H^+ ions), the unprotonated form is neutral, or nonionized.

Drug$^+$		Drug	+	H^+
cation	$\Longleftrightarrow$	neutral		proton
(protonated)				

- The protonated weak acid is neutralized by the addition of H^+ ions in an acidic environment, is nonionized, and is lipid-soluble.
- The protonated weak base gains a charge by adding H^+ ions in an acidic environment, is ionized, and is not lipid-soluble.

Figure 2-2 conceptually illustrates the principle of lipid diffusion and absorption for weak acids and bases.

Some drugs, such as ethanol, are neutral molecules and are always nonionized. They are well-absorbed into the bloodstream and across the blood-brain barrier. Other drugs, such as ipratropium bromide or d-(+)-tubocurarine, are quaternary amines, have no unshared electrons for reversible binding of H^+ ions, and are permanently positively charged. Ipratropium is not lipid soluble, and does not absorb and distribute well from the mouth or the lung with oral inhalation. A secondary or tertiary amine, such as atropine, can give up its H^+ ion, and become nonionized, increasing its absorption and distribution, and consequent side effects, in the body.

CARRIER-MEDIATED TRANSPORT

Special carrier molecules embedded in the membrane can transport some substances, such as amino acids, sugars, or naturally occurring peptides and the drugs that resemble these substances. In some instances a drug can compete with the endogenous substance normally transported by the carrier.

PINOCYTOSIS

Pinocytosis describes the incorporation of a substance into a cell by a process of membrane engulfment and transport of the substance to the cell interior in vesicles, thereby allowing translocation across a membrane barrier.

FACTORS AFFECTING ABSORPTION

The route of administration determines which barriers to absorption must be crossed by a drug. This can affect the time course of the drug's time to onset and time to peak effect. Intravenous administration bypasses the need for absorption from the gastrointestinal tract seen with oral administration, generally gives a very rapid onset and peak effect, and provides 100% availability of the drug in the bloodstream. The term *bioavailability* is used to indicate the proportion of a drug that reaches the systemic circulation. For example, the bioavailability of oral morphine is 0.24 be-

cause only about a quarter of the morphine ingested actually arrives in the systemic circulation. Bioavailability is influenced not only by absorption but also by inactivation caused by stomach acids and by metabolic degradation, which can occur before the drug reaches the main systemic compartment. Another important variable governing absorption and bioavailability is blood flow to the site of absorption.

DISTRIBUTION

To be effective at its desired site of action, a drug must have a certain concentration. For example, an antibiotic is investigated for its *minimal inhibitory concentration* (MIC). Drug distribution is the process by which a drug is transported to its sites of action, elimination, and storage. When given intravenously, most drugs distribute initially to organs that receive the most blood flow. After this brief initial distribution phase, subsequent phases of distribution occur based on the principles of diffusion and transport just outlined, as well as the drug's physical/chemical nature and ability to bind to plasma proteins. The initial distribution phase is clinically important for lipophilic anesthetics (e.g., propofol, thiopental) because they produce rapid onset of anesthesia as a function the high blood flow to the brain and their effects are quickly terminated during redistribution to other tissues. The binding of drugs to plasma proteins can also be clinically relevant in rare instances, such as when a large portion of a drug is inactive because it is bound to plasma proteins but subsequently becomes displaced (and thus active) by a second drug that binds to the same proteins.

The plasma concentration of a drug is partially determined by the rate and extent of absorption versus the rate of elimination for a given dose amount. In addition, the volume in which the drug is distributed also determines the concentration achieved in plasma. Those compartments and their approximate volumes in a 70-kg adult are given in Table 2-2.

Table 2-2

Volumes (approximate) of major body compartments

COMPARTMENT	VOLUME (L)
Vascular (blood)	5
Intersititial fluid	10
Intracellular fluid	20
Fat (adipose tissue)	14-25

Volume of Distribution

Suppose a certain drug that distributes exclusively in the plasma compartment is administered intravenously. If a 10-mg bolus of the drug is given, and the volume of the patient's plasma compartment is 5 L, then (barring degradation or elimination) the concentration in the plasma would be 2 mg/L. In this simple example, the *volume of distribution* (V_D) is the same as the volume of the plasma compartment. In practice, drug distribution is usually more complex and the actual tissue compartments occupied by the drug are not known. Nonetheless, volume of distribution describes a useful mathematical equation relating the total amount of drug in the body to the plasma concentration.

Volume of distribution (V_D) = Drug amount/plasma concentration

Example

If 350 mg of theophylline results in a concentration in the plasma of 10 mg/L (equivalent to 10 μg/mL), then the volume of distribution is calculated as:

$$V_D = 350 \text{ mg}/10 \text{ mg/L}$$
$$V_D = 35 \text{ L}$$

The drug can be absorbed and distributed into sites other than the vascular compartment, which is only approximately 5 L, and therefore the calculated volume of distribution can be much larger than the blood volume, as in the case of theophylline, which has a V_D of 35 L. For this reason the volume of distribution is referred to as the *apparent volume of distribution* to emphasize that V_D does not necessarily refer to an actual physiological space. In fact, drugs such as fluoxetine (an antidepressant) and inhaled anesthetics are sequestered in peripheral tissues, and therefore can have apparent volumes of distribution many times greater than the entire volume of the body.

In a clinical setting, V_D is rarely measured but is nonetheless important for estimating the dose needed for a given therapeutic level of drug. Rearranging the equation for V_D, the drug amount should equal the V_D multiplied by the concentration.

Example

To achieve a concentration of theophylline of 15 mg/L with a VD of 35 L, we calculate a dose of

Drug amount (drug dose) = Plasma concentration × V_D
Dose = 15 mg/L × 35 L
Dose = 525 mg

Several points should be noted. *First,* the above calculation assumes that the dose is completely available to the body. This may be true if a dose is given intravenously, but there may be less than 100% bioavailability if given orally. *Second,* this is a *loading dose,* and subsequent doses to maintain a level of concentration will depend on the rate of absorption versus the rates of metabolism and excretion, to be discussed next. *Third,* the volume of distribution may change as a function of age or disease state. *Fourth,* the concept of the volume of distribution is not directly helpful in topical drug administration and delivery of aerosolized drugs intended to act directly on the airway surface. The volume of distribution for topical deposition in the airway is not measured, and the drug is deposited locally in the respiratory tract, with some drugs absorbed from the airway into the blood.

Metabolism

The processes by which drug molecules are metabolized, or biotransformed, constitutes a complex area of biochemistry, which is beyond the scope of this text. Common pathways for the biotransformation of drugs are listed in Box 2-3. Generally, phase 1 biochemical reactions convert the active drug to a more polar (water-soluble) form, which can be excreted by the kidney. Drugs that are transformed in a phase 1 reaction also may be further transformed in a phase 2 reaction, which combines (conjugates) a substance (e.g., glucuronic acid) with the metabolite to form a highly polar conjugate. For some drugs, biotransformation is accomplished by just phase 1 or phase 2 metabolism without prior transformation by the other phase. Metabolites are often less biologically active than the parent drug. Nevertheless, some drugs are inactive until metabolized

Box 2-3	Common Pathways for Drug Metabolism

Phase 1
Oxidative hydroxylation
Oxidative dealkylation
Oxidative deamination
N-Oxidation
Reductive reactions
Hydrolytic reactions (e.g., esterase enzymes)

Phase 2
Conjugation reactions (e.g., glucuronide or sulfate)

(e.g., enalapril) or produce metabolites that are more toxic than their progenitors (e.g., breakdown products of acetaminophen).

SITE OF DRUG BIOTRANSFORMATION

The liver is the principal organ for drug metabolism, although other tissues, including the lung, intestinal wall, and endothelial vascular wall, can transform or metabolize drugs. For example, epinephrine, a weak base, will be absorbed into the intestinal wall, where sulfatase enzymes inactivate it as the drug diffuses into the circulation. The liver contains intracellular enzymes that usually convert lipophilic (lipid-soluble) drug molecules into water-soluble metabolites that are more easily excreted. The major enzyme system in the liver is the cytochrome P450 oxidase system. There are many forms of cytochrome P450, which are hemoproteins with considerable substrate versatility and the ability to metabolize new drugs or industrial compounds. The various forms of cytochrome P450 have been divided into about a dozen subcategories, termed *isoenzyme families*. The four most important isoenzyme families for drug metabolism have been designated CYP1, CYP2, CYP3, and CYP4. A given drug may be metabolized predominately by only one member of an isoenzyme family, whereas another drug may be metabolized by multiple enzymes in the same family or even several distinct enzymes across families. Knowing which particular CYP enzyme(s) metabolizes a drug can be important for predicting drug interactions, as described further below.

ENZYME INDUCTION AND INHIBITION

Chronic administration or abuse of drugs that are metabolized by the enzyme systems in the liver can induce (increase) or inhibit the levels of the enzymes (enzyme induction and inhibition). Some examples of drugs or agents that can induce or inhibit CYP enzymes are listed in Table 2-3.

Enzyme induction can affect the therapeutic doses of drugs required. For example, rifampin can induce CYP enzymes and increase the metabolism of several drugs, including warfarin and oral contraceptives. Likewise, cigarette smoking can increase the breakdown of theophylline in chronic lung patients, causing a shorter half life of the drug from approximately 7.0 hours to 4.3 hours. Dosages would need to be adjusted accordingly to maintain a suitable plasma level of theophylline. Conversely, a substantial portion

Table 2-3

Drugs causing induction or inhibition of cytochrome P (CYP) enzymes

CYTOCHROME P450 ISOENZYME	INDUCERS	INHIBITORS
CYP1A2	Phenytoin	Ciprofloxacin
	Rifampin	Diltiazem
CYP2D6		Ranitidine
		Fluoxetine
CYP3A4	Carbamazepine	Diltiazem
	Corticosteroids	Fluoxetine
	Rifampin	Erythromycin

of drug interactions involve inhibition of CYP enzymes. A given drug is not likely to inhibit all the CYP isoenzymes equally. For example, the antibiotic ciprofloxacin is a potent inhibitor of an enzyme in the CYP family, which also metabolizes theophylline. Thus coadministration of ciprofloxacin with theophylline can raise theophylline levels, the opposite effect of cigarette smoking.

FIRST-PASS EFFECT

Another clinically important effect of the liver on drug metabolism is referred to as the *first-pass effect* of elimination. When a drug is taken orally and absorbed into the blood from the stomach or intestine, the portal vein drains this blood directly into the liver. This is illustrated in Figure 2-3. The blood from the liver is then drained by the right and left hepatic veins directly into the inferior vena cava and on into the general circulation.

If a drug is highly metabolized by the liver enzymes briefly described and is administered orally, most of the drug's activity will be terminated in its passage through the liver before it ever reaches the general circulation and the rest of the body. This is the first-pass effect. Examples of drugs with a high first-pass effect are propranolol, nitroglycerin (sublingual is preferred to oral), and fluticasone propionate, an aerosolized corticosteroid. The first-pass effect causes difficulties with oral administration that must be overcome by increasing the oral dose (compared with the parenteral dosage) or by using a delivery system that circumvents first-pass metabolism. The following routes avoid first-pass circulation through the liver: injection, buccal or sublingual tablets, the transdermal (e.g., patch) or rectal (e.g., suppositories) route, and the inhalation route. These

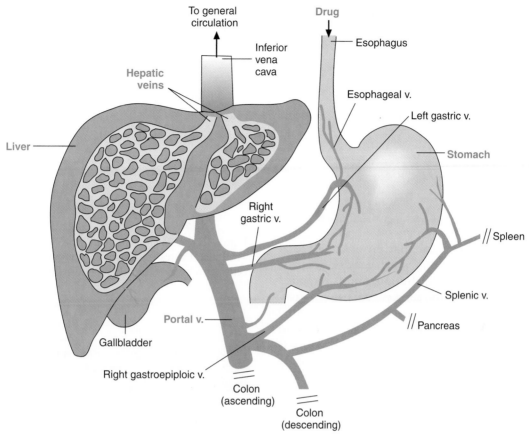

Figure 2-3   Anatomy of venous drainage from the stomach that forms the basis for the first-pass effect of orally administered drugs.

routes of administration bypass the liver's portal venous circulation, allowing drugs to be generally distributed in the body before being circulated through the liver and ultimately metabolized. They also bypass metabolic degradation occurring in the gut as a result of specific metabolic enzymes (e.g., CYP3) or bacterial flora.

ELIMINATION

The primary site of drug excretion in the body is the kidney, just as the liver is the site of much drug metabolism. The kidney is important for removing drug metabolites produced by the liver. Some drugs are not metabolized and are eliminated from the circulation entirely by the kidney. The route of elimination becomes important when choosing between alternative therapies, because liver or kidney disease can alter the clearance of a drug by these organs. In general terms, *clearance* is a measure of the body's ability to rid itself of a drug. Most often, clearance is expressed as *total systemic* or *plasma clearance* to emphasize that all of the various mechanisms by which a given drug is cleared (metabolism, excretion, etc.) are taken into account.

PLASMA CLEARANCE

Just as the term V_D is an abstraction that does not usually correspond to any real physiological volume, so the term *plasma clearance* (Cl_p) refers to a hypothetical volume of plasma that is completely cleared of all drug over a given period. Consequently, plasma clearance is usually expressed as liters per hour (L/hr), or if body weight is taken into account, liters per hour per kilogram. Because Cl_p gives an indication of the quantity of drug removed from the body over a given time, it can be used to estimate the rate at which drug must be replaced to maintain a steady plasma level.

MAINTENANCE DOSE

To achieve a steady level of drug in the body, dosing must equal the rate of elimination.

Dosing rate (mg/hr) = (Cl_p) (L/hr) × Plasma concentration (mg/L)

EXAMPLE
The clearance of theophylline is given as 2.88 L/hr/70 kg. For a 70-kg ideal adult, to maintain a plasma drug level of 15 mg/L (= 15 μg/mL), calculate a dosing rate of:

Dosing rate = 2.88 L/hr × 15 mg/L = 43.2 mg/hr

The above simplified calculation assumes total bioavailability of the drug, which may not be true for some routes of administration, and is intended for conceptual illustration only. Actual patient treatment must take other factors into account. The drug could be given by constant infusion or divided into dosing intervals (e.g., where half the daily dose is given every 12 hours). When deciding on a dosing interval, it is desirable to know the *plasma half-life.*

PLASMA HALF-LIFE

Plasma half-life $(T_{1/2})$ is a measure of how quickly a drug is eliminated from the body.

Definition: The time required for the plasma concentration of a drug to decrease by one half.

However, more pertinent to dosing schedules, plasma half-life indicates how quickly a drug can accumulate and reach steady-state plasma levels. Drugs with a short half-life (e.g., amoxicillin) reach steady-state levels quickly but must be given more frequently to maintain plasma levels, whereas the opposite is true of drugs with a long half-life, such as digoxin. Table 2-4 lists selected drugs in common use, with their plasma half-lives.

TIME-PLASMA CURVES

The concentration of a drug in the plasma over time can be graphed as a time-plasma curve (Figure 2-4). The shape of this curve describes the interplay of the kinetic factors of absorption, distribution, metabolism, and elimination. These curves can indicate whether the dose given is sufficient to reach and maintain a critical threshold of concentration needed for the desired therapeutic effect. Such a curve can also be plotted for concentrations of an aerosol drug in respiratory tract secretions. However, the duration

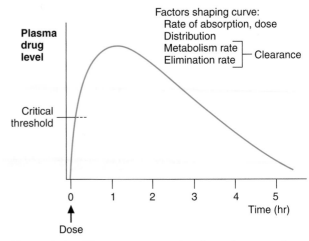

Figure 2-4   Plasma concentration for a drug over time. The critical threshold is the minimum level of drug concentration needed for a therapeutic effect.

Table 2-4

Plasma half-lives of common drugs	
DRUG	**HALF-LIFE (hr)**
Acetaminophen	2
Amoxicillin	1.7
Azithromycin	40
Digoxin	39
Gabapentin	6.5
Morphine	1.9
Paroxetine	17
Terbutaline	14

of the *clinical effect* rather than the concentration of the drug is often represented in studies of aerosol drugs, particularly bronchodilators. This is more helpful than a blood level in describing the pharmacokinetics of inhaled aerosols, which rely on topical delivery with a local effect in the airway. Figure 2-5 illustrates hypothetical curves for the peak effect and duration of three bronchodilator drugs on expiratory flow rates. The short-acting curve could represent a drug such as isoetharine, a catecholamine bronchodilator. Based on its time curve, this agent is too short-acting for maintenance therapy but could be useful for a before-and-after pulmonary function evaluation, where rapid peak effect and short duration would be desirable. The intermediate curve

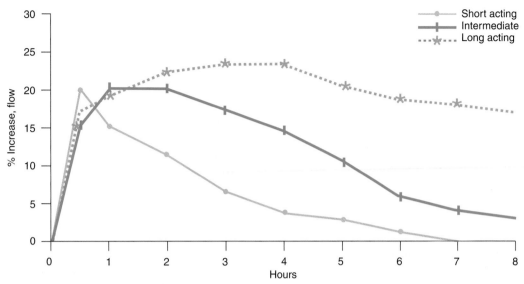

Figure 2-5   Hypothetical time-effect curves for three different bronchodilating agents, illustrating onset, peak effect, and duration.

could represent an agent such as albuterol, with a peak effect of 30 to 60 minutes by inhalation and a duration of action of approximately 4 to 6 hours. These kinetics are useful for as-required bronchodilation or for maintenance therapy if a subject uses the drug four times daily. The kinetics indicate that bronchodilation with drug B would not necessarily be maintained during an entire night. Finally, a long-acting agent such as the bronchodilator salmeterol could provide a 12-hour duration of effect, although time to peak effect is slower (>2 hours). These kinetics are useful for convenient twice-daily dosing and around-the-clock bronchodilation. This example illustrates how pharmacokinetics of an inhaled aerosol can help determine choice of a particular drug for a given clinical application, as well as the dosing schedule needed for the therapeutic effect. Other factors in the choice of a drug, whether inhaled aerosol or oral/injectable, include the side effect profile, the individual's reaction to the drug, allergies, and compliance factors (patient adherence to dosing instructions) such as delivery formulations and dose timing.

PHARMACOKINETICS OF INHALED AEROSOL DRUGS

The inhalation route used for inhaled therapeutic aerosols, together with the physical/chemical nature of the drug, will determine the absorption, distribution, metabolism, and elimination of the aerosol drug.

LOCAL VERSUS SYSTEMIC EFFECT

Inhaled aerosols are deposited on the surface of the upper or lower airway and thus are a form of topically administered drug. As topically deposited agents, inhaled aerosols can be intended for either a local effect in the upper or lower airway or a systemic effect as the drug is absorbed and distributed in the blood. A *local* effect is exemplified by a nasally inhaled vasoconstricting agent (decongestant), such as oxymetazoline (Afrin), or by an inhaled bronchodilator aerosol, such as albuterol (Proventil, Ventolin), to dilate the lower airways. A *systemic* effect might be exemplified by the administration of inhaled zanamivir (Relenza) to treat influenza, inhaled morphine for pain control, or inhaled insulin aerosol for systemic control of diabetes.[2]

INHALED AEROSOLS IN PULMONARY DISEASE

Inhaled aerosols used in the treatment of respiratory diseases such as asthma, chronic obstructive pulmonary disease (COPD), or cystic fibrosis (CF), are intended for a local, targeted effect in the lung and airway. The rationale for the inhalation route in therapy of the lung is to maximize lung deposition while minimizing body (systemic) exposure and unwanted side effects. If the ratio of drug in the lung is high relative to the amount of drug in the body overall (systemic drug level), the inhalation route offers an advantage over direct systemic administration (oral, intravenous) in treating the lung.

DISTRIBUTION OF INHALED AEROSOLS

Because a portion of an inhaled aerosol is swallowed, the inhalation route leads to gastrointestinal absorption, as well as lung absorption of drug, as illustrated in Figure 2-6. Early work by Davies[3] on the distribution of isoproterenol, an older bronchodilator, elucidated the basic paths of distribution for an inhaled drug.

After inhalation of an aerosol, in a spontaneously breathing patient with no artificial airway, a proportion of the aerosol impacts in the oropharynx and is swallowed, and a proportion is inhaled into the airway. The traditional percentages given for stomach and airway proportions, based on Stephen Newman's classic measures[4] in 1981 with an MDI, are approximately 90% and 10%, respectively. Similar percentages have been found with other aerosol delivery devices. Approximately 50% to 60% of the drug impacts in the mouth or oropharynx and contributes to the 90% reaching the stomach. These amounts are used in discussing the pathways of metabolism for an inhaled drug. Although the 10% amount is traditionally accepted as the proportion of inhaled drug reaching the lower respiratory tract with current delivery devices, the exact percentage can vary with different delivery devices or techniques of patient use from 10% to 30%. For example, lung deposition with an inhaled corticosteroid, budesonide (Pulmicort), has been reported as 15% with a pressurized MDI (pMDI) and 32% with a DPI (Turbuhaler).[5] Use of reservoir devices with MDIs or delivery through endotracheal tubes (ETTs) can significantly change oropharyngeal impaction or airway delivery (see Chapter 3).

Oral Portion (Stomach). The swallowed aerosol drug is subject to gastrointestinal absorption, distribution, and metabolism as with an orally administered drug. The aerosol drug can be absorbed from the stomach and metabolized in a first-pass effect through the liver, as shown in Figure 2-6. The drug may also be inactivated in the intestinal wall as it is absorbed into the portal circulation. Site of absorption in the gastrointestinal tract is determined by

the principles governing diffusion of drugs through lipid membranes. In general, if the first-pass metabolism is high, systemic levels will be due only to lung absorption; if first-pass metabolism is low and drug is swallowed, there will be a higher systemic level from gastrointestinal tract absorption, which may increase side effects in the body. The first-pass metabolism of several common inhaled aerosol drugs is as follows:

Albuterol: 50%
Terbutaline: 90%
Budesonide: 90%

Inhaled Portion. It is thought that aerosol drugs interact with the site of action in the airway: secretions in the lumen, nerve endings, cells (e.g., mast cells), or the bronchial smooth muscle in the airway wall. The drug may be subsequently absorbed into the bronchial circulation, which drains into both the right and left atria of the heart, and then the systemic circulation. The exact mechanism by which an aerosol drug, such as a bronchodilator, reaches the appropriate receptors to exert an effect is not well known. If inhaled drug is not removed by mucociliary action or locally inactivated, the drug may be absorbed and this will increase systemic availability of the drug.

LUNG AVAILABILITY/TOTAL SYSTEMIC AVAILABILITY (L/T) RATIO

The L/T ratio quantifies the efficiency of aerosol drug delivery to the lung and is based on the distribution to the airway and gastrointestinal tract just described.

Definition: For an aerosol drug (bronchodilator, corticosteroid, mediator antagonist) that targets the respiratory tract, the L/T ratio can be defined as the proportion of drug available from the lung, out of the total systemically available drug.

The *clinical* or *therapeutic effect* of a bronchoactive aerosol comes from the inhaled drug deposited in the airways. The *systemic* or *extrapulmonary side effects* come from the total amount of drug absorbed into the system. The total systemic drug level is due to airway absorption plus the amount absorbed from the gastrointestinal tract. As a lung/systemic ratio, the ratio can quantify and compare the efficiency of drug delivery systems targeting the respiratory tract. Any action that reduces the swallowed portion of the inhaled drug, such as a reservoir device (spacer, holding

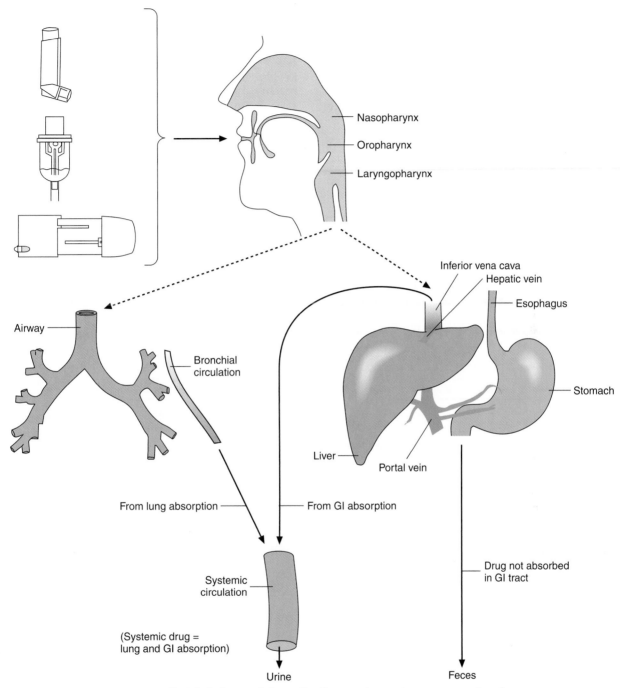

Figure 2-6   Orally inhaled aerosol drugs distribute to the respiratory tract and to the stomach through swallowing of oropharyngeally deposited drug.

chamber), or a high first-pass metabolism, can increase the L/T ratio. Factors that can increase the L/T ratio are summarized in Box 2-4. A perfectly efficient inhalation device would deliver all of the drug to the lung and none to the oropharynx or gastrointestinal tract, thus giving a ratio of 1 (lung availability = total systemic availability; all systemic drug comes only from the lung absorption).

Box 2-4   Factors Increasing the Lung Availability/ Total Systemic Availability (L/T) Ratio With Inhaled Drugs

Efficient delivery devices (high airway and low gastrointestinal delivery)
Inhaled drugs with a high first-pass metabolism
Mouthwashing, including rinsing and spitting
Use of a reservoir device (spacer, holding chamber) to decrease oropharyngeal deposition and swallowed drug amount

---

This concept was proposed in 1991 by Borgström[6] and is elaborated by Thorsson.[7] An example using the data of Thorsson for inhaled albuterol by two different delivery devices is given in Figure 2-7. Using a pMDI, approximately 30% of the inhaled drug reaches the lung, with 70% going to the stomach. With complete absorption from the stomach, half of this 70% is broken down in the liver, so that 35% reaches the systemic circulation. The total amount of the original 100% dose reaching the circulation is 65% (lung, 30%; stomach and liver, 35%). Because 30% of the 65% comes from the lung, this gives an L/T ratio of 30/65 = 0.46.

The data for the DPI, using a Rotahaler, give an L/T ratio of 0.23 (lung, 13%; stomach and liver, 44%). Based on these ratios, inhalation of albuterol using an MDI gives more efficient lung delivery with less systemic availability compared with inhalation using a DPI such as the Rotahaler. With the MDI, 46% of the systemic exposure is due to the lung, whereas using the DPI, 23% is due to the lung. A high L/T ratio is

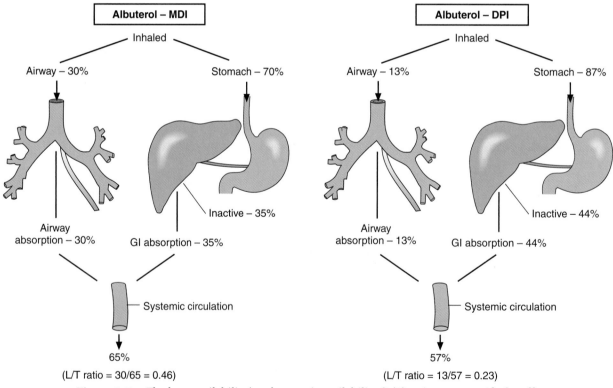

Figure 2-7   The lung availability/total systemic availability (L/T) ratio can quantify the efficiency of aerosol drug delivery to the respiratory tract by partitioning relative amounts from the gastrointestinal tract and from the respiratory tract. (See text for explanation.) (Data from Thorsson L: *J Aerosol Med* 8[suppl 3]:S29, 1995.)

desired; to indicate this, Table 2-5 gives examples of various L/T ratios, along with lung deposition for several drugs and delivery devices.

The L/T ratio is determined by the rate of first-pass metabolism and the efficiency of the inhalation device in placing drug in the airway. Note that a high L/T ratio can be achieved even with poor lung delivery and large stomach absorption if there is a high first-pass effect on swallowed drug. Comparisons of L/T ratios must be between the *same* drugs with different delivery devices. Two drugs with different first-pass metabolism rates can have different L/T ratios even if the airway deposition or delivery device is the same. A good example is provided in Table 2-5 by albuterol and terbutaline, both administered with a Turbuhaler (DPI). Albuterol and terbutaline have first-pass metabolism rates of 50% and 90%, respectively. With approximately the same lung delivery of 22% to 23% for both drug-device systems, the L/T ratio is 0.45 for albuterol but 0.79 for terbutaline. The improved L/T ratio of terbutaline compared with albuterol is not caused by a difference in device efficiency, but by the higher rate of metabolism of terbutaline that reduces systemic blood levels from gastrointestinal absorption. The L/T ratio also suggests that aerosol delivery devices should be evaluated together with the drug to be used. "Each combination of active drug and device is a unique pharmaceutical formulation, as both the drug itself and the device can influence the overall properties of the formulation."[6] The L/T ratio does not determine if systemic toxicity or side effects will occur. First, systemic effects depend on the amount of active drug absorbed into the system, whether from the lung or gastrointestinal tract. An inhaled corticosteroid such as flunisolide, is rapidly metabolized in a first-pass effect. As a result, the swallowed portion will give minimal systemic levels. However, good absorption of the aerosol drug from the lungs in sufficiently high doses could cause systemic effects. Second, delivery to the oropharynx and gastrointestinal tract with a less efficient aerosol delivery device or method may be irrelevant if the drug is largely inactivated when taken orally and causes no local oropharyngeal effects. The catecholamine bronchodilators would be examples of such a drug. The L/T ratio indicates clearly how close an aerosol drug-delivery system comes to the ideal of having all of the systemic drug exposure come from only the lung dose.

THE PHARMACODYNAMIC PHASE

Definition: The pharmacodynamic phase describes the mechanisms of drug action by which a drug molecule causes its effect in the body.

Most drugs exert their effects by binding to protein targets and subsequently modulating the normal function of these proteins, usually inducing physiological changes that affect multiple tissues and organ systems. The relevant protein targets include receptors, enzymes, ion channels, and carrier molecules. In addition, some drugs exert their main therapeutic effect by interacting with DNA rather than binding directly to proteins. For example, the

Table 2-5

The lung availability/total systemic availability (L/T) ratios for several inhaled drugs with different aerosol delivery devices*

DRUG	DEVICE	LUNG DEPOSITION (%)	L/T RATIO	SUBJECTS
Albuterol	pMDI	18.6	0.36	Patients—good coordinators
		7.2	0.17	Patients—poor coordinators
	BAI (pMDI)	20.8	0.41	Patients—poor coordinators
	Rotahaler	7.0	0.15	Healthy volunteers
	Turbuhaler	23.2	0.45	Healthy volunteers
Budesonide	pMDI	15.0	0.66	Healthy subjects
	Turbuhaler	32.0	0.87	Healthy subjects
Terbutaline	pMDI	10.7	0.57	Healthy volunteers
	Turbuhaler	22.0	0.79	Patients

Data from Borgström L: Local versus total systemic bioavailability as a means to compare different inhaled formulations of the same substance, *J Aerosol Med* 11:55, 1998.
BAI, Breath-actuated inhaler; *pMDI*, pressurized metered dose inhaler.
*All drug amounts are expressed as percentages of metered or nominal dose.

chemotherapeutic agent cisplatin inhibits cell division by binding to and disrupting cancer cell DNA, and the antiviral ganciclovir inhibits herpes virus replication by insinuating itself in the virus's DNA and stopping further transcription.

STRUCTURE-ACTIVITY RELATIONS

The matching of a drug molecule with a receptor or enzyme in the body is based on a structural similarity between the drug and its binding site. The relationship between a drug's chemical structure and its clinical effect or activity is termed the *structure-activity relation*. Isoproterenol and albuterol are examples of two aerosol bronchodilators whose differing structures cause different pharmacokinetic activity and tissue responses. The drugs' structures are illustrated in Figure 2-8, with a summary of two critical differences in their pharmacokinetic profile and one critical difference in their side effects (heart rate increase). Although the two structures are very similar, and both are in the same family of β-adrenergic bronchodilators (see Chapter 6 for a discussion of this class of drugs), they show the differences outlined. Isoproterenol is a catecholamine, which is metabolized rapidly as it is absorbed in the airway by the enzyme catechol O-methyl-transferase (COMT), giving it a very short duration of action. Albuterol is a saligenin that is not a substrate for the enzyme COMT, but is instead metabolized through sulfate conjugation, a slower process. This difference is caused by the substitution of $HOCH_2$ for the OH group at the carbon-3 position. In addition, the two side chains' structures are sufficiently different to change their receptor selectivity. Isoproterenol matches to receptors found in the airway (β_2 receptors), as well as the heart (β_1 receptors), whereas albuterol is more selective for receptors in the airway only. In recommended doses, albuterol has little or no effect on heart rate; however, isoproterenol usually will cause an increase in heart rate.

NATURE AND TYPE OF DRUG RECEPTORS

Currently, drugs having the greatest relevance to respiratory therapy act through receptor proteins, although enzymes are important targets for some antibiotics, antivirals, and antihypertensives. Receptors for many drugs have been biochemically purified and directly characterized, whereas in the past such receptors were only indirectly inferred from drug action and differences of action between similar drugs.

DRUG RECEPTORS

Most drug receptors are proteins, or polypeptides, whose shape and electric charge provide a match to a drug's corresponding chemical shape or charge. Drug receptor proteins include receptors on cell surfaces and within the cell.

The process by which attachment of a drug to its receptor results in a clinical response involves complex

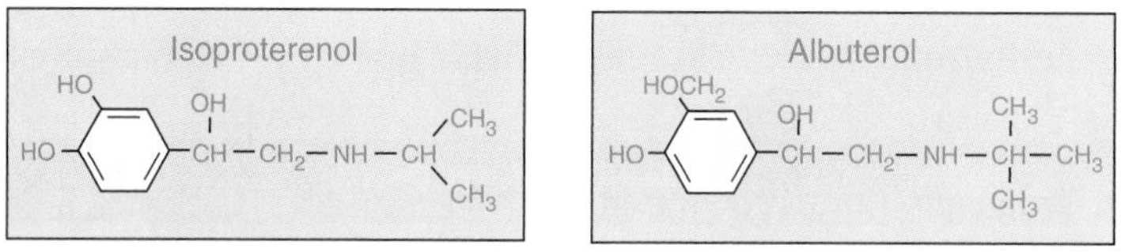

	Isoproterenol	Albuterol
Structure:	Catecholamine	Saligenin (Catecholamine analogue)
Pharmacokinetics:	Peak effect: 20 minutes Duration: 1.5-2 hours	Peak effect: 30-60 minutes Duration: 4-6 hours
Side effect:	Increased heart rate	Little/no change in heart rate
Class of drug:	Adrenergic bronchodilator	Adrenergic bronchodilator
Therapeutic effect:	Relax airway smooth muscle	Relax airway smooth muscle

Figure 2-8   Example of structure-activity relations (SAR) for two drugs in the same class of bronchodilator. Both isoproterenol and albuterol are β-adrenergic agents, with minor structural differences leading to significantly different clinical effects.

molecular mechanisms. This process translates or, better, transduces a signal from the drug chemical into an intracellular sequence that controls cell function. Usually the drug attaches to a receptor protein that spans the cell membrane, and so the process is one of "transmembrane signaling." Four mechanisms for transmembrane signaling are well understood. Each mechanism can transduce signals for a group of different drug receptors and therefore for different drugs. The four mechanisms are as follows:

1. Lipid-soluble drugs cross the cell membrane and act on intracellular receptors, to initiate the drug response. Examples: Corticosteroids, vitamin D, thyroid hormone.
2. The drug attaches to the extracellular portion of a protein receptor, which projects into the cell cytoplasm (a "transmembrane protein") and activates an enzyme system, such as tyrosine kinase, in the intracellular portion to initiate an effect. Examples: Insulin, platelet-derived growth factor (PDGF).
3. The drug attaches to a surface receptor, which regulates the opening of an ion channel. Examples: Acetylcholine receptors on skeletal muscle; γ-aminobutyric acid (GABA).
4. The drug attaches to a transmembrane receptor that is coupled to an intracellular enzyme by a G protein (guanine nucleotide–regulating protein). Examples: β-Adrenergic agents, acetylcholine at parasympathetic nerve endings.

The first, third, and fourth mechanisms are reviewed in more detail, because these are the basis for the activity of drugs commonly used in respiratory care.

LIPID-SOLUBLE DRUGS AND INTRACELLULAR RECEPTOR ACTIVATION

This process of drug signal transduction is the basis by which corticosteroids, an important class of drugs in respiratory care, cause a cell response. Examples of corticosteroid drugs are inhaled beclomethasone and flunisolide and oral prednisone. In this drug-receptor mechanism, the drug is sufficiently lipid soluble to cross the lipid bilayer of the cell membrane, diffuse into the cytoplasm, and attach to an intracellular polypeptide receptor. The drug-receptor complex translocates to the cell nucleus and binds to specific DNA sequences termed hormone response elements, which can either stimulate or repress the transcription of genes in the nucleus. An example of such drug-receptor signaling is illustrated in Figure 2-9 for glu-

cocorticoid drugs, such as inhaled flunisolide or oral prednisone. The glucocorticoid diffuses across the cell membrane and attaches to a receptor in the cytoplasm. Attachment of the drug to the receptor causes displacement of certain proteins, termed heat-shock proteins, and a change in the receptor configuration to an active state. The newly coupled drug receptor then moves or translocates to the nucleus of the cell, where the receptors form pairs that then bind to a glucocorticoid response element (GRE) of the cell's DNA. This initiates or represses transcription of target genes and cell response (see Chapter 11 for a discussion of the mechanism and effects of glucocorticoids).

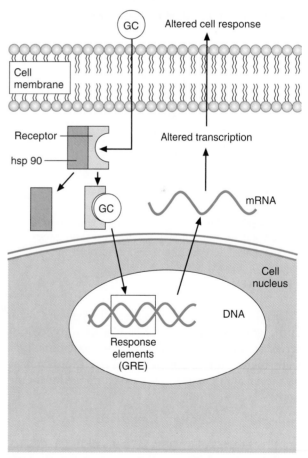

Lipid-soluble drugs and intracellular receptors

Figure 2-9 A diagram of the mechanism of action for lipid-soluble drugs such as glucocorticoids, which bind to intracellular receptors and then modify cell nuclear transcription. *GC,* Glucocorticoid; *GRE,* glucocorticoid response element; *hsp 90,* heat-shock protein.

Drug-related ion channel

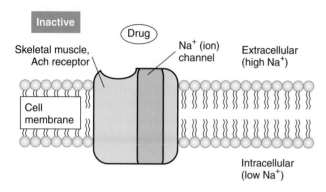

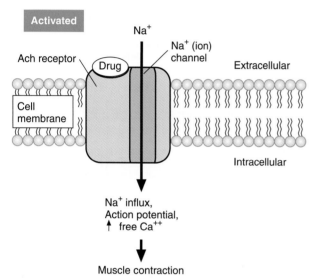

Figure 2-10   Illustration of the drug signal mechanism, which regulates ion channel flow to cause a drug response such as that of acetylcholine *(Ach)* or nicotine in stimulating skeletal muscle fibers to contract.

Drugs that act by diffusing into the cell and regulating gene responses have longer periods for observed responses, of 30 minutes to several hours. Typically there is also a persistence of effect for hours or days, even after the drug has been eliminated from the body.

DRUG-REGULATED ION CHANNELS

Another process of drug signal transduction regulates the flow of ions such as sodium or potassium through cell membrane channels. This can be seen in Figure 2-10. The drug binds to a receptor on the cell membrane surface. The receptor has a portion above or on the surface of the cell membrane and extends through the membrane into the cytoplasm of the cell. When activated by the drug (or an endogenous ligand), the receptor opens an ion channel to allow increased transmembrane conductance of an ion. An example of such a receptor is that for acetylcholine, a neurotransmitter, on skeletal muscle. This acetylcholine receptor is termed a *nicotinic* receptor because it responds to the substance nicotine, as well as acetylcholine. Attachment of acetylcholine or nicotine opens an ion channel and allows the high sodium (Na^+) concentration in extracellular fluid to flow into the lower concentration of the cell. This produces a reversal of voltage, or depolarization, and a corresponding muscle twitch. Acetylcholine is the neurotransmitter for voluntary muscle contraction and movement, and stimulation by nicotine can increase skeletal muscle tremor.

RECEPTORS LINKED TO G PROTEINS

G protein–linked receptors mediate both bronchodilation and bronchoconstriction in the airways, in response to endogenous stimulation by neurotransmitters epinephrine and acetylcholine. These same airway responses can be elicited by adrenergic bronchodilator drugs (discussed in Chapter 6) or blocked by acetylcholine blocking (anticholinergic) agents such as ipratropium bromide (discussed in Chapter 7). G proteins and G protein–linked receptors also mediate the effects of other chemicals, including those of histamine, glucagon, and the phototransduction of light in retinal rods and cones. Drug-receptor signaling with G protein–linked receptors involves three main components: the *drug receptor*, the *G protein*, and the *effector system*. When a drug attaches to a G protein–linked receptor, these three components interact to cause a cellular response to the drug. The effector system triggers the cell response ultimately by activating or inhibiting a *second messenger* within the cell. A diagram showing the main elements of a G protein–linked receptor is given in Figure 2-11. Each of the major elements in this signaling mechanism complex will be described briefly, along with the dynamics of their interaction.

Receptors that couple to G proteins have been well characterized and show a similar structure, in which there is a polypeptide chain that crosses the cell membrane seven times, giving a serpentine appearance to the receptor. The polypeptide chain has an amino (N) terminal site outside the cell membrane and a car-

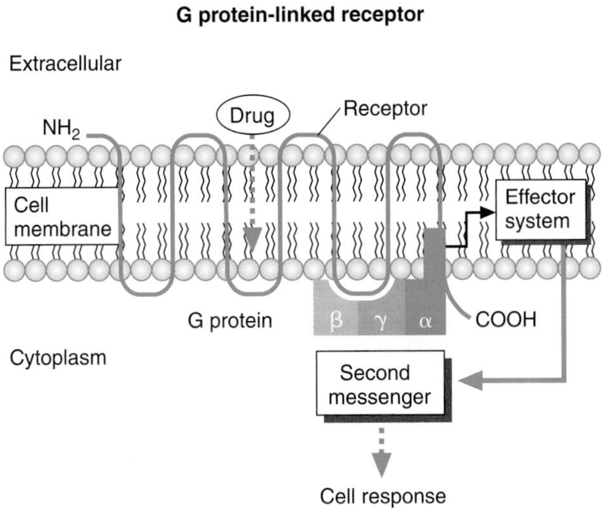

G protein-linked receptor

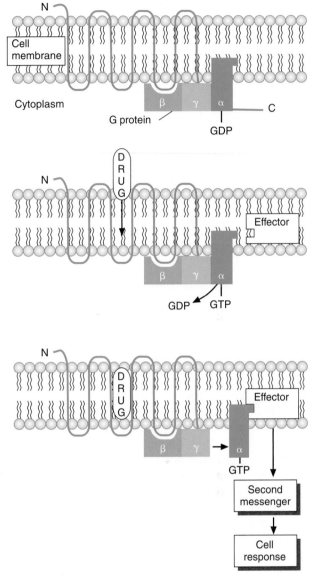

Extracellular

NH₂

Drug

Receptor

Cell membrane

G protein   β γ α   COOH

Cytoplasm

Effector system

Second messenger

Cell response

Example:	
Drug:	β-adrenergic bronchodilator
Receptor:	β-receptor
G Protein	Gₛ
Effector:	adenylyl cyclase
Second messenger:	cyclic 3,5,-AMP

Figure 2-11   Simplified diagram of the components by which a G protein–linked receptor causes a cell response: the drug receptor, the G protein, the effector system, and the second messenger. Each of these components is identified for the example of a β-adrenergic bronchodilator drug and the β-receptor, which is a G protein–linked receptor.

Extracellular
N

Cell membrane

Cytoplasm

G protein   β γ α   C

GDP

N   DRUG

Effector

β γ α

GDP   GTP

N   DRUG

Effector

β γ   α

GTP

Second messenger

Cell response

Figure 2-12   A sequential diagram of G protein–linked receptor activation and G protein function in linking a drug signal to a cell response.

boxyl terminal inside the cell. Although the seven transmembrane segments of the receptor are illustrated in Figure 2-12 as side by side, the receptor appears to form a cylindrical structure if viewed perpendicular to the surface of the cell membrane, with the transmembrane loops forming the sides of the cylinder. The drug usually couples to the receptor at a site surrounded by the transmembrane regions of the receptor protein, that is, within the interior of the cylinder. The receptor then activates a G protein on the cytoplasmic (inner) surface of the cell membrane. The site of the G protein's interaction with the receptor polypeptide is thought to be at the third cytoplasmic loop of the receptor chain.

G proteins are so termed because they are a family of guanine nucleotide–binding proteins with a three-part, or heterotrimeric structure. The three subunits of the G protein are designated by the Greek letters alpha (α), beta (β), and gamma (γ). The α subunit

differentiates members of the G protein family. Based on the α subunit, the G protein is classified into subgroups, such as Gₛ, which *stimulates* an effector system, and Gᵢ, which *inhibits* the effector system. Other types of G proteins have been identified as well; they are not reviewed in this chapter.

The activated G protein changes the activity of an *effector system*, which may be either an enzyme,

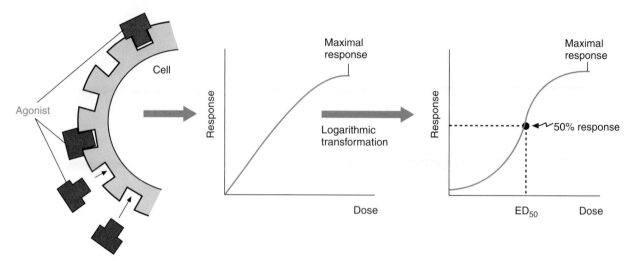

Figure 2-13   Illustration of the dose response curve, showing an increasing effect that ultimately plateaus, and its logarithmic transformation to produce a sigmoid curve.

which in turn catalyzes the formation of a second messenger, or an ion channel, which allows the outflow of K^+ ions from the cell. One of the second messengers is the well-known cyclic adenosine 3',5'-monophosphate (cyclic AMP [cAMP]). The effector enzyme for increasing cAMP is adenylyl cyclase (previously termed adenyl cyclase), which converts ATP to cAMP. The G protein that stimulates adenylyl cyclase is the G_s (for stimulatory) protein. β-Receptors, which couple with β-adrenergic bronchodilators, activate G_s proteins. Another G protein, G_i (for inhibitory), inhibits the activation of adenylyl cyclase; G_i proteins are activated by cholinergic (muscarinic) agonists such as acetylcholine or the drug methacholine.

The dynamics of cell signaling by G protein–linked receptors are illustrated schematically in Figure 2-12. When there is no drug attached to the receptor site, the α subunit of the G protein is bound to guanosine diphosphate (GDP) and the G protein is in an inactive state. When a drug attaches to the receptor, there is a change in the receptor conformation that causes the release of GDP and the binding of guanosine triphosphate (GTP) to the α subunit. This is the active state for the G protein. The GTP-bound α subunit dissociates, or unlinks, from the β-γ portion, and couples with the effector system to stimulate or inhibit a second messenger within the cell. The GTP bound to the α subunit is then hydrolyzed by a GTPase enzyme,

dissociates from the effector, and reassociates with the β-γ dimer. The G protein–linked receptor is then ready for reactivation.

Details on specific G proteins, their effector systems, and their second messengers will be presented for neurotransmitters such as epinephrine and acetylcholine in the nervous system (Chapter 5), and for those classes of drugs that link to such receptors, such as adrenergic bronchodilators (Chapter 6) and anticholinergic bronchodilators (Chapter 7).

DOSE-RESPONSE RELATIONS

Response to a drug is proportional to the drug concentration. As drug concentration increases, the number of receptors occupied increase, and the drug effect also increases up to a maximal point. This is graphed as a dose-response, or concentration-effect curve, as seen in Figure 2-13. Increasing amounts of drug will increase the response in a fairly direct fashion; however, the rate of response usually diminishes as the dose increases, until a plateau of maximal effect is reached. Such a convex, or hyperbolic, curve is normally transformed mathematically by using the logarithm of the dose, so that a sigmoid curve is obtained. The linear midportion of a sigmoid curve allows easier comparison of the dose-response for different drugs. In particular, the dose at which 50% of the response to the drug oc-

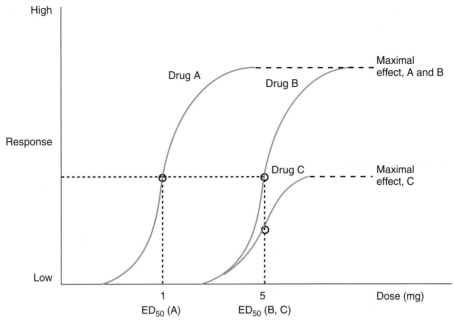

Figure 2-14   The potency of a drug is defined as the dose producing 50% of the drug's maximal effect. Drug A is more potent than drug B; however, drugs B and C are equally potent, although drug C has less maximal effect than drug B.

curs is indicated in Figure 2-13 and is referred to as the ED_{50}, the dose of drug that produces 50% of maximal effect. This may also be denoted as the EC_{50}, for effective concentration giving 50% of maximal response.

POTENCY VERSUS MAXIMAL EFFECT

Dose-response curves are the basis for defining and illustrating several concepts used to characterize and compare drugs. Two concepts that allow comparison of drugs are potency and maximal effect, both illustrated in Figure 2-14.

Potency: Refers to the concentration (EC_{50}) or dose (ED_{50}) of a drug producing 50% of that drug's maximal response. The potency of two drugs, A and B, can be compared using the ED_{50} values of the two drugs: relative potency, A and B = ED_{50}, (B)/ED_{50}(A).

Maximal effect: The greatest response that can be produced by a drug, a dose above which no further response can be elicited.

The lower the ED_{50} for a given drug, the more potent the drug is, as seen in Figure 2-14. Curves for

drug A and B show different potencies. If the ED_{50} for drug B is 5 mg and for drug A is 1 mg, then drug A is five times more potent than drug B.

$$ED_{50}(B)/ED_{50}(A) = 5 \text{ mg}/1 \text{ mg} = 5$$

Drug B requires five times the amount of drug A to produce 50% of its maximum effect. Note that potency is not the same as maximal effect, also illustrated in Figure 2-14. Potency is relatively defined using the ED_{50} of two drugs, whereas maximal effect is absolutely defined as a physiological or clinical response. Curves B and C have the same potency; that is, they have the same dose that produces 50% of maximal response. However, drug B has a greater maximal effect than drug C. Because the ED_{50} is the dose causing a response that is half of the maximal response of the *same* drug, two drugs can have different maximal responses but the same ED_{50} (and therefore the same potency), as seen in Figure 2-14.

THERAPEUTIC INDEX

The therapeutic index is also based on the dose-response curve of a drug. However, instead of

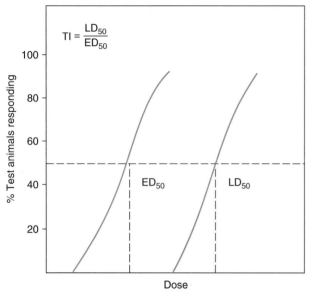

Figure 2-15   The therapeutic index (TI), defined as the ratio of the dose that is lethal for 50% of the test animals to the dose causing improvement in 50% of the test animals.

a graded clinical or physiological response such as increase in heart rate, we substitute an all-or-nothing response of improvement for each subject, or toxicity/death for each subject. In this case the ED_{50} represents the dose of the drug at which half of the test subjects improve. Similarly, the LD_{50} will be the lethal dose for 50% of the test population. Doses are established for a test population of animals (as illustrated in Figure 2-15). The therapeutic index can then be defined as follows:

Therapeutic Index (TI): The ratio of the LD_{50} to the ED_{50} for a given drug, with ED_{50} and LD_{50} indicating half of the test subjects rather than a 50% clinical response.

The ratio of the dose that is toxic to 50% of test subjects to the dose that provides relief to 50% of the subjects is the clinical therapeutic index. This index represents a safety margin of the drug. The smaller the TI, the greater is the possibility of crossing from a therapeutic effect to a toxic effect. Theophylline is an example of a drug used in respiratory care that has a narrow therapeutic margin. As a result, toxic side effects can be seen at close to therapeutic dose levels in some individuals.

AGONISTS AND ANTAGONISTS

An *agonist* is a drug or chemical that binds to a corresponding receptor (has affinity) and *initiates* a cellular effect or response (has efficacy). An *antagonist* is a drug or chemical that is able to bind to a receptor (has affinity) but causes no response (zero efficacy). Because the antagonist drug is occupying the receptor site, it can prevent other drugs or an endogenous chemical from reaching and activating the receptor site. By so doing, an antagonist *inhibits* or *blocks* the agonist at the receptor. Agonists are further divided into *full* and *partial* agonists. A full agonist is a drug that gives a higher maximal response than a partial agonist. The dose response curves for a partial and full agonist are represented in Figure 2-16. Both full and partial agonists have receptor affinity, but a partial agonist has less efficacy than a full agonist.

DRUG INTERACTIONS

The concept of drug antagonism just discussed is an example of a drug interaction in which one drug can block the effect of another. There are several mechanisms of drug antagonism, as follows:

Chemical antagonism: A direct chemical interaction between drug and biologic mediator, which inactivates the drug. An example is chelation of toxic metals by a chelating agent.

Functional antagonism: Can occur when two drugs each produce an effect, and the two effects cancel each other. For example, methacholine can stimulate parasympathetic (muscarinic) receptors in the airways, causing bronchoconstriction; epinephrine can stimulate β_2 receptors in the airways, causing bronchodilation.

Competitive antagonism: Occurs when a drug has affinity for a receptor, but no efficacy, and at the same time blocks the active agonist from binding to and stimulating the receptor. For example, fexofenadine is a competitive antagonist to histamine on specific receptors (H_1) on bronchial smooth muscle and the nasopharynx and therefore is used to treat allergies to pollens.

In addition to antagonistic drug interactions, several terms are used to describe positive interactions between two drugs.

- *Synergism:* Occurs when two drugs act on a target organ by different mechanisms of action, and the effect of the drug pair is greater than the sum of the separate effects of the drugs.

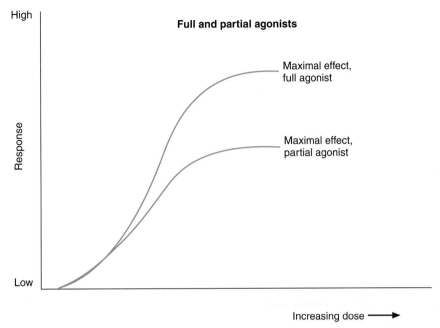

Figure 2-16   Dose response curves for a full and partial agonist, illustrating the greater maximal effect of a full agonist.

- *Additivity:* Occurs when two drugs act on the same receptors and the combined effect is the simple linear sum of the two drugs' effects, up to a maximum effect.
- *Potentiation:* A special case of synergism in which one drug has no effect but can increase the activity of the other drug.

TERMS FOR DRUG RESPONSIVENESS

Individuals exhibit variation in their responses to drugs, and the dose-response curves previously illustrated represent an average of an entire group. The following terms are encountered in pharmacology to describe individual reactions to drugs.

Idiosyncratic effect: Effect that is opposite to or unusual or no effect, compared with the usual predicted effect in an individual.

Hypersensitivity: An allergic or immune-mediated reaction to a drug, which can be serious, requiring airway maintenance or ventilatory assistance.

Tolerance: Describes a decreasing intensity of response to a drug over time.

Tachyphylaxis: Describes a rapid decrease in responsiveness to a drug.

PHARMACOGENETICS

The well-described variation between patients in their responses to drugs are being increasingly traced to hereditary differences. The study of these hereditary or genetic differences is referred to as *pharmacogenetics.* These genetic variations may not be manifested as an "abnormality" until the patient is challenged with a drug, at which time the irregularity in the pharmacokinetic or pharmacodynamic response is revealed. Genetic differences affecting drug metabolism have been most extensively studied, although variation in target proteins may be equally important.

Several examples can be given from drugs commonly seen in respiratory and critical care.

Isoniazid: An antituberculosis drug that varies in its rate of metabolism and inactivation among individuals, with rapid and slow inactivators seen. The proportion of rapid versus slow inactivators is about 50/50 in Caucasians and African Americans, but Inuit and some Asian populations tend to be rapid inactivators.

Succinylcholine: A neuromuscular paralyzing agent used during surgery that is normally metabolized by a butyrylcholinesterase enzyme (pseudocholinesterase). Approximately one in 3000 individuals have a genetically determined variant of this enzyme. As a result, a patient may take several hours to recover from the drug and begin to breathe spontaneously, rather than the several minutes usually seen. Mechanical ventilatory support will be required until spontaneous breathing is adequate.

Isoflurane: An inhalation anesthetic that (like several related anesthetics) can cause malignant hyperthermia in genetically susceptible individuals. Patients with an atypical variant of a calcium release channel can succumb to this serious complication of general anesthesia, which involves a rapid rise in body temperature and increased oxygen consumption.

SUMMARY KEY TERMS AND CONCEPTS

- Principles of drug action encompass three major topic areas: drug administration, pharmacokinetics, and pharmacodynamics.
- The *drug administration phase* identifies drug dosage forms and routes of administration. The *pharmacokinetic phase* describes the factors determining drug absorption, distribution in the body, metabolism, and breakdown of the active drug to its metabolites and elimination of active drug and inactive metabolites from the body.
- The liver is a primary site of drug metabolism and biotransformation, and the kidneys are the site of primary drug excretion, although drug and metabolites can be excreted in the feces as well.
- The inhaled route of administration can involve both gastrointestinal and lung distribution. The systemic level of an inhaled drug and possible extrapulmonary side effects depend on both gastrointestinal and lung absorption of active drug.
- The sources of total systemic drug level are quantified in the *L/T ratio*—the higher the ratio, the more the systemic drug level is from the lung, as a result of efficient lung delivery, high first-pass metabolism, or both.
- *Pharmacodynamics* describes the mechanism of activity by which drugs cause their effects in the body. The principal concept is the *drug target protein* (e.g., drug receptor).
- Two mechanisms of drug-receptor action are the basis for the effects of two drug classes in respiratory care: intracellular receptor binding and modified gene transcription by lipid-soluble drugs (glucocorticoids) and receptors linked to their effector systems by G proteins (β-adrenergic bronchodilators).
- A variety of terms describe the *dose-response* relation of drugs, as they combine with their corresponding receptors, and drug interactions. These include *potency, maxi-*

mal effect, therapeutic index, agonists and antagonists, synergism, additivity, potentiation, and reactions such as *idiosyncratic, hypersensitivity, tolerance,* and *tachyphylaxis.*
- *Pharmacogenetics* refers to hereditary differences in the way the body handles specific drugs.

SELF-ASSESSMENT QUESTIONS

1. If a drug is in liquid solution, what routes of administration are available for its delivery, considering only its dosage form?
2. Although generic drug equivalents all have the same amount of active drug, will formulations of the same drug from different manufacturers all have the same ingredients?
3. If 200 mg of a drug results in a plasma concentration of 10 mg/L, what is the calculated volume of distribution (V_D)?
4. If the V_D of a drug such as phenobarbital is 38 L/70 kg and an effective concentration is 10 mg/L, what loading dose would be needed for an average adult (assuming total bioavailability)?
5. If an inhaled aerosol has zero gastrointestinal absorption of active drug and only lung absorption, what is the L/T ratio?
6. True or False: A patient uses a reservoir device with an inhaled aerosol and there is no swallowed portion of the drug; therefore there will be no side effects systemically.
7. Which receptor system signal mechanism is responsible for the effects caused by β-receptor activation, such as those seen with adrenergic bronchodilators, terbutaline, or albuterol?

Answers to Self-Assessment Questions are found in Appendix A.

CLINICAL SCENARIO

A resident orders isoetharine (Bronkosol), a bronchodilator, to be given qid, for a 67-year-old male. The patient has been diagnosed for the past 10 years with chronic obstructive pulmonary disease (COPD) and was admitted to the hospital the previous evening with a respiratory infection. At 8:00 AM, you administer the prescribed aerosol treatment by nebulizer, with the usual recommended dose. After the treatment, the patient's respiratory rate is reduced from 22 breaths/min to 14 breaths/min and there is less use of accessory muscles. Wheezing on auscultation is also decreased, although you hear adequate breath sounds bilaterally. He seems less short of breath. At 10:30 AM, he is exhibiting moderate respiratory distress, using accessory muscles, complaining of dyspnea, and has increased wheezing on auscultation. His next aerosol treatment is due at noon. He admits to no chest pain; both wheezes and breath sounds can be auscultated over the entire thorax. You review the pharmacokinetics of isoetharine and find the following:

Onset: 1-3 minutes
Peak effect: Approximately 20 minutes
Duration: Approximately 3 hours or less

What may be a likely cause of the patient's respiratory symptoms? What solutions could you offer?

Answers to Clinical Scenario Questions are found in Appendix A.

REFERENCES

1. Ariëns EJ, Simonis AM: Drug action: target tissue, dose-response relationships, and receptors. In Teorell T, Dedrick RL, Condliffe PG, eds: *Pharmacology and pharmacokinetics*, New York, 1974, Plenum Press.

2. Laube BL, Benedict W, Dobs AS: The lung as an alternative route of delivery for insulin in controlling postprandial glucose levels in patients with diabetes, *Chest* 114:1734, 1998.

3. Davies DS: Pharmacokinetics of inhaled substances, *Postgrad Med J* 51(suppl 7):695, 1975.

4. Newman SP and others: Deposition of pressurized aerosols in the human respiratory tract, *Thorax* 36:52, 1981.

5. Thorsson L, Edsbäcker S, Conradson T-B: Lung deposition of budesonide from Turbuhaler is twice that from a pressurised metered-dose inhaler P-MDI, *Eur Respir J* 7:1839, 1994.

6. Borgström L: A possible new approach of comparing different inhalers and inhaled substances, *J Aerosol Med* 4:A13, 1991.

7. Thorsson L: Influence of inhaler systems on systemic availability, with focus on inhaled corticosteroids, *J Aerosol Med* 8(suppl 3):S29, 1995.

SUGGESTED READINGS

Chilvers ER, Sethi T: How receptors work: mechanisms of signal transduction, *Postgrad Med J* 70:813, 1994.

Katzung BG, ed: *Basic & clinical pharmacology*, ed 7, New York, 1998, Lange Medical Books/McGraw-Hill.

CHAPTER 3

Administration of Aerosolized Agents

Joseph L. Rau

*T*he term *aerosol therapy* may be defined as the delivery of aerosol particles to the respiratory tract. Currently there are three main uses of aerosol therapy in respiratory care, as follows:

- Humidification of dry inspired gases, using water aerosols
- Improved mobilization and clearance of respiratory secretions, including sputum induction, using bland aerosols of water, and hypertonic or hypotonic saline
- Delivery of aerosolized drugs to the respiratory tract

This last use of aerosol therapy is the subject of the current chapter, which offers a comprehensive consideration of the delivery of inhaled therapeutic aerosol drugs. As outlined in the previous chapter, the first prerequisite for a drug to exert a therapeutic effect at the target organ is an effective dosage form and route of administration for the target organ. Aerosol generation and delivery to the lung is a complex topic. There is ongoing development of both the technology and the scientific basis of inhaled aerosol administration. This chapter reviews physical principles of aerosol delivery to the airways and aerosol generating devices for inhalation of drugs. Research findings on aerosol delivery devices and methods of administration are summarized. The general advantages supporting the use of aerosolized drug therapy in respiratory care and the disadvantages with this method of drug delivery are summarized in Box 3-1.

PHYSICAL PRINCIPLES OF INHALED AEROSOL DRUGS

The term *aerosol* has been ascribed to a German investigator, Schmauss, who around 1920 used this label generically for dusts, fogs, clouds, mists, fumes, and smoke in the air.[1] The following definitions apply to inhaled therapeutic aerosols:

Aerosol: Suspension of liquid or solid particles between 0.001 and 100 μm in a carrier gas.[2] For pulmonary diagnostic and therapeutic applications, the particle size range of interest is 1 to 10 microns. This range of sizes is small enough to exist as a suspension and enter the lung and large enough to deposit and contain the required amount of an agent.[3,4]

Stability: Describing the tendency of aerosol particles to remain in suspension.

Penetration: Refers to the depth within the lung reached by particles.

Deposition: Process of particles depositing out of suspension to remain in the lung.

Aerosol generating devices for orally inhaled drugs have typically had an efficiency of 10% to 15%; that is, only 10% to 15% of a given dose from a device usually reaches the lower respiratory tract, regardless

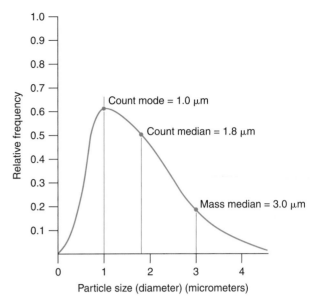

| Box 3-1 | **Advantages and Disadvantages Seen With the Aerosol Delivery of Drugs** |

Advantages
- Aerosol doses are smaller than those for systemic treatment
- Onset of drug action is rapid
- Drug delivery is targeted to the respiratory system for local pulmonary effect
- Systemic side effects are fewer and less severe than with oral or parenteral therapy
- Inhaled drug therapy is painless and relatively convenient
- The lung provides a portal to the body for inhaled aerosol agents intended for systemic effect (e.g., pain control, insulin)

Disadvantages
- The number of variables affecting the dose of aerosol drug delivered to the airways
- Difficulties in dose estimation and dose reproducibility
- Difficulty in coordinating hand action and breathing with metered dose inhalers
- Lack of physician, nurse and therapist knowledge of device use and administration protocols
- Lack of standardized technical information for practitioners on aerosol producing devices
- Number of device types and variability of use is confusing to patients and practitioners

Figure 3-1 A hypothetical skewed frequency distribution of aerosol particle sizes, illustrating the relative positions of the count mode, count median, and mass median. (From Rau JL Jr: Humidity and aerosol therapy. In Barnes TA, ed: *Core textbook in respiratory care practice,* ed 2, St Louis, 1994, Mosby.)

of the device type. Newer aerosol generating devices are proving exceptions to this lack of efficiency, with 30% to 50% or more of the dose reaching the lungs.

AEROSOL PARTICLE SIZE DISTRIBUTIONS

The aerosol particles produced for inhalation into the lung by inhalant devices such as the metered dose inhaler (MDI), small volume nebulizer (SVN), or dry powder inhaler (DPI) include a range of sizes (*polydisperse* or *heterodisperse*) rather than a single size *(monodisperse).* Several measures are used to characterize the typically skewed particle size distributions seen with bronchoactive aerosols (Figure 3-1).

Count mode: The most frequently occurring particle size in the distribution.

Count median diameter (CMD): The particle size above and below which 50% of the particles is found (i.e., the size that evenly divides the *number* of particles in the distribution).

Mass median diameter (MMD): The particle size above and below which 50% of the mass of the particles is found (i.e., the size particle that evenly divides the *mass* in the distribution).

The geometric standard deviation is the usual measure to characterize the variability, or dispersion, of particle sizes in a distribution of aerosol particle sizes.

Geometrical standard deviation (GSD): Measure of dispersion in the distribution. The ratio of particle size below which 84% of the particles occur to the particle size below which 50% occur, in a log-normal distribution.

The mass median diameter (MMD) or mass median aerodynamic diameter (MMAD) indicates where the mass of drug is centered in a distribution of particle sizes. Aerosol particles are three-dimensional and have volume. Aerosol particles are assumed to be roughly spherical, and the relation of volume (or mass if all particles have equal densities) to diameter in a sphere is given by

$$V = (4/3) \pi r^3$$

where V = volume and r = radius.

The volume increases or decreases as the third power of the radius of the particle. As a result, the bulk of drug mass will be centered in the larger particle sizes. Because it is the mass of the drug entering the lung on which the therapeutic effect is based, it is necessary to know where the mass is centered in the range of particle sizes, in order to know whether that distribution will be efficient for penetration into the respiratory tract and delivery of an adequate dose.

EXAMPLE

Two hypothetical SVNs, A and B, have the following specifications from the manufacturer:

A	B
CMD = 1.9 μm	CMD = 1.7 μm
MMAD = 3.4 μm	MMAD = 7.9 μm
GSD = 1.2 μm	GSD = 1.6 μm

Although nebulizer B has a smaller CMD than A, which appears to indicate that it gives smaller particles, it is evident from the respective MMADs that nebulizer B has more particles in a larger size range (>5 microns) compared with A. Nebulizer A produces particles whose mass centers within a lower size range (1 to 5 microns), and would be the better nebulizer to treat the lower respiratory tract.

Aerosol generators should be characterized using the MMD for the center of distribution and either the standard deviation or geometric standard deviation to indicate the range of variability of particle size.

MEASUREMENT OF PARTICLE SIZE DISTRIBUTIONS

Several physical methods are used for measuring aerosol particle size distributions, including *cascade impaction* and *laser scattering*. The *United States Pharmacopeia–National Formulary* (USP-NF) specifies that cascade impaction is the method for determining aerosol size distributions from MDIs. This is described in USP-NF Section 601, Aerosols, which gives specifications for the measuring technique. Cascade impaction devices measure what is termed the *aerodynamic diameter of aerosols*, because the measurement is based on the aerodynamic behavior (sedimentation velocity and impaction characteristics) of the particles in the cascade impactor.

Aerodynamic diameter of a particle is defined as the diameter of a unit-density (1 g/cc) spherical particle having the same terminal settling velocity as the measured particle.[4,5]

The principle by which a cascade impactor measures the particle size distribution of an aerosol cloud is illustrated in a simplified diagram in Figure 3-2.

The cascade impactor consists of a series of stages, each of which has progressively smaller orifices through which the aerosol particles must pass. A constant flow draws the particles through the stages. The fraction of particles largest in size are collected on the first stage, and particles not impacting out at this stage move on to the subsequent stages with smaller orifices in the air stream. By this method of successively smaller filtration stages, the distribution of particle sizes is separated out, or fractionated. Any particles leaving the last stage are then collected on a final filter. The amount of aerosol on each stage is then measured using weight or, preferably, spectrophotometry or high-pressure liquid chromatography (HPLC). The HPLC measure is considered the most sensitive technique for quantifying the amount of aerosol on each stage. Because each stage is calibrated for a unit density sphere of specific diameter, the distribution of aerodynamic diameters can be calculated as the percent of drug on each stage. The mass median aerodynamic diameter can be determined as the particle size dividing the drug in half. Sources of error in aerodynamic measures include particle bounce, interstage impaction, possible fragmentation of particles, and particle evaporation/condensation.[5] In addition, in vitro methods of aerosol measurement may not reflect conditions in the human lung, such as temperature, humidity, inspiratory flow rates, and exhalation phase. Dolovich[6] reviews in vitro measures used with MDI and auxiliary devices. The same method of aerosol characterization is not necessarily useful or accurate for different methods of aerosol production because of differences in the physical nature of their generation. The following have been suggested as appropriate measurement techniques for each type of generator[7]:

Metered dose inhaler (MDI): Cascade impactor with drug-specific assay

Small volume nebulizer (SVN): Light-scattering techniques, such as laser particle sizing

Dry powder inhaler (DPI): Cascade impactor (inertial impaction) calibrated for flow rates of DPI patient use if possible

PARTICLE SIZE AND LUNG DEPOSITION

One of the major factors influencing aerosol deposition in the lung is particle size. The effect of particle size on deposition in the respiratory tract is illustrated in Figure 3-3.

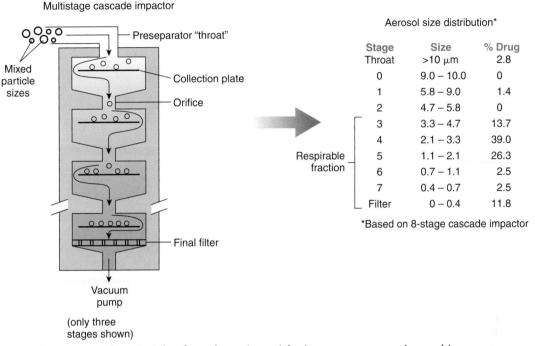

Multistage cascade impactor

Mixed particle sizes

Preseparator "throat"

Collection plate

Orifice

Final filter

Vacuum pump

(only three stages shown)

Aerosol size distribution*

Stage	Size	% Drug
Throat	>10 μm	2.8
0	9.0 – 10.0	0
1	5.8 – 9.0	1.4
2	4.7 – 5.8	0
3	3.3 – 4.7	13.7
4	2.1 – 3.3	39.0
5	1.1 – 2.1	26.3
6	0.7 – 1.1	2.5
7	0.4 – 0.7	2.5
Filter	0 – 0.4	11.8

Respirable fraction (stages 3–Filter)

*Based on 8-stage cascade impactor

Figure 3-2   The principle of aerodynamic particle size measurement using multistage cascade impaction. A series of successively smaller orifices and collection plates separate large and smaller particle sizes. Drug amounts (% drug) shown are actual measures of particle sizes for a sample of albuterol (Ventolin) through a Volumatic reservoir. (Data courtesy JP Mitchell, Trudell Medical Laboratories, London, Ontario, Canada.)

The upper airway (nose, mouth) is efficient in filtering particulate matter, so that generally there is 100% deposition in the nose and mouth of particles larger than 10 and 15 microns, respectively. Particle sizes in the 5- to 10-micron range tend to deposit out in the upper airways and the early airway generations, whereas 1- to 5-micron sizes have a greater probability of reaching the lower respiratory tract from the trachea to the lung periphery. Larger or coarser aerosol particles (>5 microns) may be useful for treating the upper airway (nasopharynx, oropharynx). It is not possible to specify exactly where a given size of particle will deposit in the lung. Particle deposition is a function of several mechanisms, including the breathing pattern, so that the site of penetration is treated probabilistically and not deterministically. For example, tables are often seen listing the percentage of droplets of a given size that will deposit in the lung at each bronchial level.[8] Yu and colleagues[9] observed that optimal deposition in the normal human lung is achieved for particles of 3 microns inhaled with low

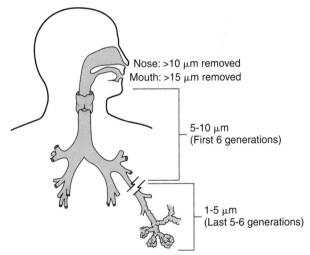

Nose: >10 μm removed
Mouth: >15 μm removed

5-10 μm (First 6 generations)

1-5 μm (Last 5-6 generations)

Figure 3-3   The effect of aerosol particle size on area of preferential deposition within the airway.

inspiratory flows of less than 1 L/sec (60 L/min) and tidal volumes of 1 L; total lung deposition is divided almost equally throughout the 23 lung generations.

FINE PARTICLE FRACTION

The labels *respirable fraction* and *respirable dose* previously were used to refer to the percentage or fraction of aerosol drug mass in a particle size range with a high probability of penetrating into the lower respiratory tract. These generally have been considered to be in the particle size range of less than 5 or 6 microns. There is rarely an absolute correspondence of lower respiratory tract deposition to this particle size range because age, disease, and breathing patterns all can affect lung deposition. At the 1997 International Society for Aerosols in Medicine (ISAM) symposium in Puerto Rico, aerosol scientists agreed that the more descriptive terms *fine particle fraction* (FPF) and *fine particle dose* (FPD) would be used in place of respirable fraction or dose.[7] Agreement was not reached on what size fraction represents the FPF. These terms may be restricted to particles in the size range of 1 to 3 microns, rather than those less than 5 or 6 microns.

PARTICLE SIZE AND THERAPEUTIC EFFECT

Because the respiratory tract appears to function as a progressive filter of successively smaller particles from the upper airway to the periphery, specific areas of the respiratory tract may be targeted by varying aerosol particle sizes. Based on the preceding considerations, the respiratory tract might be segmented by the following particle size ranges.

Particles Greater Than 10 Microns. Particles that are less than 10 microns are useful to treat the nasopharyngeal or oropharyngeal regions. An example might be a nasal spray for perennial rhinitis, such as a corticosteroid.

Particles 5 to 10 Microns. Particles in the range of 5 to 10 microns may shift deposition to the more central airways, although significant oropharyngeal deposition is expected. This may be a useful particle size for future mucokinetic drugs, although current orally inhaled bronchoactive aerosols do not fall in this size range.

Particles 2 to 5 Microns. As particle size decreases below 5 microns, deposition shifts from the orophar-

ynx and large airways to the overall lower respiratory tract (large airways to periphery).[10] This size range is considered useful for the bronchoactive aerosols currently in use. For example, β-adrenergic receptors have been identified throughout the airway, but with greater density in bronchioles. An interesting 1986 study by Clay and colleagues[11] showed greater improvement in midmaximal expiratory flow rates from a β-adrenergic bronchodilator using an MMAD size of 1.8 microns than with MMADs of 4.6 or 10.3 microns. This was confirmed subsequently in 1989 by Johnson and associates,[12] who found a greater response to the β-adrenergic bronchodilator albuterol (see Chapter 6) with an MMD of 3.3 microns compared with 7.7 microns. In contrast, cholinergic receptors are numerous in proximal bronchial smooth muscle, but rare in distal bronchioles.[13] However, in the study by Johnson and associates,[12] response to the anticholinergic agent ipratropium (see Chapter 7) was not significantly different for the two particle sizes, indicating that peripheral deposition with the smaller particle size neither decreased nor increased response.

Particles 0.8 to 3.0 Microns. Increased delivery of an aerosol to the lung parenchyma, including the terminal airways and alveolar region, could be achieved with particles less than 3 microns.[10] For example, an MMAD of 1 to 2 microns is suggested for peripheral deposition of the antiinfective drug pentamidine, to minimize deposition in and irritation of larger airways and maximize intraalveolar deposition.[14]

MECHANISMS OF DEPOSITION

Three physical mechanisms usually are considered for aerosol particle deposition in the human lung: inertial impaction, gravitational settling (sedimentation), and diffusion.

INERTIAL IMPACTION

This is a function of particle size (mass) and velocity, which increases with larger size and higher velocities. In the upper airway and early bronchial generations, particle velocity is highest, airflow tends to be turbulent, and total cross-sectional area of the airway is smallest. These factors favor inertial impaction on the airway wall, especially at airway bifurcations, for larger, fast-moving particles. Deposition by inertial impaction is expected to occur in the first 10 airway generations.[4]

GRAVITATIONAL SETTLING

This is a function of particle size and time. Settling will be greater for larger particles with slow velocities, under the influence of gravity. As particles small enough to escape inertial impaction in earlier airway generations reach the periphery, velocity probably slows and airflow is less turbulent. There is also a shorter distance to the airway wall in smaller, peripheral airways, favoring impaction resulting from settling. The probability of deposition by sedimentation is highest in the last five or six airway generations.[4] Because the process of sedimentation is time-dependent, the end-inspiratory breath-hold should maximize deposition in the periphery. The rate of settling is proportional to the square of the particle size. For a 5-micron diameter particle, the settling rate is reported to be 0.7 mm/sec.[15]

DIFFUSION (BROWNIAN MOTION)

This diffusion mechanism affects particles of less than 1 micron and is a function of time and random molecular motion. Particles between 0.1 and 1.0 micron may remain suspended or even exhaled, because the time required to diffuse to the airway surface tends to be greater than the inspiratory time of a normal breath.[16] The importance of diffusion for lung deposition of therapeutic aerosols is debatable, because the size range involved contains so little drug mass and gives such stability.

EFFECT OF TEMPERATURE AND HUMIDITY

Prediction of particle deposition with therapeutic aerosols is further complicated by the fact that the aerosol is generated at relatively dry ambient conditions and then taken into the airway, where temperature and humidity rapidly increase to saturation at 37° C. Inhaled aerosol drugs are not only heterodisperse in size but are also hygroscopic. For example, between ambient and BTPS conditions, cromolyn sodium powder particles from an MDI increased from 2.31 to 3.02 microns MMAD.[17,18] Fuller and colleagues[19] measured 50% less aerosol for ventilator delivery through an endotracheal tube using an in vitro model from a jet nebulizer in warm, humidified air compared with warm, nonhumidified air.

AEROSOL DEVICES FOR DRUG DELIVERY

Several important questions arise concerning aerosol devices. How should they be quantitatively described for clinicians? Are there differences in clinical effect

with different devices, including spacer and reservoir accessories? What is the correct or optimal use of different types of device? With all aerosol delivery devices, respiratory care personnel should carefully review instructional materials and package inserts to train patients in their correct use. Knowledge of aerosol delivery devices by medical personnel, together with the ability to teach patients in their correct use, is necessary for effective drug delivery. Respiratory care practitioners have been shown to receive formal education in the use of various aerosol devices more often than nursing staff or physicians. Both knowledge and demonstration scores with MDIs, a reservoir device, and a DPI were higher for respiratory therapists than those of registered nurses or physicians in a study by Hanania and associates.[20]

ULTRASONIC NEBULIZERS

The term *nebulizer* encompasses a variety of devices that operate on different physical principles to generate an aerosol from a drug solution. Ultrasonic nebulizers (USN) are electric-powered devices operating on the piezoelectric principle and capable of high output. Particle sizes vary by brand. A generic illustration of a USN is given in Figure 3-4. Although these devices have not been used as routinely for aerosolization of drugs as others to be described below, they have recently been reintroduced as portable, small units that can operate on DC voltage. Such units have several advantages and some disadvantages, as listed in Box 3-2.

The total output of many ultrasonic devices, especially older nonportable units, can be 1 to 2 ml/min, and is greater than that of the jet nebulizer to be discussed, which requires 2 to 8 minutes to nebulize 2 ml. The oscillator frequency of an ultrasonic device determines the particle size produced, with smaller particles sizes at higher frequencies. Frequencies greater than 1 MHz are needed to produce size ranges with an MMAD of less than 8 microns.[16]

At the frequencies used in medical devices, there are several effects with the potential for altering drug activity of the nebulizer solution. Most of the energy with ultrasonic nebulization is dissipated as heat. Protein and other thermolabile formulations can be denatured by heat, especially if the melting temperature of the protein is reached. For example, insulin was shown to be inactivated by USN delivery.[21] Most currently available inhaled drugs are stable with use of a USN.[22] However, rhDNase and tobramycin are now given as inhaled formulations, and additional drugs

Ultrasonic Nebulizer

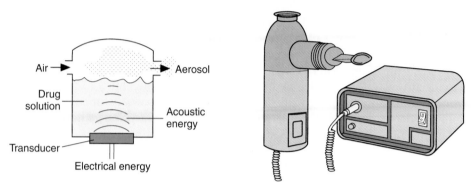

Figure 3-4   Illustration of the principle of ultrasonic nebulization, with an example of a portable device used to aerosolize medications.

Box 3-2	Advantages and Disadvantages of Portable Ultrasonic Drug Nebulizers

Advantages
- Small size
- Rapid nebulization with shorter treatment times
- Smaller drug amounts with no diluent for filling volume
- Can be used during car travel or camping

Disadvantages
- Expense
- Fragility, lack of durability
- Requires electrical source (either AC or DC)
- Possible degrading effect on drug must be determined

should be expected in aerosol delivery. The breakdown of a drug can be a cumulative effect of surface denaturation, heat, cavitation, and direct pressure effects in a USN.[22] Drug solutions must be tested with ultrasonic delivery to determine that activity is preserved, particularly when proteins or liposomes are nebulized.

SMALL PARTICLE AEROSOL GENERATOR

The small particle aerosol generator (SPAG) device is a large reservoir nebulizer, capable of holding 300 ml of solution for long periods of nebulization. It operates on a jet-shearing principle. The device was used during the clinical trials of the aerosol antiviral drug ribavirin (Virazole) and is marketed for delivery of

that drug by its manufacturer. The SPAG unit will be described more fully when ribavirin is discussed in Chapter 13.

SMALL VOLUME NEBULIZERS

Small volume nebulizer (SVN) devices are small-reservoir, gas-powered (pneumatic) aerosol generators, also referred to as *handheld nebulizers* (HHN) in the literature. A generic illustration is given in Figure 3-5. They utilize a jet-shearing principle for creation of an aerosol from the drug solution. An external source of compressed gas is directed through a narrow orifice inside the reservoir cup. The expanding gas creates a localized negative pressure, drawing the drug solution up feeder tubes. As the liquid enters the gas stream, droplets are formed from gas turbulence and impaction on baffles. Smaller particle sizes are emitted after the baffling process. Larger liquid particles are recirculated back to the reservoir. There is significant evaporation of the aqueous solution with gas-powered nebulization. Nebulizer temperatures can fall from ambient to approximately 10° C within minutes because of latent heat of vaporization. With evaporation and constant recirculation, drug solute becomes increasingly concentrated, up to 150% to 300% of the original concentration.[23] A thumb control, pictured in Figure 3-5, allows routing of gas to the nebulizer during inspiration only, although treatment time will be lengthened. Box 3-3 summarizes advantages and disadvantages with these types of nebulizing devices.

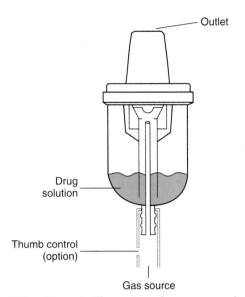

Figure 3-5 A generic illustration of a gas-powered small volume nebulizer with a thumb control attachment to allow for inspiratory nebulization only when the control port is occluded.

Box 3-3	Advantages and Disadvantages of Small Volume Nebulizers (SVNs)

Advantages
- Ability to aerosolize many drug solutions
- Ability to aerosolize drug mixtures (>1 drug) with suitable testing of drug activity
- Minimal coordination is required for inhalation
- Useful in very young or very old, debilitated patients or those in acute distress
- Effective with low inspiratory flows or volumes
- An inspiratory pause (breath-hold) is not required for efficacy
- Drug concentrations can be modified if desired
- Newer nebulizer devices are more efficient

Disadvantages
- The equipment required for use is expensive and cumbersome
- Treatment times are somewhat lengthy for traditional nebulizers compared with other aerosol devices and other routes of administration
- Variability in performance characteristics among different brands
- Contamination is possible with inadequate cleaning
- A wet, cold spray occurs with mask delivery
- Need for an external power source, either electricity or compressed gas

Because SVNs are often used with infants or with patients in acute respiratory distress, slow breathing and an inspiratory pause may not be feasible or obtainable. One of the main advantages of SVNs is that dose delivery occurs over 60 to 90 breaths, rather than in one or two inhalations. Thus a single ineffective breath will not destroy the efficacy of the treatment. Several factors must be considered with gas-powered nebulizers: residual or "dead volume," flow rate, filling volume, temperature, output rate, continuous versus inspiratory nebulization, type of power gas, length of treatment time, and physical nature of the solution to be nebulized. Some of these factors are reviewed in greater detail. Recommended use SVNs, based on the considerations reviewed and the studies available, are summarized in Appendix C.

DEAD VOLUME

Gas-powered nebulizers do not aerosolize below a minimal volume, termed the *dead volume*, which is the amount of drug solution remaining in the reservoir when the device begins to sputter, and aerosolization ceases. This volume can vary with brand of nebulizer but is on the order of 0.5 to 1.0 ml. This is primarily the reason that diluent, which is really additional volume, is added to 0.5 ml of a bronchodilator solution. One half of a milliliter does not nebulize well, al-

though the needed dose is present. Adding diluent does not alter the amount of drug (dose) in the nebulizer, but simply "expands" the solution volume. The concentration of the solution is less, not the amount of drug (see Chapter 4 for further discussion). Drug loss with nebulization can also occur into the ambient air. As a result of these factors, the amount of dose available from a nebulizer is considerably less than the dose placed into the reservoir. Kradjan and Lakshminarayan[24] found that under clinical conditions of nebulization until sputter, approximately 35% to 60% of drug solution was delivered from the nebulizer. Even with vigorous agitation, this amount increased to only 53% to 72%. A study by Shim and Williams[25] found that only 40% to 52% of total dose was delivered from gas-powered nebulizers. In a positive-pressure circuit, this efficiency may decrease further to approximately 30% of the total dose.[26] Evaporation of an aqueous solution will not only cause cooling of the nebulizer and liquid but can also increase the concentration of solute in the residual (dead) volume. If this dead volume is not discarded and the nebulizer rinsed, an increasingly concentrated solution and drug dose could be administered with subsequent treatments.

RELIABILITY

Several reports have described significant variability in performance and efficiency of this type of nebulizer, including leakage of solution.[27-29]

FILLING VOLUME AND TREATMENT TIME

Figure 3-6 demonstrates the relation of volume and flow rate with nebulizers to the time of nebulization, based on the work of Hess and associates,[30] for a pooled average of performance from 17 nebulizer brands. Increasing the volume will increase the time of effective nebulization, at any given flow rate. Below 2 ml, most pneumatic nebulizers do not perform well because the volume is close to the dead volume; that is, the residual amount that does not nebulize. At 6 ml, an excessively long time is required for treatment (>10 minutes) with most brands. Although 5 minutes seems to be a short time, even this can be inconveniently long as a way

of taking medication three or four times a day. Some patients have difficulty in taking a pill four times a day, an approximately 2- to 3-second activity. Patient compliance is directly proportional to convenience. Given the volume requirements of nebulizers for efficient operation and the need for relatively brief treatments, a volume between 3 and 5 ml of solution is recommended. Increasing the volume will also decrease the concentration of drug remaining in the dead volume when nebulization ceases.[30] This will increase the dose of drug available to the patient, although treatment times do increase also, at any given flow rate.

EFFECT OF FLOW RATE

A second practical question concerns the flow rate at which to power pneumatic nebulizers. The flow rate affects two variables: the length of treatment time and the size of the particles produced. Figure 3-6 illustrates the interaction between volume fill and flow rate in determining time of nebulization. At a flow rate of 6 L/min, a volume of 3 ml requires less than 10 minutes; at 10 L/min, a volume of 5 ml can be nebulized in approximately 10 minutes. Figure 3-7 demonstrates the effect of flow rates on particle size of the

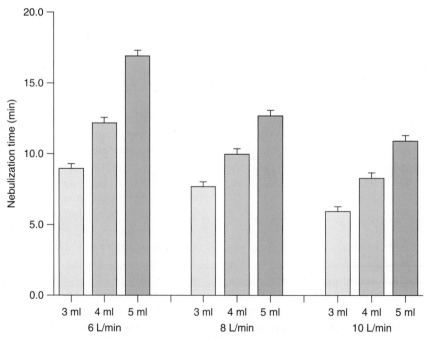

Figure 3-6   The relationship of volume and flow rate on time of nebulization averaged for 17 gas-powered nebulizers. (From Hess D and others: Medication nebulizer performance: effects of diluent volume, nebulizer flow, and nebulizer band, *Chest* 110:498, 1996.)

aerosol produced, averaged for the 17 nebulizers studied by Hess and associates.[30] With pneumatically powered nebulizers, increasing the flow rate will decrease the particle size and shift the MMAD lower. Based on Hess' results in Figures 3-6 and 3-7, an average optimum volume and flow rate for many nebulizers is a volume of 5 ml with a 10 L/min flow rate. Treatment time is kept to approximately 10 minutes or less, available drug is maximized, and MMAD is minimized. It must be emphasized that variability among different brands will affect nebulizer performance with these recommendations.

TYPE OF POWER GAS

Use of gases other than oxygen or air can change performance characteristics of a nebulizer. Hess and associates[30] showed that use of a Heliox mixture to nebulize albuterol caused particle size and inhaled drug mass to decrease, along with a more than twofold increase in nebulization time. Increasing the flow of Heliox returned output to that seen with air.[31]

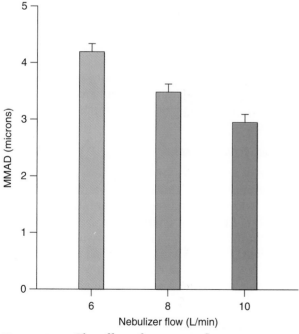

Figure 3-7 The effect of power gas flow rate on mass median aerodynamic diameter (MMAD) of aerosol particles produced on average by 17 gas-powered nebulizers. (From Hess D and others: Medication nebulizer performance: effects of diluent volume, nebulizer flow, and nebulizer band, *Chest* 110:498, 1996.)

TYPE OF SOLUTION

Droplet size of nebulized solutions is related to surface tension and viscosity of the solution, as well as partially determined by the baffles in the device.[32] Recommended filling volumes and flow rates are suitable for the aqueous bronchodilator solutions usually administered with these devices. However, the volumes and flow rates suggested may require modification for some drug solutions, such as pentamidine, or antibiotics, which have different physical characteristics and viscosities. Administration by SVN will be described when these drugs are discussed. For example, higher-viscosity antibiotic solutions of gentamicin or carbenicillin require 10 to 12 L/min power gas flow rates to produce suitably small aerosol particles for inhalation with some jet nebulizers.[33] Some disposable nebulizers may exhibit greater variability in performance or not achieve adequate output characteristics with new or nonbronchodilator drug solutions. Performance of an SVN should be tested for differing drug solutions, and newly introduced nebulizer drugs should be tested with an intended nebulizer system to ensure adequate performance. This has been done with recently introduced aerosol solutions such as dornase alfa (Pulmozyme), inhaled tobramycin (TOBI), and levalbuterol (Xopenex). Nebulizers not tested for performance with a new or unknown drug solution cannot be assumed to produce adequate output and particle sizes. As indicated in Chapter 2 in the review of L/T ratios and the pharmacokinetics of inhaled aerosol drugs, efficiency of lung delivery is a function of *both* drug and device. The drug/device combination should be tested before clinical use. Table 3-1 lists some tested and adequate drug/device combinations for nebulizer delivery. Additives to the

Table 3-1

Representative drug/device combinations tested for nebulizer drug delivery

DRUG	NEBULIZER
Tobramycin	PARI LC PLUS (with DeVilbiss Pulmo-Aide compressor)
Dornase alfa	Hudson T Updraft II, Marquest Acorn II, PARI LC Jet Plus (with Pulmo-Aide or Pari compressors)
Levalbuterol	PARI LC plus
Pentamidine	Marquest Respirgard
Ribavirin	Small particle aerosol generator

drug solution can also affect aerosol characteristics and drug delivery. Delivery of two preparations of the bronchodilator albuterol, one preservative-free and the other with the preservative benzalkonium chloride, using a Hudson T nebulizer showed significantly larger emitted doses with the addition of the preservative.[34] This was likely due to the lowering of surface tension with the benzalkonium. With the preservative, surface tension was measured as 35.0 ± 0.5 mN/m and without, as 70.5 ± 0.3 mN/m, a value close to plain water.

DEVELOPMENT OF NEWER NEBULIZER DESIGNS

The traditional jet nebulizer or SVN commonly used exhibits a large amount of drug wastage, especially within the device itself. For a traditional SVN, a typical emitted dose and loss pattern are as follows[35]:

Lung deposition, 12.4 (4.5)
Oropharynx, 1.5 (0.9)
Device loss, 66.3 (8.6)
Exhaled, 19.7 (3.9)

The data represented are for an Inspiron MiniNeb powered by compressed air at 8 L/min, using radiolabeled human serum albumin in saline. It should be noted that the overall efficiency in lung deposition of 10% to 15% of the total drug dose is not significantly better in most MDI or DPI devices that have been used clinically in the past, as will be discussed subsequently in the clinical application and equivalence of the various devices. Nebulizers, as well as MDIs and DPIs, are undergoing an evolutionary transition to greater efficiency. The spectrum of gas-powered nebulizer design and operation has been conceptualized into three categories by Dennis[23] and are illustrated in Figure 3-8.

1. *Constant Output:* This is the traditional nebulizer in which aerosol is produced constantly during inspiration or exhalation. Emitted aerosol is lost to the environment during exhalation or breathhold. This loss is the basis for using 6 inches of expiratory reservoir tubing, which reduces but does not eliminate ambient contamination. A thumb control to synchronize power to the nebulizer only on inspiration can improve efficiency but also increases treatment time substantially.
2. *Breath-enhanced:* Nebulizer operation allows more aerosol release during inspiration with decreased output during exhalation or breathhold. The PARI LC nebulizers are an example of this type. Aerosol is produced during inspiration and exhalation, but expired gas is routed through a one-way valve in the mouthpiece, with containment of aerosol in the reservoir and reduced ambient loss. Inspired gas comes through the reservoir via another one-way valve.
3. *Dosimetric:* Aerosol is only released during inspiration and all released aerosol is available for patient inhalation. In some designs, such as the AeroEclipse or the Circulaire, aerosol is generated and released only during inspiration. In these designs, no aerosol is lost during expiration and there is usually substantial reduction in the dead volume loss of drug. Based on the concept of dosimetric described by Dennis,[23] any constant-output nebulizer could be a dosimetric nebulizer if a thumb control was used, so that dose delivery occurs only on inspiration, with no nebulization during expiration.

It is evident that the direction of development in nebulizer design is toward higher efficiency in dose release and shorter treatment times, while preserving the ease of patient use traditionally seen. Greater efficiency may lessen the required drug dose in the device similar to what is seen with MDIs when compared with traditional nebulizers. In effect, a dosimetric or breath-controlled nebulizer becomes a "metered dose liquid inhaler," a term used by Dolovich.[36] Newer nebulizer devices are described briefly in Table 3-2 and include both devices in development and those available commercially (e.g., the AeroEclipse). More detailed descriptions are available elsewhere.[36-39]

METERED DOSE INHALERS

Metered dose inhalers (MDIs) were first introduced for drug delivery around 1956,[40] in response to a request by the asthmatic daughter of the president of Riker Laboratories (now 3M Pharmaceuticals) for an easier medication delivery device. These devices are small, pressurized canisters for oral or nasal inhalation of aerosol drugs and contain multiple doses of accurately metered drug. Dosage ranges of respiratory care drugs available in this type of device are from approximately 20 μg (ipratropium Br) to 800 μg (cromolyn sodium).

TECHNICAL DESCRIPTION

There are five major components found in an MDI: drug, propellant/excipient mixture, canister, metering valve, and mouthpiece/actuator. Figure 3-9 illustrates this device. The drug in an MDI is either a suspension

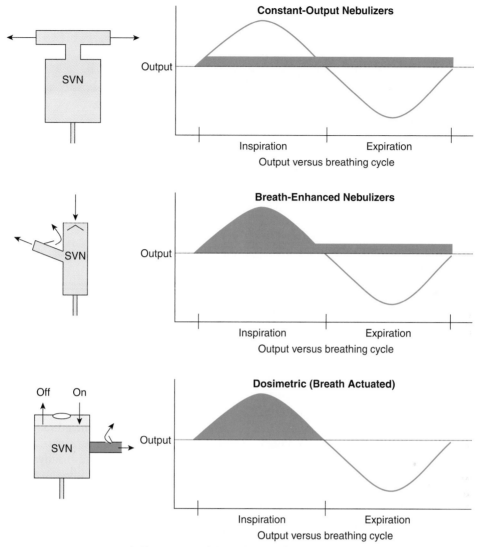

Figure 3-8 Conceptual illustration of the relation of nebulizer generation and output to the inspiratory and expiratory phases. (Based on concept introduced by Dennis JH: A review of issues relating to nebulizer standards, *J Aerosol Med* 11[suppl 1]:S73, 1998.)

of micronized powder in a liquefied propellant or a solution of the active ingredient in a cosolvent (usually ethanol) mixed with the propellant. Dispersing agents, or surfactants, are added to prevent conglomeration and coalescence of drug particles, thereby maintaining suitable particle sizes in the aerosol plume produced. Surfactants currently used include oleic acid, sorbitan trioleate (also termed *Span 85*), or soya lecithin. Flavoring agents also may be added. A detailed technical description of the complexities involved in producing an MDI is offered by Hallworth.[41]

When the canister is depressed into the actuator (see Figure 3-9), the drug-propellant mixture in the metering valve is released under pressure. The liquid propellant rapidly expands and vaporizes, or "flashes," as it ejects from the pressurized valve into ambient pressure. This expansion and vaporization shatters the liquid stream into an aerosol. The initial vaporization of propellant causes cooling of the liquid-gas aerosol suspension, which can be felt if discharged onto the skin. This also can cause users to stop inhaling as the cold aerosol hits the oropharynx.

Table 3-2

Examples of newer nebulizer designs* either available or in development with selected features and solutions tested

NEBULIZER	DESIGN FEATURES	DRUG(S) STUDIED	LUNG DEPOSITION (% OF EMITTED DOSE)
AeroEclipse	Gas-powered, breath-actuated; aerosol generated only during inspiratory effort	Various, including β-agonists	No data available
Halolite	Compressor-driven, electronically modulated aerosol delivery during inspiration only	Radiolabeled DTPA	60%
AERx	Battery powered, unit dose drug blister packs; microprocessor-controlled delivery based on inspiratory flow, volumes	Insulin, morphine	Up to 75%-80%
Respimat	Spring-powered, button-actuated multidose device, with single breath unit drug dose delivery, and "soft mist" plume	Fenoterol, flunisolide	30%-40%

Data from Dolovich M: New propellant-free technologies under investigation, *J Aerosol Med* 12(suppl 1):S9-S17, 1999.
DTPA, Diethylenetriaminepentaacetic acid.
*All of the devices would be categorized as dosimetric.

Upon release, the metering valve refills with the mixture of drug and propellant from the bulk of the canister and is ready for the next discharge. The metering valve varies from 30 to 100 μL in volume.[16]

The propellants originally used as a power source with MDIs to create an aerosol are blends of liquefied gas chlorofluorocarbons (CFCs) (e.g., Freon). This liquefied gas propellant is able to maintain a steady vapor pressure as the canister is exhausted, as long as ambient temperature does not fluctuate significantly. Dichlorodifluoromethane, or propellant 12, is used as the basic driving force for atomizing the liquid solution or suspension, and trichlorofluoromethane (propellant 11) and/or dichlorotetrafluorethane (propellant 114) are blended in to obtain the desired vapor pressure. The propellants are in a liquid state within the canister at the pressures maintained, which is around 400 kPa (approximately 58 psi).[42]

The active drug plus these other ingredients appear on the label of an MDI drug formulation. An example is provided using the label for the Proventil brand of albuterol.

Albuterol (Proventil)
Formulation: Microcrystalline suspension of albuterol
Propellants: Trichloromonofluoromethane and dichlorodifluoromethane
Surfactant (excipient): Oleic acid

The particle size of the aerosol drug released is controlled by two factors: the vapor pressure of the propellant blend and the diameter of the actuator opening.[43] Particle size is reduced as the vapor pressure increases and the diameter size of the nozzle opening decreases. Advantages and disadvantages of drug delivery by MDI are listed in Box 3-4.

CORRECT USE OF A METERED DOSE INHALER

The effectiveness of treatment with an aerosolized drug delivered by an MDI depends on correct use of the device. The major problem with MDI devices is the difficulty of patient use.[44] The most common error noted is the failure to coordinate inhalation and actuation of the inhaler (hand–breathing incoordination). Other problems include too rapid of an inspiratory flow rate, inadequate or missing breath-hold after inhalation, failure to shake and mix canister contents, cessation of inspiration as the aerosol strikes the throat, actuation of the MDI at total lung capacity, inhaling through the nose, and exhaling during actuation.[45,46] Evidence indicates that 50% to 70% of patients do not use MDIs correctly. In addition, physician knowledge of correct MDI use is often inadequate for patient education.[20,47-49]

Recommendations on use of MDIs are provided in Appendix C. These recommendations are consistent with manufacturers' instructions and are sup-

Metered Dose Inhaler

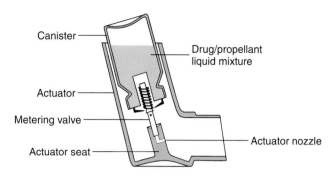

Metering Valve Function

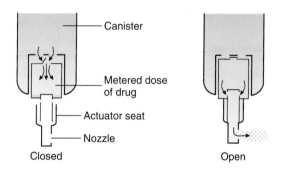

Adapters

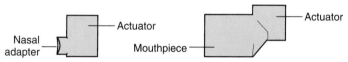

Figure 3-9   The major components of a metered dose inhaler, with an illustration of the function of the metering valve. Both an oral and nasal adapter are shown.

ported by studies by Dolovich and colleagues,[50] Newman and associates,[51] and other studies.[52-56] These studies have shown that whole-lung deposition of aerosols with an MDI is inversely proportional to inspiratory flow rate. High inspiratory flow rates, above 30 L/min, increase inertial impaction in the oropharynx and decrease aerosol reaching the lung.

FACTORS AFFECTING METERED DOSE INHALER PERFORMANCE

The accuracy and consistency of dose from MDIs may be more sensitive to handling practices than previously thought. Research on the drug content of sprays of albuterol by MDI has shown that various factors affect dose consistency.

Loss of Dose. *Loss of dose* refers to the loss of drug content in the valve even though propellant may seem to discharge a normal dose. A dose with less than the nominal amount of drug has been noted to occur on first actuating albuterol MDI when the canister is stored in the valve-down position, even after only a few hours and with shaking before discharge. The loss of dose ranged from 25% to over 50% in the studies referenced.[57,58] This was not observed with storage in a valve-up position. Other drug formulations may increase or decrease drug concentration in the first discharge, after standing unused; this would need to be determined for each product. These findings suggest keeping the canister valve-up between uses and discharging a waste dose if more than 4 hours have elapsed with the valve down, when using albuterol by MDI.

Box 3-4   **Advantages and Disadvantages of Metered Dose Inhaler (MDI) Aerosol Devices**

Advantages
- MDIs are portable and compact.
- Drug delivery is efficient.
- Treatment time is short.

Disadvantages
- Complex hand-breathing coordination is required.
- Drug concentrations are fixed.
- Canister depletion is difficult to determine accurately.
- Reactions to the propellants may occur in a small percentage of patients.
- High orophyaryngeal impaction and loss occur if an extension device is not used.
- Foreign body aspiration of coins and debris from the mouthpiece can occur.*
- CFCs are released into the environment until replacement by non-CFC propellants.

CFCs, Chlorofluorocarbons.
*From Hannan SE et al: Foreign body aspiration associated with the use of an aerosol inhaler, *Am J Respir Dis* 129:1205-1207, 1984; Schultz CH, Hargarten SW, Babbitt J: Inhalation of a coin and a capsule from a metered-dose inhaler, *N Engl J Med* 325:432, 1991 (letter).

Shaking the Canister. Many of the drugs in MDI formulation are suspensions that can separate from the propellants on standing (creaming).[59] This should not affect the dose in the valve, which was filled after the previous actuation. However, if the suspended drug is either lighter or heavier than the propellant and separation occurs, a second actuation could deliver more or less concentrated drug if the canister is not shaken to mix the propellant and drug suspension thoroughly. The MDI should be shaken *before* the first actuation after standing, so that the metering valve refills with adequately mixed suspension from the canister. Everard and colleagues[58] found that not shaking an albuterol canister before use and after the canister has been standing upright overnight led to a 25.5% reduction in total dose and a 36% reduction in particles less than 6.8 μm. This occurred despite wasting two discharges before the measurement.

Timing of Actuation Intervals. A pause of 1 to 5 minutes has been advocated between each puff of a bronchodilator from an MDI, in an attempt to improve distribution of the inhaled drug in the lung.[60] The study by Everard and colleagues[58] found that two actuations of albuterol MDI 1 second apart caused no change in total drug output, although there was a 15.8% decrease in the amount of particles below 6.8 μm. However, four actuations 1 second apart led to significant reductions in dose output. Concern over cooling of the MDI valve with rapid actuations does not seem to be supported by Everard and colleagues' results. Loss of dose probably occurs as a result of turbulence and coalescence of particles with more than two rapid actuations. Clinically, a pause between puffs from an MDI has not been found to be beneficial in routine maintenance therapy. Pedersen[61] showed no difference in forced expiratory volume in 1 second (FEV_1) with a 3- and 10-minute divided dose under nonacute basic maintenance conditions. This was found to be the case for both a β agonist (terbutaline) and a corticosteroid (budesonide) in preadolescents.[62] However, during asthma attacks with acute wheezing, a pause between puffs resulted in significantly improved bronchodilation, with greater effect using a 10-minute pause.[61]

Open-Mouth Versus Closed-Mouth Use of a Metered Dose Inhaler. Actuating the MDI several centimeters in front of the open mouth theoretically allows for slowing of the particle velocity and evaporation of aerosol droplets, resulting in less oropharyngeal impaction and loss. This maneuver further complicates the use of the MDI. Studies with both children and adults have shown no difference in lung function between an open-mouth versus a closed-mouth technique in use of a bronchodilator.[63,64] Consequently, the simpler technique should be preferred. If oropharyngeal impaction is undesirable, as in the case of inhaled corticosteroids, an extension device (spacer or holding chamber) should be used.

Loss of Prime. *Loss of prime* refers to the loss of propellant from the metering valve of the MDI.[65] When this occurs, little or no drug will be discharged on actuation; this can be felt and heard by a user. Loss of prime usually takes days or weeks to occur; regular use of the MDI should prevent this. Shaking of the canister with a waste discharge is suggested after long periods of no use, to prime the valve with propellant and drug.

Storage Temperature. Data indicate that dose delivery from CFC-propelled MDIs of albuterol decreases at lower temperatures. A significant decrease of 65% to 70% of the usual dose has been observed at $-10°$ C. An even greater drop was observed in fine particle mass (<4.7 μm), with approximately 75% of the usual dose at $10°$ C and only 25% at $-10°$ C. No medication was delivered at $-20°$ C.[66] In contrast, HFA-albuterol, discussed subsequently, remained constant in total dose over the range of $-20°$ C to $20°$ C. The fine particle mass of the CFC-free formulation decreased significantly only at $-20°$ C, delivering approximately 60% of the initial fine particle dose. Temperature effects such as these are likely to be relevant only for outdoor use of MDI canisters in extreme weather.

BREATH-ACTUATED INHALERS

A type of device to simplify MDI use is a breath-actuated adapter (Figure 3-10). In the United States the adrenergic bronchodilator pirbuterol (Maxair; see Chapter 6) is marketed as a breath-actuated inhaler. Breath-actuated inhalers offer an alternative for individuals who find it difficult to coordinate MDI actuation with inhalation. Devices such as the breath-actuated inhaler were described as early as 1971. The device is described by Newman and associates[67] and Baum and Bryant.[68]

The Autohaler. A conventional pressurized MDI (pMDI) canister is fitted within the Autohaler actuator. The MDI canister is triggered by a spring, through a triggering mechanism activated when the patient inhales. To use, the device is primed, or "cocked," by raising the lever on top of the adapter. This applies pressure to the canister. The canister cannot move downward because of a vane in the mouthpiece. As the patient inhales at flow rates of 22 to 26 L/min, the vane lifts, the spring forces the canister downward, and a metered dose is released. The device is reset by lowering the lever to its resting position, which allows the MDI valve to refill.

The SmartMist. A microprocessor-controlled MDI, the SmartMist, in effect is also breath-actuated. The device monitors the inspiratory flow and volume and fires the MDI at a predefined condition during inspiration. Lung deposition was improved to 18.6% ($\pm$ 1.42) when the device was fired early in inspiration and at a medium (90 L/min) flow rate.[69] The expense of the device ($>\$300$) at the time of this edition precludes general use clinically.[37]

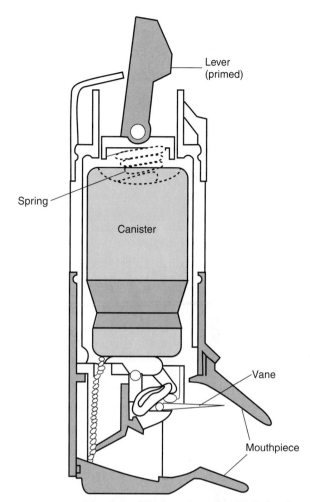

Figure 3-10   Diagram of the breath-actuated inhaler device marketed for pirbuterol (Maxair).

HYDROFLUOROALKANE (NON-CHLOROFLUOROCARBON) PROPELLANTS

The potential for damage to the protective ozone layer in the earth's atmosphere by CFCs has been noted since 1974. One CFC molecule can destroy 100,000 molecules of stratospheric ozone. The 1987 Montreal Protocol on Substances that deplete the Ozone Layer called for a phase-out of CFC *production* by the year 2000. This date was accelerated in 1992 to take effect on January 1, 1996, with the European production phase-out occurring a year earlier, on January 1, 1995.[70] Supplies of CFC propellant have been stockpiled to allow time for development of replacement propellants for MDIs. Hydrofluorocarbons (HFCs), also termed *hydrofluoroalkanes* (HFAs), have been identified as propellants that are nontoxic to the

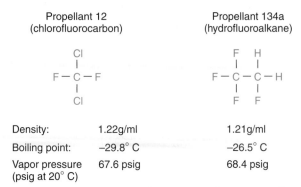

Figure 3-11   Structure and properties of CFC propellant 12 and non-CFC propellant 134a used in pressurized metered dose inhaler drug formulations.

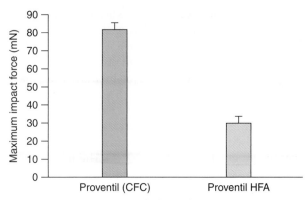

Figure 3-12   Measures of plume force exiting a metered dose inhaler for CFC- and HFA-propelled albuterol (Proventil and Proventil HFA). (Data from Ross DL, Gabrio BJ: Advances in metered dose inhaler technology with the development of a chlorofluorocarbon-free drug delivery system, *J Aerosol Med* 12:151, 1999.)

atmosphere and to the patient and have properties suitable for MDI aerosol generation. In particular, HFA 134a has a vapor pressure similar to that of CFC 12, the main CFC propellant. The structure of HFA 134a is illustrated in Figure 3-11 and compared with the CFC. HFA 134a is licensed to 3M Pharmaceuticals; it is the propellant used in the first MDI formulation of albuterol (salbutamol in Europe) and has been given the brand name Aeromir outside the United States and Proventil HFA in the United States. Replacement of the CFC propellants has led to an overall reengineering of MDI components (valve, seals, exit orifice, drug formulation), which has improved MDI performance. The differences between CFC-formulated albuterol and the newer HFA formulation are summarized in Box 3-5. Some of the differences, such as the lower plume force (Figure 3-12) and warmer plume temperature, cause patients who have used CFC-propelled MDI formulations to think there is reduced or no drug delivery occurring with the HFA formulation of albuterol.

Equivalence and Safety. HFA-formulated MDI albuterol produces a nominal dose of 120 μg of albuterol sulfate from the canister nozzle (from the valve), which is equivalent to the nominal dose of 100 μg from the valve of albuterol base found in the CFC formulation Proventil. Emitted doses average 108 μg and 90 μg, respectively, by the mouthpiece. Equivalent doses should yield equivalent clinical effects. Studies have found similar bronchodilating responses between the CFC and HFA albuterol MDI formulations.[71,72] The HFA formulation of MDI albuterol has also been shown to have a safety profile equivalent to that of the CFC formulation.[73,74] Equivalent bronchodilation has also been found with the MDI HFA

Box 3-5 | **Changes in Metered Dose Inhaler Design and Function Accompanying Hydrofluoroalkane-Albuterol Formulation (Proventil HFA)**

Formulation
- Microcrystalline suspension of albuterol sulfate (120 μg = 100 μg base)
- Propellant: HFA 134a
- Ethanol
- Oleic acid

Redesigned metering valves

Metering valve seals of elastomer developed to be compatible with HFA

Smaller valve size of approximately 25 μL

Smaller actuator spray exit orifice diameter

Smaller nozzle outer diameter compared with that for CFC (2.8 mm versus 3.2 mm)

Reshaped round mouthpiece to open patient's mouth wider

Reduced plume force at mouthpiece (softer puff)

Warmer plume than CFC formulation (no cold Freon effect)

Reliable dose delivery at low temperatures

Consistent dosing with different canister orientations (inverted, horizontal, upright)

CFC, Chlorofluorocarbons; *HFA,* hydrofluoroalkanes.

formulation of fenoterol and ipratropium bromide, both bronchodilators, compared with a conventional CFC-propelled MDI formulation.[75] Therapeutic equivalence and comparable safety was similarly found with a comparison of inhaled triamcinolone

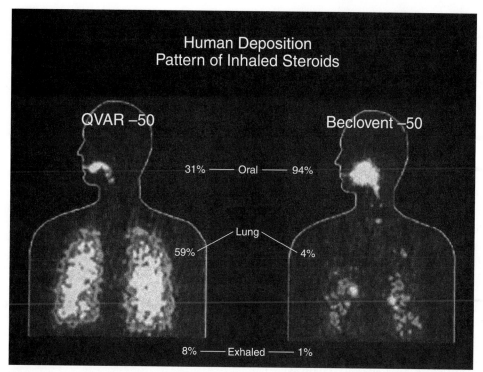

Figure 3-13 Comparison of lung deposition between the CFC and the HFA formulation of beclomethasone dipropionate by metered dose inhaler. (Scintigraph and data courtesy C. Leach, Ph.D., 3M Pharmaceuticals, Inc., St. Paul, Minn.)

acetonide (a corticosteroid) using either an HFA-propelled or a CFC-propelled formulation.[76]

Improved Drug Delivery With Hydrofluoroalkane Formulation. Although equivalent drug amounts and effects were found with the drugs noted, the reengineering of the MDI for HFA propellant can result in significant improvements in performance and in particular in lung deposition of the aerosol drug. An example is the HFA-propelled MDI formulation of beclomethasone dipropionate (BDP; a corticosteroid). The traditional amount of 10% for lung deposition has been increased more than five-fold with HFA BDP.[77] Figure 3-13 illustrates a comparison of lung delivery between HFA-based and CFC-based MDI systems. A significant increase in lung delivery is not expected to give equivalent effects between the CFC and the HFA formulations.

Equi-effective doses of the same drug such as BDP from a CFC and an HFA MDI would be different. In fact, this has been shown for HFA BDP. Gross and associates[78] found that a 400-μg/day dose of HFA BDP provided control of moderate to severe asthma equivalent to that of an 800-μg/day dose with CFC BDP.

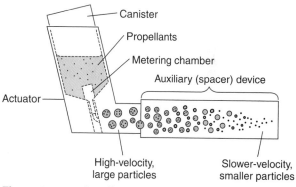

Figure 3-14 The effect of an extension device on aerosol particle size and velocity from a metered dose inhaler.

METERED DOSE INHALER RESERVOIR DEVICES

Figure 3-14 is an illustration of a generic reservoir device. Extension, or reservoir, devices were introduced primarily to simplify the complex coordination of aiming, actuation, and breathing with an MDI. Reservoir devices can modify the aerosol discharged from an MDI in the following three ways:

1. Such devices allow space and time for more vaporization of the propellants and evapora-

---

MDI, Metered dose inhaler.

tion of initially large particles to smaller sizes. The initial particle size from an MDI can exceed 35 microns at the nozzle, which must be reduced to the 1- to 5-micron range for lung penetration.[42]

2. Reservoirs allow the high initial velocity of particles released from a MDI to slow before reaching the oropharynx. Particles discharged from the actuator nozzle have velocities exceeding 30 m/sec. By holding the actuator 4 cm in front of the mouth or by using an extension device, this velocity is allowed to slow.[50]

3. As holding chambers for the aerosol cloud released, reservoir devices separate the actuation of the canister from the inhalation and simplify the coordination required for good use.

The combined effect of the first two advantages reduces oropharyngeal deposition. This will reduce the amount of drug swallowed and thereby absorbed from the gastrointestinal tract and also reduce any local oropharyngeal side effects, such as those seen with inhaled corticosteroids. The advantages and disadvantages of reservoir devices are summarized in Box 3-6.

TERMINOLOGY

A variety of reservoir devices are now available, and the size ranges from 70 to 80 ml to 750 ml for some European brands. Numerous terms are used to refer to such devices, including *spacer, reservoir, auxiliary device, extension device, holding chamber,* and *add-on device.* Some distinction of terms may be useful to denote significant design differences among these devices. The following terminology is offered, partially based on Dolovich[79]:

Reservoir device: Global term describing or referring to extension, auxiliary, add-on devices attached to MDIs for administration. This term could include both "spacer" and "holding chamber," defined as follows.

Spacer: Denotes a simple tube or extension device, with no one-way valves to contain the aerosol cloud; its purpose is simply to extend the MDI spray away from the mouth.

Holding chamber: Denotes a spacer device with the addition of one-way valve(s) to contain and hold the aerosol cloud until inspiration occurs.

DESIGN VARIABLES

Reservoir devices have several design variables, including volume, shape, direction of MDI spray, presence of one-way valves, inspiratory flow rate indicators, and presence or absence of an integral (built-in) MDI actuator. Table 3-3 summarizes these design variables for some reservoir devices available in the United States. Figure 3-15 illustrates differences in size and design of several units.

LUNG DEPOSITION WITH RESERVOIR DEVICES

The loss of drug in reservoir devices can be as much as 60% to 65% of the total dose, but this is replacing the same amount previously lost in the oropharynx.[80,81] Lung deposition can be improved, although it has not been shown to exceed 20% of the total dose and is probably in the 10% to 15% range. Variation limits for the 10% figure are clearly presented by Newman[15] in studies of various devices. With inhaled corticosteroids, reservoir devices are required to reduce oropharyngeal impaction and subsequent opportunistic throat infections, such as candidiasis, and to limit swallowed drug amount. Reservoir devices are recommended for use with an MDI when treating acute airflow obstruction[82] and offer an alternative to an SVN in acute respiratory distress. The simplified coordination of MDI actuation with inhalation given by a reservoir provides adequate doses of MDI drug even with dyspnea or tachypnea. Several articles, including a review of deposition studies and clinical aspects of

Table 3-3

Characteristics of selected reservoir devices used in the United States, exemplifying design variable differences

BRAND	VOLUME (APPROXIMATE)	INSPIRATORY VALVE	SPRAY DIRECTION*	FLOW INDICATOR	INTEGRAL ACTUATOR
Aerochamber	145 ml	One way	Forward	Yes	No†
ACE	175 ml	One way	Reverse	Yes	Yes
InspirEase	600 ml	No	Reverse	Yes	Yes
OptiHaler	70 ml	No	Reverse	No	Yes
MediSpacer	160 ml	No	Reverse	Yes	Yes

*Relative to mouth.
†Accepts mouthpiece-actuator of drug brand.

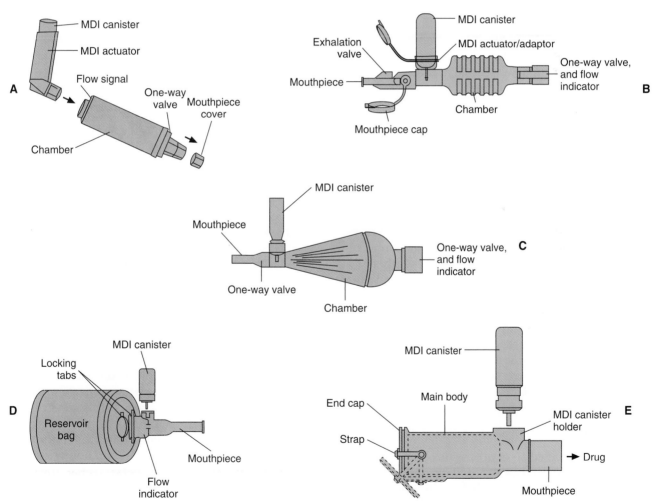

Figure 3-15 Representative metered dose inhalter auxiliary reservoir devices. **A,** Aerochamber. **B,** MediSpacer. **C,** Aerosol Cloud Enhancer, ACE. **D,** InspirEase. **E,** OptiHaler. (*A,* Courtesy Monaghan Medical Corp.; *B,* courtesy Allegiance Healthcare Inc.; *C,* courtesy Diemolding Healthcare, Inc.; *D,* courtesy Schering-Plough, Inc.; *E,* courtesy Healthscan, Inc.)

reservoir devices by Newman and Newhouse,[83] provide excellent reviews of auxiliary spacer systems with detailed references.[45,84-86]

Use of Reservoir Devices. Although reservoir devices are intended to simplify inhalation of an aerosol from an MDI, prolonged separation of MDI actuation and inhalation from the MDI can result in loss of dose. Gravitational settling can affect the aerosol dose remaining suspended in the device. Optimal dose is obtained by inhaling either simultaneously with MDI discharge or in the first second or two after discharge. The practice of discharging multiple doses of a bronchodilator into a holding chamber and then inhaling can also decrease the dose per actuation and therefore the total dose received.[86] Single discharges, each with a simultaneous inhalation or inhalation within 1 or 2 seconds, should provide an optimal dose. Unfortunately, such use minimizes or removes the separation of actuation and inhalation previously thought to be an advantage of reservoir devices.

Effect of Hydrofluoroalkane Propellant on Reservoir Dose. With many aerosol drugs, including bronchodilators, a larger reservoir volume could increase the available dose. For example, most reservoir chambers used in the United States are less than 200 ml. European versions such as the Nebuhaler or the Volumatic are 750 ml or larger. A beneficial effect with the HFA-propelled MDI of albuterol is the improved dose availability with smaller chambers.[87] Figure 3-16 illustrates the effect of chamber size on total and fine particle dose for CFC and HFA albuterol.

Although there is a significant difference in dose between the small (AeroChamber) and large (Volumatic) holding chambers using CFC albuterol, dose is increased from the small holding chamber and nearly equal to the large chamber with HFA albuterol. HFA propellants seem to decrease the importance of reservoir volume on drug delivery.

OTHER METERED DOSE INHALER AUXILIARY DEVICES

In addition to reservoir devices, which provide a holding chamber to decrease the need for close coordination between activating the MDI and inhaling, devices have been developed to improve the ease of using MDIs. One of these, represented by the Vent Ease, is illustrated in Figure 3-17. The device is essentially a lever that fits over the entire canister-actuator assembly. When the handle is squeezed, the canister is

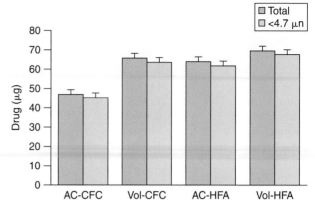

Figure 3-16   A comparison of emitted total and fine particle dose with a large- and small-volume holding chamber using either CFC or HFA-propelled metered dose inhaler albuterol. Emitted dose is the same for small or large chambers with HFA-albuterol. *AC-CFC,* AeroChamber with chlorofluorocarbon; *AC-HFA,* AeroChamber with HFA propellant; *Vol-CFC,* Volumatic with chlorofluorocarbon; *Vol-HFA,* Volumatic with HFA propellant. (Data from Mitchell JP, Nagel MW, Rau JL: Performance of large-volume versus small-volume holding chambers with chlorofluorocarbon-albuterol and hydrofluoroalkane-albuterol sulfate, *Respir Care* 44:38, 1999.)

forced down into its actuator, and a metered dose of drug is released for inhalation. The advantage offered by this device is increased ease of physically actuating the pressurized canister, particularly for elderly patients with arthritis, reduced grip strength, or problems in gripping and squeezing the small canister.

DRY POWDER INHALERS

The first dry powder inhaler (DPI) was the Spinhaler, introduced in 1971 by Bell and colleagues,[88] for the delivery of a 20-mg powder dose of cromolyn sodium. With the Spinhaler, a gelatin capsule containing a single dose of drug was placed in a propeller rotor. The sleeve of the device would slide down and cause metal needles to pierce the capsule. During a forceful inhalation the capsule revolved with the rotor and powder was dispersed. A 35-L/min flow rate was the minimum for causing dispersal of the powder mixture in the Spinhaler. The basic principle described for generation of a powder aerosol has remained the same, although devices developed after the Spinhaler, such as the Turbuhaler and Diskus (Figure 3-18), increased in sophistication. These devices are breath-actuated, with turbulent airflow from the

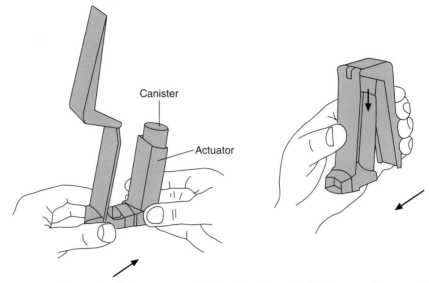

Figure 3-17   Example of a lever type of device that is intended to increase the ease of actuating a metered dose inhaler. The lever assists the user to squeeze the canister into the actuator and release the aerosol.

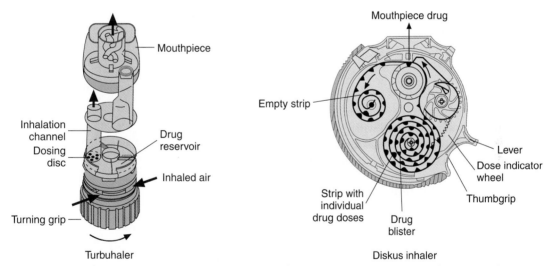

Figure 3-18   Diagrammatic representation of dry powder inhaler devices, the Turbuhaler and the Diskus inhaler.

inspiratory effort of the user providing the power to create an aerosol of microfine solid particles of drug as air is inhaled through a mouthpiece. Thus inspiration is inherently linked with generation and delivery of the aerosol, in contrast to the actuation-inhalation problem with MDIs. The drug powder consists of cohesive micronized drug particles with somewhat larger carrier particles, usually of lactose. The lactose enhances flow properties and acts as a bulking agent to provide suitable volume to the unit dose.[89,90] Table

3-4 summarizes features of powder inhaler devices available since the Spinhaler in the United States.

The use of DPIs combines the advantages of both SVNs and MDIs, that is, ease of use with small, portable efficient drug delivery while eliminating the disadvantages. The need for non-CFC aerosol delivery technology has given renewed impetus to development and use of DPIs. The primary factor in use of DPIs is the ability to generate a sufficient inspiratory flow rate to generate the powder aerosol. The advantages and

Table 3-4

List of dry powder inhaler devices and selected features

DEVICE	DRUG	PRINCIPLE	NUMBER OF DOSES	CARRIER	COUNTER
Rotahaler	Albuterol	200-μg capsule	Single dose	Lactose	N/A
Rotadisk	Fluticasone	50-, 100-, 250-μg blister pack	4 per pack	Lactose	N/A
Diskus	Salmeterol	50-μg blister strip	60 per strip	Lactose	Yes
Turbuhaler	Budesonide	200-μg doses; powder reservoir	200	None	Low-dose warning, <20

N/A, Not applicable (number of doses known by capsule count or pack).

disadvantages of DPI devices are listed in Box 3-7. Generic recommendations for use of DPI devices are provided in Appendix C.

INSPIRATORY FLOW RATE

Dispersal of drug powder from its agglomeration depends on the energy of the inspiratory flow. A moderate to high inspiratory flow is needed with DPIs to obtain an optimal dose. With inspiratory flows below 50 L/min, significant reduction in clinical response occurs with both the Rotahaler and the Spinhaler.[91,92] This affects use of these devices by young children, especially below 5 years of age, and by any patient with an acute wheezing episode associated with airflow reduction. Figure 3-19 illustrates the effect of varying inspiratory flows with three DPI devices. The Turbuhaler, illustrated in Figure 3-18, was found effective at flow rates of approximately 30 L/min, which can be achieved by many children between 3 and 6 years of age, in a study by Pedersen and colleagues.[93] In Pedersen and colleagues' study, the Turbuhaler was reported to be approximately 30% effective even with inspiratory flows as low as 13 L/min.

HUMIDITY

Another factor that can affect dose delivery from a DPI is humidity and moisture, which can reduce the fine particle mass in the dose. With the Turbuhaler, which has a bulk reservoir of drug powder, fine particle mass has been seen to decrease in approximately 2 weeks, in humid conditions (30° C, 75% relative humidity).[94] In contrast the Diskus, in which the drug dose is protected inside the blister on the foil strip, showed no change over 8 weeks of such conditions. With any DPI, it is absolutely es-

Box 3-7   Advantages and Disadvantages of Dry Powder Inhaler Devices

Advantages
- Small and portable devices
- Short preparation and administration time
- Breath-actuation removes the need for hand-breathing coordination
- No inspiratory hold or head-tilt is needed
- No CFC propellants (environmentally friendly)
- No "cold, Freon effect" to cause bronchoconstriction or inhibit full inspiration
- Count of remaining drug doses is simple

Disadvantages
- Limited range of drugs available to date
- Patients are not as aware of the dose inhaled as with an MDI and may distrust delivery
- Moderate to high inspiratory flow rates are needed for powder dispersion
- Relatively high oropharyngeal impaction and deposition can occur
- A device such as Rotahaler is single-dose and must be loaded before each use

CFC, Chlorofluorocarbon; *MDI,* metered dose inhaler.

sential that patients do not exhale into the device before inhaling; in all devices, including the Diskus and the Diskhaler, the drug powder is exposed once the device is activated.

CLINICAL EFFICACY

DPIs have been shown to be equivalent in efficacy to pressurized aerosols with MDIs.[95-99] The search for re-

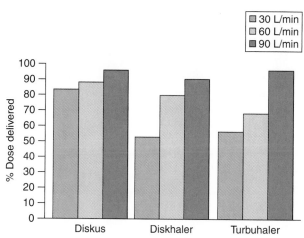

Figure 3-19   Effect of inspiratory flow rate on the percent of nominal dose delivered for three DPI devices. Data are in vitro for albuterol. (Modified from Prime D and others: A critical comparison of the dose delivery characteristics of four alternative inhalation devices delivering salbutamol: pressurized MDI, Diskus inhaler, Diskhaler, and Turbuhaler, *J Aerosol Med* 12:75, 1999).

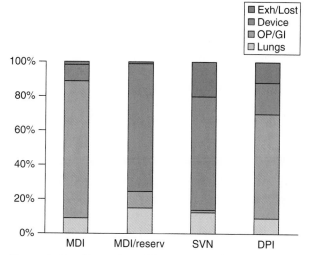

Figure 3-20   llustration of the patterns of aerosol loss for four drug delivery systems. (Data for each device are based on the following studies (see references): *DPI,* Zainudin, 1990[100]; *MDI,* Newman, 1981[52]; *MDI and spacer,* Newman, 1986[80]; *SVN,* Lewis, 1985[35].)

placements for CFC-propelled MDIs has given renewed impetus to consideration and development of DPI technology. Lung deposition has increased with more recent devices and with devices currently being developed, such as the Spiros. Lung deposition data are available for several of the DPIs currently in use:

Rotahaler (albuterol): 9.1%[100]
Diskus (fluticasone propionate): 16.6%[36]
Turbuhaler (budesonide): 32%[101]

CLINICAL APPLICATION OF AEROSOL DELIVERY DEVICES

LUNG DEPOSITION AND LOSS PATTERNS WITH TRADITIONAL AEROSOL DEVICES

Aerosol devices that have traditionally been used in respiratory care deliver approximately 10% to 15% of the total drug dose to the lung. The pattern of loss to the mouth, stomach, and apparatus and through exhalation differs among the device types. Figure 3-20 illustrates both the percentage of dose deposited in the lung and the pattern of loss with devices that have traditionally been used, based on four separate studies of the MDI, MDI and spacer, SVN, and DPI delivery systems. The four systems of aerosol delivery

each gave the following lung deposition in the studies referenced:

MDI (CFC, 99mTc Teflon): 8.8%[52]
MDI and spacer (CFC, 99mTc Teflon and IspirEase): 14.8%[81]
SVN (Inspiron Mini-Neb, 99mTc): 12.4%[35]
DPI (Rotahaler, salbutamol and 99mTc Teflon): 9.1%[100]

The average amount of lung deposition for each device varies among studies. One cannot conclude that an SVN will always deliver a higher percentage of dose to the lungs than an MDI. Spiro and associates[102] showed that an MDI delivered an average of 11.1% to the lungs, whereas a 1990 study by Zainudin and associates[100] found that an SVN delivered 9.9% of the total dose, in contrast to the percentages given above.

The MDI and the SVN show the greatest contrast in the loss pattern of aerosol drug. Most of the loss with an MDI occurs in the mouth and stomach (approximately 80%). Most of the loss with an SVN is in the delivery apparatus (66%), with most of that remaining in the nebulizer, whereas an MDI loses approximately 10% in the actuator.

Adding a spacer or holding chamber to an MDI lowers the drug amount lost in the oropharnyx and stomach.[85] In a study by Newman and others[80] in 1986 evaluating the InspirEase, use of the reservoir device shifted oropharyngeal loss from over 80% to 9.5%, with 59% lost within the reservoir.

The DPI is similar to the MDI in its pattern of aerosol loss. In the 1990 study by Zainudin and others,[100] 61% of aerosol drug was lost in the mouth or stomach and approximately 18% in the apparatus, with almost 12% apparently lost to the air during opening of the drug gelatin capsule with a Rotahaler.

EQUIVALENT DOSES AMONG DEVICE TYPES

If traditional MDI, SVN, and DPI devices all deliver approximately the same percentage of total device dose to the lungs, and the nominal dose in the devices differs, then different amounts of drug are placed within the lung. For example, the dose of albuterol, a β-adrenergic bronchodilator, by MDI versus nebulizer is:

MDI: 2 puffs, or 0.2 mg
SVN: 0.5 cc, or 2.5 mg

The ratio of MDI to SVN dose is approximately 1:12. Differences in dose between MDI and SVN formulations for various drugs are given in Table 3-5. If approximately 10% of the dose reaches the lungs, very different doses are being delivered from the three types of aerosol devices. For example, if we assume that 10% of the dose reaches the lungs using albuterol by MDI and SVN, then a lung dose of 20 µg would be given by MDI versus a lung dose of 250 µg from an SVN (10% of 200 µg versus 10% of 2.5 mg). Several studies have examined this question of equipotent doses between delivery devices.

Equipotent dose: The dose by each delivery method that produces an equivalent degree of effect (for bronchodilators, this would be bronchodilation).

The standard difference in dose between the MDI and the SVN delivery methods for albuterol is in the ratio of 1:12. However, at least two studies suggest that an MDI:SVN dose ratio of 1:3 and 1:4 to achieve equal bronchodilation or equivalent amounts of drug delivery to the lung.[103,104] This equipotent dose ratio of 1:3 or 1:4 is achieved by increasing the number of puffs from the MDI to 7 and 10, respectively, in the two studies.

One of the clearest statements on the question of delivery efficiency among traditional aerosol devices resulted from the 1990 study by Zainudin and others.[100] The study examined drug delivery by pMDI

Table 3-5

Dose differences between metered dose inhaler (MDI) and small volume nebulizer (SVN) drug formulations

DRUG	MDI	SVN	RATIO
Albuterol	0.2 mg (200 µg)	2.5 mg	1:12.5
Metaproterenol	1.3 mg	15 mg	1:11.5
Bitolterol	0.74 mg	2.5 mg	1:3.4
Ipratropium	0.04 mg (40 µg)	0.5 mg	1:12
Cromolyn	2 mg	20 mg	1:10

(CFC propellants), DPI (Rotahaler), and gas-powered SVN (Acorn). The results are particularly helpful because the investigators used the same dose of 400 µg of albuterol (salbutamol) in each of the device types. This allowed a direct microgram-for-microgram comparison of the dose from the devices. The percent of lung deposition is shown in Figure 3-21, with an MDI delivery of 11.2%, a DPI delivery of 9.1%, and an SVN delivery of 9.9%.

The clinical response, measured by the improvement in FEV$_1$, is also similar, although the change with the MDI (35.6%) is statistically significantly greater than that seen with the DPI (25.2%) or the SVN (25.8%), a result not well explained in the study. These results support the view that the amount of aerosol drug delivered to the lung is similar with any of the three device types, and the clinical response is similar. *The amount of bronchodilation obtained is a reflection of the dose of drug given and not the method of delivery.*[105,106] As discussed in the following section, the development of aerosol devices that are highly efficient for lung delivery of drug is likely to lead to changes in recommended doses. For example, the increased efficiency of HFA-propelled beclomethasone, cited in the section on HFA propellants, has resulted in use of half of the dose normally found with CFC-propelled beclomethasone, with equivalent effects. These changes will in turn affect what constitutes equivalent doses between different types of devices.

LUNG DEPOSITION WITH NEWER AEROSOL DEVICES

The development of increasingly efficient devices that was noted with MDIs, SVNs, and DPIs will cause the traditional figures of 10% to 15% for lung deposition to be revised upward. Unless newer devices com-

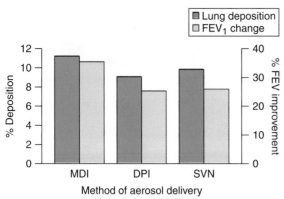

Figure 3-21 Lung deposition and response: three bronchodilator delivery methods. Comparison of lung deposition as percent of total dose, and clinical response to aerosol delivery, of the same dose of albuterol (400 μg) from three types of aerosol devices. (Data from Zainudin and others: Comparison of bronchodilator responses and deposition patterns of salbutamol inhaled from a pressurized metered dose inhaler, as a dry powder, and as a nebulized solution, *Thorax* 45:469, 1990.)

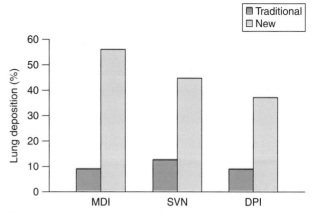

Figure 3-22 Comparison of lung deposition with older, traditional aerosol devices (CFC-MDI, Inspiron MiniNeb, Rotahaler DPI) and with newer devices (*MDI*, HFA-beclomethasone[110]; *SVN*, Respimat[109]; *New DPI*, Spiros[36] [References provide further detail.]).

pletely replace the older, traditional aerosol generators used clinically, there will be a wide variety of lung depositions seen rather than a single range of 10% to 15%. The amount of lung delivery will depend on which device is used. Figure 3-22 graphically compares lung deposition data with traditional devices (MDI, SVN, DPI) with measures from newer devices. These data are compiled from several studies and for various drugs.[36,107,108]

One implication of changing and increasing lung deposition amounts is that the total dose from a device must be reduced. With a greater percentage reaching the lung, a lower total dose is needed from the device. Without proportional reduction in total device dose, toxic effects would be possible. Ultimately, the important factor is not the device per se but rather the amount of drug reaching the lungs when treating pulmonary disease.

CLINICAL EQUIVALENCE OF METERED DOSE INHALERS AND NEBULIZERS

It is still relatively common in clinical practice to use an SVN instead of an MDI in emergent acute situations requiring aerosol bronchodilator delivery. However, a large and growing body of evidence indicates that an MDI with a spacer or holding chamber is as effective as an SVN in acute airway obstruction. Further, an MDI/reservoir has been shown as effective as an SVN with all age-groups, from nonventilated preterm infants (with addition of a face mask) to adults in emergency department treatment. Table 3-6 summarizes selected studies supporting the clinical equivalence of either an MDI or SVN in emergency treatment for various age-groups. Amirav and Newhouse[109] offer a comprehensive review of studies on this issue. A meta-analysis of studies comparing bronchodilator administration by MDI or "wet nebulizer" (SVN) concluded that either method was equivalent in treatment of acute airflow obstruction in adults.[82]

AGE GUIDELINES FOR USE OF AEROSOL DEVICES

The assumption of correct use with each type of delivery device cannot be made in every patient. However, the differences and in particular the relative advantages and disadvantages among the available devices can be used as the basis for choosing the type of device to match the patient's needs. Age is an important factor to consider when selecting an aerosol delivery system. Age guidelines have been provided in the National Asthma Education Prevention Program Expert Panel Report II (NAEPP EPR II) and are listed in Table 3-7.[114] A consideration that applies to the final decision is device/equipment cost and third party reimbursement. A consensus conference convened by the National Association

Table 3-6

Studies showing equivalence of a metered dose inhaler (MDI), with reservoir or face mask, to a small volume nebulizer (SVN) for bronchodilator administration in acute airflow obstruction for various age-groups

AGE-GROUP	DRUG	DOSE	OUTCOME VARIABLES	REFERENCE
Preterm infants, 47 ± 4.8 days	Albuterol*	MDI/spacer/mask: 2 puffs (200 μg) q4h SVN mask: 0.2 ml (200 μg) q4h	Lung compliance, resistance	Folk, 1998[110]
Infants, 16 ± 15 mo	Albuterol	MDI/HC/mask: 4 puffs (400 μg) q20min × 3 SVN: 2.5 mg q20min × 3	Respiratory rate, clinical scores, admissions	Mandelberg, 2000[111]
Children, 5-16 yr	Terbutaline	MDI/HC/mask: 3 puffs (0.75 mg) × 1 SVN/mouthpiece: 0.5 ml (2.5 mg) × 1	Lung function, clinical scores	Lin, 1995[112]
Adults, 64.6 ± 13.3 yr	Albuterol	MDI/HC: 2 puffs (200 μg) q15min × 3 SVN: 0.5 ml (2.5 mg) q15min × 3	Spirometry, asthma scores	Mandelberg, 1997[113]

First author and year of publication are given, with full citation in references.
HC, Holding chamber (valved reservoir); *spacer,* nonvalved reservoir.
*Albuterol is also known as salbutamol outside the United States.

Table 3-7

Age guidelines for use of aerosol delivery devices

AEROSOL SYSTEM	AGE
SVN	≤2 yr
MDI	>5 yr
MDI with reservoir	>4 yr
MDI with reservoir/mask	≤4 yr
MDI with ETT	≥ neonate
Breath-actuated MDI	>5 yr
DPI	≥5 yr

Data from National Institutes of Health: National Asthma Education and Prevention Program, Expert Panel Report II: *Guidelines for the diagnosis and management of asthma,* Bethesda, Md, 1997, National Institutes of Health.
DPI, Dry powder inhaler; *MDI,* metered dose inhaler; *SVN,* small volume nebulizer.

for Medical Direction of Respiratory Care (NAM-DRC) published guidelines in 1996 on the use of nebulizers outside the hospital.[115] These guidelines suggested that an MDI with a reservoir chamber is the preferred mode of aerosol delivery for individuals outside the hospital and outlined circum- stances under which an SVN would be appropriately prescribed.

PATIENT-DEVICE INTERFACE

The majority of aerosol drug administration is used with oral inhalation; that is, the subject inhales the aerosol through the open mouth. However, other types of interface occur in clinical practice and raise questions concerning efficacy and drug delivery. These are administration by positive-pressure aerosol administration with a face mask and administration of aerosolized drugs through endotracheal tubes (ETT).

ADMINISTRATION BY INTERMITTENT POSITIVE-PRESSURE BREATHING

Although administration by intermittent positive-pressure breathing (IPPB) has been a popular form of aerosol therapy in past years, the consensus of research on this method of delivery has been that IPPB delivery of aerosolized medication is no more clinically effective than simple spontaneous, unassisted inhalation from SVNs.[116-118] As a result, the use of IPPB for delivery of aerosolized drugs is not supported for general clinical or at-home use, if the patient is able to breathe spontaneously without machine support.

Table 3-8

Results of studies measuring lung deposition as a percent of total dose for both metered dose inhaler (MDI) and small volume nebulizer (SVN) aerosol administration with face mask or mouthpiece use*

AGE	METHOD	DRUG	LUNG DEPOSITION (%)	REFERENCE
21 mo (3 mo-5 yr)	MDI/HC/mask	Radiolabeled albuterol	1.97 ± 1.4	Tal, 1996[122]
2-4 yr	MDI/HC/mask	Radiolabeled	5.4 ± 2.1	Wildhaber, 1999[123]
	SVN/face mask	Albuterol	5.4 ± 1.4	
5-8 yr	MDI/HC/mouthpiece	Radiolabeled	9.6 ± 3.9	
	SVN/mouthpiece	Albuterol	11.1 ± 1.7	
1-3 yr	MDI/HC/mask	Cromolyn	0.76	Salmon, 1990[124]
	SVN/face mask		0.30	
Adults†	SVN/face mask	Cromolyn	1.5	

First author and year of publication are given, with full citation in references.
HC, Holding chamber.
*Means and standard deviations (where available) are given.
†With tidal nasal breathing.

FACE MASK ADMINISTRATION

Use of a face mask with an aerosol generator usually occurs with infant and pediatric applications or with debilitated, unresponsive patients. Clinical efficacy has been demonstrated with a face mask in a pediatric application by Conner and associates (1989)[119] and Kraemer and co-workers (1991).[120] A study published in 1992 by Lowenthal and Kattan[121] compared face mask to mouthpiece delivery with nebulized albuterol in children and adolescents ages 6 to 19 years for emergency department treatment of acute asthma. Their study found no difference in improvement on lung function measures, even in subjects with nasal congestion using the face mask. They speculated that congested nasal passages caused mouth breathing while using the mask. Greater tremor was observed with the face-mask group, implying a higher systemic level of drug compared with use of the mouthpiece.

Lung deposition of drug has also been measured for both mouthpiece and face mask administration of aerosol drugs. Most of the data available is for infants and children, because this age-group is most likely to use a face mask for aerosol delivery. Results of several studies of lung deposition are summarized in Table 3-8.[122-124] Although techniques of measuring lung deposition varied among the studies cited in Table 3-8, it is apparent that children or infants below the age of 5 years receive a lower fraction of the nominal dose with a face mask compared with older children and adults using a mouthpiece.

ENDOTRACHEAL TUBE ADMINISTRATION

Aerosolized drug delivery commonly occurs with intubated subjects, both neonatal and adult. Data have accumulated quantifying the efficiency of aerosol administration with this interface and are well summarized in a 1996 review by Dhand and Tobin.[125] Evaluation of aerosol delivery in this way is complicated by the number of variables introduced if the patient is on mechanical ventilation and by the difficulty in quantifying drug delivery accurately. Box 3-8 lists the many variables with administration of aerosol drug through an endotracheal tube (ETT) to ventilated subjects. The effect of some of these variables, with either SVN or MDI aerosol administration, has been investigated. The following list summarizes the state of knowledge represented in the literature at this time:

- The ETT seems to act as an efficient baffle to reduce drug delivery compared with the usual 10% achieved with nonintubated subjects; larger ETT size improves delivery.[126]
- Both MDI and SVN have been used, and both can produce clinical responses to bronchodilator drugs in intubated, ventilated subjects.[129-131]
- Use of an extension tube or other reservoir, or placement of the aerosol generator upstream from the ETT adapter, improves aerosol delivery.[19,130-132]
- Nebulizer (SVN) delivery of drugs to intubated, ventilated subjects may be optimized by modification or selection of the following:

Box 3-8 | **Summary of the Variables Present in Aerosol Delivery to Intubated, Mechanically Ventilated Critical Care Patients**

Ventilator	Aerosol generator
Nebulizer power system	*SVN*
Duty cycle (flow, volume, rate)	Volume of fill
Inspiratory flow pattern	Type of solution
Mode of ventilation	Brand of SVN
Breath modifications (PEEP, inflation hold)	Intraproduct reliability
Spontaneous, assisted, or controlled breaths	Continuous versus intermittent
Humidification and temperature	Power flow rate
Position of generator in circuit	
Size of endotracheal tube	*MDI*
	Timing of actuation
	Use and design of reservoir device
	Type of drug used

MDI, Metered dose inhaler; *PEEP*, positive end-expiratory pressure; *SVN*, small volume nebulizer.

Box 3-9 | **Suggested Techniques for Metered Dose Inhaler (MDI) and Small Volume Nebulizer (SVN) Aerosol Administration in Mechanically Ventilated Patients**

MDI

1. Tidal volume should be greater than 500 ml in adults, with assisted ventilation.
2. Aim for inspiratory fraction (excluding inspiratory pause) greater than 0.3 of total breathing cycle.
3. Synchronize ventilator breath with patient's inspiration.
4. Shake MDI vigorously, and use with spacer device on inspiratory limb of ventilator circuit.
5. Do not bypass the humidifier, to avoid circuit interruption, drying of the airway, and errors in reconnecting.
6. Actuate MDI simultaneously with onset of inspiration by the ventilator.
7. An end-inspiratory breath-hold will theoretically improve aerosol deposition.
8. Allow passive exhalation, and repeat every 20 to 30 seconds for desired dose.

Nebulizers

1. Use an adequate fill volume of 2 to 6 ml, based on particular brand of nebulizer used.*
2. Place nebulizer in inspiratory limb at least 30 cm from patient Y.
3. Ensure adequate power gas flow rate of 6 to 8 L/min through nebulizer.
4. Use tidal volume (>500 ml in adults) and a duty cycle of greater than 0.3 if possible.
5. Adjust ventilator volume to compensate for additional nebulizer flow if necessary.
6. Terminate flow-by or continuous flow mode on ventilator.
7. Observe nebulizer for adequate aerosol generation during use.
8. Disconnect nebulizer when aerosolization ceases, reconnect ventilator circuit, and return to original ventilator settings.

Based on Dhand R, Tobin MJ: Inhaled bronchodilator therapy in mechanically ventilated patients, *Am J Respir Crit Care Med* 156:3, 1997. (See reference for more detail on aerosol administration during mechanical ventilation.)
*Optimal filling volume varies among nebulizers.

---

1. Increased duty cycle (increased inspiratory fraction of total breath time)[133-134]
2. Use of most efficient fill volume for nebulizer[133]
3. Selection of efficient SVN brands[133]
4. Selection of ventilator with adequate power system for SVN, because ventilator brands differ in their efficiency of SVN drive systems, or use of an alternative system (external power flow, MDI/reservoir)[135]

- Bypassing the humidification system to allow lower temperature and humidity increases aerosol delivery through a ventilator circuit and ETT.[19,133]

Table 3-9

Selected in vivo and in vitro studies quantifying lung delivery of aerosolized drugs with intubated, mechanically ventilated lung models and human or animal subjects

STUDY	AEROSOL SYSTEM	ETT SIZE (mm)	LUNG DEPOSITION (%)
IN VITRO			
Crogan, 1989[126]	MDI and ETT adapter	6.0	3.0
		7.5	4.7
		9.0	6.5
Fuller, 1992[19]	MDI and 700-ml reservoir	8.0	30.3
	MDI and 167-ml reservoir		27.7
	SVN 70 cm upstream		4.6
	Ultravent SVN		1.3
O'Doherty, 1999[134]	SVN (System 22 Acorn) and 3-ml volume	9.0	
	Between Y and ETT		5.4
	Just proximal to Y		8.0
	With 600-ml reservoir		10.3
Rau, 1992[131]	MDI and ETT adapter	8.0	7.3
	MDI and reservoir (Aerovent)		32.1
Everard, 1996[139]	DPI on ETT (Turbohaler, budesonide)	9.0	20.6
Cameron, 1990[140]	SVN	3.5	0.22-1.52
	SPAG		0.15
	USN		0.60
Rau, 1992[26]	SVN before Y	3.0	0.97
	SVN and 13 cm tubing added		1.78
	Manual inflation		1.03
IN VIVO			
Fuller, 1990[141]	MDI and reservoir	Varied (adult)	5.65
	SVN 70 cm upstream		1.22
Fuller, 1994[132]	MDI and reservoir		6.33
	MDI and 167-ml reservoir		5.53
	MDI and inline T		1.67
	MDI and ETT adapter		3.89

First author and year of publication are given, with full citation in references.
DPI, Dry powder inhaler; *ETT,* endotracheal tube; *MDI,* metered dose inhaler; *SPAG,* small particle aerosol generator; *SVN,* small volume nebulizer; *USN,* ultrasonic nebulizer.

- In vitro studies overestimate aerosol delivery compared with in vivo results, but the relative differences of aerosol delivery seen in vitro have been found to be predictive of differences in vivo.[136]

Application of the findings summarized for nebulizer delivery resulted in an optimized dose with an SVN to mechanically ventilated adult patients with a variety of diagnoses.[137] Both nebulizers and MDIs can be effective when suitable techniques are used. Box 3-9 gives guide-lines from Dhand and Tobin[138] to optimize drug delivery from both SVNs and MDIs with mechanically ventilated, intubated patients. Results of several studies quantifying lung deposition with both adult and neonatal, and in vivo as well as in vitro models, are given in Table 3-9.*

The studies indicate that less aerosol is delivered with smaller-size ETTs, and this would be consistent with increased inertial baffling of particles.

*References 19, 26, 126, 131, 132, 134, 139-141.

The larger delivery efficiencies seen with bench studies than with human or in vivo methods may be due to the fact that the amount of control over extraneous variables, such as coordination with respiratory patterns, is far greater in the laboratory than with an actual patient and this tends to maximize delivery.

SUMMARY KEY TERMS AND CONCEPTS

- An *aerosol* is a suspension of solid or liquid particles whose *deposition* in the respiratory tract is determined by *inertial impaction, sedimentation (gravitational settling)* and perhaps less importantly, *diffusion.*
- A major factor in lung *penetration* by aerosols is particle size, which is best characterized by the *mass median aerodynamic diameter (MMAD)* for inhaled drugs, because particle mass is a function of the third power of particle radius. The particle size of interest for pulmonary applications is in the range of 1 to 10 μm, and the *fine particle fraction* is considered to be particles below 5 μm.
- Common devices for the delivery of inhaled aerosol drugs include *nebulizers, metered dose inhalers,* and *dry powder inhalers. Reservoir devices,* such as spacers and holding chambers, can reduce oropharyngeal deposition of drug and simplify hand-breathing coordination with MDIs. Proper use of these aerosol generating devices is absolutely necessary to ensure adequate lung delivery, and correct use should be understood by practitioners. Traditional aerosol generating devices all deliver about 10% to 15% of the dose produced to the lung, although different types of devices vary in their loss patterns.
- Most of the loss with an SVN occurs in the device, whereas an MDI and a DPI lose drug in the mouth and gastrointestinal tract. Addition of a reservoir device to an MDI shifts loss from the throat to the reservoir.
- Because traditional aerosol device delivers approximately 10% to 15% of the total dose to the airway and total dose amounts vary among type of device for the same drug, the different device types do not necessarily deliver equivalent amounts to the lung. Newer and ongoing developments in aerosol devices have increased their efficiency, with resultant lung depositions of 30% to 50% or greater. The improved efficiency in lung delivery will necessitate dose modifications.
- *Patient-device interface* is another variable in aerosol delivery to the lung and includes *IPPB administration, face mask administration,* and *delivery to intubated, ventilated patients,* which is complicated by numerous variables.

SELF-ASSESSMENT QUESTIONS

1. What are the three most common aerosol generating devices used to deliver inhaled drugs?
2. Describe the inspiratory pattern you would instruct a patient to use with an MDI.
3. What are three advantages offered by a reservoir device used with an MDI?
4. Would a DPI be appropriate for a 3-year-old child with asthma?
5. What is meant by the term *dead volume* in an SVN?
6. What is the optimal filling volume and power gas flow rate to use with an SVN?

Answers to Self-Assessment Questions are found in Appendix A.

CLINICAL SCENARIO

A 17-year-old adolescent male with a history of allergic asthma is given a prescription for MDI albuterol, a bronchodilator used as a rescue agent. The HFA formulation of albuterol (Proventil HFA) is prescribed. After using the MDI a few times, the patient complains to you that he can feel drug in the canister when he shakes it before using, but it feels as if "very little spray" is coming out when he inhales a puff. He believes the MDI is not functioning properly and that he is not getting the regular inhaled dose.

What would you do to analyze this situation and ensure that the MDI is functioning properly?

Assuming the MDI appears functional based on the preceding check, how would you explain the situation with HFA albuterol to the patient?

Answers to Clinical Scenario Questions are found in Appendix A.

REFERENCES

1. Morrow PE: An evaluation of the physical properties of monodisperse and heterodisperse aerosols used in the assessment of bronchial function, *Chest* 80(suppl.):809, 1981.
2. Kohler D, Fleischer W: Established facts in inhalation therapy: a review of aerosol therapy and commonly used drugs, *Lung Respir* VI:1, 1989.
3. Morrow PE: Aerosol characterization and deposition, *Am Rev Respir Dis* 110(suppl.):88, 1974.
4. Lourenco RV, Cotromanes E: Clinical aerosols. I, Characterization of aerosols and their diagnostic uses, *Arch Intern Med* 142:2163, 1982.

5. Hiller C and others: Aerodynamic size distribution of metered-dose bronchodilator aerosols, *Am Rev Respir Dis* 118:311, 1978.

6. Dolovich M: In vitro measurements of delivery of medications from MDIs and spacer devices, *J Aerosol Med* 9(suppl 1):S49, 1996.

7. Clark AR, Gonda I, Newhouse MT: Towards meaningful laboratory tests for evaluation of pharmaceutical aerosols, *J Aerosol Med* 11(suppl 1):S1, 1998.

8. Lippman M: Regional deposition of particles in the human respiratory tract. In Lee DHK, Falk HL, Murphy SD, eds: *Handbook of physiology,* section 9, Bethesda, Md, 1977, American Physiological Society.

9. Yu CP, Nicolaides P, Soong TT: Effect of random airway sizes on aerosol deposition, *Am Ind Hyg Assoc J* 40:999, 1979.

10. Consensus Conference on Aerosol Delivery, *Respir Care* 9:916, 1991.

11. Clay MM, Pavia D, Clarke SW: Effect of aerosol particle size on bronchodilation with nebulised terbutaline in asthmatic subjects, *Thorax* 41:364, 1986.

12. Johnson MA and others: Delivery of albuterol and ipratropium bromide from two nebulizer systems in chronic stable asthma: efficacy and pulmonary deposition, *Chest* 96:1, 1989.

13. Barnes PJ, Basbaum CB, Nadel JA: Autoradiographic localization of autonomic receptors in airway smooth muscle, *Am Rev Respir Dis* 127:758, 1983.

14. Corkery KJ, Luce JM, Montgomery AB: Aerosolized pentamidine for treatment and prophylaxis of *Pneumocystis carinii* pneumonia: an update, *Respir Care* 33:676, 1988.

15. Newman SP: Aerosol deposition considerations in inhalation therapy, *Chest* 88(suppl):152S, 1985.

16. Dolovich M: Physical principles underlying aerosol therapy, *J Aerosol Med* 2:171, 1989.

17. Smith G and others: Aerodynamic size distribution of cromolyn sodium at ambient and airway humidity, *Am Rev Respir Dis* 121:513,1980.

18. Hiller FC and others: Physical properties, hygroscopicity and estimated pulmonary retention of various therapeutic aerosols, *Chest* 77(suppl.):318, 1980.

19. Fuller HD and others: Aerosol delivery during mechanical ventilation: a predictive in-vitro lung model, *J Aerosol Med* 5:251, 1992.

20. Hanania NA and others: Medical personnel's knowledge of and ability to use inhaling devices: metered-dose inhalers, spacing chambers, and breath-actuated dry powder inhalers, *Chest* 105:111, 1994.

21. Wigley FM and others: Insulin across respiratory mucosae by aerosol delivery, *Diabetes* 20:552, 1971.

22. Niven RW and others: Some factors associated with the ultrasonic nebulization of proteins, *Pharmaceut Res* 12:53, 1995.

23. Dennis JH: A review of issues relating to nebulizer standards, *J Aerosol Med* 11(suppl 1):S73, 1998.

24. Kradjan WA, Lakshminarayan S: Efficiency of air compressor-driven nebulizers, *Chest* 87:512, 1985.

25. Shim CS, Williams MH Jr: Effect of bronchodilator therapy administered by canister versus jet nebulizer, *J Allergy Clin Immunol* 73:387, 1984.

26. Rau JL Jr, Harwood RJ: Comparison of nebulizer delivery methods through a neonatal endotracheal tube: a bench study, *Respir Care* 37:1233, 1992.

27. Alvine GF and others Disposable jet nebulizers: how reliable are they? *Chest* 101:316, 1992.

28. Hess D, Horney D, Snyder T: Medication-delivery performance of eight small-volume, hand-held nebulizers: effects of diluent volume, gas flowrate, and nebulizer model, *Respir Care* 34:717, 1989.

29. Hollie MC and others: Extreme variability in aerosol output of the DeVilbiss 646 jet nebulizer, *Chest* 100:1339, 1991.

30. Hess D and others: Medication nebulizer performance: effects of diluent volume, nebulizer flow, and nebulizer brand, *Chest* 110:498, 1996.

31. Hess DR and others: The effect of Heliox on nebulizer function using a β agonist bronchodilator, *Chest* 115:184, 1999.

32. O'Callaghan C, Barry PW: The science of nebulised drug delivery, *Thorax* 52(suppl 2):S31, 1997.

33. Newman SP and others: Evaluation of jet nebulisers for use with gentamicin solution, *Thorax* 40:671, 1985.

34. MacNeish CF and others: A comparison of pulmonary availability between Ventolin (albuterol) Nebules and Ventolin (albuterol) respirator solution, *Chest* 111:204, 1997.

35. Lewis RA, Fleming JS: Fractional deposition from a jet nebulizer: how it differs from a metered dose inhaler, *Br J Dis Chest* 79:361, 1985.

36. Dolovich M: New propellant-free technologies under investigation, *J Aerosol Med* 12(suppl 1):S9, 1999.

37. Ganderton D: Targeted delivery of inhaled drugs: current challenges and future goals, *J Aerosol Med* 12(suppl 1):S3, 1999.

38. Farr SJ and others: AERx: development of a novel liquid aerosol delivery system: concept to clinic. In Dalby RN, Byron PR, Farr SJ, eds: *Respiratory drug delivery V,* Buffalo Grove, Ill, 1996, Interpharm Press, Inc.

39. Zierenberg B: Optimizing the in vitro performance of Respimat, *J Aerosol Med* 12(suppl 1):S19, 1999.

40. Freedman T: Medihaler therapy for bronchial asthma: a new type of aerosol therapy, *Postgrad Med* 20:667, 1956.

41. Hallworth GW: The formulation and evaluation of pressurized metered-dose inhalers. In Ganderton D, Jones T, eds: *Drug delivery to the respiratory tract,* Chichester, England, 1987, Ellis Horwood, Ltd.

42. Clarke SW, Newman SP: Differences between pressurized aerosol and stable dust particles, *Chest* 80(suppl):907, 1981.

43. Moren F: Pressurized aerosols for oral inhalation, *Int J Pharm* 8:1, 1981.

44. McFadden ER Jr: Improper patient techniques with metered dose inhalers: clinical consequences and solutions to misuse, *J Allergy Clin Immunol* 96:278, 1995.

45. Sackner MA, Kim CS: Auxiliary MDI aerosol delivery systems, *Chest* 88(suppl.):161S, 1985.

46. Tobin MJ and others: Response to bronchodilator drug administration by a new reservoir aerosol delivery system and a review of other auxiliary delivery systems, *Am Rev Respir Dis* 126:670, 1982.

47. Kelling JS and others: Physician knowledge in the use of canister nebulizers, *Chest* 83:612, 1983.

48. Epstein SW and others: Survey of the clinical use of pressurized aerosol inhalers, *Can Med Assoc J* 120:813, 1979.

49. Lee HS: Proper aerosol inhalation technique for delivery of asthma medications, *Clin Pediatr* 22:440-443, 1983.

50. Dolovich M and others: Optimal delivery of aerosols from metered dose inhalers, *Chest* 80(suppl):911, 1981.

51. Newman SP, Pavia D, Clarke SW: Improving the bronchial deposition of pressurized aerosols, *Chest* 80(suppl):909, 1981.

52. Newman SP and others: Deposition of pressurized aerosols in the human respiratory tract, *Thorax* 36:52, 1981.

53. Newman SP and others: Effects of various inhalation modes on the deposition of radioactive pressurized aerosols, *Eur J Respir Dis* 119(suppl):57, 1982.

54. Newman SP, Clarke SW: Inhalation technique with aerosol bronchodilators: does it matter? *Pract Cardiol* 9:157, 1983.

55. Blake KV, Harman E, Hendeles L: Evaluation of a generic albuterol metered-dose inhaler: importance of priming the MDI, *Ann Allergy* 68:169, 1992.

56. Newman SP, Pavia D, Clarke SW: How should a pressurized beta-adrenergic bronchodilator be inhaled? *Eur J Respir Dis* 62:3, 1981.

57. Cyr TD and others: Low first-spray drug content in albuterol metered-dose inhalers, *Pharmaceut Res* 8:658, 1991.

58. Everard ML and others: Factors affecting total and "respirable" dose delivered by a salbutamol metered dose inhaler, *Thorax* 50:746, 1995.

59. Berg E: *In vitro* properties of pressurized metered dose inhalers with and without spacer devices, *J Aerosol Med* 8(suppl. 3):S3, 1995.

60. Heimer D, Shim C, Williams MH Jr: The effect of sequential inhalation of metaproterenol aerosol in asthma, *J Allergy Clin Immunol* 66:75, 1980.

61. Pedersen S: The importance of a pause between the inhalation of two puffs of terbutaline from a pressurized aerosol with a tube spacer, *J Allergy Clin Immunol* 77:505, 1986.

62. Pedersen S, Steffensen G: Simplification of inhalation therapy in asthmatic children, *Allergy* 41:296, 1986.

63. Unzeitig JC, Richards W, Church JA: Administration of metered-dose inhalers: comparison of open- and closed-mouth techniques in childhood asthmatics, *Annals Allergy* 51:571, 1983.

64. Chhabra SK: A comparison of "closed" and "open" mouth techniques of inhalation of a salbutamol metered-dose inhaler, *J Asthma* 31:123, 1994.

65. Schultz RK: Drug delivery characteristics of metered-dose inhalers, *J Allergy Clin Immunol* 96:284, 1995.

66. Ross DL, Gabrio BJ: Advances in metered dose inhaler technology with the development of a chlorofluorocarbon-free drug delivery system, *J Aerosol Med* 12:151, 1999.

67. Newman, SP and others: Improvement of drug delivery with a breath actuated pressurised aerosol for patients with poor inhaler technique, *Thorax* 46:712, 1991.

68. Baum EA, Bryant AM: The development and laboratory testing of a novel breath-actuated pressurized inhaler, *J Aerosol Med* 1:219, 1988.

69. Farr SJ and others: Aerosol deposition in the human lung following administration from a microprocessor controlled pressurised metered dose inhaler, *Thorax* 50:639, 1995.

70. Partridge MR: Metered-dose inhalers and CFCs: what respiratory physicians need to know, *Respir Med* 99:645, 1994.

71. Kleerup EC and others: Cumulative dose-response study of non-CFC propellant HFA 134a salbutamol sulfate metered-dose inhaler in patients with asthma, *Chest* 109:702, 1999.

72. Bleeker ER and others: Proventil HFA provides bronchodilation comparable to Ventolin over 12 weeks of regular use in asthmatics, *Chest* 113:283, 1998.

73. Tinkelman DG and others: Proventil HFA and Ventolin have similar safety profiles during regular use, *Chest* 113:290, 1998.

74. Ramsdell JW and others: Safety of long-term treatment with HFA albuterol, *Chest* 115:945, 1999.

75. Maesen FPV and others: Therapeutic equivalence of a novel HFA 134a-containing metered-dose inhaler and the conventional CFC inhaler (Berodual) for the delivery of a fixed combination of fenoterol/ipratropium bromide, *Respiration* 64:273, 1997.

76. Welch M and others: Azmacort HFA Study Group: A controlled trial of chlorofluorocarbon-free triamcinolone acetonide inhalation aerosol in the treatment of adult patients with persistent asthma, *Chest* 116:1304, 1999.

77. Donnell D: Development of a CFC-free glucocorticoid metered-dose aerosol system to optimize drug delivery to the lung, *Pharm Sci Tech Today* 3:183, 2000.

78. Gross G and others: Hydrofluoroalkane-134a beclomethasone dipropionate, 400 μg, is as effective as chlorofluorocarbon beclomethasone dipropionate, 800 μg, for the treatment of moderate asthma, *Chest* 115:343,1999.

79. Dolovich M: Spacer design II: holding chambers and valves. Oral presentation at the International Symposium on Spacer Devices, Boston, 1995, Drug Information Association.

80. Newman SP and others: Effect of InspirEase on the deposition of metered-dose aerosols in the human respiratory tract, *Chest* 89:551, 1986.

81. Kim CS, Eldridge MA, Sackner MA: Oropharyngeal deposition and delivery aspects of metered-dose inhaler aerosols, *Am Rev Respir Dis* 135:157, 1987.

82. Turner MO and others: Bronchodilator delivery in acute airflow obstruction: a meta-analysis, *Arch Intern Med* 157:1736, 1997.

83. Newman SP, Newhouse MT: Effect of add-on devices for aerosol drug delivery: deposition studies and clinical aspects, *J Aerosol Med* 9:55, 1996.

84. König P: Spacer devices used with metered-dose inhalers: breakthrough or gimmick? *Chest* 88:276, 1985.

85. Newman SP and others: Deposition of pressurized suspension aerosols inhaled through extension devices, *Am Rev Respir Dis* 124:317,1981.

86. Rau JL, Restrepo R, Deshpande V: Inhalation of single vs multiple metered-dose bronchodilator actuations from reservoir devices: an *in vitro* study, *Chest* 109:969, 1996.

87. Mitchell JP, Nagel MW, Rau JL: Performance of large-volume versus small-volume holding chambers with chlorofluorocarbon-albuterol and hydrofluoroalkane-albuterol sulfate, *Respir Care* 44:38, 1999.

88. Bell JH, Hartley PS, Cox JSG: Dry powder aerosols. I, A new powder inhalation device, *J Pharm Sci* 60:1559, 1971.

89. Vidgren M and others: Effect of powder inhaler design on drug deposition in the respiratory tract, *Int J Pharmaceut* 42:211, 1988.

90. Brown K: The formulation and evaluation of powders for inhalation. In Ganderton D, Jones T, eds: *Drug delivery to the respiratory tract*, Chichester, England, 1987, Ellis Horwood, Ltd.

91. Pedersen S: How to use a rotahaler, *Arch Dis Child* 61:11, 1986.

92. Richards R and others: Inhalation rate of sodium cromoglycate determines plasma pharmacokinetics and protection agonist AMP-induced bronchoconstriction in asthma, *Eur Respir J* 1:896, 1988.

93. Pedersen S, Hansen OR, Fuglsang G: Influence of inspiratory flow rate upon the effect of a Turbuhaler, *Arch Dis Child* 65:308, 1990.

94. Fuller R: The Diskus: a new multi-dose powder device—efficacy and comparison with Turbuhaler, *J Aerosol Med* 8(suppl 2):S11, 1995.

95. Hetzel MR, Clark TJH: Comparison of salbutamol Rotahaler with conventional pressurized aerosol, *Clin Allergy* 7:563, 1977.

96. Chambers S, Dunbar J, Taylor B: Inhaled powder compared with aerosol administration of fenoterol in asthmatic children, *Arch Dis Child* 55:73, 1980.

97. Towns SJ and others: Bronchodilator effects of salbutamol powder administered via Rotahaler and of terbutaline aerosol administered via Misthaler, *Med J Aust* 1:633, 1983.

98. Vilsvik J and others: Comparison between Bricanyl Turbuhaler and Ventolin metered dose inhaler in the treatment of exercise-induced asthma in adults, *Ann Allergy* 67:315, 1991.

99. Chapman KR and others: Albuterol via Turbuhaler versus albuterol via pressurized metered-dose inhaler in asthma, *Ann Allergy Asthma Immunol* 78:59, 1997.

100. Zainudin BMZ and others: Comparison of bronchodilator responses and deposition patterns of salbutamol inhaled from a pressurised metered dose inhaler, as a dry powder, and as a nebulised solution, *Thorax* 45:469, 1990.

101. Thorsson L, Edsbäcker S, Conradson T-B: Lung deposition of budesonide from Turbuhaler is twice that from a pressurized metered-dose inhaler P-MDI, *Eur Respir J* 7:1839, 1994.

102. Spiro SG and others: Direct labelling of ipratropium bromide aerosol and its deposition pattern in normal subjects and patients with chronic bronchitis, *Thorax* 39:432, 1984.

103. Tarala RA, Madsen BW, Paterson JW: Comparative efficacy of salbutamol by pressurized aerosol and wet nebulizer in acute asthma, *Br J Clin Pharmaceut* 10:393, 1980.

104. Blake KV and others: Relative amount of albuterol delivered to lung receptors from a metered-dose inhaler and nebulizer solution, *Chest* 101:309, 1992.

105. Mestitz H, Copland JM, McDonald CF: Comparison of outpatient nebulized vs metered dose inhaler terbutaline in chronic airflow obstruction, *Chest* 96:1237, 1989.

106. Newhouse M, Dolovich M: Aerosol therapy: nebulizer vs metered dose inhaler *Chest* 91:799, 1987 (editorial).

107. Newman SP and others: Lung deposition of fenoterol and flunisolide delivered using a novel device for inhaled medicines: comparison of RESPIMAT with conventional metered-dose inhaler with and without spacer devices, *Chest* 113:957, 1998.

108. Leach CL, Davidson PJ, Boudreau RJ: Improved airway targeting with the CFC-free HFA-beclomethasone metered-dose inhaler compared with CFC-beclomethasone, *Eur Respir J* 12:1346, 1998.

109. Amirav I, Newhouse MT: Metered-dose inhaler accessory devices in acute asthma: efficacy and comparison with nebulizers: a literature review, *Arch Pediatr Adolesc Med* 151:876, 1997.

110. Fok TF and others: Delivery of salbutamol to nonventilated preterm infants by metered-dose inhaler, jet nebulizer, and ultrasonic nebulizer, *Eur Respir J* 12:159, 1998.

111. Mandelberg A and others: Is nebulized aerosol treatment necessary in the pediatric emergency department? Comparison with a metal spacer device for metered-dose inhaler, *Chest* 117:1309, 2000.

112. Lin YZ, Hsieh KH: Metered dose inhaler and nebuliser in acute asthma, *Arch Dis Child* 72:214, 1995.

113. Mandelberg A and others: Nebulized wet aerosol treatment in emergency department: is it essential? Comparison with large spacer device for metered-dose inhaler, *Chest* 112:1501, 1997.

114. National Institutes of Health: National Asthma Education and Prevention Program, Expert Panel Report II: *Guidelines for the diagnosis and management of asthma*, Bethesda, Md, 1997, National Institutes of Health.

115. O'Donohue WJ Jr: National Association for Medical Direction of Respiratory Care (NAMDRC) Consensus Group: Guidelines for the use of nebulizers in the home and at domiciliary sites, *Chest* 109:814, 1996.

116. Chester EH and others: Bronchodilator therapy: comparison of acute response to three methods of administration, *Chest* 62:394, 1972.

117. Dolovich MB and others: Pulmonary aerosol deposition in chronic bronchitis: intermittent positive pressure breathing versus quiet breathing, *Am Rev Respir Dis* 115:397, 1977.

118. Loren M and others: Comparison between simple nebulization and intermittent positive-pressure in asthmatic children with severe bronchospasm, *Chest* 72:145, 1977.

119. Conner WT and others: Reliable salbutamol administration in 6- to 36-month-old children by means of a metered dose inhaler and aerochamber with mask, *Pediatr Pulmonol* 6:263, 1989.

120. Kraemer R and others: Short-term effect of albuterol, delivered via a new auxiliary device, in wheezy infants, *Am Rev Respir Dis* 144:347, 1991.

121. Lowenthal D, Kattan M: Facemasks versus mouthpieces for aerosol treatment of asthmatic children, *Pediatr Pulmonol* 14:192, 1992.

122. Tal A and others: Deposition pattern of radiolabeled salbutamol inhaled from a metered-dose inhaler by means of a spacer with mask in young children with airway obstruction, *J Pediatr* 128:479, 1996.

123. Wildhaber JH and others: Inhalation therapy in asthma: nebulizer or pressurized metered-dose inhaler with holding chamber? In vivo comparison of lung deposition in children, *J Pediatr* 135:28, 1999.

124. Salmon B, Wilson NM, Silverman M: How much aerosol reaches the lungs of wheezing infants and toddlers? *Arch Dis Child* 65:401, 1990.

125. Dhand R, Tobin MJ: Bronchodilator delivery with metered-dose inhalers in mechanically-ventilated patients, *Eur Resp J* 9:585, 1996.

126. Crogan SJ, Bishop MJ: Delivery efficiency of metered dose aerosols given via endotracheal tubes. *Anesthesiol* 70:1008, 1989.

127. Gay PC and others: Metered dose inhalers for bronchodilator delivery in intubated, mechanically ventilated patients, *Chest* 99:66, 1991.

128. Duarte AG, Momii K, Bidani A: Bronchodilator therapy with metered-dose inhaler and spacer versus nebulizer in mechanically ventilated patients: comparison of magnitude and duration of response, *Respir Care* 45:817, 2000.

129. Dhand R, Jubran A, Tobin MJ: Bronchodilator delivery by metered-dose inhaler in ventilator-supported patients, *Am J Respir Crit Care Med* 151:1827, 1995.

130. Hughes JM, Saez J: Effects of nebulizer mode and position in a mechanical ventilator circuit on dose efficiency, *Respir Care* 32:1131, 1987.

131. Rau JL, Harwood RJ, Groff JL: Evaluation of a reservoir device for metered-dose bronchodilator delivery to intubated adults: an in vitro study, *Chest* 102:924, 1992.

132. Fuller HD and others: Efficiency of bronchodilator aerosol delivery to the lungs from the metered dose inhaler in mechanically ventilated patients: a study comparing four different actuator devices, *Chest* 105:214, 1994.

133. O'Riordan TG and others: Nebulizer function during mechanical ventilation, *Am Rev Respir Dis* 145:1117, 1992.

134. O'Doherty MJ and others: Delivery of a nebulized aerosol to a lung model during mechanical ventilation, *Am Rev Respir Dis* 146:383, 1992.

135. McPeck M, O'Riordan TG, Smaldone GC: Choice of mechanical ventilator: influence on nebulizer performance, *Respir Care* 38:887, 1993.

136. O'Riordan TG and others: Predicting aerosol deposition during neonatal ventilation: feasibility of bench testing, *Respir Care* 39:1162, 1994.

137. O'Riordan TG, Palmer LB, Smaldone GC: Aerosol deposition in mechanically ventilated patients: optimizing nebulizer delivery, *Am J Respir Crit Care Med* 149:214, 1994.

138. Dhand R, Tobin MJ: Inhaled bronchodilator therapy in mechanically ventilated patients, *Am J Respir Crit Care Med* 156:3,1997

139. Everard ML, Devadason SG, Le Souef PN: In vitro assessment of drug delivery through an endotracheal tube using a dry powder inhaler delivery system, *Thorax* 51:75, 1996.

140. Cameron D, Clay M, Silverman M: Evaluation of nebulizers for use in neonatal ventilator circuits, *Crit Care Med* 18:866, 1990.

141. Fuller HD and others: Pressurized aerosol versus jet aerosol delivery to mechanically ventilated patients, *Am Rev Respir Dis* 141:440, 1990.

CHAPTER 4

Calculating Drug Doses

Joseph L. Rau

CHAPTER OUTLINE

*C*hapter 4 presents calculations of drug doses. Systems of measure are reviewed briefly. Dose calculations from prepared-strength formulations such as liquids, tablets, and capsules are presented with examples. The calculation of doses from solutions whose concentrations are expressed as a percentage-strength, along with intravenous dose calculations, are presented with examples. Practice problems and answers are included.

SYSTEMS OF MEASURE

THE METRIC SYSTEM

Table 4-1 provides metric units of measure for length, volume, and weight. Primary units in the metric system are as follows:

Length: Meter
Volume: Liter
Mass: Gram

Fractional parts, or multiples of these primary (base) units, are expressed by adding Latin prefixes for sizes smaller than the primary unit, and Greek prefixes for sizes larger than the primary unit. Examples of both Latin and Greek prefixes found in Table 4-1 are as follows:

Increasing prefixes—Latin:

Micro = $^1/_{1,000,000}$
Milli = $^1/_{1000}$
Centi = $^1/_{100}$
Deci = $^1/_{10}$

Increasing prefixes—Greek:

Deca = 10
Hecto = 100
Kilo = 1000

In calculating drug doses, the metric units for volume and mass (weight) are needed. A commonly encountered unit of volume in respiratory care pharmacology is the milliliter (ml) or 0.001 L. Common units of weight are the kilogram (kg), the gram (g), the milligram (mg) and with aerosolized drugs, the microgram (µg). Blood levels of drug amounts within the body may be in nanograms per milliliter (ng/ml). Conversions within the metric system should be familiar, such as converting 1 mg to 0.001 g, 500 ml to 0.5 L, or 0.4 mg to 400 µg. Facility with decimal fractions and with the other basic rules of arithmetic are necessary for drug dose calculations.

The gram is defined as the weight of 1 milliliter of distilled water at 4° C *in vacuo*. Under these

Table 4-1

The metric system of length, volume and mass (weight)

LENGTH

1 Kilometer (km)	=	10^3 meters	=	1000 meters
1 Hectometer (hm)	=	10^2 meters	=	100 meters
1 Decameter (dm)	=	10^1 meters	=	10 meters
1 Meter (m)		**Base unit**		
1 Decimeter (dm)	=	10^{-1} meter	=	0.1 meter
1 Centimeter (cm)	=	10^{-2} meter	=	0.01 meter
1 Millimeter (mm)	=	10^{-3} meter	=	0.001 meter
1 Micrometer (μm)	=	10^{-6} meter	=	0.000001 meter

VOLUME (CAPACITY)

1 Kiloliter (kl)	=	10^3 liters	=	1000 liters
1 Hectoliter (hl)	=	10^2 liters	=	100 liters
1 Decaliter (dl)	=	10^1 liters	=	10 liters
1 Liter (L)		**Base unit**		
1 Deciliter (dl)	=	10^{-1} liter	=	0.1 liter
1 Centiliter (cl)	=	10^{-2} liter	=	0.01 liter
1 Milliliter (ml)	=	10^{-3} liter	=	0.001 liter
1 Microliter (μl)	=	10^{-6} liter	=	0.000001 liter

MASS

1 Kilogram (kg)	=	10^3 grams	=	1000 grams
1 Hectogram (hg)	=	10^2 grams	=	100 grams
1 Decagram (dg)	=	10^1 grams	=	10 grams
1 Gram (g)		**Base unit**		
1 Decigram (dg)	=	10^{-1} gram	=	0.1 gram
1 Centigram (cg)	=	10^{-2} gram	=	0.01 gram
1 Milligram (mg)	=	10^{-3} gram	=	0.001 gram
1 Microgram (μg)	=	10^{-6} gram	=	0.000001 gram
1 Nanogram (ng)	=	10^{-9} gram	=	0.000000001 gram
1 Picogram (pg)	=	10^{-12} gram	=	0.000000000001 gram

conditions, 1 g of water and 1 ml of water are equal. This should not be used to convert from weight to volume, however, because a gram of liquid is not always equal to a milliliter of liquid, depending on the temperature, pressure, and nature of the substance.

Appendix B provides a summary of scientific notation, metric and SI units, and temperature scales with conversions. Although three different systems of measure have been used in drug calculations, metric units of measure are currently employed with formulations in the United States. Therefore all of the examples in this chapter will be based on the metric system. For completeness as a reference, the older apothecary system, the avoirdupois system, and a set of equivalents between these systems and the metric system are provided in Appendix B.

THE INTERNATIONAL SYSTEM OF UNITS

The International System of Units, or *Systeme International* (SI) was adopted in 1960 and is the modern metric system (see Appendix B). The SI system is well presented by Chatburn,[1] with conversion factors between older metric units for volume and the English system of measurement units. The SI system is based on the meter-kilogram-second (MKS) system, with volume as a derived unit of length. The primary units of interest in pharmacology calculations are as follows:

Mass: Kilogram (kg)
Volume: Cubic meter (m^3)

Although the base unit of measure in the SI system for volume is the cubic meter (m^3), the liter (L) and its fractions or multiples are currently accepted in measures of liquid volume.

Equivalence: $10^{-3}m^3 = 1$ liter (L)

DROPS AS UNITS OF VOLUME

Orders in respiratory care may often involve *drops*, such as 4 drops of racemic epinephrine, with 2.5 cubic centimeters (cc) of distilled water. The following equivalence is used:

16 drops (gtts) = 1 milliliter (ml)

In this example, then, 4 drops would equal $\frac{1}{4}$ milliliter (1 ml/16 drops $\times$ 4 drops = $\frac{4}{16}$ ml). Therefore $\frac{1}{4}$ ml is drawn up into a small accurate syringe, such as a tuberculin syringe, to obtain the 4 drops. One cubic centimeter (cc) is equivalent to 1 milliliter (ml): 1 cc = 1 ml.

It should be noted that drops are not standardized and can vary in size because of the physical properties of the particular fluid (specific gravity, viscosity) and the orifice of the dropper. Because drops can vary in amount delivered, physicians should be diplomatically cautioned to prescribe in metric units (cubic centimeters or milliliters) unless a dropper calibrated specifically for the particular medication is supplied by the manufacturer.

HOUSEHOLD UNITS OF MEASURE

Household units of measure are useful when instructing patients to take medications at home, and are based on common kitchen measures, such as the teaspoon, tablespoon, and cup. Metric equivalents to these household measures are given in Appendix B. Although the teaspoon is equivalent to 5 ml, not every teaspoon used for eating will actually equal 5 ml. However, measuring spoons and cups will more accurately give the volumes indicated, such as 5 ml per teaspoon, 15 ml per tablespoon, or 240 ml per cup.

CALCULATING DOSES FROM PREPARED-STRENGTH LIQUIDS, TABLETS, AND CAPSULES

Once the clinician is able to freely convert within the metric system, it is possible to begin calculating drug doses. In general, such calculations will be of the following three types:

1. Those involving fluids, tablets, or capsules of a given strength (e.g., 5 mg per milliliter)

2. Those involving solutions of a percentage strength (e.g., 0.5 ml of a 0.5% solution)
3. Those involving intravenous infusion rates (e.g., 10 µg/min)

Each type of dose calculation will be treated separately.

CALCULATING WITH PROPORTIONS

When using a prepared-strength liquid, tablet, or capsule, you are always trying to determine how much liquid or how many tablets or capsules are needed to give the amount, or dose, of the drug ordered. For example, if one tablet of a drug contains 5 mg and you want to give 2.5 mg, you immediately realize that half a tablet must be given. The simplest and therefore probably the most accurate, error-free method of calculation when using a vial of a prepared-strength drug (or a tablet or capsule) involves two steps at most, as follows:

1. Convert to consistent units of measure
2. Set up a straight-forward proportion:

$$\frac{\text{Original dose}}{\text{Per amount}} = \frac{\text{Desired dose}}{\text{Per amount}}$$

or, original dose:per amount :: desired dose:per amount.

In step 1, this conversion may be from grams to milligrams within the metric system, or even from apothecary to metric, if an apothecary dosage strength has been ordered. In step 2, either format for the proportion is correct. In the second form, the extremes and means are each multiplied together. If one arrangement is intuitively clearer, that should be preferred by the user.

EXAMPLE 1

You have oxytetracycline tablets, each 250 mg strength. If you need 0.5 g of the drug, either convert 250 mg to 0.25 g, or 0.5 g to 500 mg (preferred). Once the units are consistent, set up the proportion to find the unknown, which is how many tablets are needed to deliver the desired dose to the patient. Using the above formula,

$$\text{Original drug dose} = 250 \text{ mg}$$
$$\text{Per amount} = \text{Per tablet}$$
$$\text{Desired drug dose} = 0.5 \text{ g} = 500 \text{ mg}$$
$$\text{Per amount} = \text{Unknown}$$
$$\frac{250 \text{ mg}}{1 \text{ tab}} = \frac{500 \text{ mg}}{x \text{ tab}}$$
$$500 \times 1 = 250 \times x$$
$$x \text{ tab} = \frac{500}{250} = 2 \text{ tablets}$$

Whereas this calculation is trivially clear and can be performed mentally, others may require calculation for the sake of accuracy.

EXAMPLE 2
You have 120 mg of phenobarbital in 30 ml of phenobarbital elixir. How many milliliters of elixir will you use to give a 15 mg dose?

$$\frac{120 \text{ mg (original dose)}}{30 \text{ ml (per amount)}} = \frac{15 \text{ mg (desired dose)}}{x \text{ (per amount)}}$$

Cross-multiplying:

$$120 \text{ mg} \times x = 15 \text{ mg (30 ml)}$$
$$x \text{ ml} = 3.75 \text{ ml}$$

Simplification is possible, such as reducing 120 mg/30 ml to 4 mg/ml. Then knowing that there are 4 mg in every milliliter, simply divide 4 mg/ml into 15 mg, to determine how many milliliters are needed. Often, reducing a liquid to its dosage strength per 1 ml allows quick mental computation of the dose. Caution and care should be observed in the initial reduction, however. An error at that point causes a subsequent dosage error. *Do not hesitate to write out a calculation:* In a busy clinical setting, a patient's well-being should take precedence over a practitioner's mathematical pride.

DRUG AMOUNTS IN UNITS

It should be noted that some drugs are manufactured in units (U) rather than in grams or milligrams. Examples are penicillin, insulin, and heparin. Solving dose problems for these drugs is exactly the same as for the other dosage units previously mentioned.

EXAMPLE 3
A brand of sodium heparin is available in 1000 U/ml. How many milliliters do you need for 500 U of the drug? Using the second form of the proportion (extremes and means), we set up:

Original dose:amount :: Desired dose:amount
1000 U:1 ml :: 500 U:x ml

By multiplying the extremes and the means, we obtain:

$$1000 \ (x) = 500$$
$$x \text{ ml} = 0.5 \text{ ml}$$

ANSWER: The amount required for 500 U, given the prepared-strength liquid, is 0.5 ml.

There is no universal equivalence between units as a measure of amount and the metric weight system. Units are used with biological standardization and are defined for each drug by a standard preparation of that drug, when the drug is measured in units. For example, there is a standard preparation of digitalis, consisting of dried, powdered digitalis leaves, and 100 mg of this preparation equals one United States Pharmacopeia (USP) unit of activity. In this way, when drugs are extracted from animals, plants, or minerals, there is a standard reference preparation. Note that 100 mg is not 1 U for every drug with units; for example, insulin has a standard preparation of 0.04 mg = 1 U. When a drug is isolated as a pure chemical form, either extracted as the active substance in a natural source or synthesized in the laboratory, biological standardization based on a standard preparation from the natural source is no longer necessary. The specific chemical amount is given in metric weight or volume measure.

CALCULATIONS WITH A DOSAGE SCHEDULE

There are times when the dose of a drug must be obtained from a *schedule*, which may be based on the size of a person. For example, a suggested schedule for albuterol syrup in children 2 to 6 years old is 0.1 mg/kg of body weight. This means that the *dose* must first be calculated after the body weight is obtained, and then the amount of the drug preparation needed for treatment can be calculated.

EXAMPLE 4
Using a schedule of 0.1 mg/kg for albuterol syrup, and a prepared-strength mixture of 2 mg/5 ml, how much of the syrup is needed for a 20-kg child?

1. Calculate the dose needed:

$$\text{Dose} = 0.1 \text{ mg/kg} \times 20 \text{ kg} = 2.0 \text{ mg}$$

2. Calculate the amount of the preparation:

$$\frac{2 \text{ mg}}{5 \text{ ml}} = \frac{2 \text{ mg}}{x \text{ ml}}$$

Simplifying,

$$2 \ (x) = 10$$
$$x \text{ ml} = 5 \text{ ml}$$

ADDITIONAL EXAMPLES OF CALCULATIONS WITH PREPARED-STRENGTH DRUGS

EXAMPLE 5
An injectable solution of glycopyrrolate with a prepared-strength of 0.2 mg/ml is used for nebulization. How many milliliters are needed for a 1.5 mg dose?

Solution:

Original dose per amount: 0.2 mg per ml
Desired dose: 1.5 mg
Amount needed: x ml

Substituting:

$$\frac{0.2 \text{ mg}}{1 \text{ ml}} = \frac{1.5 \text{ mg}}{x \text{ ml}}$$

Using cross-multiplication to simplify:

$$0.2 \text{ mg} (x) = 1.5 \text{ mg} (1 \text{ ml})$$
$$x = 1.5/0.2$$
$$x \text{ ml} = 7.5 \text{ ml}$$

ANSWER: An amount of 7.5 ml will contain the desired dose of 1.5 mg, using the prepared-strength given.

EXAMPLE 6

You have terbutaline 1 mg/ml in an ampule for injection. How much do you need, to give a 0.25 mg dose subcutaneously?

Solution:

Original dose per amount: 1 mg per ml
Desired dose: 0.25 mg
Amount needed: x ml

Substituting:

$$\frac{1 \text{ mg}}{1 \text{ ml}} = \frac{0.25 \text{ mg}}{x \text{ ml}}$$

Solving for x:

$$1 \text{ mg} (x) = 0.25 \text{ mg} (1 \text{ ml})$$
$$x = 0.25 \text{ ml}$$

ANSWER: Give 0.25 ml for the desired dose of 0.25 mg.

EXAMPLE 7

A dosage schedule of a surfactant calls for 5 ml per kilogram of body weight. If a premature infant weighs 1200 g, how many milliliters are needed?

Solution:
Convert body weight to kilograms.

$$1 \text{ kg}/1000 \text{ g} \times 1200 \text{ g} = 1.2 \text{ kg}$$

Multiply the weight in kilograms by the schedule of 5 ml/kg.

$$1.2 \text{ kg} \times 5 \text{ ml/kg} = 6 \text{ ml}$$

ANSWER: Based on the dosage schedule and weight, 6 ml should be given.

EXAMPLE 8

The prepared-strength of a drug is 100 mg per 4 ml. The dosage schedule is 100 mg per kilogram of birth weight. A premature newborn weighs 1100 g. Based on the weight, what dose is needed? How many milliliters of the drug should be given to achieve this dose?

Solution: Dose needed:
Convert birth weight to kilograms.

$$1 \text{ kg}/1000 \text{ g} \times 1100 \text{ g} = 1.1 \text{ kg}$$

Multiply the birth weight by the dosage schedule.

$$100 \text{ mg/kg} \times 1.1 \text{ kg} = 110 \text{ mg}$$

The dose needed is 110 mg of drug.
Solution: Amount needed for dose:

Original dose per amount: 100 mg per 4 ml
Desired dose: 110 mg
Amount needed: x ml

Substituting:

$$\frac{100 \text{ mg}}{4 \text{ ml}} = \frac{110 \text{ mg}}{x \text{ ml}}$$
$$100 \text{ mg} (x) = 110 \text{ mg} (4 \text{ ml})$$
$$x = 110 \text{ mg} (4 \text{ ml})/100 \text{ mg}$$
$$x \text{ ml} = 4.4 \text{ ml}$$

ANSWER: Based on the dosage schedule, weight of the newborn, and the prepared-strength, 4.4 ml will give the needed dose of 110 mg.

CALCULATING DOSES FROM PERCENTAGE-STRENGTH SOLUTIONS

Because an area of expertise for respiratory therapists is solutions for aerosolization, solutions and percentage strengths will often be needed to calculate a drug dose. A *solution* contains a *solute*, which is dissolved in a *solvent*, giving a homogeneous mixture. The *strength* of a solution is expressed in percentage of solute to total solvent and solute. *Percentage* means parts of the active ingredient (solute) in a preparation contained in 100 parts of the total preparation (solute *and* solvent).

TYPES OF PERCENTAGE PREPARATIONS

WEIGHT TO WEIGHT

Percent in weight (W/W) expresses the number of grams of a drug or active ingredient in 100 g of a mixture:

W/W: Grams per 100 g of mixture

WEIGHT TO VOLUME

Percent may be expressed for the number of grams of a drug or active ingredient in 100 ml of a mixture:

W/V: Grams per 100 ml of mixture

VOLUME TO VOLUME

Percent volume in volume (V/V) expresses the number of milliliters of drug or active ingredient in 100 ml of a mixture:

V/V: Milliliters per 100 ml of mixture

SOLUTIONS BY RATIO

Frequently when diluting a medication for use in an aerosol or intermittent positive-pressure breathing (IPPB) treatment, a solute to solvent ratio is given (e.g., isoproterenol 1:200 or Bronkosol 1:8).

RATIO BY GRAMS TO MILLILITERS

In the isoproterenol example, the following is indicated:

1 g per 200 ml of solution = 0.5% strength

This is what is indicated with traditional examples such as epinephrine 1:100, which is a 1% strength solution.

RATIO BY SIMPLE PARTS

In the Bronkosol example, actual parts medication to parts solvent are indicated, as follows:

1:8 = 1 part to 8 parts, which is the same as:
¼ cc to 2 cc

However, part-to-part ratios do not indicate actual amounts or specific units, although usually milliliters to milliliters are meant. It is assumed you know that ¼ cc or ½ cc of Bronkosol is given as the usual dose, and not a 1 cc amount. An order such as Bronkosol 1:8 is not precise without further specifications of the amount of drug (whether 0.25 ml, 0.5 ml, etc.) to be given.

SOLVING PERCENTAGE-STRENGTH SOLUTION PROBLEMS

For solutions in which the active ingredient itself is pure (undiluted, 100% strength), the following equation can be used:

EQUATION 1

$$\text{Percent strength (in decimals)} = \frac{\text{Solute (in grams or cubic centimeters)}}{\text{Total amount (solute and solvent)}}$$

Alternatively, a ratio format can be used:

EQUATION 2

$$\frac{\text{Amount of solute}}{\text{Total amount}} = \frac{\text{Amount of solute}}{\text{100 parts (grams or cubic centimeters)}}$$

When the active ingredient, or solute, is already diluted and less than pure, the following equation can be used:

EQUATION 3

$$\text{Percent strength (in decimals)} = \frac{\text{(Dilute solute)} \times \text{(Percent strength of solute)}}{\text{Total amount (solution)}}$$

In equation 3 the solute (active ingredient) multiplied by the percent strength gives the amount of pure ac-

tive ingredient in the dilute solution. This equation adds only one modification to the formula given in equation 1. This is to multiply the dilute solute by its actual percentage strength, with the result indicating the amount of active ingredient at a 100% (pure) strength. For example, 10 ml of 10% solute means you have 1 ml of pure (100%) solute. Put another way, you would need 10 ml of dilute solute to have 1 ml of pure solute (active ingredient). When used in equation 3, the unknown is usually how much of the dilute solute, or active ingredient, is needed in the total solution to give the desired strength. The preceding equations are illustrated in the following two examples.

EXAMPLE 9
Undiluted active ingredient: How many milligrams of active ingredient are there in 2 cc of 1:200 isoproterenol?

Percent strength: 1:200 = 0.5% = 0.005
Total amount of solution: 2 cc
Active ingredient: x

Substituting in equation 1:

$$0.005 = x \, \text{g}/2 \, \text{cc}$$
$$x \, \text{g} = 0.005 \times 2$$
$$x \, \text{g} = 0.01 \, \text{g}$$

ANSWER: Converting 0.01 g to milligrams gives 10 mg. In 2 cc of 1:200 solution there are 10 mg.

EXAMPLE 10
Diluted active ingredient: How much 20% Mucomyst (brand of acetylcysteine) is needed to prepare 5 cc of 10% Mucomyst? Using the equation for dilute active ingredients (here the acetylcysteine is only 20% strength, not pure), the following is obtained:

Desired percentage strength: 10% = 0.10
Total solution amount: 5 cc
Active ingredient percentage strength: 20% = 0.20
Amount of active ingredient needed: x

Substituting in equation 3:

$$0.10 = x(0.20)/5 \, \text{cc}$$
$$x = 5(0.10)/0.20$$
$$x \, \text{cc} = 2.5 \, \text{cc of the 20% Mucomyst}$$

ANSWER: The 2.5 cc of the 20% Mucomyst is then mixed with enough normal saline to give a total of 5 cc of solution. This 5 cc will be a 10% strength solution.

Although diluting a 20% solution to a 10% solution is obviously a "half and half" procedure and need not require use of an equation, less intuitive dilutions may need to be calculated. The reader might try diluting 20% Mucomyst to obtain 5 cc of a 5% strength solution, using the preceding approach.

SUMMARY

Calculations with solutions of drugs using percentage-strengths can be summarized as follows:

1. Convert to metric units and decimal expressions.
2. Substitute knowns in the appropriate equation (undilute or dilute active ingredient).
3. Use grams or milliliters in the percentage equation.
4. Express answer in units requested.

NOTE ON MIXING SOLUTIONS

In mixing solutions, determine the amount of active ingredient needed for the percent strength desired, and then add enough solvent to "top off" to the total solution amount needed. When ordering a solution this is indicated by *quantity sufficient (qs)*, for the total needed. For example, to obtain 30 cc of 3% procaine HCl, we calculate 0.9 cc of the active ingredient, and water qs for 30 cc of solution. Do not merely give the difference between solute and total solution (30 cc − 0.9 cc = 29.1 cc), because certain solutes can change volume (e.g., alcohol "shrinks" in water).

PERCENTAGE-STRENGTHS IN MILLIGRAMS PER MILLILITER

The basic definition of percentage strength in solutions involves grams or milliliters. However, the amount of active ingredient in most nebulized drug solutions is in milligrams. It may be a useful clinical reference, and one that is easily remembered, to define percentage strengths in terms of milligrams per single milliliter, using a 1% strength reference point. Recall that 1% strength is 1 g per 100 ml. Using the formula for percentage strength, you have:

$$0.01 = \frac{1\,g}{100\,ml}$$

For 1 ml of a 1% strength, you would have:

$$0.01 = \frac{x\,g}{1\,ml}$$
$$xg = 0.01\,g$$

and 0.01 g × 1000 mg/gram = 10 mg. Because 0.01 g equals 10 mg, you then have 10 mg per 1 ml in a 1% solution. The 1% strength is an easily learned reference point. Table 4-2 lists some common percentage strengths, giving amounts in milligrams per milliliter, in reference to the 1% concentration.

Note the relationship of 1% to 10%: If there are 10 mg/ml in a 1% solution, there would be 10 times that

Table 4-2

Drug amounts in milligrams per milliliter for common percentage strengths

PERCENTAGE STRENGTH (%)	DRUG AMOUNT (mg/ml)
20	200
10	100
5	50
1	**10**
0.5	5
0.1	1
0.05	0.5

amount in a 10% solution, or 100 mg/ml. Likewise, a 0.5% solution has one-half as much active ingredient as 1%: One half of 10 mg/ml would be 5 mg/ml. This amount of 5 mg/ml could have been used to solve example 9, of an undiluted active ingredient percentage problem. In example 9, it was found that a 1:200 solution (a 0.5% strength) has 10 mg per 2 ml, which is the same as 5 mg in 1 ml.

Equations 1 and 3 should be known and represent a more general statement of percentage strengths for solving any problem. However, knowledge of milligrams per milliliters for a 1% solution can be very helpful in many problems, to know how many milligrams of the active ingredient are being given. Examples of drug solutions with the strengths listed in Table 4-2 can be given. Metaproterenol is available as a 5% solution or 50 mg/ml, and an ampule of terbutaline (1 mg/cc) is a 0.1% strength.

DILUENTS AND DRUG DOSES

A common misconception persists that the amount of diluent added to a liquid drug to be aerosolized by nebulization is intended to "weaken" the dose or strength delivered to the patient. This is not necessarily the case. One-half cc of a 1% drug solution has the same amount (5 mg) of active ingredient, whether it is diluted with 2 cc or 10 cc of normal saline. The amount of diluent affects the time required to nebulize a given solution but not the amount of active ingredient in a nebulizer reservoir. Practicality dictates that 2.5 cc of solution nebulizes in a reasonable time limit of 10 minutes or so, whereas 10 cc may take much longer. The diluent also is needed because disposable nebulizers cannot create an aerosol with less than approximately 1 ml of solution in the reservoir (the "dead volume"). Theoretically, given a suitable nebulizing device, there is no reason that the original 0.5 cc of 1% drug could not be nebulized undiluted in order to deliver the dose of 5 mg. It is the amount of the active ingredient, determined by the percentage strength and quantity in cubic centimeters of the drug that gives a dose amount. Although technically the percentage strength of the resulting solution in the reservoir is weaker, the dose remains unchanged at 5 mg. It is the dose in milligrams that should be of concern to the clinician.

ADDITIONAL EXAMPLES OF CALCULATIONS WITH SOLUTIONS

EXAMPLE 11

How many milligrams of active ingredient are in 3 cc of a 2% solution of procaine HCl?

Use the percentage formula of equation 1, pure-strength ingredient.

$$\% \text{ (in decimals)} = \frac{\text{Solute}}{\text{Total amount}}$$

Convert percentage to decimals and substitute the known values:

$$0.02 = \frac{x\,\text{g}}{3\,\text{cc}}$$
$$0.02\,(3\,\text{cc}) = x\,\text{g}$$
$$x\,\text{g} = 0.06\,\text{g}$$

In milligrams:

$$0.06\,\text{g} \times 1000\,\text{mg/g} = 60\,\text{mg}$$

ANSWER: 60 mg

EXAMPLE 12

A resident wants to dilute 20% acetylcysteine to a strength of 6% for a research study.

How many milliliters of 20% drug solution are needed to have 10 ml of 6% strength?

Use the modified equation 3 for dilute active ingredient:

$$\% \text{ (decimals)} = \frac{(\text{Dilute solute}) \times (\% \text{ strength})}{\text{Total solution}}$$

Solution:

> % desired: 6% = 0.06
> Dilute solute: Unknown = x ml
> Percentage strength: 20% = 0.20
> Total solution: 10 ml

Substituting and solving:

$$0.06 = \frac{(x\,\text{ml}) \times (0.20)}{10\,\text{ml}}$$
$$0.06\,(10\,\text{ml}) = x\,\text{ml}\,(0.20)$$
$$x = 0.06\,(10)/0.20$$
$$x\,\text{ml} = 3\,\text{ml}$$

ANSWER: Draw up 3 ml of the 20% strength and add saline, quantity sufficient, for a total of 10 ml. Check your calculation for correctness: 3 ml of 20% strength solution has 600 mg of active ingredient (20% = 200 mg/ml); 600 mg is 0.6 g; and 0.6 g per 10 ml (or 6 g per 100 ml) is in fact a 6% strength. So you obtained the needed amount of drug with 3 ml of the 20% solution.

EXAMPLE 13

The usual dose of albuterol sulfate is 0.5 ml of a 0.5% strength solution. How many milligrams is this?

Using equation 1 for percentage strength:

> Percentage in decimals: 0.5% = 0.005
> Active ingredient: unknown (x)
> Total solution: 0.5 ml

Substituting:

$$0.005 = \frac{x\,\text{g}}{0.5\,\text{ml}}$$
$$x\,\text{g} = 0.005\,(0.5) = 0.0025\,\text{g}$$

Converting:

$$0.0025\,\text{g} = 2.5\,\text{mg}$$

ANSWER: 2.5 milligrams of active ingredient.

EXAMPLE 14

Albuterol sulfate is also available as a unit dose, with 3 ml and a percentage strength of 0.083%. If the entire amount of 3 ml is given, is this the same as the usual dose of 2.5 mg?

Using equation 1 for percentage strength:

> Percentage in decimals: 0.083% = 0.00083
> Active ingredient: unknown = x
> Total solution: 3 ml

Substituting:

$$0.00083 = \frac{x\,\text{g}}{3\,\text{ml}}$$
$$x\,\text{g} = 3\,(0.00083) = 0.00249\,\text{g}$$

and

$$0.00249\,\text{g} = 2.49\,\text{mg}$$

ANSWER: The result is approximately 2.5 mg, the usual dose.

EXAMPLE 15

Terbutaline sulfate is available as 1 mg in 1 ml of solution. What percentage strength is this?

Solution:

Convert 1 mg to 0.001 g (1 mg × 1 g/1000 mg = 0.001 g)

$$x = \frac{0.001\,\text{g}}{1\,\text{ml}}$$

$$x = 0.001 = 0.1\%$$

ANSWER: The result is 0.1%.

CALCULATING INTRAVENOUS INFUSION RATES

The previous knowledge of prepared strength drug units and solutions allows relatively straightforward calculation of intravenous (IV) infusion rates. IV infusion incorporates calculation of the *rate* of drug administration per unit time (e.g., milligrams per minute). Ultimately an infusion rate in drops per minute will be needed on the IV infusion set. This requires knowing the Standard Drop Factor for that IV administration set, which gives the number of drops that equal 1 ml in the drip chamber. This information can be found when the IV set is opened. The following formulas can be used, depending on the type of order to be followed.

TOTAL SOLUTION OVER TIME

The simplest IV infusion calculation involves administering a volume of solution over a period of time. In this case, the flow rate is expressed in milliliters per minute, using the solution amount in milliliters and time in minutes.

$$\text{Flow rate (ml/min)} = \frac{\text{Total solution (ml)}}{\text{Time (min)}}$$

The flow rate can be converted into drops per minute using the Standard Drop Factor, which gives the number of drops in each milliliter.

EQUATION 4

$$\text{Flow rate (drops/min)} = \frac{\text{Drops}}{\text{Milliliter}} \times \frac{\text{Milliliter}}{\text{Minute}}$$

EXAMPLE 16

You wish to give 1 L of solution in a 3-hour period. What is the flow rate in drops per minute, if the Standard Drop Factor for your IV set is 15 drops per milliliter?

$$1 \text{ L of solution} = 1000 \text{ ml}$$
$$3 \text{ hr} = 180 \text{ min}$$

Calculate the flow rate in milliliters per minute from the volume of solution and the time given:

$$\text{Flow rate (in ml/min)} = \frac{1000 \text{ ml}}{180 \text{ min}} = 5.56 \text{ ml/min}$$

Calculate flow rate as drops per minute, using equation 4:

Flow rate (in drops/min) = 15 drops/ml × 6 ml/min = 90 drops/min

ANSWER: An infusion rate of 90 drops/min should deliver the desired 1 L in about 3 hours.

AMOUNT OF DRUG PER UNIT OF TIME

An IV drug may be administered as an amount per unit of time (usually minutes). For example, epinephrine can be given as micrograms per minute (μg/min). The drug amount per minute must be converted into a drip rate of drops per minute, for proper drug infusion. In this case the concentration of the drug solution is used to calculate the drug amount in 1 ml.

EQUATION 5

$$\text{Concentration (in amount/ml)} = \frac{\text{Total drug amount}}{\text{Total solution (in milliliters)}}$$

The rate of flow in milliliters per minute can then be calculated from the needed drug amount per minute and the concentration of drug per milliliter.

EQUATION 6

$$\text{Flow rate (in ml/min)} = \frac{\text{Amount}}{\text{Minute}} \times \frac{\text{Milliliter}}{\text{Amount}}$$

The flow rate can then be converted from milliliters per minute to drops per minute needed to give the desired amount of drug per unit of time, as before, using the Standard Drop Factor, as shown in equation 4.

Flow rate (in drops/min) = Drop factor (in drops/ml) × ml/min

The last two equations can be combined to allow direct calculation of drops per minute, from the known concentration in amount per milliliter and the desired delivery rate in amount per unit of time.

EQUATION 7

$$\text{Flow rate (in drops/min)} = \frac{\text{Amount}}{\text{Minute}} \times \frac{\text{Milliliter}}{\text{Amount}} \times \frac{\text{Drops}}{\text{Milliliter}}$$

EXAMPLE 17

What infusion rate is needed to deliver 10 μg/min of a drug that comes in a solution of 500 μg/250 ml? The Standard Drop Factor for the IV administration set is 15 drops/ml.

Concentration of drug (in μg/ml) = 500 μg/250 ml = 2 μg/ml
Rate of flow (in ml/min) = 10 μg/min × 1 ml/2 μg = 5 ml/min
Rate of flow (in drops/min) = 15 drops/ml × 5 ml/min
$$= 75 \quad \text{drops/min}$$

ANSWER: An infusion rate of 75 drops per minute will deliver the desired drug dose of 10 μg/min.

The maximum dose of drug to be delivered will determine how long the infusion continues. For example, if the maximum dose is 1 mg, this dose would be reached in 100 minutes with the infusion rate of 10 μg/min:

$$1 \text{ mg} = 1000 \text{ μg}$$
$$\text{Time (min)} = 1000 \text{ μg} \times 1 \text{ min}/10 \text{ μg}$$
$$\text{Time} = 100 \text{ minutes or 1 hour and 40 minutes}$$

The rate of drug administration, in amount per minute, is used to calculate how long it will take to deliver a set amount of drug. In general, equations 4, 5, and 6 or 7 can be used to solve for any unknown factor in IV drug administration, as shown in the additional examples below.

ADDITIONAL EXAMPLES OF INTRAVENOUS DOSE CALCULATIONS

EXAMPLE 18
In advanced cardiac life support (ACLS), dopamine is given IV to increase cardiac output. If you add a 200 mg ampule of dopamine to 250 ml of 5% dextrose in water (D_5W), what drip rate is needed to deliver a dose of 10 μg/kg/min for the average adult of 70 kg? Assume that the drop factor is 15 drops/ml.

Dose needed (in μg/min): 70 kg × 10 μg/kg/min = 700 μg/min
Concentration available: 200 mg per 250 ml, or 0.8 mg/ml
$$= 800 \text{ μg/ml}$$

Using the combined equation 7 for amount per minute, milliliters per amount, and drops per milliliter (Drop Factor), we would calculate:

$$\text{Flow rate (in drops/min)} = \frac{700 \text{ μg}}{\text{Minute}} \times \frac{1 \text{ ml}}{800 \text{ μg}} \times \frac{15 \text{ drops}}{1 \text{ ml}}$$
$$= 13.125 \text{ drops/min}$$

ANSWER: A drip rate of 13 drops/min will deliver approximately 693 μg/min total, or about 10 μg/kg/min to the patient.

EXAMPLE 19
Phenobarbital may be given in status epilepticus as an IV infusion, with a dose of 10 mg/kg. The rate of infusion should not exceed 50 mg/min. The Drop Factor is 15 drops/ml, and you have a solution of 650 mg in 10 ml. What is the total dose for a 65-kg adult?

$$\text{Total dose} = 10 \text{ mg/kg} \times 65 \text{ kg} = 650 \text{ mg}$$

How long will it take for the dose to be given, using the maximal allowed rate of infusion (50 mg/min)?

$$\text{Time (in min)} = 650 \text{ mg} \times 1 \text{ min}/50 \text{ mg} = 13 \text{ min}$$

What is the maximum rate of drip (drops per minute) allowed?

First calculate the drug concentration available in milligrams/milliliter, using equation 5:

$$\text{Concentration (in mg/ml)} = 650 \text{ mg}/10 \text{ ml} = 65 \text{ mg/ml}$$

Then you can use the combined equation 7 to calculate flow rate in milliliters per minute and convert to drops per minute using the Drop Factor:

$$\text{Flow rate (drops/min)} = 50 \text{ mg/min} \times 1 \text{ ml}/65 \text{ mg} \times 15 \text{ drops/ml}$$
$$= 750 \text{ drops}/65 \text{ min}$$

or,

$$\text{Flow rate (drops/min)} = 11.5 \text{ drops/min}$$

EXAMPLE 20
If a drug concentration is 500 μg/250 ml, and the Standard Drop Factor is 15 drops/ml, how long will it take to deliver the 500 μg using a drip rate of 30 drops/min?

Calculate the drug concentration in a single milliliter:

$$\text{Concentration (in μg/ml)} = 500 \text{ μg}/250 \text{ ml} = 2 \text{ μg/ml}$$

Convert the flow rate from drops per minute to milliliters per minute using the Drop Factor and given drip rate of 30 drops/min:

$$\text{Flow rate (in ml/min)} = 30 \text{ drops/min} \times 1 \text{ ml}/15 \text{ drops} = 2 \text{ ml/min}$$

Convert this flow rate into a drug amount per unit of time using the concentration (amount per milliliter):

$$\text{Drug amount (per min)} = 2 \text{ ml/min} \times 2 \text{ μg/ml} = 4 \text{ μg/min}$$

and,

$$\text{Time (in min)} = 1 \text{ min}/4 \text{ μg} \times 500 \text{ μg} = 125 \text{ min, or 2 hours}$$
$$\text{and 5 minutes}$$

Or, more simply, the flow rate in ml/min and the total amount of solution (250 ml) could be used to calculate the time the infusion would take:

$$\text{Time (in min)} = 250 \text{ ml} \times 1 \text{ min}/2 \text{ ml} = 125 \text{ min}$$

EXAMPLE 21
If an IV dose is ordered at 5 μg/min, how long will it take to reach a maximum dose of 0.375 mg?

Convert 0.375 mg to micrograms:

$$0.375 \text{ mg} = 375 \text{ μg}$$

Calculate the total time for delivery from the rate of delivery and the total amount of drug:

$$\text{Time (in min)} = 1 \text{ min}/5 \text{ μg} \times 375 \text{ μg} = 75 \text{ min}$$

EXAMPLE 22
If an IV dose is given at 30 drops/min and the drug solution is 100 μg/2 ml, how much drug in micrograms per minute is being given? Standard Drop Factor = 15 drops/ml

$$\text{Concentration (in amount/ml)} = 100 \text{ μg}/2 \text{ ml} = 50 \text{ μg/ml}$$

Calculate the flow rate in milliliters per minute, from the Drop Factor and the drops per minute:

$$\text{Flow rate (in ml/min)} = \frac{30 \text{ drops}}{1 \text{ min}} \times \frac{1 \text{ ml}}{15 \text{ drops}}$$
$$= 2 \text{ ml/min}$$

The drug amount per minute is obtained from the flow rate in milliliters per minute and the concentration in µg/ml:

$$x \text{ µg/min} = 2 \text{ ml/min} \times 50 \text{ µg/ml} = 100 \text{ µg/min}$$

SUMMARY KEY TERMS AND CONCEPTS

- Drug calculations use the metric system of measurement.
- Volume and weight measures are the most common.
- Household measures (cup, teaspoon, etc.) are also used in administering medication.
- The three types of drug calculations are prepared-strength doses, doses from solutions with a concentration expressed as a percentage, and intravenous dose calculations.
- Prepared-strength doses involve calculating how many tablets, capsules, or milliliters of a liquid are needed to administer a given amount of drug and are most easily solved using a proportion, after units are made consistent, as follows:

$$\frac{\text{Original dose}}{\text{Per amount}} = \frac{\text{Desired dose}}{\text{Per amount}}$$

- Calculating doses based on a percentage-strength concentration of a solution can be done using the following equation:

$$\frac{\text{Percentage strength}}{\text{(in decimals)}} = \frac{\text{Solute (in grams or cubic centimeters)}}{\text{Total amount (solute and solvent)}}$$

- An easy reference point for the amount of drug contained in a solution, in milligrams per milliliter is a 1% strength, which is 10 mg/ml.
- Intravenous (IV) drug dose calculations are based on solutions and solution concentrations. Given the concentration of the drug solution in milliliters per amount of drug, calculate how many milliliters per minute are needed. Convert this flow rate of milliliters per minute into drops per minute, using the Standard Drop Factor obtained from the IV administration set.

$$\text{Flow rate (in drops/min)} = \frac{\text{Amount}}{\text{Minute}} \times \frac{\text{Milliliter}}{\text{Amount}} \times \frac{\text{Drops}}{\text{Milliliter}}$$

SELF-ASSESSMENT QUESTIONS

PREPARED-STRENGTH DOSE CALCULATIONS

Answers to the practice problems are in Appendix A. The solution to each problem is set up and the answer given. Details of the algebraic solution are not given.

1. A bottle is labeled Demerol (meperidine) 50 mg/cc. How many cc are needed to give a 125 mg dose?
2. Promazine HCl comes as 500 mg/10 ml. How many milliliters are needed to give a 150 mg dose?
3. Hyaluronidase comes as 150 U/cc. How many cc are needed for a 30 U dose?
4. Morphine sulfate 4 mg is ordered. You have a vial with 10 mg/ml. How much do you need?
5. A dosage schedule for the surfactant poractant calls for 2.5 ml/kg birth weight. How much drug will you need for a 800-g baby?
6. Diphenhydramine (Benadryl) elixir contains 12.5 mg of diphenhydramine HCl in each 5 ml of elixir. How many milligrams are there in one half teaspoonful dose (1 tsp = 5 ml)?
7. A pediatric dose of oxytetracycline 100 mg is ordered. The dosage form is an oral suspension containing 125 mg/5 cc. How much of the suspension contains a 100 mg dose?
8. How much heparin is in 0.2 ml, if you have 1000 U/ml?
9. Albuterol syrup is available as 2 mg/5 ml. If a dose schedule of 0.1 mg/kg is used, how much syrup is needed for a 30-kg child? How many teaspoons is this?
10. Terbutaline is available as 2.5 mg tablets. How many tablets do you need for a 5 mg dose?
11. If Tempra is available as 120 mg/5 ml, how much dose is there in ½ teaspoon?
12. Theophylline is available as 250 mg/10 ml and is given intravenously as 6 mg/kg body weight. How much solution do you give for a 60-kg woman?
13. Terbutaline sulfate is available as 1 mg/ml in an ampule. How many milliliters are needed for a 0.25 mg dose?
14. A patient is told to take 4 mg of albuterol four times daily. The medication comes in 2 mg tablets. How many tablets are needed for one 4 mg dose?
15. Metaproterenol is available as a syrup with 10 mg/5 ml. How many teaspoons should be taken for a 20 mg dose?
16. If you have 3 mg/ml of d-(+)-tubocurarine, how many milliliters are needed for a dose of 9 mg?
17. If a dosage schedule requires 0.25 mg/kg of body weight, what dose is needed for an 88-kg person?
18. If theophylline is available as 80 mg/15 ml, how much is needed for a 100 mg dose?
19. How much drug is needed for a 65-kg adult, using 0.5 mg/kg?
20. Pediatric dosage of an antibiotic is 0.5 g/20 lb of body weight, not to exceed 75 mg/kg/24 hr.
    a. What is the dose for a 40-lb child?
    b. If this dose is given twice in 1 day, is the maximum dose exceeded?

PERCENTAGE-STRENGTH SOLUTIONS

1. How many grams of calamine are needed to prepare 120 g of an ointment containing 8% calamine?
2. One milliliter of active enzyme is found in 147 ml of solution. What is the percentage strength of active enzyme in the solution?

3. If theophylline is available in a 250 mg/10 ml solution, what percentage strength is this?
4. You have epinephrine 1:100. How many milliliters of epinephrine would be needed to contain 30 mg of active ingredient?
5. A dose of 0.4 ml of epinephrine HCl 1:100 is ordered. This dose contains how many milligrams of epinephrine HCl? (the active ingredient?)
6. If you administer 3 ml of a 0.1% strength solution, how many milligrams of active ingredient have you given?
7. A drug is available as a 1:200 solution and the maximum dose that may be given by aerosol for a particular patient is 3 mg. What is the maximal amount of solution (in milliliters) that may be used?
8. Epinephrine 1:1000 contains how many milligrams per milliliter?
9. How many milligrams per milliliter are there in 0.3 ml of 5% strength metaproterenol?
10. How many milligrams of sodium chloride are needed for 10 ml of a 0.9% solution?
11. If you have 5 mg/ml of Xylocaine, what percentage strength is this?
12. A 0.5% strength solution contains how many milligrams in 1 ml?
13. Cromolyn sodium contains 20 mg in 2 ml of water. What is the percentage strength?
14. How much active ingredient of acetylcysteine (Mucomyst) have you given with 4 cc of a 20% solution?
15. You have 20% acetylcysteine; how many milliliters do you need of this to form 4 ml of an 8% solution?
16. The recommended dose of metaproterenol 5% is 0.3 cc. How many milligrams of solute are there in this amount?
17. Mucomyst brand of acetylcysteine was marketed as 10% acetylcysteine with 0.05% isoproterenol. How many milligrams of each ingredient were in a 4 cc dose of solution?
18. Which contains more drug: ½ cc of 1% drug solution with 2 ml of saline, or ½ cc of 1% drug solution with 5 ml of saline?
19. How many milligrams per milliliter are in a 20% solution?
20. On an emergency cart, you have sodium bicarbonate solution ($NaHCO_3$), 44.6 mEq/50 ml.

    A physician orders an aerosol of 5 cc and 3.25% strength. How many milliliters of the bicarbonate solution do you need?

    1 mEq = 1/1000 GEW; GEW = Gram formula wt/valence
    Atomic weights: Na, 23; H, 1; C, 12; O, - 16

INTRAVENOUS INFUSION RATES

Assume a Drop Factor of 15 drops = 1 ml.

1. You wish to give a solution of 500 mg/L of dobutamine, at a rate of 10 µg/kg/min, to a 50-kg woman. What drip rate will you need?
2. If you have 2 mg of isoproterenol in 500 ml of solution, and you wish to deliver 5 µg/min intravenously, what drip rate is needed?
3. You have 250 mg of dobutamine in 1 L of solution. You want to deliver 5 µg/kg/min to a 60-kg man. What infusion rate in milliliters per minute and in drops per minute is needed?
4. You have 250 ml of D_5W and a drip rate of 15 drops/min. How long will the bag of solution last?
5. You have epinephrine solution, 1 mg/250 ml. What drip rate is needed to deliver 4 µg/min?
6. If you wish to deliver 500 ml of a solution in 1 hour and 40 minutes, what drip rate should you set?
7. A recommended dose of epinephrine IV is 15 ml/hr, using a solution of 4 µg/ml. What drip rate is needed to achieve the recommended infusion rate?

Answers to Self-Assessment Questions are found in Appendix A.

CLINICAL SCENARIO

You have a 1 Normal (N) solution of saline (NaCl), and you need isotonic saline 0.9%, also called "normal saline," for diluent in a nebulizer solution.

Can you use the 1 N solution as diluent, unchanged?

Answers to Clinical Scenario Questions are found in Appendix A.

REFERENCE

1. Chatburn RL: Measurement, physical quantities, and le Systeme International d'Unites (SI units), *Respir Care* 33:861, 1988.

SUGGESTED READING

Fitch GE, Larson MA, Mooney MP: *Basic arithmetic review and drug therapy*, ed 4, New York, 1977, Macmillan.

Richardson LI, Richardson JK: *The mathematics of drugs and solutions with clinical applications*, New York, 1976, McGraw-Hill.

Saxton DF, Walter JF: *Programmed instruction in arithmetic, dosages and solutions*, ed 3, St Louis, 1974, Mosby.

CHAPTER 5

The Central and Peripheral Nervous System

Joseph L. Rau

The goal of Chapter 5 is to provide a clear introduction to and understanding of the peripheral nervous system; its control mechanisms, especially neurotransmitter function; and its physiological effects in the body. The control mechanisms and physiological effects form the basis for a subsequent understanding of drug actions and drug effects, both for agonists and antagonists that act at various points in the nervous system. The chapter concludes with a summary of autonomic and other neural control mechanisms and effects in the pulmonary system.

THE NERVOUS SYSTEM

There are two major control systems in the body: the *nervous system* and the *endocrine system*. Both systems of control can be manipulated by drug therapy, which either mimics or blocks the usual action of the control system, to produce or inhibit physiological effects. The endocrine system will be considered separately, when discussing the corticosteroid class of drugs. The nervous system is divided into the central nervous system and the peripheral nervous system, both of which

offer sites for drug action. The overall organization of the nervous system can be outlined as follows:

Central nervous system
    Brain
    Spinal cord
Peripheral nervous system
    Sensory (afferent) neurons
    Somatic (motor) neurons
    Autonomic nervous system
        Parasympathetic branch
        Sympathetic branch

Figure 5-1 indicates a functional, but not anatomically accurate, diagram of the central and peripheral nervous system. The *sensory* branch of the nervous system consists of afferent neurons from heat, light, pressure, and pain receptors in the periphery, to the central nervous system. The *somatic* portion of the nervous system is under voluntary, conscious control and innervates skeletal muscle for motor actions such as lifting, walking, or breathing. This portion of the nervous system is manipulated by neuromuscular blocking agents, to induce paralysis in surgical procedures or during

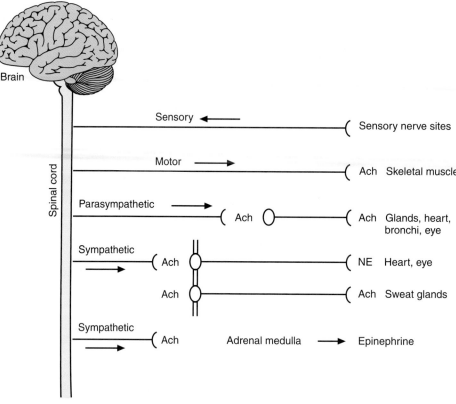

Figure 5-1   A functional diagram of the central and peripheral nervous system, indicating the somatic branches (sensory, motor) and the autonomic branches (sympathetic, parasympathetic), with their neurotransmitters. *Ach*, Acetylcholine; *NE*, norepinephrine.

mechanical ventilation. The *autonomic nervous system* is the involuntary, unconscious control mechanism of the body, sometimes said to control vegetative or visceral functions. For example, the autonomic nervous system regulates heart rate, pupillary dilation and contraction, glandular secretion such as salivation, and smooth muscle in blood vessels and the airway. It is divided into the *parasympathetic* and *sympathetic* branches.

ANATOMICAL DESCRIPTION OF THE AUTONOMIC BRANCHES

Neither the motor nor the sensory branches have synapses outside of the spinal cord before reaching the muscle or sensory receptor site. The motor neuron extends without interruption from the CNS to the skeletal muscle, and its action is mediated by a neurotransmitter, acetylcholine. This is in contrast to the synapses occurring in the sympathetic and parasympathetic divisions of the autonomic system. The multiple synapses of the autonomic system offer potential sites for drug action, in addition to the terminal neuroeffector sites.

The parasympathetic branch arises from the craniosacral portions of the spinal cord and consists of two neurons—a preganglionic fiber leading from the

vertebrae to the ganglionic synapse outside the cord and a postganglionic fiber from the ganglionic synapse to the gland or smooth muscle being innervated. The parasympathetic branch has good specificity, with the postganglionic fiber arising very near the effector site (gland, smooth muscle). As a result, stimulation of a parasympathetic preganglionic neuron causes activity limited to individual effector sites, such as the heart or the eye. Figure 5-2 illustrates the portions of the spinal cord where the parasympathetic and sympathetic nerve fibers originate.

The sympathetic branch arises from the thoracolumbar portion of the spinal cord and has a short preganglionic fiber and a long postganglionic fiber. Sympathetic neurons from the spinal cord terminate in ganglia that lie on either side of the vertebral column. In the ganglia, or the ganglionic chain, the preganglionic fiber makes contact with postganglionic neurons. As a result, when one sympathetic preganglionic neuron is stimulated, the action passes to many or all of the postganglionic fibers. The effect of sympathetic activation is further widened because sympathetic fibers innervate the adrenal medulla and cause

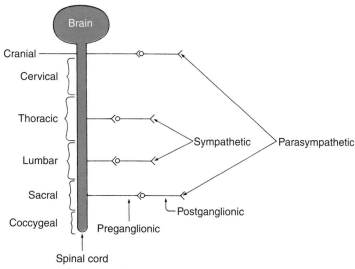

Figure 5-2   Parasympathetic nerve fibers arise from the cranial and sacral portions of the spinal cord, whereas sympathetic fibers primarily leave the cord from the thoracic and lumbar regions.

the release of epinephrine into the general circulation. Circulating epinephrine stimulates all receptors responding to norepinephrine, even if no sympathetic nerves are present. Where the parasympathetic system allows discrete control, the design of the sympathetic system causes a widespread reaction in the body.

CONTRASTS BETWEEN PARASYMPATHETIC AND SYMPATHETIC REGULATION

There are general differences between the parasympathetic and sympathetic branches of the autonomic nervous system, which can be contrasted. The parasympathetic control is essential to life and is considered a more discrete, finely regulated system than the sympathetic. Parasympathetic effects control day-to-day body functions of digestion, bladder and rectum discharge, and basal secretion of bronchial mucus. Overstimulation of the parasympathetic branch would prevent violent action for the body and would result in what is termed the *SLUD syndrome: s*alivation, *l*acrimation, *u*rination, and *d*efecation. These reactions are definitely counterproductive to fleeing or fighting!

By contrast the sympathetic branch reacts as a general-alarm system and does not exercise discrete controls. This is sometimes characterized as a "fight-or-flight" system: heart rate and blood pressure increase, blood flow shifts from the periphery to muscles and the heart, blood sugar rises, and bronchi dilate. The organism prepares for maximum physical exertion. The sympathetic branch is not essential to life; sympathectomized animal models can survive but of course are not prepared to cope with violent stress.

NEUROTRANSMITTERS

Another general feature of the autonomic nervous system, both sympathetic and parasympathetic branches, is the mechanism of neurotransmitter control of nerve impulses. Nerve propagation is both electrical and chemical (electrochemical). A nerve signal is carried along a nerve fiber by *electrical* action potentials, caused by ion exchanges (sodium, potassium). At gaps in the nerve fiber (synapses), the electrical transmission is replaced by a chemical neurotransmitter. This is the *chemical* transmission of the electrical impulse at the ganglionic synapses and at the end of the nerve fiber, termed the *neuroeffector site.* Identification of the chemical transmitters dates back to Loewi's experiments in 1921, and is fundamental to understanding autonomic drugs and their classifications. The usual neurotransmitters in the peripheral nervous system, including the ganglionic synapses and terminal sites in the autonomic branches, are indicated in Figure 5-1, where *Ach* is acetylcholine and *NE* is norepinephrine.

The neurotransmitter conducting the nerve impulse at skeletal muscle sites is acetylcholine, and this site is referred to as the *neuromuscular* junction, or the *myoneural* junction. In the parasympathetic branch, the neurotransmitter is also acetylcholine at both the ganglionic synapses and at the terminal nerve site, referred to as the *neuroeffector* site. In the sympathetic branch, acetylcholine is the neurotransmitter at the ganglionic synapse; however, norepinephrine is the neurotransmitter at the neuroeffector site. There are two exceptions to this pattern, both in the sympathetic branch.

Sympathetic fibers to sweat glands release acetylcholine instead of norepinephrine, and preganglionic sympathetic fibers directly innervate the adrenal medulla, where the neurotransmitter is acetylcholine. Sympathetic fibers that have acetylcholine at the neuroeffector sites are *cholinergic* (for acetylcholine) *sympathetic* fibers. This would be an apparent contradictory combination of terms if not for the exceptions to the rule of norepinephrine as the sympathetic neurotransmitter. Sweating can be caused by giving a cholinergic drug such as pilocarpine, although this effect is under sympathetic control. "Breaking out in a sweat," along with sweaty palms and increased heart rate resulting from circulating epinephrine, are common effects of stress or fright mediated by sympathetic discharge.

Although it is an oversimplification, an easy way to initially learn the various neurotransmitters is to remember that acetylcholine is the neurotransmitter *everywhere* (skeletal muscle, all ganglionic synapses, and parasympathetic terminal nerve sites) *except* at sympathetic terminal nerve sites where norepinephrine is the neurotransmitter. Then the exceptions provided by sympathetic fibers releasing acetylcholine can be remembered as exceptions to the general rule.

EFFERENT AND AFFERENT NERVE FIBERS

The autonomic system is generally considered an *efferent* system; that is, impulses in the sympathetic and parasympathetic branches travel *from* the brain and spinal cord out *to* the various neuroeffector sites, such as the heart, gastrointestinal tract, or lungs. However, *afferent* nerves run alongside the sympathetic and parasympathetic efferent fibers and carry impulses *from* to the periphery to the cord. The afferent fibers convey impulses resulting from visceral stimuli and can form a reflex arc of stimulus input–autonomic output analogous to the well-known somatic reflex arcs, such as the knee-jerk reflex. The mechanism of a vagal reflex arc mediating bronchoconstriction will be further discussed in Chapter 7, in conjunction with drugs used to block the parasympathetic impulses.

TERMINOLOGY OF DRUGS AFFECTING THE NERVOUS SYSTEM

Terminology of drugs and drug effects on the nervous system can be confusing and seem inconsistent. The confusion is due to the fact that drugs and drug effects are derived from the type of nerve fiber (parasympathetic or sympathetic) or, alternatively, the type of neurotransmitter and receptor (acetylcholine, norep-

inephrine). The following terms are based on the anatomy of the nerve fibers, to describe stimulation or inhibition.

Parasympathomimetic: An agent causing stimulation of the parasympathetic nervous system sites
Parasympatholytic: An agent blocking or inhibiting effects of the parasympathetic nervous system
Sympathomimetic: An agent causing stimulation of the sympathetic nervous system
Sympatholytic: An agent blocking or inhibiting the effect of the sympathetic nervous system

Additional terms are used, based on the type of neurotransmitter and receptor. *Cholinergic* refers to acetylcholine, and *adrenergic* is derived from adrenalin, another term for epinephrine, which is similar to norepinephrine and can stimulate sympathetic neuroeffector sites. Because acetylcholine is the neurotransmitter at more sites than just parasympathetic sites, and because receptors exist on smooth muscle or blood cells without any nerve fibers innervating them, these terms denote a wider range of sites than the anatomically based terms such as parasympathomimetic, defined above. For example, *cholinergic* can refer to a drug effect at a ganglia, a parasympathetic nerve ending site, or the neuromuscular junction. *Adrenergic* describes receptors on bronchial smooth muscle or on blood cells, where there are no sympathetic nerves. For this reason, cholinergic and adrenergic are not strictly synonymous with parasympathetic or sympathetic. *Cholinoceptor* and *adrenoceptor* are alternative terms for cholinergic and adrenergic receptors, respectively.

Cholinergic (cholinomimetic): Refers to a drug causing stimulation of a receptor for acetylcholine
Anticholinergic: Refers to a drug blocking a receptor for acetylcholine
Adrenergic (adrenomimetic): Refers to a drug stimulating a receptor for norepinephrine or epinephrine
Antiadrenergic: Refers to a drug blocking a receptor for norepinephrine or epinephrine

PARASYMPATHETIC BRANCH

CHOLINERGIC NEUROTRANSMITTER FUNCTION

In the parasympathetic branch, the neurotransmitter *acetylcholine* conducts the nerve transmission at the ganglionic site, as well as at the parasympathetic effector site at the end of the postganglionic fiber. This action is illustrated in Figure 5-3. The term *neurohor-*

mone has also been used in place of *neurotransmitter.* Acetylcholine (Ach) is concentrated in the presynaptic neuron (both at the ganglia and the effector site). Acetylcholine is synthesized from acetyl CoA and choline, catalyzed by the enzyme choline acetyltransferase. The acetylcholine is stored in vesicles as quanta of 1000 to 50,000 molecules per vesicle. When a nerve impulse (action potential) reaches the presynaptic neuron site, an influx of calcium is triggered into the neuron. Increased calcium in the neuron causes exocytosis of the vesicles containing acetylcholine in the end of the nerve fiber. After release, the acetylcholine attaches to receptors on the postsynaptic membrane and initiates an effect in the tissue or organ site.

Acetylcholine is then inactivated through hydrolysis by cholinesterase enzymes, which split the acetylcholine molecule into choline and acetate, terminating stimulation of the postsynaptic membrane. In effect the nerve impulse is "shut off." There are also receptors on the presynaptic neuron, termed *autoreceptors,* that

can be stimulated by acetylcholine, to regulate and inhibit further neurotransmitter release from the neuron. The effects of the parasympathetic branch of the autonomic system are listed for various organs in Table 5-1. Drugs can mimic or block the action of the neurotransmitter acetylcholine, to stimulate parasympathetic nerve ending sites (parasympathomimetics) or to block

Table 5-1

Effects of parasympathetic stimulation on selected organs or sites

ORGAN/SITE	PARASYMPATHETIC (CHOLINERGIC) RESPONSE
Heart	
SA node	Slowing of rate
Contractility	Decreased atrial force
Conduction velocity	Decreased AV node conduction
Bronchi	
Smooth muscle	Constriction
Mucous glands	Increased secretion
Vascular smooth muscle	
Skin and mucosa	No innervation*
Pulmonary	No innervation*
Skeletal muscle	No innervation†
Coronary	No innervation*
Salivary glands	Increased
Skeletal muscle	None
Eye	
Iris radial muscle	None
Iris circular muscle	Contracts (miosis)
Ciliary muscle	Contracts for near vision
Gastrointestinal tract	Increased motility
Gastrointestinal sphincters	Relaxation
Urinary bladder	
Detrusor	Contraction
Trigone sphincter	Relaxation
Glycogenolysis	
Skeletal muscle	None
Sweat glands	None‡
Lipolysis	None
Renin secretion	None
Insulin secretion	Increased

*No direct parasympathetic nerve innervation; response to exogenous cholinergic agonists is dilation.
†Dilation occurs as a result of sympathetic cholinergic discharge or as a response to exogenous cholinergic agonists.
‡Sweat glands are under sympathetic control; receptors are cholinergic, however, and response to exogenous cholinergic agonists is increased secretion.

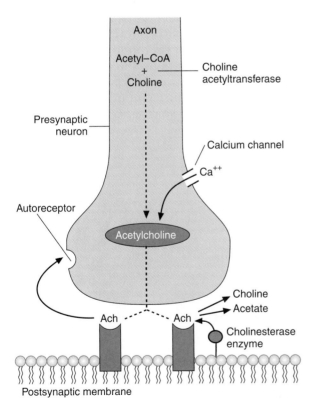

Figure 5-3   Cholinergic nerve transmission mediated by the neurotransmitter acetylcholine *(Ach).* The action of the neurotransmitter is terminated by cholinesterase enzymes; attachment of acetylcholine to presynaptic autoreceptors inhibits further neurotransmitter release.

the transmission of such impulses (parasympatholytics). Both categories of drugs affecting the parasympathetic branch are commonly seen clinically. The effects of the parasympathetic system on the heart, bronchial smooth muscle, and exocrine glands should be mentally reviewed before considering parasympathetic agonists or antagonists (blockers).

Heart: Slows rate (vagus)
Bronchial smooth muscle: Constriction
Exocrine glands: Increased secretion

MUSCARINIC AND NICOTINIC RECEPTORS AND EFFECTS

Two additional terms are used to refer to stimulation of receptor sites for acetylcholine; they are derived from the action in the body of two substances, the alkaloids *muscarine* and *nicotine*. Receptor sites that are stimulated by these two chemicals are illustrated in Figure 5-4.

MUSCARINIC EFFECTS

Muscarine, from the mushroom plant *Amanita muscaria*, stimulates acetylcholine (cholinergic) receptors at the parasympathetic terminal sites: exocrine glands (lacrimal, salivary, bronchial mucous glands), cardiac muscle, smooth muscle (gastrointestinal tract). Acetylcholine receptors at these sites, and the effects of parasympathetic stimulation at these sites, are therefore termed *muscarinic*. A muscarinic effect well known to respiratory care clinicians is the increase in airway

secretions after administration of acetylcholine-like drugs such as neostigmine. There is also a fall in blood pressure caused by slowing of the heart and vasodilation. *In general, a parasympathomimetic effect is the same as a muscarinic effect, and a parasympatholytic effect is referred to as an* antimuscarinic *effect.*

NICOTINIC EFFECTS

Nicotine, a substance in tobacco products, stimulates acetylcholine (cholinergic) receptors at autonomic ganglia (both parasympathetic and sympathetic) and at skeletal muscle sites. Acetylcholine receptors at autonomic ganglia and at the skeletal muscle are termed *nicotinic*, as are the effects on these sites of stimulation. Practical effects of stimulating these nicotinic receptors include a rise in blood pressure resulting from stimulation of sympathetic ganglia, causing vasoconstriction when the postganglionic fibers discharge, and muscle tremor caused by skeletal tissue stimulation.

SUBTYPES OF MUSCARINIC RECEPTORS

Parasympathetic receptors, and cholinergic receptors in general with or without corresponding nerve fibers, are further classified into subtypes. These differences among cholinergic or *muscarinic* (M) receptors are based on different responses to different drugs, or recognition through use of DNA probes. There are five subtypes of muscarinic receptor identified: M_1, M_2, M_3, M_4, and M_5, all of which are G protein linked (see

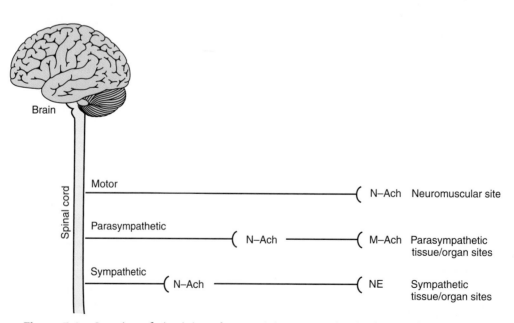

Figure 5-4   Location of nicotinic and muscarinic receptor sites in the peripheral nervous system. *M–Ach,* Muscarinic site; *N–Ach,* nicotinic site; *NE,* norepinephrine.

Chapter 2). As G protein–linked receptors, these five subtypes of muscarinic receptors share a structural feature common to such receptors—a long, "serpentine" polypeptide chain that crosses the cell membrane seven times, as previously illustrated for G protein receptors in Chapter 2. Table 5-2 summarizes muscarinic receptor subtypes, with their predominant location and the type of G protein with which they are coupled. Additional detail on muscarinic receptor location and function in the pulmonary system is presented in the final section of this chapter, which summarizes nervous control and receptors in the lung.

CHOLINERGIC AGENTS

Cholinergic drugs mimic the action caused by acetylcholine at receptor sites in the parasympathetic or neuromuscular system. Such agents can cause stimulation at the terminal nerve site (neuroeffector junction) by two distinct mechanisms, leading to their classification as direct or indirect acting. Table 5-3 lists cholinergic agents, categorized as direct or indirect acting, and their clinical uses. The terms *cholinergic, cholinoceptor stimulant,* and *cholinomimetic* are broader than *parasympathomimetic* and denote agents stimulating acetylcholine receptors located in the parasympathetic system (muscarinic) or other sites, such as the neuromuscular junction (nicotinic). A cholinergic drug can activate muscarinic or nicotinic receptors.

Table 5-2

Muscarinic receptor subtypes, location, and G-protein linkage

RECEPTOR TYPE	LOCATION	G-PROTEIN SUBTYPE
M_1	Parasympathetic ganglia, nasal submucosal glands	G_q
M_2	Heart, postganglionic parasympathetic nerves	G_i
M_3	Airway smooth muscle, submucosal glands	G_q
M_4	Postganglionic cholinergic nerves, possible CNS	G_i
M_5	Possible CNS	G_q

CNS, Central nervous system.

Table 5-3

Examples of direct- and indirect-acting cholinergic agents, with their generic names, brand names, and clinical uses

CATEGORY	GENERIC NAME	BRAND NAME	USES
DIRECT ACTING			
	Acetylcholine Cl	Miochol	Ophthalmic miotic, glaucoma
	Carbachol	Carboptic	Ophthalmic miotic, glaucoma
	Pilocarpine HCl	Pilocar, various	Ophthalmic miotic, glaucoma
	Methacholine	Provocholine	Diagnostic, asthma
	Bethanechol	Urecholine	Treat urinary retention
INDIRECT ACTING			
	Physostigmine	Eserine Sulfate	Ophthalmic miotic, glaucoma
	Echothiophate	Phospholine	Ophthalmic miotic, glaucoma
	Demecarium	Humorsol	Ophthalmic miotic, glaucoma
	Pyridostigmine	Mestinon	Improve muscle function
	Ambenonium	Mytelase	Improve muscle function
	Neostigmine	Prostigmin	Improve muscle function
	Edrophonium	Tensilon	Diagnostic, myasthenia gravis

DIRECT ACTING

Direct-acting drugs in this group are structurally similar to acetylcholine. As shown in Figure 5-3, direct-acting cholinergic agents mimic acetylcholine and bind and activate muscarinic or nicotinic receptors directly. Examples of this group include methacholine, carbachol, bethanechol, and pilocarpine. Methacholine has been used in bronchial challenge tests by inhalation to assess the degree of airway reactivity in asthmatics and others. The parasympathetic effect is bronchoconstriction. Methacholine is a useful diagnostic agent to detect differences in degree of airway reactivity between asthmatics with hyperreactive airways and nonasthmatic individuals.

INDIRECT ACTING

Indirect-acting cholinergic agonists inhibit the cholinesterase enzyme, as seen in Figure 5-3. Because cholinesterase usually inactivates the acetylcholine neurotransmitter, inhibiting this enzyme results in accumulation of endogenous acetylcholine at the neuroeffector junction of parasympathetic nerve endings or the neuromuscular junction. This makes more acetylcholine available to attach to receptor sites and stimulate cholinergic responses. If acetylcholine receptors have been blocked, this increase in neurotransmitter can reverse the block by competing with the blocking drug for the receptors. Nerve transmission can then resume, either at the parasympathetic terminal site or the neuromuscular junction.

The drug physostigmine, listed in Table 5-2, stimulates autonomic muscarinic receptors in the iris sphincter and ciliary muscle of the eye, to produce pupillary constriction (miosis) and lens thickening. The increase in the neurotransmitter acetylcholine at the neuromuscular junction makes drugs such as neostigmine useful in reversing neuromuscular blockade caused by paralyzing agents such as pancuronium or doxacurium (see Chapter 18). Neostigmine and edrophonium are also useful in increasing muscle strength in a neuromuscular disease such as myasthenia gravis, in which the cholinergic receptor is blocked by autoantibodies. The drug edrophonium (Tensilon) is used in the Tensilon test, to determine if muscle weakness is caused by overdosing with an indirect-acting cholinergic agent (causing ultimate receptor fatigue and blockade) or undertreatment with insufficient drug. Because edrophonium is short-acting (5 to 15 minutes, depending on dose), it is useful as a diagnostic agent, rather than as a maintenance treatment in neuromuscular disease.

When using indirect-acting cholinergic agents such as neostigmine to increase nerve function at the neuromuscular junction, acetylcholine activity at parasympathetic sites such as salivary and nasopharyngeal glands also increases. These undesirable muscarinic effects can be blocked by pretreating with a parasympatholytic or antimuscarinic drug such as atropine or its derivatives.

CHOLINESTERASE REACTIVATOR (PRALIDOXIME)

Organophosphates such as parathion and malathion, and the drug echothiophate (Phospholine), form an irreversible bond with acetylcholinesterase. The organophosphates are used as insecticides, and occasionally patients are seen with toxic exposure and absorption. The effects of these agents can be lethal, and because of this, they have also been used as "nerve gas." Because they affect acetylcholine, they have an effect on neuromuscular function as well as muscarinic receptors; there is initial stimulation, then blockade if a high enough dosage is absorbed. Muscle weakness and paralysis can result.

The bonding of irreversible inhibitors with the cholinesterase is slow, taking up to 24 hours. However, once formed, the duration is limited only by the body's ability to produce new cholinesterase, which takes 1 to 2 weeks. A drug such as *pralidoxime (Protopam)*, a cholinesterase reactivator, can be used in the treatment of organophosphate toxicity, in the first 24 hours. After this time, the bond of cholinesterase and cholinesterase inhibitors cannot be reversed, but atropine (a parasympatholytic) can be used to block the overly available acetylcholine neurotransmitter at the receptor sites. Support of ventilation and airway maintenance would be required for the duration of the effects.

ANTICHOLINERGIC AGENTS

Anticholinergic agents block acetylcholine receptors and act as cholinergic antagonists. Parasympatholytic (antimuscarinic) agents such as atropine, as well as drug classes such as neuromuscular blockers and ganglionic blockers, are all anticholinergic because they all block acetylcholine at their respective sites. However, a neuromuscular or ganglionic blocking agent would *not* be considered a parasympatholytic or antimuscarinic agent, because the site of action is not within the parasympathetic system. The parasympatholytic agents are antimuscarinic because of the limitation to parasympathetic terminal fiber sites.

ATROPINE AS A PROTOTYPE PARASYMPATHOLYTIC AGENT

Atropine is usually considered the prototype parasympatholytic, and there is renewed interest in use of aerosolized analogues to atropine in respiratory care. This is discussed more fully in Chapter 7. Atropine occurs naturally as the levoisomer in the plant *Atropa belladonna*, the nightshade plant, and also in *Datura stramonium*, or jimsonweed. The drug is referred to as a *belladonna alkaloid*. Atropine is a *competitive antagonist* to acetylcholine at muscarinic receptor sites (glands, gastrointestinal tract, heart, eyes), and can form a reversible bond with these cholinergic receptors. It is nonspecific for muscarinic receptor subtypes and blocks M_1, M_2, and M_3 receptors. Atropine blocks salivary secretion and causes dry mouth. In the respiratory system, atropine decreases secretion by mucous glands, and relaxes bronchial smooth muscle by blocking parasympathetically maintained basal tone. Atropine blocks vagal innervation of the heart to produce increased heart rate. There is no effect on blood vessels because these do not have parasympathetic innervation, only the acetylcholine receptors. Vascular resistance would not increase with atropine. Of course, if a parasympathomimetic *were* given, then atropine would block the dilating effect on blood vessel receptor sites. Pupillary dilation (mydriasis) occurs as a result of blockade of the circular iris muscle, and the lens is flattened (cycloplegia) by blockade of the ciliary muscle. In the gastrointestinal tract, atropine decreases acid secretion, tone, and mobility. Bladder wall smooth muscle is relaxed and voiding is slowed. Sweating is inhibited by atropine, which blocks acetylcholine receptors on sweat glands. Sweat glands are innervated by sympathetic cholinergic fibers.

In usual clinical doses, atropine has a low level of central nervous system stimulation, with a slower sedative effect in the brain. Scopolamine, another classic antimuscarinic agent, can produce drowsiness and even amnesia. In larger doses, atropine can cause toxic effects in the central nervous system, including hallucinations.

The anticholinergic (antimuscarinic) effect on the vestibular system can inhibit motion sickness. Scopolamine was used for this, and antihistamine drugs such as dimenhydrinate (Dramamine) that have anticholinergic effects are commonly used to prevent motion sickness. The dry mouth and drowsiness that also occur with a drug such as dimenhydrinate are typical antimuscarinic effects.

Box 5-1	Uses and Effects of Parasympatholytic (Antimuscarinic) Agents

- Bronchodilation
- Preoperative drying of secretions
- Antidiarrheal agent
- Prevention of bed-wetting in children (increase urinary retention)
- Treatment of peptic ulcer
- Treatment of organophosphate poisoning
- Treatment of mushroom (*Amanita muscaria*) ingestion
- Treatment of bradycardia

PARASYMPATHOLYTIC (ANTIMUSCARINIC) EFFECTS

If the basic effects of the parasympathetic system are known, the effects of an antagonist such as atropine can be deduced. For example, if the parasympathetic (vagus) slows the heart rate, a parasympatholytic should increase heart rate by blocking that innervation. Box 5-1 lists the effects and uses of parasympatholytic agents.

SYMPATHETIC BRANCH

As noted in the general description of the parasympathetic and sympathetic branches of the autonomic nervous system, sympathetic (adrenergic) effects are mediated by both by neurotransmitter release from sympathetic nerves and the release of circulating catecholamines, norepinephrine and epinephrine, from the adrenal medulla. Circulating catecholamines stimulate adrenergic receptors throughout the body, not just receptors with nerve fibers present. Sympathetic activation results in stimulation of the heart, increased cardiac output, increased blood pressure, mental stimulation, accelerated metabolism, and bronchodilation in the pulmonary system.

ADRENERGIC NEUROTRANSMITTER FUNCTION

In the sympathetic branch of the autonomic nervous system, the usual neurotransmitter at the terminal nerve sites is norepinephrine, with the exceptions described previously (sweat glands, adrenal medulla). Figure 5-5 illustrates neurotransmitter function with norepinephrine. In the presnaptic neuron, tyrosine is converted to dopa and then dopamine, which is then converted by dopamine β-hydroxylase to norepinephrine, in the storage vesicle. An action potential

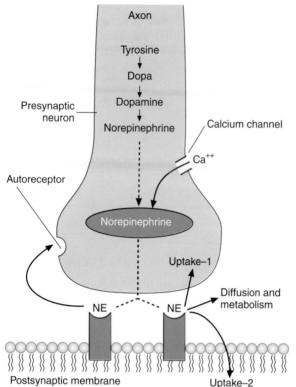

Figure 5-5 Adrenergic nerve transmission mediated by the neurotransmitter norepinephrine *(NE)*. The action of the neurotransmitter is terminated primarily by a reuptake mechanism (uptake-1), as well as by enzyme metabolism and a second uptake mechanism into tissue sites (uptake-2). Norepinephrine attaches to autoreceptors sites on the presynaptic neuron to inhibit further neurotransmitter release.

in the nerve opens calcium channels, allowing an influx of calcium. Increased intracellular calcium leads to exocytosis of the vesicles containing norepinephrine, which then attaches to receptors on the postsynaptic membrane. The exact physiological effect depends on the site of innervation and the type of sympathetic receptor, which can also vary, as described below.

The primary method of terminating the action of norepinephrine at the postsynaptic membrane is through a reuptake process, back into the presynaptic neuron. This is termed *uptake-1*. The neurotransmitter action can be ended by two other mechanisms as well: uptake into tissue sites around the nerve terminal, a process termed *uptake-2* to distinguish it from reuptake into the nerve terminal itself, and diffusion of excess norepinephrine away from the receptor site,

to be metabolized in the liver or plasma. In addition, norepinephrine can stimulate *autoreceptors* on the presynaptic neuron, which inhibits further neurotransmitter release. This receptor is identified as an α_2-receptor (discussed later in this chapter).

The distinction between two types of uptake processes is due to research published by Iversen in 1965.[1] The uptake-2 process is a mediated uptake of exogenous amines (chemicals such as norepinephrine) in *nonneuronal* tissues; for example, cardiac muscle cells. Iversen distinguished the following details of the uptake-2 process[2]:

- It is a mediated transport system
- It is a low-affinity but high-capacity system
- It is not as stereochemically specific as uptake-1
- It is specific to catecholamines
- The order of affinity for uptake of specific agents, in *decreasing* order, is: isoproterenol > epinephrine > norepinephrine
- Certain corticosteroids can inhibit the uptake-2 process, thereby potentiating catecholamines

The last effect of uptake-2 inhibition by corticosteroids is discussed more fully in Chapter 11. The physiological effects of sympathetic activation are listed in Table 5-4. The effects in the table are given for the same organs as those listed in Table 5-1 for the parasympathetic system, for comparison.

ENZYME INACTIVATION

The enzymes that metabolize norepinephrine, epinephrine, and chemicals similar to these neurotransmitters are important for understanding differences in the action of the adrenergic bronchodilator group. Chemicals structurally related to epinephrine are termed *catecholamines,* and their general structure will be outlined in Chapter 6 in the discussion of sympathomimetic (adrenergic) bronchodilators. Two enzymes are available that can inactivate catecholamines such as epinephrine. These are catechol O-methyltransferase (COMT) and monoamine oxidase (MAO). The action of both enzymes on epinephrine (Figure 5-6) is of importance because COMT is responsible for ending the action of catecholamine bronchodilators.

CATECHOL O-METHYLTRANSFERASE

The name of the catechol O-methyltransferase (COMT) enzyme describes its action: a methyl group is transferred to the oxygen at the carbon-3 site of the catechol nucleus. To avoid being vulnerable to COMT, catecholamine bronchodilators would have to be modified. This is of clinical interest because COMT is very rapid in inactivating drugs such as epinephrine or isoproterenol. For example, it is estimated that isoproterenol by aerosol using 1:200 strength solution in therapeutic dosages, peaks in 20 minutes, and total duration is on the average of 1.5 hours. These kinetics are not useful for long-term maintenance therapy.

MONOAMINE OXIDASE

A second enzyme monoamine oxidase (MAO) is also capable of degrading catecholamines, as seen in Figure 5-6. When there is a single amine group (NH) on a terminal carbon atom in the side chain, MAO can deaminate, or remove, the amine group, leaving an acid. MAO is found in the gastrointestinal tract, together with additional sulfatase enzymes, which makes oral use of catecholamines such as epinephrine or isoproterenol very ineffective. Catecholamines are primarily metabolized by COMT, but also by MAO, and these enzymes ultimately convert the catecholamines to a product, 3-methoxy-4-hydroxymandelic acid, which is excreted in urine.

SYMPATHETIC (ADRENERGIC) RECEPTOR TYPES

The effects of adrenergic receptors are mediated by coupling with G proteins, and they are identified as G protein–linked receptors. A summary of adrenergic receptor subtypes, with examples of their location and the type of G protein with which they are coupled, is given in Table 5-5.

α AND β RECEPTORS

In 1948, Ahlquist distinguished *alpha* (α) and *beta* (β) sympathetic receptors on the basis of differing responses to a variety of adrenergic drugs, all of which were similar to norepinephrine, with minor structural differences.[3] These drugs included phenylephrine, norepinephrine, epinephrine, and isoproterenol. The two types of sympathetic receptors were distinguished as follows:

α Receptors: Generally *excite*, with the exception of the intestine and central nervous system receptors where inhibition or relaxation occurs

β Receptors: Generally inhibit or *relax*, with the exception of the heart where stimulation occurs

Table 5-4

Effects of sympathetic (adrenergic) stimulation on selected organs or sites in the body*

ORGAN/SITE	SYMPATHETIC (ADRENERGIC) RESPONSE
Heart	
SA node	Increase in rate
Contractility	Increase in force
Conduction velocity	Increased
Bronchi	
Smooth muscle	Relaxation and dilation of airway diameter
Mucous glands	Increased secretion
Vascular smooth muscle	
Skin and mucosa	Vasoconstriction
Pulmonary	Dilation/constriction (two types of sympathetic receptors)
Skeletal muscle	Dilation predominates
Coronary	Dilation/constriction (two types of sympathetic receptors)
Salivary glands	Decreased
Skeletal muscle	Increased contractility
Eye	
Iris radial muscle	Contracts (mydriasis)
Iris circular muscle	None
Ciliary muscle	Relaxes for far vision†
Gastrointestinal tract	Decreased motility
Gastrointestinal sphincters	Contraction
Urinary bladder	
Detrusor	Relaxation
Trigone sphincter	Contraction
Sweat glands	Increased secretion‡
Glycogenolysis	
Skeletal muscle	Increased
Lipolysis	Increased
Renin secretion	Increased
Insulin secretion	Decreased

*Effects of sympathetic activation are mediated by direct innervation of nerve fibers, as well as by released circulating epinephrine from the adrenal medulla.

†Relaxes as a result of circulating epinephrine, with sympathetic activation.

‡Innervated by sympathetic nerves with *acetylcholine* neurotransmitter (cholinergic receptors); response to exogenous cholinergic agent is increased sweating.

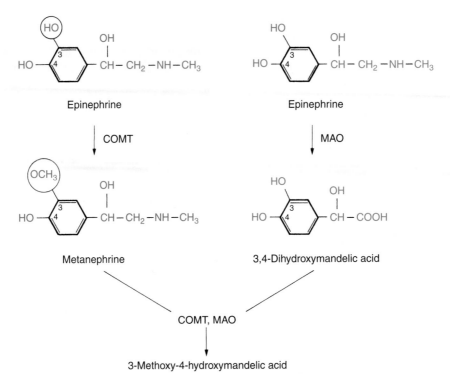

Figure 5-6   Metabolic pathways for the transformation of epinephrine by the enzymes catechol *O*-methyl-transferase (COMT) and monoamine oxidase (MAO) to an inactive form.

Table 5-5

Adrenergic receptor subtypes: location and G-protein linkage

RECEPTOR TYPE	LOCATION	G-PROTEIN SUBTYPE
Alpha-1 (α_1)	Peripheral blood vessels	G_q
Alpha-2 (α_2)	Presynaptic sympathetic neurons (autoreceptor), CNS	G_i
Beta-1 (β_1)	Heart	G_s
Beta-2 (β_2)	Smooth muscle (including bronchial), cardiac muscle	G_s
Beta-3 (β_3)	Lipocytes	G_s

CNS, Central nervous system.

α-Sympathetic receptors are found on peripheral blood vessels, and stimulation results in vasoconstriction. α-Adrenergic agonists are frequently used for topical vasoconstriction of the nasal mucosa, to treat symptoms of nasal congestion caused by the common cold. β-Adrenergic receptors are found on airway smooth muscle and in the heart. Drug activity of adrenergic stimulants (sympathomimetics) ranges along the spectrum seen in Figure 5-7.

As illustrated in Figure 5-7, phenylephrine is one of the purest α stimulants, and isoproterenol is an almost pure β stimulant. It is stressed that "pure" reactions do not occur with any drug; that is, even phenylephrine may affect other sites. Epinephrine

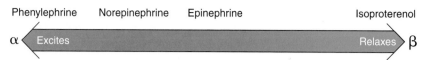

Figure 5-7 The spectrum of activity of adrenergic agonists, ranging from excitatory effects to inhibitory effects, by which α and β receptors are distinguished.

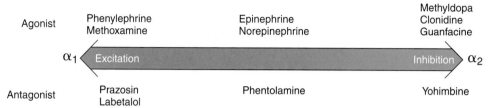

Figure 5-8 The spectrum of activity of α-receptor agonists and antagonists, from excitatory to inhibitory. Epinephrine and norepinephrine can stimulate both α_1 and α_2 receptor sites. A drug such as phenylephrine stimulates α_1 receptors and causes vasoconstriction, whereas methyldopa stimulates α_2 receptors and can lower blood pressure, although both are α-receptor agonists. Prazosin is a selective α_1-blocking agent, and yohimbine a selective α_2-blocking agent.

stimulates both α and β sites equally, but norepinephrine has more of an α than β effect.

β_1 AND β_2 RECEPTORS

In 1967, Lands further differentiated β receptors into β_1 and β_2.[4] The β_1 receptors are found in cardiac muscle, and β_2 are all other β receptors, including those of bronchial, vascular, and skeletal muscle. The distinction among types of β receptors is as follows:

β_1: Increases the rate and force of cardiac contraction

β_2: Relaxes bronchial smooth muscle and vascular beds of skeletal muscle

The β_1 receptors constitute the exception to the general rule that β receptors cause relaxation. The β_2 receptors form the basis for the class of adrenergic bronchodilators, which act to relax bronchial smooth muscle by stimulation of these receptors. The β receptor, briefly characterized as an example of a G protein–linked receptor in Chapter 2 in the introduction of *pharmacodynamics* (drug-receptor interaction), will be discussed in more detail in Chapter 6, which discusses β-adrenergic bronchodilators. A third type of β receptor, the β_3 receptor, has also been distinguished as a β receptor type found on lipocytes (fat cells) and whose stimulation results in lipolysis.

α_1 AND α_2 RECEPTORS

The α receptors have also been differentiated into α_1 and α_2 receptor types. This classification has been on a *morphological* basis (location of the receptors) and a *pharmacological* basis (response differences to various drugs). The pharmacological differentiation of α_1 and α_2 receptors is similar to the distinction of α and β receptors (Figure 5-8). This differentiation is based on a response continuum ranging from excitation (α_1) to inhibition (α_2) as different drugs are administered. For example, phenylephrine causes vasoconstriction, as previously mentioned, whereas clonidine (Catapres) causes a lowering of blood pressure and sympathetic activity. *Both* agents are considered α-receptor agonists. Other agents such as prazosin (Minipress) or labetalol (Normodyne) cause a lowering of blood pressure, but yohimbine causes a rise in blood pressure. Yet these agents are *all* considered α-receptor antagonists. However, blockade of α_1 excitatory receptors by prazosin would prevent vasoconstriction and lower blood pressure, whereas blockade of α_2 inhibitory receptors by yohimbine would prevent vasodilation and increase blood pressure. Because different α agonists can cause opposite effects, and different α blockers do the same, α receptors were subdivided into the two types given. The location, or morphologic differentiation, of α_1 and α_2 receptors is

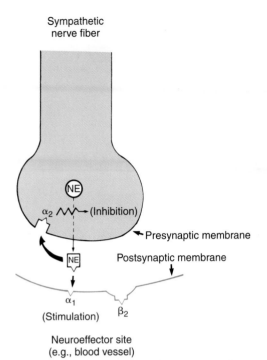

Sympathetic
nerve fiber

α_2 (Inhibition)

NE

Presynaptic membrane

NE

Postsynaptic membrane

α_1
(Stimulation) β_2

Neuroeffector site
(e.g., blood vessel)

Figure 5-9   Location and effect of α_2 receptors, designated
autoreceptors. Stimulation of α_2 receptors by norepinephrine
on the presynaptic neuron inhibits further neurotransmitter
release and nerve action.

more complex. In *peripheral* nerves, α_1 receptors are
located on postsynaptic sites such as vascular smooth
muscle and α_2 receptors are presynaptic (Figure 5-9).
Stimulation of these peripheral α_1 receptors causes excitation and vasoconstriction; activation of peripheral
(presynaptic) α_2 receptors causes inhibition of further
neurotransmitter release. Peripheral α_2 receptors
thereby perform a negative feedback control mechanism, referred to as *autoregulation,* which has been
demonstrated with sympathetic (adrenergic) neurons;
they are referred to as *autoreceptors* (see Figure 5-5).[5]
Norepinephrine released from the nerve ending can
activate both α_1 (postsynaptic) and α_2 (presynaptic)
receptors. The postsynaptic stimulation causes the cell
response such as vasoconstriction, but the presynaptic
stimulation leads to inhibition of further neurotransmitter release. In the central nervous system, α_2 receptors are generally considered to be on postsynaptic
sites; this is the reverse of their location peripherally,
where they are presynaptic. These central postsynaptic
α_2 receptors are the site of action for antihypertensive
agents such as clonidine (Catapres) or methyldopa
(Aldomet). These are further discussed and illustrated
in Chapter 20.

To summarize, α_1 and β_1 receptors *excite,* and α_2
and β_2 receptors *inhibit.* This consistency of subscripts
for excitation (1) versus inhibition (2) aids in re-
membering their effects.

DOPAMINERGIC RECEPTORS

There are other receptors in the central nervous system (brain) that respond to dopamine, a chemical
precursor of norepinephrine, and are therefore termed
dopaminergic. Because dopamine is chemically similar
to epinephrine and stimulates α and β receptors,
dopaminergic receptors are classified as a type of
adrenergic receptor.

SYMPATHOMIMETIC (ADRENERGIC) AND SYMPATHOLYTIC (ANTIADRENERGIC) AGENTS

Drugs that stimulate the sympathetic system and produce adrenergic effects (sympathomimetics) and
drugs that block adrenergic effects (sympatholytics)
will be discussed in greater detail in separate chapters.
In this text, emphasis is placed on β-adrenergic agonists used for bronchodilating effect (see Chapter 6)
and for adrenergic agonists used for cardiovascular effects such as cardiac stimulation (see Chapter 19) or
vasoconstriction (Chapter 20). Adrenergic blocking
agents will be considered for their antihypertensive
and antianginal effect (see Chapter 20). To exemplify
both sympathomimetic and sympatholytic agents,
Table 5-6 provides selected examples of drugs categorized as agonists or antagonists of the sympathetic system, with generic names, brand names, and common
clinical uses.

NEURAL CONTROL OF LUNG FUNCTION

Both branches of the autonomic nervous system, sympathetic and parasympathetic, exert control of lung
function. Currently, the two branches form the basis
for two classes of respiratory care drugs that modify
airway smooth muscle tone: the adrenergic bronchodilator group and the anticholinergic bronchodilator group.

Lung function includes more than just airway
smooth muscle tone. Multiple sites and tissues are involved in lung function, as follows:

Airway smooth muscle
Submucosal and surface secretory cells
Bronchial epithelium
Pulmonary and bronchial blood vessels

Table 5-6

Examples of adrenergic agonists and antagonists, with their generic names, brand names, and common clinical uses

CATEGORY	GENERIC NAME	BRAND NAME	USES
SYMPATHOMIMETIC			
	Epinephrine	Adrenalin Cl	Bronchodilator, cardiac stimulant, vasoconstrictor
	Ephedrine	Sudafed, various	Nasal decongestant
	Amphetamine	Dexedrine	CNS stimulant (obesity)
	Methoxamine	Vasoxyl	Vasopressor
	Dopamine	Intropin	Shock syndrome
	Albuterol	Proventil, Ventolin	Bronchodilator
	Salmeterol	Serevent	Bronchodilator
	Ritodrine	Ritodrine, Yutopar	Uterine relaxation in preterm labor
SYMPATHOLYTIC			
	Phentolamine	Regitine	Pheochromocytoma
	Prazosin	Minipress	Antihypertensive
	Labetalol	Normodyne, Trandate	Antihypertensive
	Metoprolol	Lopressor	Antihypertensive, antianginal
	Propranolol	Inderal	Antiarrhythmic (PAT)
	Timolol	Blocadren	Treat glaucoma
	Esmolol	Brevibloc	Antiarrhythmic

CNS, Central nervous system; *PAT,* paroxysmal atrial tachycardia.

In addition to autonomic nerve fibers and the receptors associated with them, sites in the lung (smooth muscle, glands, vascular beds) may be affected by release of mediators from inflammatory cells, such as mast cells and platelets, or by release of epithelial factors, such as a relaxant factor, which can reduce airway contractility to spasmogens such as histamine, serotonin, or even acetylcholine.[6] Receptors in the lung and airways for mediators released by inflammatory cells include the following:

Histamine receptors: Especially the H_1 type
Prostaglandin receptors: Such as prostacyclin, prostaglandin D_2 (PGD_2), prostaglandin $F_{2\alpha}$ ($PGF_{2\alpha}$), and thromboxane A_2
Leukotriene receptors: Such as B_4 and the C_4-D_4-E_4 series that comprise what was formerly termed *slow-reacting substance of anaphylaxis* (SRS-A)
Platelet-activating factor (PAF) receptors
Adenosine receptors: Such as A_1 and A_2
Bradykinin receptors

The mediators of inflammation and their receptors (e.g., histamine, prostaglandins) will be discussed in the review of corticosteroids and other antiasthmatic drugs intended to inhibit or prevent an inflammatory response in the lung.

SYMPATHETIC INNERVATION AND EFFECTS

The sympathetic nervous system exerts its effects by both direct and indirect means, as outlined in previous sections. *Direct effects* refer to direct innervation of tissue sites by nerve fibers. *Indirect effects* are mediated by the release of circulating catecholamines epinephrine and norepinephrine.

Sympathetic nerve fibers form ganglionic synapses outside the lung. Postganglionic sympathetic nerve fibers from the cervical and upper thoracic ganglia form plexuses at the hilar region of the lung and enter the lung mingled with parasympathetic nerves. Histochemical and ultrastructural studies show a relatively high density of sympathetic nerve fibers to submucosal glands and bronchial arteries, but little or no nerve fibers to airway smooth muscle in human lung.[7] Figure 5-10 illustrates sympathetic innervation and effects mediated by direct nerve action and indirectly by circulating epinephrine, in the human lung.

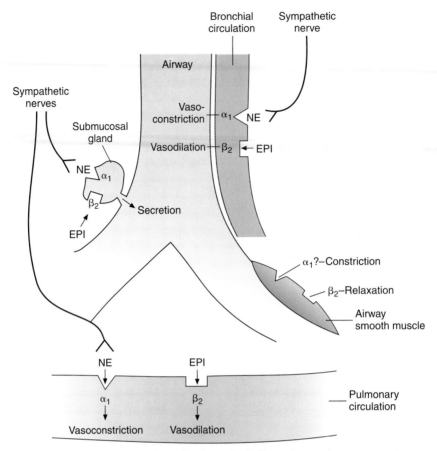

Figure 5-10 Adrenergic control mechanisms, including adrenergic receptor subtypes and effects in the pulmonary system. Sites of direct sympathetic nerve innervation, such as the pulmonary vasculature, are indicated. Other sites such as airway smooth muscle lack nerve innervation but respond to circulating epinephrine released by the adrenal medulla with sympathetic activation and can also respond to exogenous catecholamines. *EPI,* Epinephrine; *NE,* norepinephrine.

AIRWAY SMOOTH MUSCLE

There is little or no direct sympathetic innervation of airway smooth muscle in human lung.[8] The sympathetic nervous system controls bronchial smooth muscle tone by circulating epinephrine and norepinephrine, which act on α and β receptors on airway smooth muscle. Recall that epinephrine stimulates both α and β receptors, whereas norepinephrine acts primarily on α receptors.

β Receptors. The β receptors mediate relaxation of airway smooth muscle. This action is mimicked by the class of β-adrenergic bronchodilators, introduced in Chapter 6. The β receptors are distributed from the trachea to the terminal bronchioles, and the density

of these receptors increases as airway diameter becomes smaller. The β agonists can therefore cause relaxation of small airways.

The β_2 receptors traditionally have been identified as the β-receptor subtype on the airway smooth muscle. This has been further verified for human lung by autoradiographic studies and molecular gene studies.[9] There is species variation for the presence of β-receptor subtypes, however, with β_1 and β_2 receptors present in guinea pig and dog airways.

The β_1 and β_2 receptors in the lung have also been distinguished as *neuronal* and *hormonal* receptors, respectively. This is based on the concept that β_1 receptors are β receptors for sites where norepinephrine is released from sympathetic nerve terminal fibers (neuronal); β_2 receptors are β receptors responsive to circulating epinephrine (hormonal). Both cause airway smooth muscle relaxation when stimulated, either by sympathetic nerve release of norepinephrine or by circulating epinephrine, in species such as the dog or guinea pig, which have β_1 receptors on airway smooth muscle.[10] In the human lung, which has no sympathetic innervation of the airway smooth muscle, adrenergic receptors are all of the β_2 type; β_1 receptors have been identified by radioligand binding and autoradiographic studies in alveolar walls in the lung periphery.[9] Using this terminology, relaxation of human airway smooth muscle would be accomplished by stimulation of hormonal β receptors, by circulating or exogenous catecholamines. The β_3 receptors, which have also been identified on lipocytes, have no known function in the human airway.[11]

α Receptors. The α receptors exist in human lung in less quantity than β receptors and with no difference in distribution between large and small airways. Norepinephrine stimulates α receptors, but their effect in the airway appears to be minor. Evidence for α-sympathetic induced bronchoconstriction has been provided by studies in which lung tissue was treated with a β-blocker, or antagonist, such as propranolol, and then exposed to epinephrine, which stimulates both α and β receptors.[12] Because β receptors were blocked, the epinephrine attached to the free α receptors, and the result was contraction of the smooth muscle, thus providing evidence for the existence of α receptors and showing a contractile effect. The clinical use of α-receptor blocking agents such as dibenamine, thymoxamine, and phentolamine in cases of status asthmaticus has been reported for over 40 years, lending support to the role of α receptors in bronchial contraction.[13] The role of α receptors in controlling airway smooth muscle remains the subject of investigation.

Lung Blood Vessels

Blood flow in the lung is made up of two different systems: the *pulmonary* and the *bronchial* circulations. The pulmonary circulation receives the body's venous return from the right heart and is critical for gas exchange. The bronchial circulation is an arterial supply and perfuses lung tissue, to supply nutrients and remove metabolic by-products.

The pulmonary circulation is innervated by both parasympathetic and sympathetic nerves. Sympathetic nerves release norepinephrine to stimulate α recep-

tors and cause vascular contraction. The β receptors on pulmonary blood vessels cause relaxation and are stimulated by circulating epinephrine. An exogenous catecholamine can cause vasoconstriction, dilation, or no effect, depending on the relative stimulation of receptor types.

The bronchial circulation is innervated predominantly by sympathetic nerves. Activation of sympathetic nerves causes vasoconstriction, mediated by α receptors. Stimulation of β receptors by circulating epinephrine causes relaxation and vasodilation in bronchial blood vessels.

Mucous Glands

Human bronchial submucosal glands are innervated by both sympathetic and parasympathetic nerves. There are α and β receptors on tracheal submucosal glands. Stimulation of these receptors causes an increase in secretion of fluid and mucus. Epithelial cells on the airway lining do not have direct sympathetic innervation, but do possess β_2 receptors whose stimulation can also increase secretion of fluid. Mucociliary clearance is enhanced, removing trapped particulate matter.[14]

Parasympathetic Innervation and Effects

The lung is supplied by vagus nerves, with the recurrent laryngeal nerve (part of the thoracic vagus) innervating the trachea; other branches of the vagus enter the lung at the hilum and innervate the intrapulmonary airways. In the trachea and remaining airways, parasympathetic nerves supply airway smooth muscle and glands. The vagus nerves in the lung release acetylcholine and are therefore termed cholinergic. Acetylcholine couples with muscarinic acetylcholine receptors on airway smooth muscle to cause bronchoconstriction and on submucosal glands to stimulate secretion. The action of acetylcholine is limited by the enzyme acetylcholinesterase, or cholinesterase, which breaks down acetylcholine.

Cholinergic nerve fibers in the lung are densest in the hilar region and decrease toward the airway periphery. Cholinergic muscarinic receptors also decrease in density in distal airways. Electrical stimulation of vagus nerves in dog studies causes more contraction in the intermediate bronchi than in the main bronchi or trachea.[15]

Muscarinic Receptors in the Airway

The genes for five subtypes of acetylcholine, or muscarinic, receptors have been identified, designated

M_1 through M_5. Only four of these subtypes, M_1 to M_4, have been identified by chemical (ligand) binding studies pharmacologically. Three of these muscarinic receptor subtypes have been identified in human lung: M_1, M_2, and M_3. Their location is illustrated in Figure 5-11, and the function of each will be discussed.

M_1 Receptors. M_1 receptors are present at the parasympathetic ganglion, on the postjunctional membrane. Usually, acetylcholine ganglionic receptors are nicotinic, as described previously. However, the M_1 receptor may facilitate nicotinic receptor activity and nerve transmission, with an overall excitatory effect.

M_2 Receptors. M_2 receptors are localized to the parasympathetic neuron ending site on the presynaptic membrane. These receptors are thought to be autoregulatory receptors whose stimulation by acetylcholine inhibits further acetylcholine release from the nerve ending, thereby limiting the cholinergic stimulation. This is analogous to the α_2 receptor inhibiting further release of norepinephrine from sympathetic nerve endings and was identified as an autoreceptor in the discussion of cholinergic neurotransmitter function earlier in the chapter. Stimulation of prejunctional M_2 receptors in human airways in vitro results in strong inhibition of cholinergic parasympathetic-induced bronchoconstriction. Pilo-

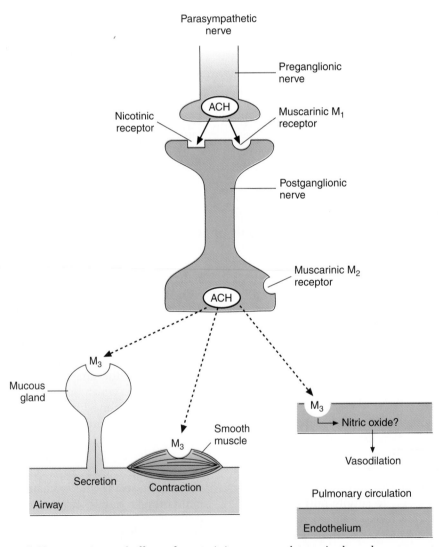

Figure 5-11   Location and effects of muscarinic receptor subtypes in the pulmonary system. *Ach,* Acetylcholine.

carpine, a direct-acting cholinergic agonist (parasympathomimetic) is a selective stimulant of M_2 receptors.[16] Inhalation of pilocarpine blocks cholinergic reflex bronchoconstriction caused by sulfur dioxide in *nonasthmatic* human subjects, verifying that M_2 receptor stimulation can block cholinergic bronchoconstriction.[17]

In *asthmatic* subjects, pilocarpine does not inhibit bronchoconstriction. This suggests the possibility of M_2 receptor dysfunction in asthma, resulting in increased cholinergic bronchoconstriction. If M_2 receptors fail to provide their normal inhibition of acetylcholine release and bronchial contraction, this may explain why blockade of β receptors can cause such severe bronchoconstriction in asthmatics. The normal balance of acetylcholine inhibition by M_2 receptors is lacking, and β blockade by drugs such as propranolol leaves acetylcholine stimulation of airway smooth muscle unchecked.

M_3 Receptors. M_3 receptors are present on submucosal glands and airway smooth muscle and possibly on surface goblet cells. Stimulation of M_3 receptors causes bronchoconstriction of smooth muscle and exocytosis and glandular secretion from submucosal mucous glands. M_3 receptors may also be present on airway epithelial cells, to increase ciliary beat. Antagonism of M_3 receptors is the basis for a class of bronchodilator agents, the anticholinergic bronchodilators (Chapter 7).

MUSCARINIC RECEPTORS ON BLOOD VESSELS

Muscarinic M_3 receptors are located on endothelial cells of both the bronchial and pulmonary vasculature. Stimulation of M_3 receptors causes release of an endothelial-derived relaxant factor.[18] This relaxant factor, which produces vasodilation and is mediated by an increase in intracellular cyclic guanosine monophosphate (cGMP), has been identified as nitric oxide (NO) or a very similar nitrosocompound.[19]

NONADRENERGIC, NONCHOLINERGIC INHIBITORY NERVES

There is evidence for a branch of nerves that are neither parasympathetic (cholinergic) nor sympathetic (adrenergic), which can cause relaxation of airway smooth muscle. These nerves have been termed *nonadrenergic, noncholinergic* (NANC) *inhibitory nerves.*[20] They are also referred to as simply *nonadrenergic inhibitory nerves* because adrenergic activity relaxes airway smooth muscle, and this is an additional but nonadrenergic neural method of relaxing such

smooth muscle. Evidence for NANC inhibitory nerves is based on the following type of experimentation. When parasympathetic (cholinergic) receptors are blocked with an antagonist, such as atropine, and sympathetic (adrenergic) receptors are also blocked with a β blocker, such as propranolol, electric field stimulation of the lung will produce relaxation of bronchial smooth muscle. A more detailed description of this methodology and evidence is given by Diamond and Altiere.[21] Figure 5-12 illustrates this inhibitory system that is neither adrenergic nor cholinergic and its possible neurotransmitter substances. A nonadrenergic inhibitory nervous system found in the gastrointestinal tract is primarily responsible for the relaxation of peristalsis and the internal anal sphincter. In the gastrointestinal tract, this system develops in conjunction with the parasympathetic branch. Embryologically, the gastrointestinal and respiratory tracts share a common origin, and the separation of the trachea and gut occurs around the fourth or fifth week of gestation. This adds plausibility to the presence of a nonadrenergic inhibitory system in the lungs similar to that in the gastrointestinal tract. The clinical relevance of such a system for pharmacology awaits development of drugs capable of modifying its usual function.

The exact neurotransmitter responsible for relaxation responses mediated by NANC inhibitory nerves is under investigation. A possible neurotransmitter that has been proposed is vasoactive intestinal peptide. Vasoactive intestinal peptide can relax mammalian airway smooth muscle. Another possible neurotransmitter causing airway smooth muscle relaxation is NO. The enzyme responsible for NO synthesis, nitric oxide synthase (NOS), has been found in nerve terminals around airway smooth muscle, and NO produces effects similar to those caused by NANC inhibitory nerve activation. Definitive identification of a NANC inhibitory neurotransmitter substance remains to be accomplished.

NONADRENERGIC, NONCHOLINERGIC (NANC) EXCITATORY NERVES

The existence of nonadrenergic, noncholinergic *excitatory* nervous control of airway smooth muscle has also been demonstrated using electrical field stimulation (EFS) techniques. This system is also referred to as simply *noncholinergic excitatory nervous control*, because cholinergic activity contracts airway smooth muscle, and this is an additional but noncholinergic neural

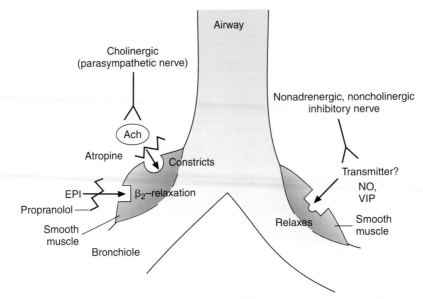

Figure 5-12 Illustration of the nonadrenergic inhibitory nervous system in the lung, which can cause relaxation of airway smooth muscle. Relaxation of smooth muscle occurs in the presence of cholinergic blockade by atropine and adrenergic blockade by propranolol. *Ach*, Acetylcholine; *EPI*, epinephrine; *NO*, nitric oxide; *VIP*, vasoactive intestinal peptide.

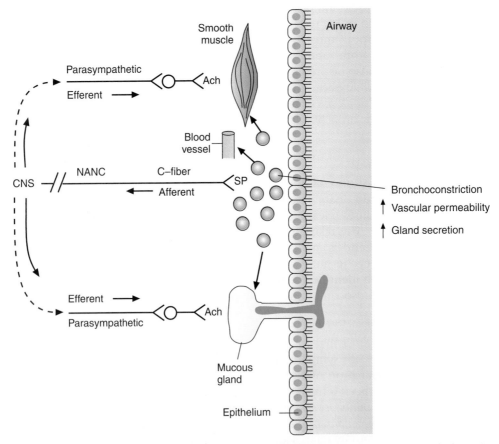

Figure 5-13 Illustration of afferent C-fibers making up the nonadrenergic, noncholinergic (NANC) excitatory nervous system in the lung. Activation of C-fibers causes both an afferent impulse with a reflex parasympathetic activity and release of substance P, causing local effects in the airway. *Ach*, Acetylcholine; *CNS*, central nervous system; *SP*, substance P.

method of exciting and constricting such smooth muscle. Stimulation of NANC excitatory nerves causes bronchial contraction. There are sensory *afferent* nerves termed *C-fibers* present in the airways, as well as around bronchial blood vessels and submucosal glands and within airway epithelium. These afferent fibers follow vagal nerve tracts into the central nervous system, as shown in Figure 5-13.

Sensory C-fiber nerves contain substance P, which is a tachykinin (a family of small peptide mediators). Substance P is also referred to as a *neuropeptide*. Sensory C-fibers can be stimulated by noxious substances such as capsaicin, found in chili peppers. When stimulated, C-fibers conduct impulses to the central nervous system that result in reflexes of cough and parasympathetic-induced bronchoconstriction. Sensory C-fibers also release their neuropeptides such as substance P at the local site of the nerve fiber. Substance P and other tachykinins cause bronchoconstriction in the airways and vasodilation, increased vascular permeability, mucous gland secretion, and enhanced mucociliary activity. The NANC excitatory C-fiber system has been considered as a possible cause of the hyperreactive airway seen in asthma. The presence of C-fibers is less marked in human airways than in rodent species.

SUMMARY KEY TERMS AND CONCEPTS

- One of the major control systems in the body is the *nervous system,* comprising *sensory* afferent nerves, *motor* efferent nerves, and the *autonomic nervous system,* which is further divided into the *sympathetic* and *parasympathetic* branches.
- Nerve impulses are conducted by both electrical and chemical means; the chemical portion of nerve transmission is referred to as a *neurotransmitter.* The neurotransmitter is *acetylcholine* at the *myoneural (neuromuscular)* junction, at *ganglia,* and at *parasympathetic end sites.* The neurotransmitter at *sympathetic end sites* is generally *norepinephrine,* except at sweat glands and the adrenal medulla, where acetylcholine is the neurotransmitter.
- *Sympathetic effects* are widespread, mediated by norepinephrine at nerve endings, as well as by circulating epinephrine released from the adrenal medulla.
- The terms *cholinergic* or *cholinoceptor* and *adrenergic* or *adrenoceptor* are used, respectively, for acetylcholine and norepinephrine/epinephrine receptors in the two autonomic branches.

- The neurotransmitter acetylcholine is terminated by the enzyme *cholinesterase,* and norepinephrine and sympathetic transmission is terminated by neurotransmitter *reuptake* into the presynaptic neuron *(uptake-1),* as well as by the enzymes *COMT* and *MAO.*
- *Parasympathetic effects on the cardiopulmonary system* are decreased heart rate, lower blood pressure, bronchoconstriction, and mucous secretion in the airways.
- *Sympathetic effects on the cardiopulmonary system* are increased heart rate and contractile force, increased blood pressure, bronchodilation, and probable increased secretion from mucous glands in the airway.
- The term *nicotinic* refers to cholinergic receptors on ganglia and at the neuromuscular junction.
- *Muscarinic* refers to cholinergic receptors at parasympathetic end sites. Muscarinic receptors are distinguished into subtypes: M_1 through M_5, with M_2 receptors in the heart, and M_3 receptors on airway smooth muscle, mediating bronchoconstriction.
- Parasympathomimetic, or cholinergic, agonists are divided into *direct-acting* agents (e.g., methacholine), which resemble acetylcholine and stimulate cholinergic receptors directly, and *indirect-acting* agents (e.g., neostigmine), which inhibit the enzyme cholinesterase, to allow increased acetylcholine transmission. A typical *parasympatholytic,* or *anticholinergic,* agent is atropine.
- Receptors at sympathetic end sites are subdivided into α and β, with α receptors mediating excitatory effects (e.g., vasoconstriction) and β receptors mediating inhibitory effects (e.g., smooth muscle relaxation).
- The α receptors are subdivided into α_1, which are excitatory, and α_2, which are inhibitory, and found on the presynaptic neuron to inhibit further neurotransmitter release.
- The β receptors are divided into β_1, which are excitatory and found in the heart, and β_2, which are found elsewhere and mediate inhibitory responses.
- In the human lung, glands and blood vessels are innervated by sympathetic nerve fibers, but airway smooth muscle has few if any such fibers, responding instead to circulating epinephrine by means of β receptors. Parasympathetic vagal nerves innervate the lung as well, supplying the airway smooth muscle and mucous glands.
- In addition to sympathetic and parasympathetic nerves in the lung, there is evidence for a *nonadrenergic, noncholinergic (NANC)* system. This system has both an inhibitory and excitatory branch.
- *Inhibitory effects* on airway smooth muscle cause bronchodilation and may be mediated by the neurotransmitter vasoactive intestinal peptide (VIP) or even nitric oxide (NO).
- *Excitatory effects* such as bronchoconstriction are produced by afferent sensory fibers that have substance P as a neurotransmitter; these effects are caused by local release of substance P, as well as by afferent-efferent reflex arcs, involving efferent cholinergic transmission.

SELF-ASSESSMENT QUESTIONS

1. Which portion of the nervous system is under voluntary control: the autonomic or the skeletal muscle motor nerve portion?
2. What is the neurotransmitter at each of the following sites: neuromuscular junction, autonomic ganglia, most sympathetic end sites?
3. Where are muscarinic receptors found?
4. What is the effect of cholinergic stimulation of airway smooth muscle?
5. What is the effect of adrenergic stimulation on the heart?
6. Classify the drugs pilocarpine, physostigmine, propranolol, and epinephrine.
7. How do indirect-acting cholinergic agonists (parasympathomimetics) produce their action?
8. What effect would the drug atropine have on the eye and on airway smooth muscle?
9. What is the general difference between α and β receptors in the sympathetic nervous system?
10. What is the primary mechanism for terminating the neurotransmitters acetylcholine and norepinephrine?
11. What is the predominant sympathetic receptor type found on airway smooth muscle?
12. Identify the adrenergic receptor preference for phenylephrine, norepinephrine, epinephrine, and isoproterenol.
13. What is the autoregulatory receptor on the sympathetic presynaptic neuron?
14. Classify the following drugs by autonomic class and receptor preference: dopamine, ephedrine, albuterol, phentolamine, propranolol, prazosin.
15. What is the autoregulatory receptor on the parasympathetic presynaptic neuron at the terminal nerve site?
16. Contrast α_1 and α_2 receptor effects, in general.
17. What substance may be the neurotransmitter in the NANC inhibitory nervous system in the lung?
18. What substance is the neurotransmitter in the NANC excitatory nervous system in the lung?

Answers to Self-Assessment Questions appear in Appendix A.

CLINICAL SCENARIO

A 42-year-old Caucasian female with a long-standing history of asthma presents to the emergency department (ED) of a local acute care hospital. She states that she has been feeling as if her "heart were racing" today. She currently uses a β-adrenergic bronchodilator (albuterol) as needed and inhales an anticholinergic bronchodilator (ipratropium bromide) before bedtime, both drugs administered by metered dose inhaler (MDI) inhalation.

On admission to the ED, she has the following vital signs: P, 155 beats/min and regular; BP, 146/90 mm Hg; and RR, 22 breaths/min, with mild distress.

Her breath sounds are clear to auscultation, and a chest radiograph (PA) shows no abnormalities. A lead II electrocardiogram (ECG) reveals supraventricular tachycardia (SVT). Pulse oximetry reveals an SpO_2 of 90%. A resident orders oxygen at 2 L/min by nasal cannula, and intravenous propranolol for her SVT, which is given. Approximately 5 minutes later, her heart rate is reduced to 110 beats/min, but she begins to wheeze audibly and complains of severe shortness of breath (SOB), and her respiratory pattern is labored at 26 breaths/min. She is anxious, and her pulse oximetry reading drops from 92% back to 72%.

What may have led to the wheezing and dyspnea of the patient? What changes in the therapeutic approach would you suggest in a case such as this?

Answers to Clinical Scenario Questions appear in Appendix A.

REFERENCES

1. Iversen LL: The uptake of catecholamines at high perfusion concentrations in the rat isolated heart: a novel catecholamine uptake process, *Br J Pharmacol* 25:18, 1965.
2. Iversen LL, Salt PJ: Inhibition of catecholamine uptake2 by steroids in the isolated rat heart, *Br J Pharmacol Chemother* 40:528, 1970.
3. Ahlquist RP: Study of adrenotropic receptors, *Am J Phsyiol* 153:586, 1948.
4. Lands AM and others: Differentiation of receptor systems activated by sympathomimetic amines, *Nature (London)* 214:597, 1967.
5. Langer SZ: Presynaptic regulation of the release of catecholamines, *Pharmacol Rev* 32:337, 1980.
6. Barnes PJ: Airway receptors, *Postgrad Med J* 65:532, 1989.
7. Partanen M and others: Catecholamine- and acetylcholinesterase-containing nerves in human lower respiratory tract, *Histochemistry* 76:175, 1982.
8. Barnes PJ: Neural control of human airways in health and disease, *Am Rev Respir Dis* 134:1289, 1986.
9. Carstairs JR, Nimmo AJ, Barnes PJ: Autoradiographic visualization of beta-adrenoceptor subtypes in human lung, *Am Rev Respir Dis* 132:541, 1985.
10. Ariens EJ, Simonis AM: Physiological and pharmacological aspects of adrenergic receptor classification, *Biochem Pharmacol* 32:1539, 1983.
11. Emorine L, Blin N, Strosberg AD: The human 3-adrenoceptor: the search for a physiological function, *Trends Pharmacol Sci* 15:3, 1994.

12. Adolphson RL, Abern SB, Townley RG: Human and guinea pig respiratory smooth muscle: demonstration of alpha adrenergic receptors, *J Allergy* 47:110, 1971 (abstract).

13. Falliers CJ, Tinkelman DG: Alternative drug therapy for asthma, *Clin Chest Med* 7:383, 1986.

14. Altiere RJ, Lindsay G: Sympathetic innervation. In Leff AR, ed: *Pulmonary and critical care pharmacology and therapeutics,* New York, 1996, McGraw-Hill.

15. Jacoby DB, Fryer AD: Parasympathetic innervation of the airways. In Leff AR, ed: *Pulmonary and critical care pharmacology and therapeutics,* New York, 1996, McGraw-Hill.

16. Barnes PJ: Muscarinic receptor subtypes in airways, *Life Sci* 52:521, 1993.

17. Minette PAH and others: A muscarinic agonist inhibits reflex bronchoconstriction in normal but not in asthmatic subjects, *J Appl Physiol* 67:2461, 1989.

18. Cuss FM, Barnes PJ: Epithelial mediators, *Am Rev Respir Dis* 136:S32-S35, 1987.

19. Wylam ME: Pulmonary vascular pharmacology. In Leff AR, ed: *Pulmonary and critical care pharmacology and therapeutics,* New York, 1996, McGraw-Hill.

20. Richardson JB, Beland J: Nonadrenergic inhibitory nervous system in human airways, *J Appl Physiol* 41:764, 1976.

21. Diamond L, Altiere RJ: The airway nonadrenergic, noncholinergic inhibitory nervous sytem. In Leff AR, ed: *Pulmonary and critical care pharmacology and therapeutics,* New York, 1996, McGraw-Hill.

DRUGS USED TO TREAT THE RESPIRATORY SYSTEM

Adrenergic (Sympathomimetic) Bronchodilators

Joseph L. Rau

Chapter 6 presents adrenergic drugs used as inhaled bronchodilators. The specific agents and the clinical indication for this class of drugs is summarized, along with their mechanism of action as mediated by β receptors. Structure-activity relations of available agents are presented as a basis for their differences in receptor selectivity and duration of action. Differences among routes of administration are discussed, and side effects are reviewed. A brief summary of the β agonist debate over possible harmful effects with these agents is given.

HISTORY AND DEVELOPMENT

The class of drugs known as *adrenergic bronchodilators* are all analogues of epinephrine, the naturally occurring neuromediator. The subcutaneous use of epinephrine was reported as early as 1903, and the use of epinephrine as an aerosol in asthma dates to at least 1910, making this one of the oldest sympa-

thomimetic agents in current use. Ephedrine, a very weak bronchodilator, was introduced into the United States in 1926 and used in asthma as early as 1927.[1] Today, ephedrine is used in cold medications based on its α-sympathetic, decongestant effect, rather than as a bronchodilator. In 1940, isoproterenol was reported as a "broncholytic" agent. Another commonly used bronchodilator, isoetharine, was synthesized in 1936, and its use in asthma was reported in 1951. The early, less specific short-acting adrenergic agents were replaced beginning in the 1970s with longer-acting β2-specific aerosol drugs. Metaproterenol, known to exist since the late 1930s, was reported for the treatment of asthma as early as 1961 and was released for general clinical use in the United States by Boehringer Ingelheim, Inc., in 1973 in a metered dose inhaler (MDI). In January, 1981, a solution for nebulization was marketed. Other β2-specific inhaled agents followed in the 1980s, including an MDI form of terbutaline, albuterol (known as salbutamol in Europe), the prodrug bitolterol, and pirbuterol. Several of these agents have been available in multiple dosage forms, including inhaled (MDI and/or nebulizer), oral, and injectable. The first long-acting bronchodilator, salmeterol, was released in the United States in 1994 in MDI form. In March, 1999, the first synthetically produced single-isomer β_2 agonist was released as levalbuterol for general clinical use.

Overall, the class of adrenergic bronchodilators has progressed from short-acting, nonspecific agents, such as epinephrine or isoproterenol; to intermediate-acting, β_2-specific drugs, such as albuterol; to long-acting drugs, such as salmeterol or formoterol; and to pure isomers in place of racemates. A good overview of the clinical pharmacology of β-adrenergic drugs can be found in recent reviews.[2,3]

CLINICAL INDICATION FOR ADRENERGIC BRONCHODILATORS

The general indication for use of an adrenergic bronchodilator is relaxation of airway smooth muscle in the presence of reversible airflow obstruction associated with acute and chronic asthma (including exercise-induced asthma), bronchitis, emphysema, bronchiectasis, and other obstructive airway diseases. Differences in the rate of onset, peak effect, and duration led to a distinction in use between short-acting and long-acting agents. Appendix D outlines recommendations and guidelines for use of β agonists in chronic obstructive pulmonary disease (COPD) and asthma.

INDICATION FOR SHORT-ACTING AGENTS

Short-acting β_2 agonists such as albuterol, levalbuterol, or pirbuterol are indicated for relief of *acute* reversible airflow obstruction in asthma or other obstructive airway diseases.

Short-acting agents are termed "rescue" agents in the 1997 National Asthma Education and Prevention Program Expert Panel II (NAEPP EPR II) guidelines.[4]

INDICATION FOR LONG-ACTING AGENTS

Long-acting agents, such as salmeterol or formoterol, are indicated for maintenance bronchodilation and control of bronchospasm and control of nocturnal symptoms in asthma or other obstructive diseases.

NAEPP EPR II guidelines consider salmeterol a "controller"; its slow time to peak effect makes it a poor rescue drug. In asthma, a long-acting bronchodilator is usually combined with antiinflammatory medication for control of airway inflammation and bronchospasm.

Even though formoterol has a rapid onset of action, similar to that of albuterol, its slower peak effect and prolonged activity make it a better maintenance drug than an acute reliever or rescue agent.

INDICATION FOR RACEMIC EPINEPHRINE

Racemic epinephrine is often used either by inhaled aerosol or direct lung instillation for its strong α-adrenergic vasoconstricting effect, to reduce airway swelling after extubation or during epiglottitis, croup, or bronchiolitis or to control airway bleeding during endoscopy.

SPECIFIC ADRENERGIC AGENTS AND FORMULATIONS

Table 6-1 lists the adrenergic bronchodilators currently approved for general clinical use in the United States at the writing of this edition. Practitioners are urged to read package inserts on a drug before administration. Such inserts give details of dosage strengths and frequencies, adverse effects, shelf life, and storage requirements, all of which are needed for safe application. Table 6-1 is not intended to replace more detailed information supplied by the manufacturer on each of the bronchodilator agents. There are three subgroups of adrenergic bronchodilators based on distinct differences in duration of action:

Ultra–short-acting (<3 hours' duration): Epinephrine, isoproterenol, isoetharine

Short-acting (4 to 6 hours' duration): Metaproterenol, terbutaline, albuterol, bitolterol, pirbuterol, levalbuterol

Long-acting (12 hours' duration): Salmeterol, formoterol

CATECHOLAMINES

The sympathomimetic bronchodilators are all either catecholamines or derivatives of catecholamines. In Figure 6-1 the basic catecholamine structure is seen to be composed of a benzene ring with hydroxyl groups at the third and fourth carbon sites and an amine side chain attached at the first carbon position.

Catecholamine: One of a group of similar compounds having a sympathomimetic action, the aromatic portion of whose molecule is a catechol and the diphatic portion an amine.

The terminal amine group (NH_2) and the benzene ring are connected by two carbon atoms, designated as

Table 6-1

Inhaled adrenergic bronchodilator agents currently available in the United States

DRUG	BRAND NAME	RECEPTOR PREFERENCE	ADULT DOSAGE	TIME COURSE (ONSET, PEAK, DURATION)
Epinephrine	Adrenalin Cl	α, β	SVN: 1% solution (1:100), 0.25-0.5 ml (2.5-5.0 mg) qid MDI: 0.2 mg/puff, puffs as ordered or needed	*Onset:* 3-5 min *Peak:* 5-20 min *Duration:* 1-3 hr
Racemic epinephrine	Micro-Nefrin, Asthma Nefrin, various	α, β	SVN: 2.25% solution, 0.25-0.5 ml (5.63-11.25 mg) qid	*Onset:* 3-5 min *Peak:* 5-20 min *Duration:* 0.5-2 hr
Isoproterenol	Isuprel, Isuprel Mistometer	β	SVN: 0.5% solution (1:200), 0.25-0.5 ml (1.25-2.5 mg) qid MDI: 103 µg/puff, 2 puffs qid	*Onset:* 2-5 min *Peak:* 5-30 min *Duration:* 0.5-2 hr
Isoetharine	Isoetharine HCl	β_2	SVN: 1% solution, 0.25-0.5 ml (2.5-5.0 mg) qid	*Onset:* 1-6 min *Peak:* 15-60 min *Duration:* 1-3 hr
Terbutaline	Brethaire	β_2	MDI: 200 µg/puff, 2 puffs q4-6h Tab: 2.5 or 5 mg, 5 mg q6h Inj: 1 mg/ml, 0.25 mg SC	*Onset:* 5-30 min *Peak:* 30-60 min *Duration:* 3-6 hr
Metaproterenol	Alupent	β_2	SVN: 5% solution, 0.3 ml (15 mg) tid, qid MDI: 650 µg/puff, 2-3 puffs tid, qid Tab: 10 or 20 mg, 20 mg tid, qid Syrup: 10 mg/5 ml, 2 tsp tid, qid	*Onset:* 1-5 min *Peak:* 60 min *Duration:* 2-6 hr
Albuterol	Proventil, Proventil HFA, Ventolin	β_2	SVN: 0.5% solution, 0.5 ml (2.5 mg) tid, qid MDI: 90 µg/puff, 2 puffs tid, qid DPI: 200 µg capsule, 1 capsule q4-6h Tab: 2 mg, 4 mg tid, qid Syrup: 2 mg/5 ml, 1-2 tsp tid, qid	*Onset:* 15 min *Peak:* 30-60 min *Duration:* 5-8 hr
Bitolterol	Tornalate	β_2	SVN: 0.2% solution, 1.25 ml (2.5 mg) bid-qid MDI: 370 µg/puff, 2 puffs q8h	*Onset:* 3-4 min *Peak:* 30-60 min *Duration:* 5-8 hr
Pirbuterol	Maxair	β_2	MDI: 200 µg/puff, 2 puffs q4-6h	*Onset:* 5 min *Peak:* 30 min *Duration:* 5 hr
Levalbuterol	Xopenex	β_2	SVN: 0.63 mg/3 ml tid; or 1.25 mg/3 ml tid	*Onset:* 15 min *Peak:* 30-60 min *Duration:* 5-8 hr
Salmeterol	Serevent	β_2	MDI: 25 µg/puff, 2 puffs bid DPI: 50 µg/blister bid	*Onset:* 20 min *Peak:* 3-5 hr *Duration:* 12 hr
Formoterol	Foradil	β_2	DPI: 12 µg/inhalation bid	*Onset:* 15 min *Peak:* 30-60 min *Duration:* 12 hr

DPI, Dry powder inhaler; *MDI,* metered dose inhaler; *SVN,* small volume nebulizer.

α and β, a notation not to be confused with α and β receptors in the sympathetic nervous system. Examples of catecholamines are dopamine, epinephrine, norepinephrine, isoproterenol, and isoetharine. The first three occur naturally in the body. Catecholamines, or sympathomimetic amines, mimic the actions of epinephrine more or less precisely, causing tachycardia, elevated blood pressure, smooth muscle relaxation of bronchioles and skeletal muscle blood vessels, glycogenolysis, skeletal muscle tremor, and central nervous system stimulation.

ADRENERGIC BRONCHODILATORS AS STEREOISOMERS

Adrenergic bronchodilators can exist in two different spatial arrangements, producing isomers. Rotation about the β carbon on the ethylamine side chain of the basic molecule structure seen in Figure 6-1 produces two non-superimposable mirror images, termed *enan-*

Catecholamines
{
Benzene ring
Two hydroxyl groups
Amine side chain
}

Structure:

Catechol nucleus | Side chain

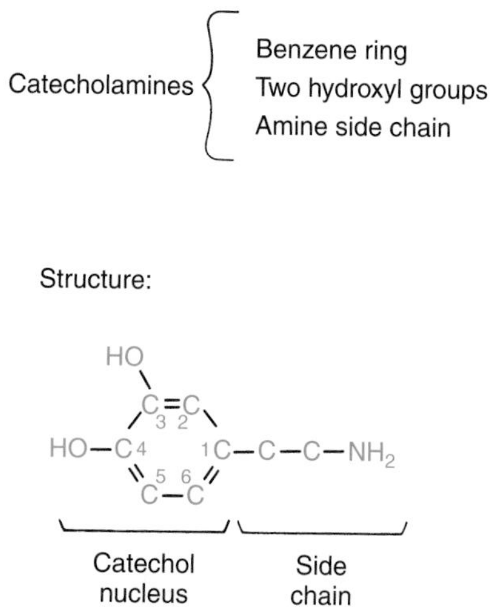

Figure 6-1   The basic catecholamine structure showing the catechol nucleus connected to an amine side chain.

tiomers or simply *isomers.* Figure 6-2 illustrates epinephrine as a stereoisomer, showing the R- and S-isomers as the mirror image of each other. Enantiomers have similar physical and chemical properties, but not the same physiological effects. The R-isomer, or levoisomer, is active on airway β receptors to produce bronchodilation and on extrapulmonary adrenergic receptors. The S-isomer, or dextroisomer, is not active on adrenergic receptors such as β receptors, and until recently the S-isomer was considered physiologically inert. The two mirror images of the isomers rotate light in opposite directions, and this is the basis for designating them as dextrorotatory (*d*, +) or levorotatory (*l*, −). Using their actual spatial configuration, the levoisomer and the dextroisomer are referred to as the *R-isomer* (for rectus, right) or *S-isomer* (for sinister, or left), respectively. Adrenergic bronchodilators such as epinephrine, albuterol, or salmeterol have been produced synthetically as racemic mixtures, or 50:50 equimolar mixes of the R-isomers and S-isomers. Natural epinephrine found in the adrenal gland occurs as the R-(levo)isomer only. Levalbuterol, released in 1999, represents the first *synthetic* inhaled solution available as the single R-isomer of racemic albuterol. The structures of the currently available inhaled β agonists to be discussed are shown in Figure 6-3. Only a single isomer form is shown, for simplification and clarity.

Epinephrine is a potent catecholamine bronchodilator that stimulates both α and β receptors. Because epinephrine lacks β_2-receptor specificity, there is a high prevalence of side effects such as tachycardia, blood pressure increase, tremor, headache, and insomnia. Epinephrine occurs naturally in the adrenal medulla and has a rapid onset but a short duration because of metabolism by COMT. It is used both by inhalation and subcutaneously to treat patients with acute asthmatic

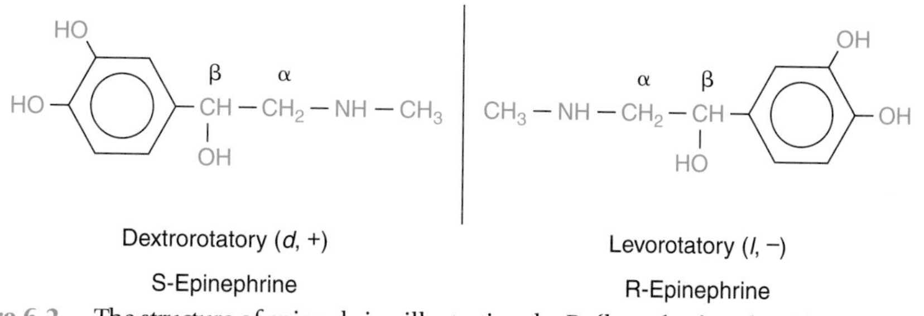

Dextrorotatory (*d*, +)

S-Epinephrine

Levorotatory (*l*, −)

R-Epinephrine

Figure 6-2   The structure of epinephrine illustrating the R- (levo, *l*, −) and S- (dextro, *d*, +) isomers as mirror images of each other, termed *enantiomers.* Natural epinephrine is R-epinephrine. Synthetic formulations for inhalation are racemic (50:50) mixtures of R- and S-isomers.

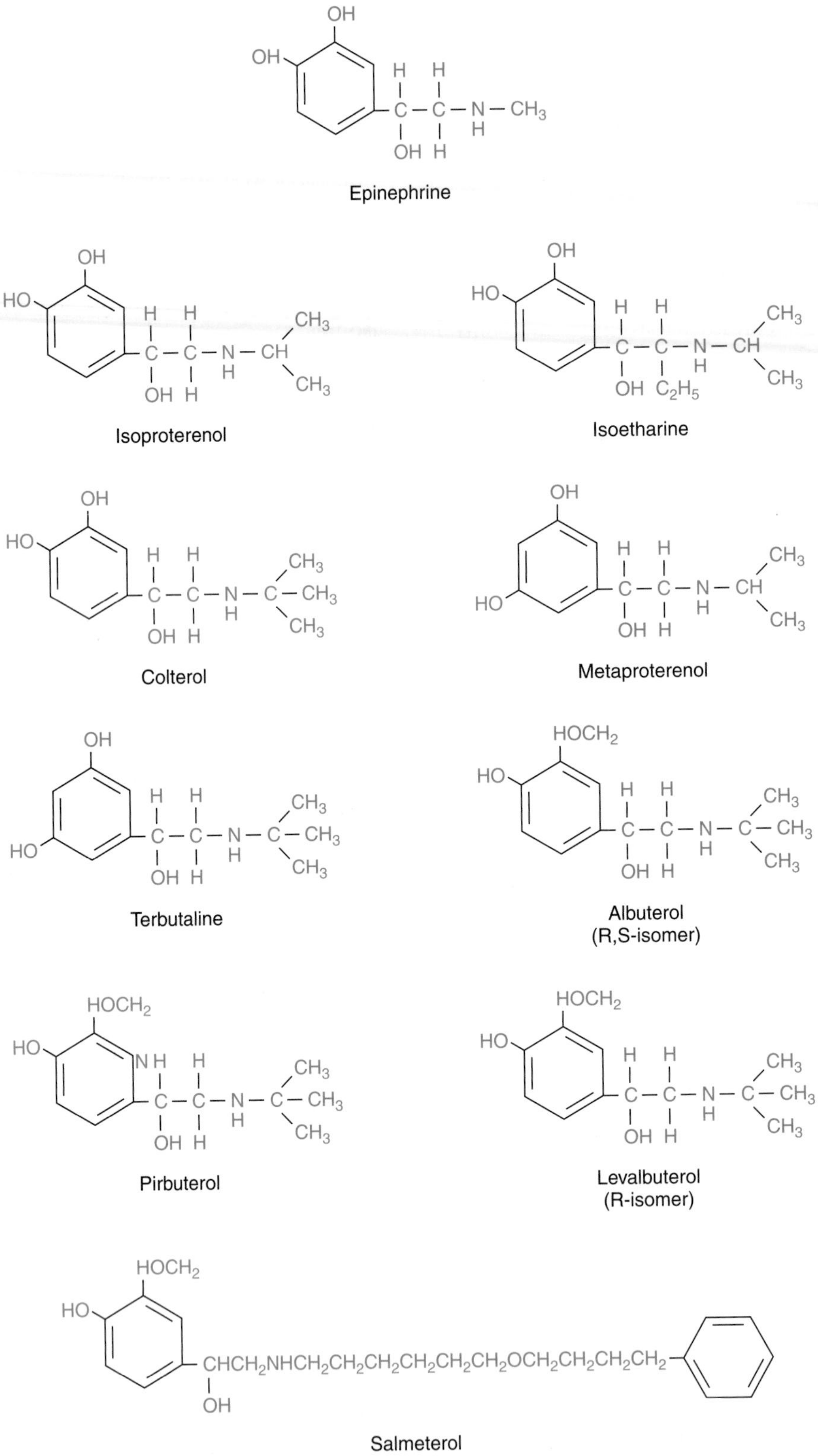

Figure 6-3 Chemical structures of currently available inhaled adrenergic bronchodilators in the United States. With the exception of natural epinephrine and levalbuterol, all formulations are racemic mixtures and are shown in the same orientation for clarity. The isomers of racemic albuterol and levalbuterol are labeled to indicate the difference in these two drugs. Formoterol, not shown, is illustrated in Figure 6-8. (From Rau JL: Inhaled adrenergic bronchodilators: historical development and clinical application, *Respir Care* 45:854, 2000.)

episodes. It is also used as a cardiac stimulant, based on its strong β_1 effects. Self-administered, intramuscular injectable doses of 0.3 and 0.15 mg are marketed to control systemic hypersensitivity (anaphylactoid) reactions. This drug is more useful for management of acute asthma rather than for daily maintenance therapy because of its pharmacokinetics and side effect profile. The parenteral form of epinephrine is a natural extract, consisting of only the R-(levo)isomer. The synthetic formulation of epinephrine for nebulization, micro-Nefrin or Asthma Nefrin, is a racemic mixture of the R-(levo) and the S-(dextro) isomers. The mode of action of racemic epinephrine is the same as with natural epinephrine, giving both α and β stimulation. Because only the R-isomer is active on adrenergic receptors, a 1:100 strength formulation of natural epinephrine (injectable formulation) is used for nebulization, whereas a 2.25% strength racemic mixture is used in nebulization.

Isoproterenol is a potent catecholamine bronchodilator that stimulates both β_1 (cardiac) and β_2 receptors. The drug was widely used for nebulization until the advent of the more β_2-specific agents such as isoetharine and later the resorcinols, saligenins, and others. The main disadvantages of isoproterenol are its short duration because of COMT breakdown and its strong cardiac (β_1) effects, causing tachycardia. Isoproterenol is metabolized to a weak β-blocker, 3-methoxyisoproterenol, which has been thought to cause resistance to its bronchodilating effects. This is probably not clinically important as a cause of reduced response to the drug.[5]

Isoetharine was one of the first β_2-specific adrenergic bronchodilators in the United States. It is considered obsolete as an inhaled bronchodilator. As a catecholamine, it has a short duration of action, but a rapid onset. Cardiac (β_1) stimulation is minimal compared with isoproterenol or epinephrine. Originally the brand of isoetharine was marketed with two other active ingredients: thenyldiamine, which is an antihistamine, and phenylephrine, a strong α stimulant for reducing mucosal swelling. Both have been deleted for lack of efficacy. Theoretically, α stimulation may antagonize the relaxing effect of β_2 stimulation if α receptors are present in human airways.

KEYHOLE THEORY OF β_2 SPECIFICITY

The three catecholamine drugs differ in their receptor preference, ranging from α *and* β (epinephrine), to β nonspecific (isoproterenol), and finally to β_2 specific (isoetharine). The theory that explains the shift from α activity to β_2 specificity has been termed the *keyhole theory* of β sympathomimetic receptors: The larger the side-chain attachment to a catechol base, the greater is the β_2 specificity. If the catecholamine structural pattern is seen as a keylike shape, the larger the "key" (side chain), the more β_2 specific is the drug. The increase in side chain substitutions can be seen in the drug structures presented in Figure 6-3, for the three catecholamines and subsequent β_2-selective agents to be discussed.

Epinephrine has a methyl group attached to the terminal amine group and equally activates α and β receptors. *Isoproterenol* adds an additional methyl group with strong β stimulation and very little α stimulation. *Isoetharine* further increases the bulk of the amine side chain and adds an ethyl group, modifying the structure of isoproterenol and producing β_2-preferential activity. Actually, bronchodilator activity is reduced by an approximate factor of 10 compared with that of isoproterenol, but cardiovascular stimulation is less by a factor of 300.

METABOLISM OF CATECHOLAMINES

Despite the increase in β_2 specificity with increased side-chain bulk, all of the previously mentioned catecholamines are rapidly inactivated by the cytoplasmic enzyme COMT. This enzyme is found in the liver and kidneys, as well as throughout the body. Figure 6-4, *A*, illustrates the action of COMT as it transfers a methyl group to the carbon-3 position on the catechol nucleus. The resulting compound, metanephrine, is inactive on adrenergic receptors. Because the action of COMT on circulating catecholamines is very efficient, the *duration* of action of these drugs is severely limited, with a range of 1.5 to at most 3 hours.

Catecholamines are also unsuitable for *oral* administration because they are inactivated in the gut and liver by conjugation with sulfate or glucuronide at the carbon-4 site. Because of this action, they have no effect taken by mouth, limiting their route of administration to inhalation or injection. Catecholamines are also readily inactivated to inert adrenochromes by heat, light, or air (Figure 6-4, *B*). For this reason, racemic epinephrine, isoetharine, and isoproterenol are stored in amber bottles. The residue from nebulizer rain-out in tubing may appear pinkish after treatment, and a patient's sputum may even appear pink-tinged after using aerosols of catecholamines.

RESORCINOL AGENTS

Because the limited duration of action with catecholamines is hardly suitable for maintenance therapy

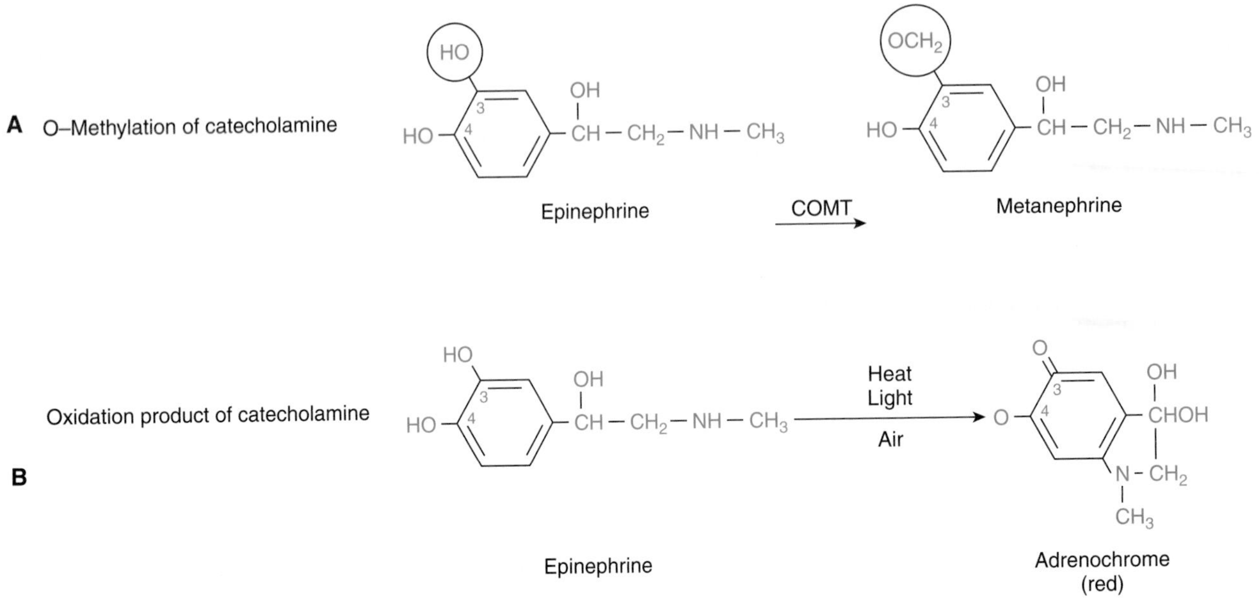

A O–Methylation of catecholamine

Epinephrine → COMT → Metanephrine

B Oxidation product of catecholamine

Epinephrine → Heat Light Air → Adrenochrome (red)

Figure 6-4   **A,** Inactivation of the catecholamine epinephrine by the enzyme COMT. **B,** Conversion of a catecholamine such as epinephrine to an adrenochrome.

of bronchospastic airways, drug researchers sought to modify the catechol nucleus, which is so vulnerable to inactivation by COMT. As a result, the hydroxyl attachment at the carbon-4 site was shifted to the carbon-5 position, producing a resorcinol nucleus (see Figure 6-3). This change resulted in *metaproterenol* (named for the 3,5-attachments in the meta position) and *terbutaline* (for the tertiary butyl group). Because neither drug is acted upon by COMT, both have a significantly longer duration of action of 4 to 6 hours compared with the short-acting catecholamine bronchodilators. Because of its bulky side chain, terbutaline is β_2-preferential, thus possessing minimal cardiac (β_1) effects. Both drugs can be taken orally because they resist inactivation by the sulfatase enzymes in the gastrointestinal tract and liver. For these reasons, the newer generation of resorcinols and other catecholamine derivatives were much better suited for maintenance therapy than the older catecholamine agents. Metaproterenol and terbutaline are slower to reach a peak effect (30 to 60 minutes) than epinephrine, isoproterenol, or isoetharine.

SALIGENIN AGENTS

A different modification of the catechol nucleus at the carbon-3 site resulted in the saligenin *albuterol*, referred to as *salbutamol* in Europe (see Figure 6-3). Albuterol is available in a variety of pharmaceutical ve-hicles in the United States. These include oral tablets, syrup, nebulizer solution, MDI, extended-release tablet, and DPI capsule. As with the resorcinol bronchodilators, this drug has a β_2-preferential effect, is effective by mouth, and has a duration of up to 6 hours, with a peak effect in 30 to 60 minutes.

PIRBUTEROL

Pirbuterol is another noncatecholamine adrenergic agent currently available as pirbuterol acetate (Maxair) in an MDI formulation with a breath-actuated inhaler delivery device (see Chapter 3). The strength is 0.2 mg per puff, and the usual dose is 2 puffs. The MDI canister contains 400 inhalations. Pirbuterol is structurally similar to albuterol except for a pyridine ring in place of the benzene ring (see Figure 6-3). The onset of activity by aerosol is 5 to 8 minutes, with a peak effect at 30 minutes and a duration of action of approximately 5 hours. When pirbuterol is given orally, the pharmacokinetics differ, with onset of action within 1 hour, time to peak activity around 2 hours, and duration of 5 to 6 hours. Aerosol inhalation results in undetectable plasma concentrations with a maximum dose of 0.8 mg. The drug has a plasma half-life of 2 to 3 hours, measured with oral doses, and is primarily metabolized by sulfate conjugation. Around 60% of an oral dose is excreted in urine. Pirbuterol is said to be less potent on a weight

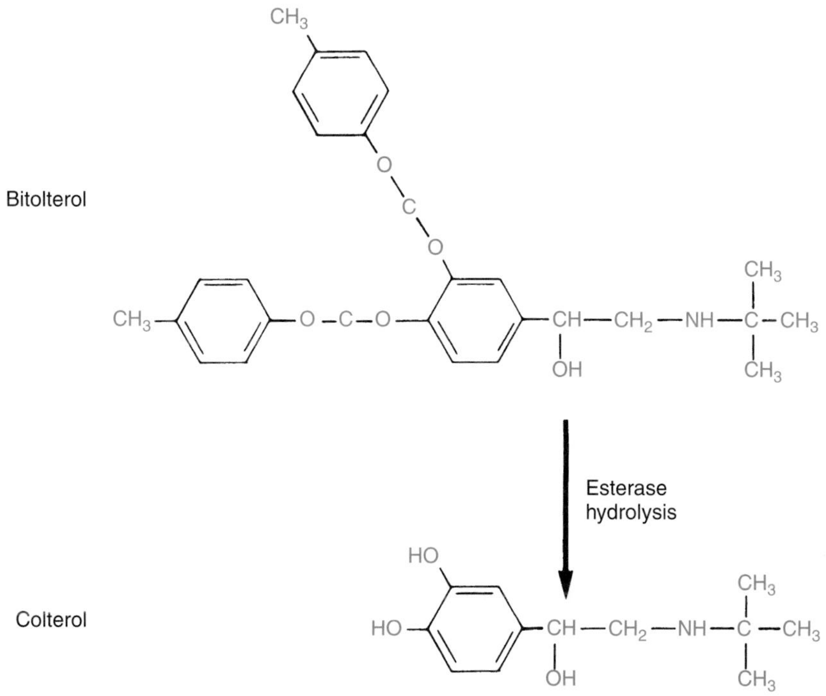

Figure 6-5   Illustration of the structure of bitolterol, showing conversion by esterase enzymes to its active catecholamine form, colterol, a β_2-preferential agonist.

basis than albuterol and similar in both efficacy and toxicity to metaproterenol.[6] The side effect profile is the same as with other β_2 agonists. An oral dose of 10 to 15 mg has effectively produced bronchodilation in asthmatic patients, and a syrup of 7.5 mg/5 ml has been used in pediatric patients.

A PRODRUG: BITOLTEROL

Bitolterol (Tornalate) differs from the previous agents discussed in that the administered form must be converted in the body to the active drug. Because of this, bitolterol is referred to as a *prodrug*. The sequence of activation is seen in Figure 6-5.

The bitolterol molecule consists of two toluate ester groups on the aromatic ring at the carbon-3 and carbon-4 positions. These attachments protect the molecule from degradation by COMT. The large *N*-tertiary butyl substituent on the amine side chain prevents oxidation by MAO. Bitolterol is administered by inhalation using an MDI, and once in the body, the bitolterol molecule is hydrolyzed by esterase enzymes in the tissue and blood to the active bronchodilator colterol. The process of activation begins when the drug is administered and gradually continues over time. This results in a prolonged duration or sustained-release effect of up to 8 hours. Onset and peak effect

are similar to those of noncatecholamine agents such as metaproterenol or terbutaline by inhalation. The active form, colterol, is a catecholamine and will be inactivated by COMT like any catecholamine. The speed of this inactivation is offset by the gradual hydrolysis of bitolterol, to provide the prolonged duration of activity. The bulky side chain gives a preferential β_2 effect, to the active form, colterol.[7]

In animal studies, bitolterol given orally or intravenously selectively distributed to the lungs. The inhalation route in humans seems preferable to treat the lungs locally, and the hydrolysis of bitolterol to colterol proceeds faster in the lungs than elsewhere, giving a selective effect and accumulation in the lungs. Colterol is excreted in urine and feces as free and conjugated colterol and metabolites of colterol. The drug was originally marketed in MDI form, and a nebulizer solution was subsequently released. Although interesting from a pharmacological viewpoint, bitolterol was not widely accepted for clinical use.

LEVALBUTEROL: THE R-ISOMER OF ALBUTEROL

Previous inhaled formulations of adrenergic bronchodilators were all synthetic racemic mixtures, containing both the R-isomer and the S-isomer in equal amounts. Levalbuterol is the pure R-isomer of racemic

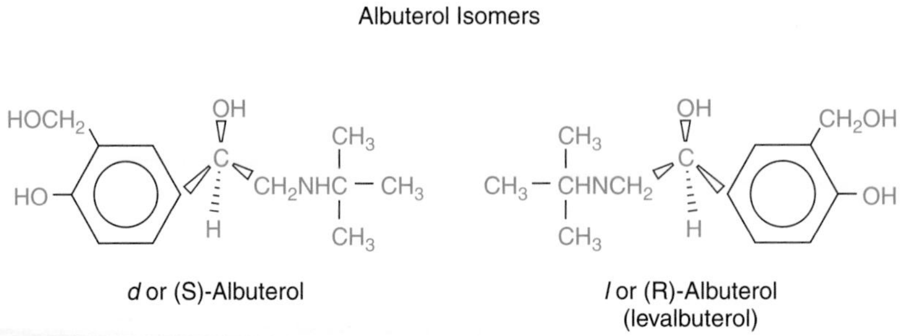

Albuterol Isomers

d or (S)-Albuterol   *l* or (R)-Albuterol
                                        (levalbuterol)

Figure 6-6   The R- and S-isomers of racemic albuterol. Levalbuterol is the single, R-isomer form of racemic albuterol and contains no S-isomer.

Box 6-1	Effects and Characteristics of the S-Isomer of Albuterol

- Increases intracellular calcium concentration in vitro[8]
- Activity is blocked by the anticholinergic agent atropine[8]
- Does not produce pulmonary or extrapulmonary β_2-mediated effects[9]
- Enhances experimental airway responsiveness in vitro[10]
- Increases contractile response of bronchial tissue to histamine or leukotriene C_4 (LTC_4) in vitro[11]
- Enhances eosinophil superoxide production with interleukin-5 (IL-5) stimulation[12]
- Slower metabolism than R-albuterol in vivo[13]
- Preferential retention in the lung when inhaled by MDI (in vivo)[14]

albuterol. Both stereoisomers of albuterol are shown in Figure 6-6 with the single-isomer (R-isomer) form of levalbuterol. Although the S-isomer is physiologically inactive on adrenergic receptors, there is accumulating evidence that the S-isomer is *not* inactive completely. Box 6-1 lists some of the physiological effects of S-albuterol noted in the literature.[8-14] The effects noted would antagonize the bronchodilating effects of the R-isomer of an adrenergic drug and promote bronchoconstriction. In addition, the S-isomer is more slowly metabolized than the R-isomer. Levalbuterol is the single R-isomer form of racemic albuterol, and was released as a nebulization solution in two strengths: a 0.63 mg and a 1.25 mg unit dose. In a study by Nelson and associates,[15] the 0.63 mg dose has been found comparable to the 2.5 mg racemic albuterol dose in onset and duration (Figure 6-7).

Side effects of tremor and heart rate changes were less with the single-isomer formulation. The 1.25 mg dose showed a higher peak effect on FEV_1 with an 8-hour duration compared with racemic albuterol. Side effects with this dose were equivalent to those seen with racemic albuterol. It is significant that an equivalent clinical response was seen with one fourth of the racemic dose (0.63 mg) using the pure isomer, although the racemic mixture contains 1.25 mg of the R-isomer (one half of the total 2.5 mg dose). A detailed review of levalbuterol and differences between the R-isomer and S-isomer of albuterol is available.[16]

LONG-ACTING β-ADRENERGIC AGENTS

The trend in adrenergic bronchodilators has been a development from nonspecific, short-acting agents such as epinephrine, to β_2-specific agents with an action lasting 4 to 6 hours such as terbutaline or albuterol. A major limitation with previous β adrenergic bronchodilators developed after isoproterenol and isoetharine was their 4- to 6-hour duration of action, which limited their usefulness in controlling nocturnal asthma symptoms and necessitated a less convenient four-times-daily dosing schedule. Longer-acting agents offer the advantages of less frequent dosing and protection through the night for asthmatic patients. These agents include sustained-release forms of albuterol and newer drugs such as salmeterol (Serevent) and formoterol.

Long-acting bronchodilators are contrasted with short-acting agents. Short-acting agents include albuterol or pirbuterol, although these agents at one time were considered longer-acting in comparison with the ultra–short-acting catecholamines such as isoetharine.

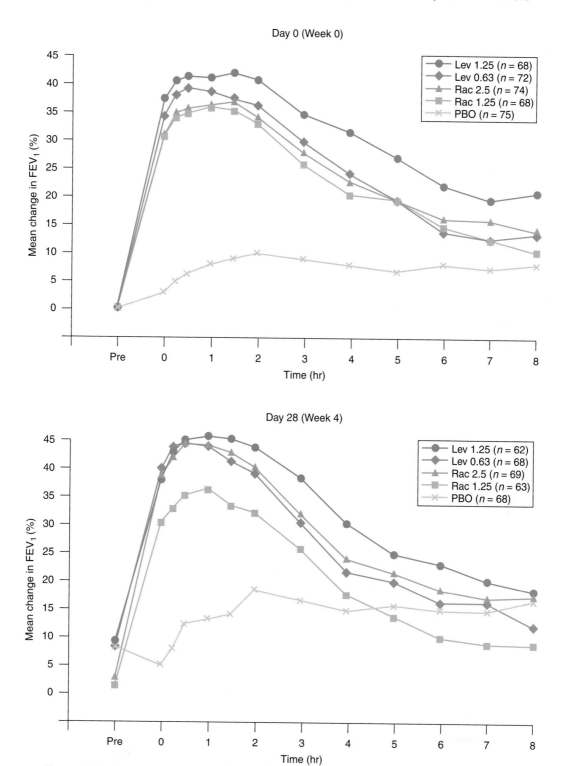

Figure 6-7 Mean percent change in FEV_1 from baseline at the beginning (week 0) and end (week 4) with different doses of levalbuterol, racemic albuterol, and placebo. (From Nelson HS and others: Improved bronchodilation with levalbuterol compared with racemic albuterol in patients with asthma, *J Allergy Clin Immunol* 102:943, 1998.)

SUSTAINED-RELEASE ALBUTEROL

A sustained-released form of albuterol is available as either Proventil Repetabs or Volmax. This is a 4 mg or 8 mg tablet taken orally with extended activity up to 12 hours. The extended activity of Repetabs is achieved with a tablet formulation that contains 2 mg of drug in the coating for immediate release and 2 mg in the core for release after several hours. The Volmax product uses an osmotic gradient to draw water into the tablet, dissolve the albuterol, and gradually release active drug through a pin-hole in the tablet. Thus the 6-hour duration can be extended for 8 to 12 hours and mimics the effect of taking two doses.

SALMETEROL

Salmeterol, a β_2-selective receptor agonist, is available as a pressurized MDI (pMDI) for oral inhalation. It contains a microcrystalline suspension of salmeterol xinafoate, with a chlorofluorocarbon (CFC) propellant (trichlorofluoromethane or CFC-11, and dichlorodifluoromethane or CFC-12) and lecithin as a dispersing agent. It is also available in a dry powder formulation in the Diskus Inhaler. Salmeterol xinafoate is a racemic mixture of two enantiomers, with the R-isomer containing the predominant β_2 activity.[17] Salmeterol xinafoate is the 1-hydroxy-2-naphthoic salt of salmeterol base, with 36.25 μg of the salt equivalent to 25 μg of salmeterol base. The MDI formulation of Serevent releases 25 μg of salmeterol base as the xinafoate salt from the canister valve per actuation; of this amount, 21 μg of salmeterol base is delivered from the mouthpiece actuator. The canister contains 120 actuations and the Diskus 60 doses.

Bronchodilator Effect. Salmeterol represents a new generation of long-acting β_2-specific bronchodilating agents, whose bronchodilating profile differs from the agents previously discussed. The median time to reach an increase of 15% in FEV$_1$ above baseline (considered as the onset of bronchodilation) in asthmatic subjects is longer with salmeterol than albuterol and has been reported between 14 and 22 minutes in different studies[18-19] and generally is greater than 10 minutes.[20] The slower onset of action with salmeterol is significant for its clinical application, discussed subsequently. The time to peak bronchodilating effect is generally 3 to 5 hours, and its duration of action in maintaining an FEV$_1$ 15% above pretreatment baseline is 12 hours or longer. At each point (onset, peak effect, duration), salmeterol exhibits slower, longer times for effect compared with shorter-acting bronchodilators such as albuterol.

With inhaled salmeterol xinafoate, an initial peak plasma concentration of 1 to 2 μg/L is seen 5 minutes after inhalation, with a second peak of 0.07 to 0.2 μg/L at 45 minutes; the second peak is probably due to absorption of swallowed dose. The drug is metabolized by hydroxylation, with elimination primarily in the feces.[21] The increased duration of action of salmeterol is due to its increased lipophilicity conferred by the long side chain. The "tail" of the molecule anchors at an exosite in the cell membrane, allowing continual activation of the β receptor. The mode of action is discussed more fully below.

FORMOTEROL

Formoterol is another β_2-selective agonist with a long-acting bronchodilatory effect of up to 12 hours' duration. A racemic mixture of RR-, SS-formoterol was approved by the Food and Drug Administration (FDA) as Foradil for maintenance treatment of asthma in children and adults 5 years or older and for acute prevention of exercise-induced bronchospasm in adults and children 12 years or older. Racemic formoterol is available as dry powder aerosol using the Aerolizer Inhaler. A single isomer form (RR-formoterol) is in development by Sepracor, Inc. at the time of this edition. Outside the United States, the drug is available as racemic eformoterol in both a pressurized MDI (pMDI) and DPI form. The name *eformoterol* has been used in an effort to distinguish formoterol from fenoterol, another β agonist not currently available in the United States. Current recommended dose for adults and children 5 years or older is 12 μg twice daily by Aerolizer (a DPI).

The chemical structure of formoterol is seen in Figure 6-8. As with salmeterol, the extensive side chain or tail makes formoterol more lipophilic than the shorter-acting bronchodilators and is the basis for its longer duration of effect. The increased lipophilicity of both salmeterol and formoterol allows the drugs to remain in the lipid cell membrane. Even if a tissue preparation containing the drugs is perfused or washed, the drug activity persists. Salmeterol is more lipophilic than formoterol, and this with its anchoring capability may explain why salmeterol is less washable than formoterol.[20]

Bronchodilator Effect. Like salmeterol, formoterol has a prolonged duration of bronchodilating effect of up to 12 hours. *Unlike* salmeterol, the

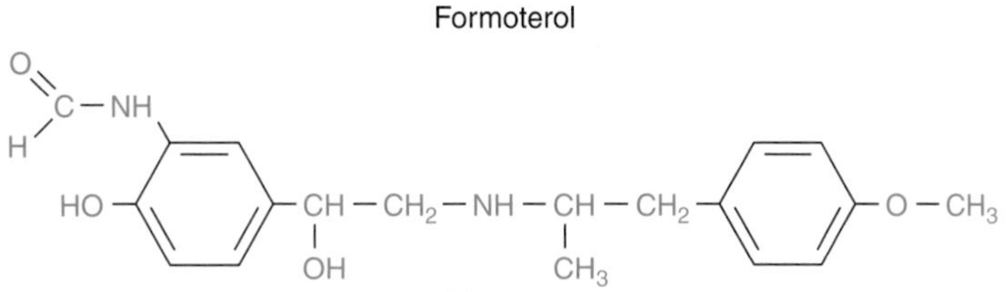

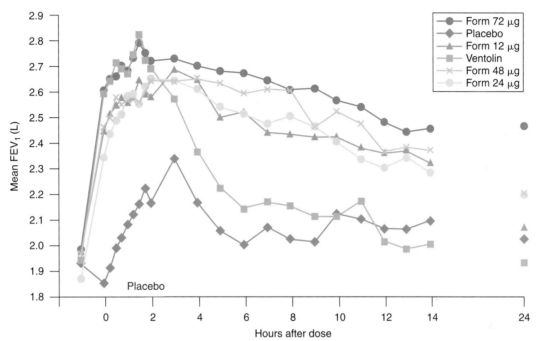

Formoterol

Figure 6-8   The chemical structure of formoterol, a long-acting lipophilic β_2 agonist.

Figure 6-9   A single-dose crossover study of (R,R)-formoterol in the treatment of asthmatic adults. Dose-proportional FEV_1 responses and duration of action for the single isomer of RR-formoterol, a long-acting β_2 agonist. (Courtesy Sepracor, Inc. Data from Vaickus L, Claus R: (R,R)-Formoterol: rapid onset and 24 hour duration of response after a single dose, *Am J Respir Crit Care Med* 161:A191, 2000.)

onset of action for formoterol is significantly faster. The time from inhalation to significant bronchodilation is similar to that of albuterol. It has been reported that 1 minute after inhalation of formoterol there was a significant increase in specific airway conductance (sGaw).[22] The onset of bronchodilation is generally considered to be 2 to 3 minutes with formoterol, compared with 10 minutes or longer with salmeterol. Figure 6-9 shows the dose-proportional response to inhaled RR-formoterol, the single isomer of RR-, SS-formoterol compared with inhaled racemic albuterol.[23] In a study by van Noord and colleagues[24] comparing racemic formoterol 24 µg, salmeterol 50

µg, and albuterol 200 µg, the increase in airway conductance after 1 minute was 44%, less than 16%, and 44%, respectively. The time to maximal increase in airway conductance was 2 hours, 2 to 4 hours, and 30 minutes, respectively, for the three drugs. The maximal increase was 135%, 111%, and 100%, respectively.[22,24]

The efficacy of formoterol in relaxing airway smooth muscle (its maximal effect) is higher than that of albuterol, which is higher than that of salmeterol. The lower intrinsic efficacy of salmeterol would make it a better agent than formoterol for patients with cardiovascular disease.[20]

ANTIINFLAMMATORY EFFECTS

Both the short-acting and the long-acting β agonists show antiinflammatory effects in vitro. Salmeterol and formoterol inhibit human mast cell activation and degranulation in vitro, prevent an increase in vascular permeability with inflammatory mediators, and generally diminish the attraction and accumulation of airway inflammatory cells.[20] Despite these in vitro antiinflammatory effects, salmeterol and formoterol have not been shown to inhibit accumulation of inflammatory cells in the airway or the rise in inflammatory markers in vivo. Neither drug is considered to have a sufficient effect on airway inflammation in patients with asthma to replace antiinflammatory drugs such as corticosteroids.

CLINICAL USE

Long-acting β agonists are indicated for maintenance therapy of asthma, which is not controlled by regular low-dose inhaled corticosteroids, and for chronic obstructive lung disease needing daily inhaled bronchodilator therapy for reversible airway obstruction. National guidelines recommend introduction of salmeterol in Step 3 asthma (asthma not controlled by lower doses of antiinflammatory medications).[4] Use of the long-acting β agonist may prevent the need to increase the inhaled dose of corticosteroid. Several points should be noted in the clinical use of long-acting agents, because of their differences from shorter-acting β agonists.

- Long-acting $β_2$ agonists are not recommended for rescue bronchodilation because repeated administration with their longer duration and increased lipophilic property risk accumulation and toxicity[20]; however, product literature with racemic formoterol (Oxis, Turbuhaler) suggests up to two additional inhalations (a maximum of 72 μg per day) for acute relief of symptoms.
- A shorter-acting $β_2$ agonist, such as albuterol or other agents previously discussed, should be prescribed and available for asthmatics for treatment of breakthrough symptoms if additional bronchodilator therapy is needed between scheduled doses of a long-acting $β_2$ agonist; Asthmatics must be well educated in the appropriate use of the two types of β agonists (shorter-acting versus long-acting).
- Although they have antiinflammatory effects, short-acting or long-acting β agonists are not a substitute for inhaled corticosteroids in asthma

maintenance or for other antiinflammatory medications if such are required.
- The difference in rate of onset between salmeterol and formoterol may require classifying $β_2$ agonists as "fast" and "slow" in addition to "short" and "long" acting, with salmeterol being a slow and long-acting bronchodilator versus formoterol as a fast and long-acting bronchodilator.[25]

The addition of a long-acting $β_2$ agonist to inhaled corticosteroids can lead to improved lung function and a decrease in symptoms.[26] A combination product of salmeterol and fluticasone in a Diskus inhaler (Advair) demonstrated superior asthma control and better lung function than either drug taken alone.[27] Because of their prolonged bronchodilation, long-acting $β_2$ agonists taken twice daily have a greater area under the FEV_1 curve compared with short-acting agents taken four times daily. This can be seen in Figure 6-10, which illustrates dose-response curves for albuterol and salmeterol. Unlike albuterol, which tends to return to baseline in 4 to 6 hours, salmeterol provides a more sustained level of bronchodilation, giving a higher baseline of lung function.[28] The same effect has been found in comparing twice-daily salmeterol with four-times-daily inhaled ipratropium bromide, a shorter-acting anticholinergic bronchodilator discussed in Chapter 7.[29]

MODE OF ACTION

The bronchodilating action of the adrenergic drugs is due to stimulation of $β_2$ receptors located on bronchial smooth muscle. Distinctions among types of adrenergic receptors were identified in Chapter 5. In addition to $β_2$ receptors, some adrenergic bronchodilators can stimulate α and $β_1$ receptors, with the following clinical effects:

Receptor stimulation: Causes vasoconstriction and a vasopressor effect; in the upper airway (nasal passages) this can provide decongestion

$β_1$-*Receptor stimulation:* Causes increased myocardial conductivity and increased heart rate, as well as increased contractile force

$β_2$-*Receptor stimulation:* Causes relaxation of bronchial smooth muscle, with some inhibition of inflammatory mediator release and stimulation of mucociliary clearance

Both α and β receptors are examples of G protein–linked receptors. Table 6-2 lists each of the

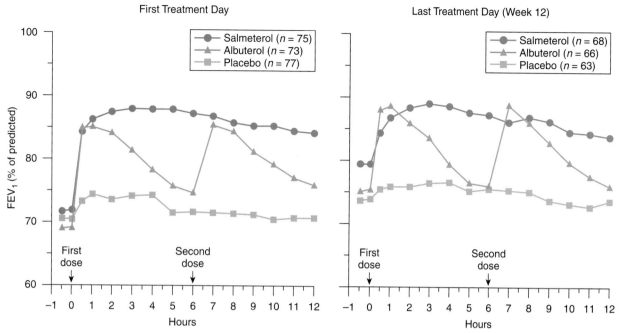

Figure 6-10   Mean FEV_1 response and duration of effect for inhaled salmeterol 42 μg twice daily, albuterol 180 μg four times daily, and placebo. (Modified from Pearlman DS and others: A comparison of salmeterol with albuterol in the treatment of mild-to-moderate asthma, *N Engl J Med* 327:1420, 1992.)

Table 6-2

Adrenergic receptor types, with their G proteins, effector systems, second messengers and examples of cell responses

RECEPTOR	G PROTEIN	EFFECTOR	SECOND MESSENGER	RESPONSE
α_1	G_q	Phospholipase C (PLC)	Inositol trisphosphate (IP_3), diacylglycerol (DAG)	Vasoconstriction
α_2	G_i	Adenylyl cyclase (inhibits)	cAMP (inhibits)	Inhibition of neuro-transmitter release
β (β_1, β_2, β_3)	G_s	Adenylyl cyclase (stimulates)	cAMP (increases)	Smooth muscle relaxation

cAMP, cyclic adenosine-3′, 5′-monophosphate.

adrenergic receptor types, along with its particular type of G protein, effector system, and second messenger and an example of cell response in the lungs. As described in Chapter 2, the G protein is a heterotrimer whose α subunit differentiates the type of G protein. The G protein couples the adrenergic receptor to the effector enzyme, which in turn initiates the cell response by means of a particular intracellular second messenger. The mode of action with β-receptor, α_2-receptor, and α_1-receptor stimulation are each described.

β- AND α_2-RECEPTOR ACTIVATION

The mode of action of β agonists and the β receptor have been well characterized, although the activity of α receptors is not as well understood. The mode of

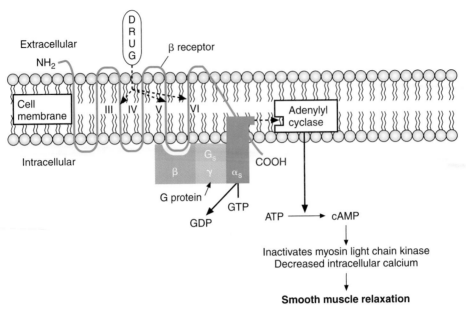

Figure 6-11   Diagram illustrating the mode of action by which stimulation of the G protein–linked β receptor by a β agonist causes smooth muscle relaxation.

action for relaxation of airway smooth muscle when a β_2 receptor is stimulated is illustrated in Figure 6-11. Adrenergic agonists such as albuterol or epinephrine attach to β receptors that are polypeptide chains that traverse the cell membrane seven times and have an extracellular NH_2 terminal and an intracellular carboxyl (COOH) terminal. This causes activation of the stimulatory G protein designated G_S. The actual binding site of a β agonist is within the cell membrane, inside the "barrel" or circle formed by the transmembrane loops of the receptor chain. The β agonist forms bonds with elements of the third, fifth, and sixth transmembrane loops. When stimulated by a β agonist, the receptor undergoes a conformational change, which reduces the affinity of the α subunit of the G protein for guanosine diphosphate (GDP). The GDP is replaced by GTP, and the α subunit dissociates from the receptor and the β-γ portion of the G protein to link with the effector system. The effector system for the β receptor is adenylyl cyclase, a membrane-bound enzyme. Activation of adenylyl cyclase by the G_S protein causes an increased synthesis of the second messenger, cyclic adenosine-3',5'-monophosphate (cAMP). cAMP may cause smooth muscle relaxation by increasing the inactivation of myosin light chain kinase, an enzyme initiating myosin-actin interaction and subsequent smooth muscle contraction. An in-

crease in cAMP also leads to a decrease in intracellular calcium.

A similar sequence of events is responsible for the action of α_2-receptor stimulation, which can inhibit further neurotransmitter release from the presynaptic neuron when stimulated by norepinephrine in a feedback, autoregulatory fashion (see Chapter 5). However, stimulation of α_2 receptors (not shown in Figure 6-11) results in activation of an inhibitory G protein, designated G_i, whose α subunit serves to inhibit the enzyme adenylyl cyclase, thereby lowering the rate of synthesis for intracellular cAMP.

α_1-RECEPTOR ACTIVATION

Stimulation of an α_1 receptor by an agonist such as phenylephrine or epinephrine (which has affinity for both α and β receptors) results in vasoconstriction of peripheral blood vessels, including those in the airway. The mode of action for this effect as mediated by the G protein–linked α_1 receptor is illustrated in Figure 6-12. Stimulation of the α_1 receptor causes a conformational change in the receptor, which in turn activates the G protein designated G_q. With activation, GDP dissociates from the G protein, GTP binds to the α subunit of the G protein, and the α subunit dissociates from the β-γ dimer, to activate the effector phospholipase C (PLC). Activation of the effector,

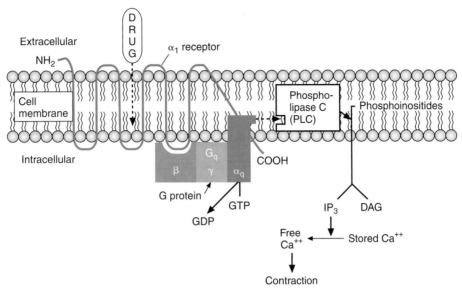

Figure 6-12   Diagram illustrating the mode of action by which the G protein–linked α_1 receptor causes smooth muscle contraction, which can result in vasoconstriction in blood vessels.

PLC, leads to the conversion of membrane phosphoinositides into inositol 1,4,5-trisphosphate (IP_3) and diacylglycerol (DAG). IP_3 stimulates release of intracellular stores of calcium into the cytoplasm of the cell, and DAG activates protein kinase C. Contraction of vascular smooth muscle results.

SALMETEROL: MECHANISM OF ACTION

The action of salmeterol in providing sustained protection from bronchoconstriction differs to a degree from that of the previously described adrenergic bronchodilators. The difference in salmeterol's pharmacodynamics is reflected in its pharmacokinetics with a slower onset and time to peak effect and a longer duration of action compared with previous adrenergic agents.

The structure of salmeterol is seen in Figure 6-3, along with that of other β agonists for comparison. The drug is a modification of the saligenin, albuterol, with a long *lipophilic* nonpolar N-substituted side chain. Salmeterol thus consists of a polar, or *hydrophilic*, phenyl ethanolamine "head," with a large lipophilic "tail" or side chain. As a result of this structure, salmeterol is lipophilic, unlike most β agonists, which are hydrophilic and approach the β receptor directly from the aqueous extracellular space. In contrast, salmeterol, as a lipophilic molecule, diffuses into the cell membrane phospholipid bilayer and approaches the β receptor laterally, as shown in Figure 6-13. The lipophilic nonpolar side chain then binds to an area of the β receptor referred to as the *exosite*. With the side chain (tail) anchored in the exosite, a hydrophobic region of the receptor, the active saligenin head binds to and activates the β receptor at the same location as albuterol.

The binding properties of salmeterol differ from those of albuterol and other β agonists. Because the side chain is anchored at the exosite, the active head portion continually attaches to and detaches from the active receptor site. This provides ongoing stimulation of the β receptor and is the basis for the persistent duration of action of salmeterol. This model of activity is supported by studies of the effect of β antagonists on the β agonist action of salmeterol, as well as molecular binding studies. If albuterol is attached to the β receptor, the smooth muscle relaxation can be fully reversed by a β-blocking agent such as propranolol or sotalol, indicating a competitive blockade. When the β-blocking agent is removed, there is no further relaxation of smooth muscle. The drug is displaced and the action of albuterol is terminated. If salmeterol stimulates a receptor, a β antagonist such as propranolol will also reverse the effect of relaxation. However, when the propranolol is removed from the tissue, the relaxant effect of salmeterol is reestablished. This indicates that the salmeterol remains anchored

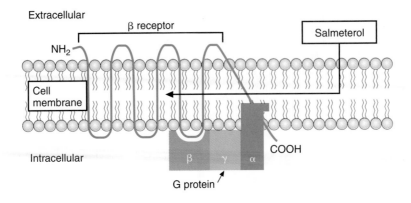

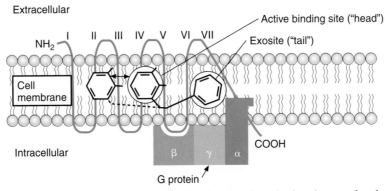

Figure 6-13   An illustration of the mode of action by which salmeterol, a long-acting β_2-specific bronchodilator, interacts with the β receptor by means of an exosite anchor with the lipophilic side chain, allowing continual stimulation of the active receptor site.

in the receptor and is available to continually stimulate the β receptor once the blocking agent is removed.[17]

The prolonged activity of formoterol is also thought to be due to its lipophilicity, although formoterol is less lipophilic than salmeterol. Formoterol, which is moderately lipophilic, enters the bilipid cell membrane, where it is retained, with the lipid layer acting as a depot and giving a long-acting effect. At the same time, formoterol can approach the β receptor from the aqueous phase, giving it a rapid onset of action.[22]

ROUTES OF ADMINISTRATION

β-Adrenergic bronchodilators are currently available in inhaled form (MDI, nebulizer solution, or DPI), orally (tablets or syrup), and parenterally, although not all agents are found in each form. Regardless of the route of administration, there are three general patterns to the time course of bronchodilation with drugs in this group. The *catecholamines* show a rapid onset of 1 to 3 minutes, a peak effect around 15 to 20 minutes, and a rapid decline in effect after 1 hour. The *noncatecholamines* (resorcinols, saligenins), with the exception of salmeterol, show an onset of 5 to 15 minutes, a peak effect of 30 to 60 minutes, and a duration of 4 to 6 hours. Salmeterol differs significantly, with a slower onset (>20 minutes) and peak effect (about 3 hours), and a 12-hour duration. Formoterol is similar in duration to salmeterol but with an onset as rapid as albuterol. Aside from these general patterns, which depend on the type of drug used, the route of administration will further affect the time course of a drug. Inhaled and injected adrenergic bronchodilators have a quicker onset than orally administered agents.

INHALATION ROUTE

All of the β-adrenergic bronchodilators marketed in the United States are available for inhalational delivery, either using an MDI, a nebulizer (including intermittent positive-pressure breathing nebulization), or a DPI. Catecholamines must be given by inhalation because they are ineffective orally. Inhalation is the preferred route for administering β-adrenergic drugs for all of the following reasons:

1. Onset is rapid.
2. Smaller doses are needed compared with those for oral use.
3. Side effects such as tremor and tachycardia are reduced.
4. Drug is delivered directly to the target organ (i.e., lung).
5. Inhalation is painless and safe.

The use of aerosol delivery *during* an acute attack of airway obstruction has been questioned. However, several studies have failed to show substantial differences between inhaled and parenteral β-adrenergic agents in acute severe asthma.[30,31] There is no reason to avoid these bronchodilators as inhaled aerosols during acute episodes.[32] The inhaled route targets the lung directly. In fact, combining the oral delivery with additional inhalation has been shown to produce good additive effects with albuterol.[33]

The major difficulties with aerosol administration are the time needed for nebulization (5 to 10 minutes), the possible embarrassment of using an MDI in public or at school, and inability to use an MDI correctly. Difficulty in correctly using an MDI can be remedied by using spacer devices or, alternatively, by using a gas-powered handheld nebulizer. A DPI eliminates problems associated with both nebulizers and MDIs, and both albuterol and salmeterol are currently available in DPI form in the United States.

CONTINUOUS NEBULIZATION

The administration of inhaled adrenergic agents by continuous nebulization has been used for management of severe asthma, in an effort to avoid respiratory failure, intubation, and mechanical ventilation. The *Guidelines for the Diagnosis and Management of Asthma* released by the National Heart, Lung, and Blood Institute panel of experts II (NAEPP EPR II) also recommend 2.5 to 5 mg of albuterol by nebulizer every 20 minutes for three doses, as well 10 to 15 mg/hr by continuous nebulization.[4] Because a nebulizer treatment takes approximately 10 minutes, giv-

ing three treatments every 20 minutes requires repeated therapist attendance. Continuous administration by nebulizer may simplify such frequent treatments. The use of continuous nebulization of β-agonist bronchodilators was recently reviewed by Fink and Dhand.[34] A summary of studies, including dosages used, is given. With continuous nebulization, there are no general standards for doses other than the recommendation from the NAEPP EPR II; in the studies cited in Fink and Dhand,[34] dosages vary from 2.5 mg/hr to 15 mg/hr and include schedules based on milligrams per kilogram per hour.

The impact and optimal use of continuous nebulization versus intermittent nebulization is not clear. In the five randomized controlled trials from 1993 to 1996 cited by Fink and Dhand,[34] there was similar improvement between continuous versus intermittent nebulization. One study by Lin and associates[35] showed faster improvement in patients with FEV_1 less than 50% of predicted, using continuous nebulization. A study by Shrestha and colleagues[36] compared a high (7.5 mg) and low dose (2.5 mg) of albuterol with both continuous and intermittent nebulization. FEV_1 improved more with continuous than intermittent nebulization, and the low dose of 2.5 mg was as effective as the higher dose of 7.5 mg with continuous administration. These and other results suggest that there is a benefit to continuous nebulization in severe airflow obstruction, but a dose less than 10 to 15 mg/hr may be effective, with less toxicity. Less clinician time is required for the administration of continuous nebulization. Fink and Dhand[34] suggest that for emergency department patients with severe airway obstruction, who do not respond sufficiently after an hour of intermittent nebulization of β agonists, continuous nebulization offers a practical approach to optimal dosing in a cost-effective manner.

Delivery Methods. Several delivery methods to accomplish continuous nebulization have been tried and reported. These include the following:

- Measured refilling of a small-volume nebulizer (SVN)
- Volumetric infusion pump with an SVN[37]
- Large-reservoir nebulizer such as the HEART or HOPE

Toxicity and Monitoring. Continuous nebulization of β2 agonists is not standard therapy, and patients receiving this treatment have serious airflow obstruction. Potential complications include cardiac arrhythmias, hypokalemia, and hyperglycemia. Unifocal premature ventricular contractions were reported in one patient by Portnoy and associates.[38] Significant tremor may also occur. Subsensitivity to continuous therapy was not observed by Portnoy and colleagues. Close monitoring of patients receiving continuous β agonists is necessary and includes observation, along with cardiac and electrolyte monitoring. Selective β_2 agonists, such as terbutaline and albuterol, should be used to reduce side effects.

ORAL ROUTE

The oral route has the advantages of ease, simplicity, short time required for administration, and exact reproducibility and control of dosage. However, in terms of clinical effects, this is not the preferred route. The time course of oral β agonists differs from that of the inhaled route. Onset of action begins in about 1.5 hours, with a peak effect reached after 1 to 2 hours and a duration of action between 3 and 6 hours.[39] Larger doses are required than with inhalation, and the frequency and degree of unwanted side effects increase substantially. The catecholamines are ineffective by mouth, as previously discussed. Noncatecholamine bronchodilators in the adrenergic group seem to lose their β_2 specificity with oral use, possibly because of the reduction of the side chain bulk in a first pass through the liver.[40] Patient compliance on a three- or four-times-daily schedule may be better than with a nebulizer. If this is the case with an individual patient and the side effects are tolerable, then oral use may be indicated for bronchodilator therapy. The introduction of an oral tablet of albuterol with extended-action properties (Repetabs, Volmax) offers the possibility of protection from bronchoconstriction for longer than 8 hours. However, inhaled salmeterol and formoterol now offer a 12-hour duration. Either the extended-release tablet or a long-acting β agonist is advantageous in preventing nocturnal asthma and deterioration of flow rates in the morning.

PARENTERAL ADMINISTRATION

β-Adrenergic bronchodilators have been given subcutaneously as well as intravenously, usually in the emergency management of acute asthma. Subcutaneously, epinephrine 0.3 mg (0.3 ml of 1:1000 strength) every 15 to 20 minutes up to 1 mg in 2 hours and terbutaline 0.25 mg (0.25 ml of a 1 mg/ml solution) repeated in 15 to 30 minutes, not exceeding 0.5 mg in 4 hours, have been used. Shim[41] suggests that for practical purposes both aerosolized and subcutaneous routes should be used to manage acute obstruction, although there may be little difference in effect with the two routes. No difference in effect between epinephrine and terbutaline has been found when given subcutaneously.

The intravenous route has been used most commonly with isoproterenol and also with albuterol. Intravenous administration of these agents was thought useful during severe obstruction because these agents would be distributed throughout the lungs, whereas aerosol delivery would not allow them to penetrate the periphery. This is questionable for both subcutaneous and intravenous bronchodilator therapy because aerosols do exert an effect with obstruction. Intravenous isoproterenol is not clearly advantageous as a bronchodilator, although this route is used for cardiac stimulation in shock and bradycardia. The dose-limiting factor is tachycardia. Intravenous therapy is a last resort and requires an infusion pump, cardiac monitor, and close attention. Children's dosages range from 0.1 to 0.8 μg/kg/min, and adult dosages range from 0.03 to 0.2 μg/kg/min, until bronchial relaxation or side effects occur.[41] However, the combination of myocardial stimulation and hypoxia can cause serious arrhythmias, and intravenous isoproterenol should be avoided in acute asthma, in favor of β_2-specific agents. Albuterol has been given intravenously as a bolus between 100 to 500 μg or by infusion between 4 and 25 μg/min.[42] Although albuterol is more β_2-specific by aerosol than is isoproterenol, the usefulness of intravenous administration compared with oral, aerosol, or subcutaneous is not clearly established.

ADVERSE SIDE EFFECTS

Just as the adrenergic bronchodilators exert a therapeutic effect by stimulation of α-, β_1-, or β_2-adrenergic receptors, they can likewise cause unwanted effects as a result of stimulation of these receptors. Generally, the term *side effect* indicates any effect other than the intended therapeutic effect. The most common clinically observed side effects of adrenergic bronchodilators are listed in Box 6-2 and are briefly discussed. It must be emphasized that the number and severity of these side effects vary from patient to patient; not every side effect is seen with each patient. It must be remembered that the later adrenergic agents (terbutaline, albuterol, bitolterol, pirbuterol, levalbuterol, or salmeterol) are much more β_2-specific than previ-

Box 6-2 Side Effects Seen With β Agonist Use

Tremor
Palpitations and tachycardia
Headache
Insomnia
Rise in blood pressure
Nervousness
Dizziness
Nausea
Tolerance to bronchodilator effect
Loss of bronchoprotection
Worsening ventilation-perfusion ratio (decrease in PaO_2)
Hypokalemia
Bronchoconstrictor reaction to solution additives (SVN) and propellants (MDI)

ous agents such as ephedrine, epinephrine, or isoproterenol. Because of this, there is greater likelihood of cardiac stimulation causing tachycardia and blood pressure increases with the last three agents than with the newer drugs. The more recent agents are safe, and the side effects listed are more of a nuisance than a danger and are easily monitored by clinicians. The introduction of single isomer β agonists such as levalbuterol may show a further specificity and decrease in side effects, which are potentially due to the detrimental effects of the S-isomer of β agonists.

TREMOR

The annoying effect of muscle tremor with β agonists is due to stimulation of $β_2$ receptors in skeletal muscle, is dose related, and is the dose-limiting side effect of the $β_2$-specific agents, especially with oral administration. The adrenergic receptors mediating muscle tremor have been shown to be of the $β_2$ type.[43,44] As shown previously, this side effect is much more noticeable with oral delivery, which provides a rationale for aerosol administration of these agents. Tolerance to the side effect of tremor usually develops after a period of days to weeks with the oral route, and patients should be reassured of this when beginning to use these drugs.

CARDIAC EFFECTS

The older adrenergic agents with strong $β_1$- and α-stimulating effects were considered dangerous in the presence of congestive heart failure. The dose-limiting side effect with these agents was tachycardia. They increase cardiac output and oxygen consumption by stimulating $β_1$ receptors, leading to a decrease in cardiac efficiency, which is the work relative to the oxygen consumption. Newer agents have a preferential $β_2$ effect to minimize cardiac stimulation. However, tachycardia may also follow use of the newer agents, and there is evidence that this is due to the presence of $β_2$ receptors even in the heart.[45] $β_2$-Agonists cause vasodilation, and this can also cause a reflex tachycardia. Despite this effect, agents such as terbutaline or albuterol can actually improve cardiac performance. Albuterol and terbutaline can cause peripheral vasodilation and increase myocardial contractility without increasing oxygen demand by the heart.[30] The net effect is to reduce afterload and improve cardiac output with no oxygen cost. These agents are therefore attractive for use with airway obstruction combined with congestive heart failure. Seider and colleagues[46] reported that neither heart rate nor frequency of premature beats were significantly affected by inhaled terbutaline or ipratropium bromide (an anticholinergic bronchodilator) in 14 patients with chronic obstructive pulmonary disease (COPD) and ischemic heart disease.

TOLERANCE TO BRONCHODILATOR EFFECT

Adaptation to a drug with repeated use is a concern because use of the drug is actually reducing its effectiveness. With β agonists, there is in vitro evidence of an acute desensitization of the β receptor within minutes of exposure to a β agonist, as well as a longer-term desensitization. This is illustrated in Figure 6-14, which shows both an acute decrease in response *during* sustained exposure of the receptor to the agonist and a long-term decrease in maximal response with subsequent drug exposure. This decrease in bronchodilator response has been observed with both short-acting and long-acting β agonists.

Exposure of cells with β receptors to isoproterenol causes a short-term, acute reduction in adenylyl cyclase activity and production of cAMP. The immediate desensitization is caused by an "uncoupling" of the receptor and the effector enzyme adenylyl cyclase.[47] A model for desensitization of the β receptor is diagrammed in Figure 6-15. When stimulated by a β agonist, the β receptor goes into a low-affinity binding state (i.e., has reduced affinity for binding with a β agonist). Simultaneously, the β agonist causes an increase in cAMP, which increases protein kinase A, also referred to as β-*adrenergic receptor kinase*, or β-*ARK*. β-ARK causes phosphorylation (transfer of

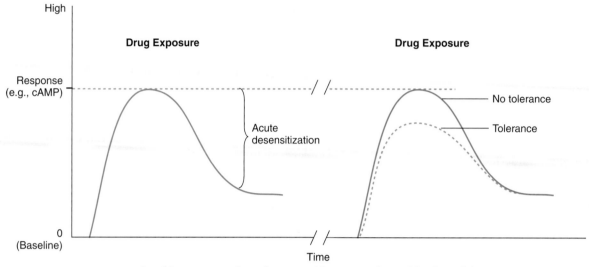

Figure 6-14   Graphic representation of acute and long-term desensitization of the β receptor response to β agonists. Cell response during actual receptor stimulation by agonist immediately declines *(left side)*; subsequent exposure to drug will produce a lower peak initial response if tolerance or long-term desensitization occurs *(right side)*.

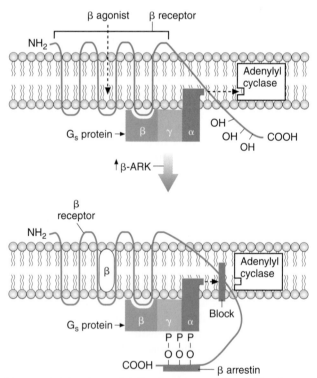

Figure 6-15   A model for β receptor desensitization through phosphorylation of the β receptor at the carboxyl terminal site by β-adrenergic receptor kinase (β-ARK), blocking the action of the α_2 subunit on the effector enzyme adenylyl cyclase.

phosphate groups, P) of the hydroxyl groups (OH) on the carboxyl terminal portion of the β receptor. This phosphorylation induces binding of a protein named β-arrestin (β-arr), which prevents the receptor from interacting with G_s and disrupts the coupling of G_s with the effector enzyme, adenylyl cyclase. Removal of the β agonist allows the dissociation of both β-arrestin and the phosphate from the receptor, and the receptor returns to a fully active state.

Long-term desensitization is considered to be caused by a reduction in number of β receptors. This is termed *downregulation*. Both norepinephrine and albuterol have caused a reduction of almost 50% in vitro in the number of β adrenergic receptors in airway smooth muscle of guinea pigs.[47] Exposure of isolated human bronchus to isoproterenol or terbutaline produces similar desensitization.[48] Long-term desensitization is also illustrated in Figure 6-14, as indicated by the lower peak response to subsequent administration of an adrenergic agonist.

Although use of an inhaled β agonist does cause a reduction in peak effect, the bronchodilator response is still significant and stabilizes within several weeks with continued use.[20] Such tolerance is not generally considered clinically important and does not contraindicate the use of these agents. The same phenomenon of tolerance is also responsible for diminished side effects such as muscle tremor for patients on regular use of inhaled β-agonist bronchodilators.

In addition to loss of receptors (downregulation) by exposure to a β agonist, altered β-receptor function may be caused secondary to inflammation. Increased levels of phospholipase A_2 (PLA$_2$) may destabilize membrane support of the β receptor, changing its function. Cytokines such as interleukin 1β (IL-1β) may cause desensitization, and platelet-activating factor (PAF) inhibits the relaxing effect of isoproterenol on human tracheal tissue.

Corticosteroids can reverse the desensitization of β receptors and are said to be able to potentiate the response to β agonists.[49] Corticosteroids have the following effects, in relation to β-agonist and β-receptor function:

- Increase the proportion of β receptors expressed on the cell membrane (upregulation)
- Increase the proportion of β receptors in the high-affinity binding state
- Inhibit the release and action of inflammatory mediators such as PLA$_2$, cytokines, or PAF

β Agonists may in turn have a positive effect on corticosteroid function and activity. A recent review by Anderson explores possible mechanisms for the beneficial interaction of β agonists and corticosteroids.[26]

LOSS OF BRONCHOPROTECTION

A distinction was found by Ahrens and colleagues to exist between *bronchodilation* and the *bronchoprotective* effect of β agonists.[50] The bronchodilating effect of a β agonist can be measured in airflow changes, such as FEV_1 or peak expiratory flows (PEFR). The bronchoprotective effect refers to the reaction of the airways to challenge by provocative stimuli such as allergens or irritants and is measured with doses of histamine, methacholine, or cold air. Ahrens and colleagues[50] found that the protective effect with agonists such as metaproterenol or albuterol declines more rapidly than the bronchodilating effect. Not only is there a difference in time between these effects, tolerance occurs with the protective effect of a β agonist, just as with the bronchodilator response. Results from a study by O'Connor and associates[51] are shown in Figure 6-16. The difference in dose of adenosine (AMP) and methacholine required for a 20% decline in FEV_1 (PC$_{20}$) after the inhalation of terbutaline compared with placebo is seen before and after 7 days of steady treatment with terbutaline. Airway response to

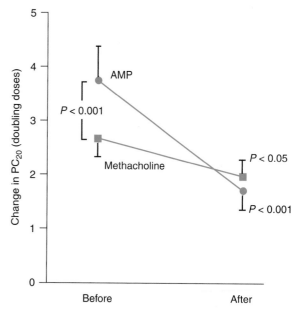

Figure 6-16   Data of O'Connor and colleagues showing a decrease in the provocational dose of adenosine (AMP) and methacholine after inhaling 500 μg of terbutaline compared with placebo, before and after a 7-day treatment period with terbutaline, indicating a loss of protection against airway stimuli with regular terbutaline use, especially with the inflammatory agent AMP. The higher the number of doubling doses needed for bronchoconstriction, the lower is the airway responsiveness, that is, the greater the airway protection. (From O'Connor BJ, Aikman SL, Barnes PJ: Tolerance to the nonbronchodilator effects of inhaled β$_2$-agonists in asthma, *New Engl J Med* 327:1204, 1992.)

challenge is seen to occur with a significantly lower dose of either AMP (adenosine) or methacholine in subjects with mild asthma, *after* 7 days of β agonist exposure, showing tolerance to the protective effect of terbutaline. The development of tolerance to the bronchoprotective effect of the long-acting β agonist salmeterol was shown to occur both in the absence of corticosteroid therapy by Bhagat and colleagues and with concomitant inhaled corticosteroid treatment by Kalra and associates.[52-53] After the first 4 weeks of regular treatment with salmeterol, there was no increase in bronchial hyperresponsiveness or loss of bronchoprotection, in a study by Rosenthal and associates.[54] Sustained improvements were seen in pulmonary function and asthma symptom control.[54]

The mechanism underlying the increase in bronchial hyperresponsiveness with use of β agonists is not clear. Evidence accumulating on the effects of the S-isomer of β agonists suggests a possible cause.[55] The same effects could conceivably be implicated in the reduction in maximal bronchodilator effect with repeated use.

CENTRAL NERVOUS SYSTEM EFFECTS

Commonly reported side effects of the adrenergic bronchodilators include headache, nervousness, irritability, anxiety, and insomnia, which are caused by central nervous system stimulation. Feelings of nervousness or anxiety may be due to the muscle tremor seen with these drugs, rather than to direct central nervous system stimulation. Excessive stimulation of the central nervous system, or at least symptoms of such, should be noted by clinicians and can warrant evaluation of the dosage used.

FALL IN PaO$_2$

A fall in PaO$_2$ has been noted with isoproterenol administration during asthmatic bronchospasm, as the ventilation improves and the attack is relieved. The same effect has subsequently been noted with newer β agonists such as albuterol and salmeterol.[56] The mechanism for this seems to be an increase in perfusion of poorly ventilated portions of the lung. It is known that regional alveolar hypoxia produces regional pulmonary vasoconstriction in an effort to shunt perfusion to lung areas of higher oxygen tension. This vasoconstriction is probably accomplished by α-sympathetic receptors.[57]

Administration of inhaled β agonists may reverse hypoxic pulmonary vasoconstriction by β$_2$-stimulation, increasing perfusion to underventilated lung regions.[58] Preferential delivery of the inhaled aerosol to better ventilated lung regions increases the ventilation-perfusion mismatch. It has been noted that such PaO$_2$ drops are statistically significant but physiologically may be negligible.[56,59] Oxygen tension falls most in subjects with the highest initial PaO$_2$. Decreases in arterial PO$_2$ rarely exceed 10 mm Hg, and the PaO$_2$ values tend to be on the flat portion of the oxyhemoglobin curve, so that drops in saturation (SaO$_2$) are minimized. Oxygen tensions usually return to baseline within 30 minutes.

METABOLIC DISTURBANCES

Adrenergic bronchodilators can increase blood glucose and insulin levels, as well as decrease serum potassium levels. This is a normal effect of sympathomimetics. In diabetic patients, clinicians should be aware of a possible effect on glucose and insulin levels. Hypokalemia has also been reported after par-

enteral administration of albuterol and epinephrine.[60] The clinical importance of this is controversial and would mainly be of concern in patients with cardiac disease or in interpreting serum potassium levels obtained shortly after use of adrenergic bronchodilators. The mechanism of the effect on potassium is probably activation of the sodium-potassium pump by the β receptor, with enhanced transport of potassium from the extracellular to the intracellular compartment. Such metabolic effects are minimized with inhaled aerosols of β-adrenergic agents, because plasma levels of the drug remain low.

PROPELLANT TOXICITY AND PARADOXICAL BRONCHOSPASM

The use of Freon-powered (CFC) MDIs can cause bronchospasm from hyperreactive airways. This reaction to the propellant was shown by Yarbrough and colleagues.[61] They found that 7% of 175 subjects who used placebo MDI with propellant alone experienced a decrease of 10% or more in their FEV$_1$. The incidence was about 4% using an MDI with metaproterenol and propellant, probably because of the bronchodilating effect overcoming the propellant effect. In most cases, bronchospasm lasts less than 3 minutes. A dry powder formulation is an ideal alternative formulation to an MDI if sensitivity to propellants exists, assuming drug availability and adequate inspiratory flow rate. Use of a nebulizer instead of an MDI can also be considered if bronchospasm occurs with a patient. Finally, the oral route offers an alternative to the inhalation route of administration. Cocchetto and associates[62] review the literature on paradoxical bronchospasm with use of inhalation aerosols.

SENSITIVITY TO ADDITIVES

An increasingly publicized problem for those with hyperreactive airways is sensitivity to sulfite preservatives, with resulting bronchospasm. Sulfiting agents are used as preservatives for food and are also used as antioxidants for bronchodilator solutions to prevent degradation and inactivation. Sulfites include sodium or potassium sulfite, bisulfite, and metabisulfite. When a sulfite is placed in solution, at warm temperature in an acid pH such as saliva, it converts to sulfurous acid and sulfur dioxide. Sulfur dioxide is known to cause bronchoconstriction in asthmatic patients. Solutions of Bronkosol, Isuprel, Vaponefrin, and microNefrin all contain sulfites as preservatives. There have been reports of coughing and wheezing, as well as pruritus, after use of sulfite-containing bronchodilators. Other additives and preservatives that can potentially have an effect on airway smooth muscle include benzalkonium chloride (BAC), ethylenediamine tetraacetic acid (EDTA), and hydrochloric or sulfuric acid to adjust pH of the solution. Asmus and colleagues[63] recommend that only additive-free, sterile-filled unit dose bronchodilator solutions be used for nebulizer treatment of acute airflow obstruction, especially if doses are given hourly or continuously. Clinicians should check aerosol formulations for BAC or EDTA, and if symptoms of bronchoconstriction occur, consider these as a possible cause.

THE β AGONIST CONTROVERSY

The *asthma paradox* is a descriptive phrase for the increasing incidence of asthma morbidity and especially asthma mortality despite advances in the understanding of asthma and availability of improved drugs to treat asthma. Several events and studies have implicated use of β agonists as a potential culprit. These are noted, with analysis based on the literature.

- In the mid-1960s, Speizer and associates[64] reported an increase in deaths among patients with asthma and chronic bronchitis in countries including England, New Zealand, Australia, and Norway, where a high-dose formulation of isoproterenol, termed isoprenaline-forte, was available. Removal of the formulation was followed by a decrease in deaths from asthma. Isoprenaline-forte had a concentration two to eight times greater than standard isoprenaline (isoproterenol) in other countries. Other countries (United States, Canada, Germany) did not show the same mortality increase.[55]

- Asthma mortality again increased in the 1970s in New Zealand,[65] and a series of three case-control studies found an increased risk of asthma deaths in patients who were prescribed inhaled fenoterol (an adrenergic bronchodilator not available in the United States) but not other asthma medications such as albuterol.[66-68] However, a later study by Haas and colleagues[69] found no correlation between asthma mortality in New Zealand and inhaled β₂ agonist use with fenoterol and albuterol for the years 1970 to 1989. Yet, similar to the experience with isoprenaline-forte, the asthma mortality rate fell with warnings and restriction of fenoterol in New Zealand.[55] Isoproterenol and fenoterol both have greater β-receptor intrinsic activity and *less* β₂-selectivity than other β agonists such as albuterol and terbutaline. This high in-

trinsic activity was associated with worsening of asthma severity and does not necessarily generalize to other β agonists.[55]

- A Canadian case-control study by Spitzer and associates[70] published in 1992 reported an association between the use of β₂-agonist bronchodilators and asthma mortality. Use of two or more canisters per month of fenoterol or albuterol was linked to an increased risk of death. Both the case-control study and a subsequent cohort study found that prescription of high-dose fenoterol was associated with an increased risk of death compared with use of albuterol.[55,71] Whether the increased use of β agonists is simply a marker for increased asthma severity and therefore risk or whether β agonists are causing an adverse reaction is not resolved by these data.

- In 1990, Sears and colleagues[72] published data suggesting that intermittent rather than regular use of fenoterol was superior in controlling asthma and that regular use may even lead to a worsening of asthma. In contrast, a National Institutes of Health (NIH) study in patients with mild asthma found neither benefit nor detriment with use of regular inhaled albuterol.[73] Again, the difference in intrinsic activity of fenoterol compared with other β agonists may be related to the worsening of asthma in Sears' study.

CONCLUSION

Short-acting drugs, such as albuterol, and long-acting agents, such as salmeterol, have not in general been associated with a significant worsening of asthma.[74] The evidence indicates that regular use of *fenoterol* and *isoproterenol*, but not other β agonists, may lead to worsening asthma control.[55] Tolerance to the bronchodilator effect does occur, although this stabilizes and does not progress. There is an increase in bronchial hyperreactivity after institution of regular β-agonist therapy, which is not well explained. There is currently evidence to suggest that this effect may be caused or enhanced by the S-enantiomer of β agonists, which has a range of proinflammatory effects.

ASTHMA MORBIDITY AND MORTALITY

A complete analysis of the relation between β-agonists and worsening asthma based on the literature seems to indicate that there is *not* a class effect of these drugs causing deterioration of asthma.[55] Although it is not clear that β-agonist use increases risk of morbidity or death from asthma, asthma mortality is reported to be rising in the United States and worldwide, despite more available treatment options, including β_2-specific and longer-acting adrenergic bronchodilators.[75] There are several causes, not all involving β-agonist therapy, that may potentially lead to worsening asthma severity.

- Use of β agonists may allow allergic individuals to expose themselves to allergens and stimuli, with no immediate symptoms to warn them, but with development of progressive airway inflammation and increasing bronchial hyperresponsiveness.
- Repeated self-administration of β agonists gives temporary relief of asthma symptoms through bronchodilation, which may cause underestimation of severity and delay in seeking medical help. The β agonists do not block progressive airway inflammation, which can lead to death from lethal airway obstruction and hypoxia.
- Insufficient use, through poor patient education, poor patient compliance, or both, of antiinflammatory therapy with the use of β agonists, to control the basic inflammatory nature of asthma, while β agonists target the symptoms of wheezing and resistance.
- Accumulation of the S-isomer with racemic β agonists could exert a detrimental effect on asthma control.
- There is increased airway irritation with environmental pollution and lifestyle changes.[76]

Discussion of the relation of β agonist use to asthma morbidity and mortality should review the use of β agonists in the context of the National Asthma Education and Prevention Program guidelines. Both the 1991 and the 1997 documents stress that asthma is a disease of chronic airway inflammation. Treatment with regular β-agonist therapy in severe asthma (asthma of step 2 or greater severity) does not address the underlying inflammatory process. In evaluating β-agonist therapy in asthma, one must evaluate concomitant antiinflammatory therapy (or the lack of it), as well as environmental management of the asthma.

RESPIRATORY CARE ASSESSMENT OF β-AGONIST THERAPY

- Assess effectiveness of drug therapy based on the indication(s) for the aerosol agent: Presence of reversible airflow resulting from primary bronchospasm or obstruction secondary to an inflammatory response or secretions, either acute or chronic.
- Monitor flow rates using bedside peak flow meters, portable spirometry, or laboratory reports of pulmonary function before and after bronchodilator studies, to assess reversibility of airflow obstruction.
- Perform respiratory assessment: Breathing rate and pattern, and breath sounds by auscultation, before and after treatment.
- Assess pulse before, during, and after treatment.
- Assess patient's subjective reaction to treatment, for any change in breathing effort or pattern.
- Assess arterial blood gases or pulse oximeter saturation, as needed, for acute states with asthma or COPD, to monitor changes in ventilation and gas exchange (oxygenation).
- Note effect of β agonists on blood glucose (increase) and K^+ (decrease) laboratory values, if high doses, such as with continuous nebulization or emergency department treatment, are used.
- Long term: Monitor pulmonary function studies of lung volumes, capacities, and flows.
- Instruct asthmatic patients in use and interpretation of disposable peak flow meters to assess severity of asthmatic episodes and ensure there is an action plan for treatment modification.
- Patient education should emphasize that β agonists do not treat underlying inflammation nor prevent progression of asthma, and additional antiinflammatory treatment or more aggressive medical therapy may be needed if there is a poor response to the rescue β agonist.
- Instruct and then verify correct use of aerosol delivery device (SVN, MDI, reservoir, DPI).
- Instruct patients in use, assembly, and especially cleaning of aerosol inhalation devices.

For long-acting β agonists:

- Assess ongoing lung function, including predose FEV_1 over time and variability in peak expiratory flows.
- Assess amount of rescue β agonist use and nocturnal symptoms.
- Assess number of exacerbations, unscheduled clinic visits, and hospitalizations.
- Assess days of absence resulting from symptoms.
- Assess ability to reduce the dose of concomitant inhaled corticosteroids.

SUMMARY KEY TERMS AND CONCEPTS

- The adrenergic bronchodilator group is indicated for the treatment of reversible airway obstruction in diseases such as asthma and COPD. These agents produce bronchodilation by stimulating β_2 receptors on airway smooth muscle.
- The *structure-activity relations* of the *catecholamines* such as isoproterenol are reviewed. Their short duration of action is due to metabolism by the enzyme COMT; β_2-specificity is considered to be due to side chain bulk *(keyhole theory)*.
- Modification of the catecholamine structure produces *noncatecholamines* such as metaproterenol, albuterol, and terbutaline, which have a 4- to 6-hour duration and are β_2-preferential.
- *Salmeterol* and *formoterol* represent a long-acting agonist, with 12-hour duration resulting from their unique pharmacodynamics (drug-receptor interaction).
- Routes of administration for β agonists can include inhaled aerosol, oral, or parenteral, with minimal side effects seen with inhalation.
- Adverse side effects can occur with β agonists and include tremor (very common), headache, insomnia, bronchospasm with MDI use, palpitations, and some tolerance.
- The β agonists have been questioned as a possible factor in the increase in asthma mortality, leading to the "β agonist controversy."

SELF-ASSESSMENT QUESTIONS

1. Identify three adrenergic bronchodilators used clinically that are catecholamines.
2. Which of the catecholamine bronchodilators given by aerosol is β_2-specific?
3. What is the duration of action of the catecholamine bronchodilators?
4. Identify two advantages introduced with the modifications of the catecholamine structure in adrenergic bronchodilators.
5. Identify the usual dose by aerosol for an SVN for metaproterenol and albuterol.
6. What is an extremely common side effect with β_2-adrenergic bronchodilators?
7. Identify the approximate duration of action for isoetharine, pirbuterol, and salmeterol.
8. Identify the generic drug for each of the following brand names: Alupent, Tornalate, Maxair, Serevent, Brethaire, Ventolin.
9. Which route of administration is more likely to have greater severity of side effects with a β agonist, oral or inhaled aerosol?
10. You notice a pinkish tinge to aerosol rain-out in the large-bore tubing connecting a patient's mouthpiece to a nebulizer after a treatment with racemic epinephrine; what has caused this?
11. A patient exhibits paradoxical bronchoconstriction from the Freon propellant when using his albuterol by MDI. Suggest an alternative for the patient.
12. If you are working with an asthmatic with occasional symptoms of wheezing and chest tightness, which respond well to an inhaled β agonist, would you suggest using salmeterol?
13. Suggest a β agonist that would be appropriate for the patient in question 12.

Answers to Self-Assessment Questions are found in Appendix A.

CLINICAL SCENARIO

A 24-year-old white male moved to the metropolitan Atlanta area in Fall of the previous year. He presents to your outpatient clinic with a complaint of difficulty in breathing. He has no history of asthma or other previous pulmonary disease. He is an accountant with a medium-size firm. He noticed a few "chest colds" from October through January, but these resolved with over-the-counter cold medications such as decongestants and cough suppressants. It is now late May, and during a golf game he had difficulty breathing. He described a tightness in his chest and the sound of wheezing on interview. The course had recently been mown. The pollen count was quite high at the time, and there was an increased ozone concentration, leading to a smog alert on the day of his game. He also complained of waking up several times during the night with mild shortness of breath.

His RR is 14 breaths/min, with no obvious distress at rest; BP is 128/74 mm Hg; HR is 76 beats/min; and T is within normal limits. His SpO_2 is 93% on room air. On auscultation you detect mild expiratory wheezing bilaterally.

How could you assess the presence of airflow obstruction in this patient?
Given his symptoms, your physical findings, and a reduced peak flow, would you recommend a β agonist?
If you recommend a bronchodilator, suggest an appropriate agent.
How could you assess his response to a β-agonist bronchodilator?
At this point, suggest a β agonist to prescribe for his use at home or work when he leaves the clinic.
What type of instructions and follow-up would you suggest for this patient?

Answers to Clinical Scenario Questions are found in Appendix A.

REFERENCES

1. Weinberger MM: Use of ephedrine in bronchodilator therapy, *Ped Clin North Am* 22:121, 1975.
2. Aranson R, Rau JL: The evolution of beta-agonists, *Respir Care Clin North Am* 5:479, 1999.
3. Rau JL: Inhaled adrenergic bronchodilators: historical development and clinical application, *Respir Care* 45:854, 2000.
4. National Asthma Education and Prevention Program, Expert Panel Report II: *Guidelines for the diagnosis and management of asthma*, Bethesda, Md, 1997, National Institutes of Health.
5. Patterson JW and others: Isoprenaline resistance and the use of pressurized aerosols in asthma, *Lancet* 2:426, 1968.
6. Richards DM, Brogden RN: Pirbuterol: a preliminary review of its pharmacological properties and therapeutic efficacy in reversible bronchospastic disease, *Drugs* 30:7, 1985.
7. Orgel HA and others: Bitolterol and albuterol metered-dose aerosols: comparison of two long-acting beta-2 adrenergic bronchodilators for treatment of asthma, *J Allergy Clin Immunol* 75:55, 1985.
8. Mitra S and others: (S)-Albuterol increases intracellular free calcium by muscarinic receptor activation and a phospholipase C-dependent mechanism in airway smooth muscle, *Molec Pharmacol* 53:347, 1998.
9. Lipworth BJ and others: Pharmacokinetics and extrapulmonary β_2 adrenoceptor activity of nebulised racemic salbutamol and its R and S isomers in healthy volunteers, *Thorax* 52:849, 1997.
10. Johansson FJ and others: Effects of albuterol enantiomers on in vitro bronchial reactivity, *Clin Rev Allergy Immunol* 14:57, 1996.
11. Templeton AGB and others: Effects of S-salbutamol on human isolated bronchus, *Pulmon Pharm Ther* 11:1, 1998.
12. Volcheck GW, Gleich GJ, Kita H: Pro- and anti-inflammatory effects of beta adrenergic agonists on eosinophil response to IL-5, *J Allergy Clin Immunol* 101:S35, 1998.
13. Schmekel B and others: Stereoselective pharmacokinetics of S-salbutamol after administration of the racemate in healthy volunteers, *Eur Respir J* 13:1230, 1999.
14. Dhand R and others: Preferential pulmonary retention of (S)-albuterol after inhalation of racemic albuterol, *Am J Respir Crit Care Med* 160:1136, 1999.
15. Nelson HS and others: Improved bronchodilation with levalbuterol compared with racemic albuterol in patients with asthma, *J Allergy Clin Immunol* 102:943, 1998.
16. Rau JL: Introduction of a single isomer beta agonist, *Respir Care* 45:962, 2000.
17. Johnson M and others: The pharmacology of salmeterol, *Life Sci* 52:2131, 1993.
18. Kemp JP, Bierman CW, Cocchetto DM: Dose-response study of inhaled salmeterol in asthmatic patients with 24-hour spirometry and Holter monitoring, *Ann Allergy* 70:316, 1993.
19. Boyd G, Anderson K, Carter R: Placebo controlled comparison of the bronchodilator performance of salmeterol and salbutamol over 12 hours, *Thorax* 45:340P, 1990.
20. Moore RH, Khan A, Dickey BF: Long-acting inhaled β_2-agonists in asthma therapy, *Chest* 113:1095, 1998.
21. Brogden RN, Faulds D: Salmeterol xinafoate: a review of its pharmacological properties and therapeutic potential in reversible obstructive airways disease, *Drug Eval* 42:895, 1991.
22. Bartow RA, Brogden RN: Formoterol: an update of its pharmacological properties and therapeutic efficacy in the management of asthma, *Drugs* 56:303, 1998.
23. Vaickus L, Claus R: (R,R)-Formoterol: rapid onset and 24 hour duration of response after a single dose, *Am J Respir Crit Care Med* 161:A191, 2000.
24. van Noord JA and others: Salmeterol versus formoterol in patients with moderately severe asthma: dose and duration of action, *Eur Respir J* 9:1684, 1996.
25. Politiek MJ, Boorsma M, Aalbers R: Comparison of formoterol, salbutamol and salmeterol in methacholine-induced severe bronchoconstriction, *Eur Respir J* 13:988, 1999.
26. Anderson GP: Interactions between corticosteroids and β-adrenergic agonists in asthma disease induction, progression, and exacerbation, *Am J Respir Crit Care Med* 161:S188, 2000.
27. Shapiro G and others: Combined salmeterol 50 μg and fluticasone propionate 250 μg in the Diskus device for the treatment of asthma, *Am J Respir Crit Care Med* 161:527, 2000.
28. Pearlman DS and others: A comparison of salmeterol with albuterol in the treatment of mild-to-moderate asthma, *N Engl J Med* 327:1420, 1992.
29. Mahler DA and others: Efficacy of salmeterol xinafoate in the treatment of COPD, *Chest* 115:957, 1999.
30. McFadden ER Jr: Clinical use of β-adrenergic agonists, *J Allergy Clin Immunol* 76:352, 1985.
31. Robertson C, Levison H: Bronchodilators in asthma, *Chest* 87:64S, 1985.
32. Tinkelman DG and others: Comparison of nebulized terbutaline and subcutaneous epinephrine in the treatment of acute asthma, *Ann Allergy* 50:398, 1983.
33. Fernandez E: Beta-adrenergic agonists, *Semin Respir Med* 8:353, 1987.
34. Fink J, Dhand R: Bronchodilator resuscitation in the emergency department. II, Dosing strategies, *Resp Care* 45:497, 2000.
35. Lin RY and others: Continuous versus intermittent albuterol nebulization in the treatment of acute asthma, *Ann Emerg Med* 22:1847, 1993.
36. Shrestha M and others: Continuous vs intermittent albuterol, at high and low doses, in the treatment of severe acute asthma in adults, *Chest* 110:42, 1996.
37. Moler F, Hurwitz M, Custer J: Improvement of clinical asthma scores and Paco$_2$ in children with severe asthma treated with continuously nebulized terbutaline, *J Allergy Clin Immunol* 81:1101, 1988.

38. Portnoy J and others: Continuous nebulization for status asthmaticus, *Ann Allergy* 69:71, 1992.

39. Popa V: Beta-adrenergic drugs, *Clin Chest Med* 7:313, 1986.

40. Leifer KN, Wittig HJ: The beta-2 sympathomimetic aerosols in the treatment of asthma, *Ann Allergy* 35:69, 1975.

41. Shim C: Adrenergic agonists and bronchodilator aerosol therapy in asthma, *Clin Chest Med* 5:659, 1984.

42. Popa V: Clinical pharmacology of adrenergic drugs, *J Asthma* 21:183, 1984.

43. Larsson S, Svedmyr N: Studies of muscle tremor induced by beta-adrenostimulating drugs, *Scand J Respir Dis* 88(suppl):54, 1974.

44. Marsden CD and others: Peripheral beta-adrenergic receptors concerned with tremor, *Clin Sci* 33:53, 1967.

45. Brown JE, McLeod AA, Shand DG: Evidence for cardiac adrenoreceptors in man, *Clin Pharmacol Ther* 33:424, 1983.

46. Seider N, Abinader EG, Oliven A: Cardiac arrhythmias after inhaled bronchodilators in patients with COPD and ischemic heart disease, *Chest* 104:1070, 1993.

47. Jenne JW: Beta2-adrenergic receptor-agonist interaction. In Leff AR, ed: *Pulmonary and critical care pharmacology and therapeutics*, New York, 1996, McGraw-Hill.

48. Avner BP, Jenne JW: Desensitization of isolated human bronchial smooth muscle to beta receptor agonists, *J Allergy Clin Immunol* 68:51, 1981.

49. Svedmyr N: Action of corticosteroids on beta-adrenergic receptors: clinical aspects, *Am Rev Respir Dis* 141:S31, 1990.

50. Ahrens RC and others: Use of bronchial provocation with histamine to compare the pharmacodynamics of inhaled albuterol and metaproterenol in patients with asthma, *J Allergy Clin Immunol* 79:876, 1987.

51. O'Connor BJ, Aikman SL, Barnes PJ: Tolerance to the non-bronchodilator effects of inhaled β2-agonists in asthma, *N Engl J Med* 327:1204, 1992.

52. Bhagat R and others: Rapid onset of tolerance to the bronchoprotective effect of salmeterol, *Chest* 105:1235, 1995.

53. Kalra S and others: Inhaled corticosteroids do not prevent the development of tolerance to the bronchoprotective effect of salmeterol, *Chest* 109:953, 1996.

54. Rosenthal RR and others: Effect of long-term salmeterol therapy compared with as-needed albuterol use on airway hyperresponsiveness, *Chest* 116:595, 1999.

55. Beasley R and others: β-Agonists: what is the evidence that their use increases the risk of asthma morbidity and mortality? *J Allergy Clin Immunol* 103:S18, 1999.

56. Khoukaz G, Gross NJ: Effects of salmeterol on arterial blood gases in patients with stable chronic obstructive pulmonary disease: comparison with albuterol and ipratropium, *Am J Respir Crit Care Med* 160:1028, 1999.

57. Hales CA, Kazemi H: Hypoxic vascular response of the lung: effect of aminophylline and epinephrine, *Am Rev Respir Dis* 110:126, 1974.

58. Chick TW, et al: Effects of bronchodilators on the distribution of ventilation and perfusion in asthma, *Chest* 63:11S, 1973.

59. Sharp JT: Workshop No. 2: bronchodilator therapy and arterial blood gases, *Chest* 73(suppl):980, 1978.

60. Kung M: Parenteral adrenergic bronchodilators and potassium, *Chest* 89:322, 1986.

61. Yarbrough J, Mansfield LE, Ting S: Metered dose inhaler induced bronchospasm in asthmatic patients, *Ann Allergy* 55:25, 1985.

62. Cocchetto DM, Sykes RS, Spector S: Paradoxical bronchospasm after use of inhalation aerosols: a review of the literature, *J Asthma* 28:49, 1991.

63. Asmus MJ, Sherman J, Hendeles L: Bronchoconstrictor additives in bronchodilator solutions, *J Allergy Clin Immunol* 104:S53, 1999.

64. Speizer FE and others: Investigation into use of drugs preceding death from asthma, *Br Med J* 1:339, 1968.

65. Jackson R and others: International trends in asthma mortality: 1970-1985, *Chest* 94:914, 1988.

66. Crane J and others: Prescribed fenoterol and death from asthma in New Zealand, 1981-1983: case-control study. *Lancet* 1:917, 1989.

67. Pearce N and others: Case-control study of prescribed fenoterol and death from asthma in New Zealand 1977-81, *Thorax* 45:170, 1990.

68. Granger J and others: Prescribed fenoterol and death from asthma in New Zealand, 1981-1987: a further case-control study, *Thorax* 46:105, 1991.

69. Haas JF, Staudinger HW, Schuijt C: Asthma deaths in New Zealand, *Br Med J* 304:1634, 1992.

70. Spitzer WO and others: The use of β-agonists and the risk of death and near death from asthma, *N Engl J Med* 326:501, 1992.

71. Suissa S and others: A cohort analysis of excess mortality in asthma and the use of inhaled beta agonists, *Am J Respir Crit Care Med* 149:604, 1994.

72. Sears MR and others: Regular inhaled beta-agonist treatment in bronchial asthma, *Lancet* 336:1391, 1990.

73. Drazen JM and others: Comparison of regularly scheduled with as-needed use of albuterol in mild asthma, *N Engl J Med* 335:841, 1996.

74. Williams C and othersl: A case-control study of salmeterol and near fatal attacks of asthma, *Thorax* 53:7, 1998.

75. Sears MR: Worldwide trends in asthma mortality, *Bull Int Union Tuberc Lung Dis* 66:79, 1991.

76. Platts-Mills TAE and others: Changing concepts of allergic disease: the attempt to keep up with real changes in lifetyles, *J Allergy Clin Immunol* 98:S297, 1996.

CHAPTER 7

Anticholinergic (Parasympatholytic) Bronchodilators

Joseph L. Rau

*C*hapter 7 discusses a second class of bronchodilators, the anticholinergic agents. Anticholinergic drugs given by inhaled aerosol can block cholinergic-induced airway constriction. Their mode of action is reviewed along with their pharmacologic effects, based on their structural differences. Specific agents are profiled, and their clinical effect in chronic obstructive pulmonary disease (COPD) and asthma is discussed.

HISTORY AND DEVELOPMENT

The prototype anticholinergic (parasympatholytic) agent is atropine, which is an alkaloid found naturally in the plants *Atropa belladonna* (the nightshade plant) and *Datura* species (*D. stramonium, D. metel*, and *D. innoxa*). Scopolamine (hyoscine) is also extracted from the belladonna plant, and both atropine and scopolamine are therefore referred to as *belladonna alkaloids*.

There is evidence that these alkaloid ingredients have been ingested in one form or another for thousands of years for their effects on the central nervous system. An excellent historical review of these agents is given by Gandevia.[1] Of interest for respiratory care is the fact that fumes from burning the *Datura* species of plants were inhaled as a treatment for respiratory disorders as early as the seventeenth century in India.

The earliest documentation of this is in the Ayurvedic literature, in which *Datura* is mentioned specifically for asthma or for cough with dyspnea. By 1802, inhalation of *Datura* fumes to treat asthma had reached Britain, brought from India by British medical officers. In the mid-nineteenth century, inhalational therapy with alkaloids was advocated in America. Cigars, cigarettes, and pipes of various design were employed to smoke a preparation of *Datura* leaves. In Australia, severe patients were placed inside a tent of sheets, inside of which stramonium leaves were burned.

Even aerosols of liquid with *Datura* were noted in the nineteenth century, and the respiratory route for delivery of medications began to be appreciated. A variety of inhalational devices appeared for delivering liquids and gases, far predating the incorporation of respiratory therapy as a profession. In 1833, the alkaloid daturine was identified as atropine by Geiger and Hesse. Controversy surrounded the inhalational use of parasympatholytic agents. Many physicians attacked their use in Britain and America in the nineteenth century as quackery, but use of *Datura* was widely accepted by patients who often obtained the ingredient without their physician's knowledge. Physician disagreement on the use of *Datura* probably rested on several issues: (1) difficulty in accurate dosage with smoking or aerosol therapy (a familiar contention); (2) irritant effects of smoke especially when other ingredients were added to the *Datura*; and (3), probably most of all, confusion over diagnosing and clinically differentiating asthma, bronchitis, emphysema, occupational diseases, and mediastinal gland dysfunction in the nineteenth and early twentieth centuries. The last factor led to inappropriate use of the *Datura* alkaloids.

By the 1930s, adrenaline and ephedrine, both sympathomimetics, had been introduced and had largely replaced stramonium and belladonna extracts for treatment of asthma. However, parasympatholytic (anticholinergic) agents never completely disappeared in treatment of asthma and other obstructive diseases. Anticholinergics were used as an adjunct to the β-adrenergic drugs, and in the 1980s, interest in anticholinergic drugs was renewed, based on two factors: (1) new understanding of the role of the parasympathetic system in airway obstruction, and (2) introduction of atropine derivatives with fewer obnoxious side effects. In 1987, ipratropium bromide, previously known by the code name SCH 1000, was released in the United States as an aerosol with the brand name Atrovent. A long-acting anticholinergic bronchodilator, tiotropium, with a duration of action up to 24 hours after a single inhaled dose, is under investigation. Anticholinergic bronchodilators have been recently reviewed by Witek.[2]

CLINICAL INDICATION FOR USE

A summary of recommendations and guidelines for use of anticholinergic (antimuscarinic) bronchodilators in treatment of COPD and asthma can be found in Appendix D.

INDICATION FOR ANTICHOLINERGIC BRONCHODILATOR

Ipratropium or other anticholinergic agents are indicated as a bronchodilator for maintenance treatment in COPD, including chronic bronchitis and emphysema.

INDICATION FOR COMBINED ANTICHOLINERGIC AND β-AGONIST BRONCHODILATORS

A combination anticholinergic and β agonist, such as ipratropium and albuterol (Combivent), is indicated for use in patients with COPD on regular treatment who require additional bronchodilation for relief of airflow obstruction.

Ipratropium is also commonly used in severe asthma in addition to β agonists, especially in acute bronchoconstriction that does not respond well to β-agonist therapy.

ANTICHOLINERGIC NASAL SPRAY

A nasal spray formulation is indicated for symptomatic relief of allergic and nonallergic perennial rhinitis and the common cold.

SPECIFIC ANTICHOLINERGIC (PARASYMPATHOLYTIC) AGENTS

Parasympatholytic (anticholinergic, or antimuscarinic) agents that have been given by aerosol include atropine sulfate, ipratropium, a combination of ipratropium and albuterol, glycopyrrolate, oxitropium (outside the United States at this time), and the investigational drug tiotropium. Dose and administration for each agent are given in Table 7-1.

Atropine sulfate has been administered as a nebulized solution, using either the injectable solution or preferably solutions marketed for aerosolization, such as Dey-Dose. Both duration of bronchodilation and the incidence of side effects are dose dependent. Dosages for children based on dose-response curves have been given as 0.05 mg/kg three or four times daily.[3] Dosages for adults are based on a schedule of 0.025 mg/kg three or four times daily.[4] Although greater bronchodilation and duration are seen with dosage schedules of 0.05 or 0.1 mg/kg for adults, the side effects of dry mouth, blurred vision, and tachycardia become unacceptable. Because it is a tertiary ammonium compound and not fully ionized, atropine is readily absorbed from the gastrointestinal tract and respiratory mucosa. Systemic side effects (which are discussed subsequently) are seen in doses required for effective bronchodilation when given as an inhaled aerosol. The drug is not recommended for inhalation as a bronchodilator because of its widespread distribution in the body and the availability of the approved agent ipratropium.

Ipratropium bromide (Atrovent) is a nonselective antagonist of M_1, M_2, and M_3 receptors. Ipratropium is currently available in two formulations for bronchodilator use: an MDI with 18 μg/puff, and a nebulizer solution of 0.02% concentration in a 2.5-ml vial, giving a 500 μg dose per treatment. This agent is an *N*-isopropyl derivative of atropine. As a quaternary ammonium derivative of atropine, ipratropium is fully ionized and does not distribute well across lipid membranes, limiting its distribution more to the lung when inhaled. Ipratropium is approved specifically for the maintenance treatment of airflow obstruction in COPD.

Table 7-1

Inhaled anticholinergic bronchodilator agents*

DRUG	BRAND NAME	ADULT DOSAGE	TIME COURSE (ONSET, PEAK, DURATION)
Ipratropium bromide	Atrovent	MDI: 18 μg/puff, 2 puffs qid SVN: 0.02% solution (0.2 mg/ml), 500 μg tid, qid Nasal spray: 0.03%, 0.06%; 2 sprays per nostril 2 to 4 times daily (dosage varies)	*Onset:* 15 min *Peak:* 1-2 hr *Duration:* 4-6 hr
Ipratropium bromide and albuterol	Combivent	MDI: ipratropium 18 μg/puff and albuterol 90 μg/puff, 2 puffs qid	*Onset:* 15 min *Peak:* 1-2 hr *Duration:* 4-6 hr
	DuoNeb	SVN: ipratropium 0.5 mg and albuterol 3.0 mg (equal to 2.5 mg albuterol base)	
Oxitropium bromide†		MDI: 100 μg/puff , 2 puffs bid, tid	*Onset:* 15 min *Peak:* 1-2 hr *Duration:* 8 hr
Tiotropium bromide‡	Spiriva	DPI: 18 μg/inhalation, 1 inhalation daily	*Onset:* 30 min *Peak:* 3 hr *Duration:* 24 hr

*Ipratropium bromide is the only agent currently approved for use in the United States as an inhaled bronchodilator. A holding chamber is recommended with MDI administration to prevent accidental eye exposure.
†Available outside the United States.
‡Investigational.
DPI, Dry powder inhaler; *MDI,* metered dose inhaler; *SVN,* small volume nebulizer.

Ipratropium is poorly absorbed into the circulation from either the nasal mucosa when given by nasal spray or from the airway when inhaled orally by aerosol. Approximately 20% of the nasal dose and the MDI dose is absorbed, with only 2% of the larger nebulizer solution absorbed into the bloodstream. Ipratropium is partially metabolized by ester hydrolysis to inactive products. It is minimally bound to plasma proteins such as albumin (<9%), and the elimination half-life is around 1.6 hours.

The profile of clinical effect for ipratropium differs from inhaled β-adrenergic agonists. The onset of bronchodilation begins within minutes but proceeds more slowly to a peak effect 1 to 2 hours after inhalation. The β-agonists can peak between 20 to 30 minutes depending on the agent. In asthma, the duration of bronchodilator effect is about the same for ipratropium as for β agonists. However, in COPD the duration is longer by 1 to 2 hours.[5]

Ipratropium bromide (Atrovent Nasal Spray) is also available for treatment of rhinopathies and rhinorrhea, including nonallergic perennial rhinitis, viral infectious rhinitis (colds), and allergic rhinitis, if intranasal corticosteroids fail to control symptoms.[6] The nasal spray is available in two strengths, with a 0.03% solution delivering 21 μg/spray, and the 0.06% solution delivering 42 μg/spray. The 0.03% strength is given as two sprays per nostril two or three times daily, and the 0.06% strength is given as two sprays per nostril, three or four times daily. Optimal dosage varies. Intranasal ipratropium has been shown to significantly reduce the volume of nasal secretions and symptoms in both patients with allergic rhinitis and those with nonallergic rhinitis.[6] Side effects with the nasal spray are largely local and have included nasal dryness, itching, and epistaxis in a few patients. Dry mouth and dry throat have also occurred. Systemic symptoms such as blurred vision or urinary hesitancy are rare.

Ipratropium and albuterol (Combivent) is a combination MDI product, with the usual doses of each agent (18 μg/puff of ipratropium, 90 μg/puff of albuterol). The combination therapy has been shown to be more effective in stable COPD than either agent alone.[7] A combination product of ipratropium (0.04

mg per puff) and fenoterol (0.1 mg per puff) is marketed in Great Britain as Duovent, to provide the additive effective of anticholinergic and β-adrenergic activity.

Glycopyrrolate is a quaternary ammonium derivative of atropine that, like ipratropium, does not distribute well across lipid membranes in the body. It is usually administered parenterally as an antimuscarinic agent during reversal of neuromuscular blockade, as an alternative to atropine, with fewer ocular or central nervous system side effects. The injectable solution has been nebulized in a 1 mg dose for bronchodilation. Gal and colleagues[8] reported a comparison of glycopyrrolate with atropine and established dose-response curves. Glycopyrrolate has an onset of action of approximately 15 to 30 minutes, a peak effect of 0.5 to 1 hour, and a duration of approximately 6 hours. Although the injectable formulation of glycopyrrolate is used as a less expensive alternative to the Atrovent brand of ipratropium, it is not approved for inhalation.

Oxitropium bromide (Ba 235) is a quaternary derivative of scopolamine, available outside the United States as an aerosolized anticholinergic bronchodilator in subjects with chronic obstructive airway disease. A 200 μg dose by MDI provided a peak effect on forced expiratory volume in 1 second (FEV_1) within 1 to 2 hours, with a duration of 6 to 8 hours.[9-11] It is considered to be more potent than ipratropium by a ratio of approximately 2:1, with one inhalation of oxitropium equivalent in effect to two inhalations of ipratropium. The onset has also been reported as more rapid than ipratropium.[12] Oxitropium is available as Oxivent in Great Britain in a 200-dose pressurized MDI (pMDI), with 100 μg/puff. The usual dose is 2 actuations two or three times daily. Systemic anticholinergic effects are rare, and side effects include local irritation of the throat and nose, dry mouth, nausea, wheeze, cough, and chest tightness in a small proportion of patients.

Tiotropium bromide (Ba 679 BR; Spiriva) is a muscarinic receptor antagonist that has been investigated as a long-acting bronchodilator. It is a quaternary ammonium compound structurally related to ipratropium. Like ipratropium, tiotropium is poorly absorbed after inhalation. Inhalation of a single dose gives a peak plasma level within 5 minutes, with a rapid decline to very low levels within 1 hour.[2,13] Tiotropium exhibits receptor subtype selectivity for M_1 and M_3 receptors. The drug binds to all three muscarinic receptors (M_1, M_2, and M_3) but dissociates much more slowly than ipratropium from the M_1 and M_3 receptors. This results in a selectivity of action on M_1 and M_3 receptors. Atropine and ipratropium both block all three types of muscarinic receptor. The M_2 receptor is an autoreceptor inhibiting further release of acetylcholine, so that blockade can increase acetylcholine release and may offset the bronchodilating effect of atropine or ipratropium.[13] In patients with COPD, tiotropium gives a bronchodilating effect for up to 24 hours, with adequate dose. The drug also gives a prolonged, dose-dependent protection against inhaled methacholine challenge.[14]

Several studies have examined the bronchodilating effect of different doses of tiotropium, in comparison with both placebo and ipratropium.[14-16] A single dose of 18 μg inhaled once daily from a dry powder inhaler (DPI), the HandiHaler,[17] provided significant bronchodilation for up to 24 hours, with a low side effect profile. An increase of 15% from baseline FEV_1 occurred 30 minutes after inhalation, with a peak effect around 3 hours. By 3 hours after inhalation, improvement in FEV_1 was greater for tiotropium than for ipratropium. After a dose of tiotropium, the trough, or lowest, value for FEV_1 remained above that of ipratropium, because of the prolonged action of tiotropium. Ipratropium had a more rapid onset of action than tiotropium, but after the initial dosing this difference loses relevance because tiotropium maintains a higher level of baseline bronchodilation.

CLINICAL PHARMACOLOGY

STRUCTURE-ACTIVITY RELATIONS

Chemical structures of the two naturally occurring belladonna alkaloids, atropine and scopolamine (also called hyoscine), are illustrated in Figure 7-1. Atropine, including its sulfate (atropine sulfate), and scopolamine are both tertiary ammonium compounds that differ from each other only by an oxygen bridging the carbon-6 and carbon-7 positions. Quaternary ammonium derivatives of atropine include atropine methylnitrate (not available in the United States), ipratropium, and tiotropium. Another quaternary atropine derivative, which has been administered experimentally as a bronchodilator by aerosol, is glycopyrrolate (Robinul) (not shown in Figure 7-1). Oxitropium, an experimental agent, is a quaternary ammonium derivative of scopolamine.

Tertiary ammonium forms such as atropine sulfate or scopolamine are easily absorbed into the bloodstream, distribute throughout the body, and

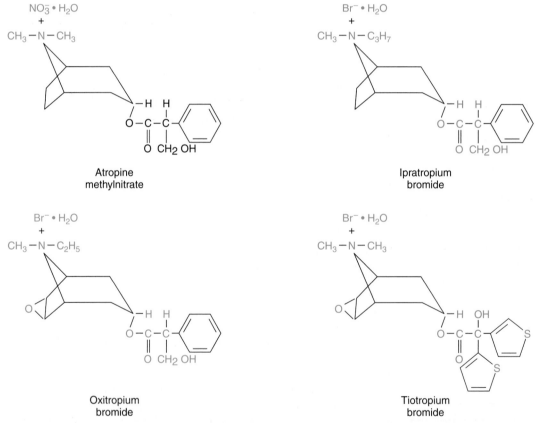

Anticholinergic (Parasympatholytic) Agents
TERTIARY AMMONIUM COMPOUNDS

Atropine

Scopalamine
(Hyoscine)

QUATERNARY AMMONIUM COMPOUNDS

Atropine
methylnitrate

Ipratropium
bromide

Oxitropium
bromide

Tiotropium
bromide

Figure 7-1   Chemical structures of both tertiary compounds such as atropine and scopo-lamine, and quaternary compounds such as ipratropium.

in particular cross the blood-brain barrier to cause central nervous system changes. Quaternary ammonium forms (such as ipratropium, tiotropium, the methylnitrate form of atropine, glycopyrrolate, or oxitropium) are fully ionized and poorly absorbed into the bloodstream or central nervous system. As a result, the systemic side effects seen with aerosol administration of the tertiary ammonium atropine sulfate do not occur or are minimal with a quaternary ammonium such as ipratropium. Generally, quaternary ammonium agents given by inhalation are poorly absorbed from the lung, not rapidly removed from the aerosol deposition site, and do not cross the blood-brain barrier, as atropine sulfate does, giving them a wider therapeutic margin in relation to side effects.

PHARMACOLOGICAL EFFECTS OF ANTICHOLINERGIC (ANTIMUSCARINIC) AGENTS

The general effects of cholinergic (muscarinic) stimulation and the corresponding effects produced by anticholinergic (antimuscarinic) action are listed in Table 7-2. Specific effects differ for tertiary and quaternary ammonium compounds because of their absorption differences as previously outlined for their structure-activity relations. These effects and their differences are summarized in Table 7-3 and discussed below.

Table 7-2

Comparison of cholinergic antagonism (antimuscarinic effects) to cholinergic effects (muscarinic effects)

CHOLINERGIC EFFECT	ANTICHOLINERGIC EFFECT
Decreased heart rate	Increased heart rate
Miosis (contraction of iris, eye)	Mydriasis (pupil dilatation)
Contraction (thickening) of lens, eye	Cycloplegia (lens flattened)
Salivation	Drying of upper airway
Lacrimation	Inhibition of tear formation
Urination	Urinary retention
Defecation	Antidiarrheal or constipation
Secretion of mucus	Mucociliary slowing
Bronchoconstriction	Inhibition of constriction

Table 7-3

Pharmacological effects of tertiary versus quaternary anticholinergic agents given by inhaled aerosol

	TERTIARY (e.g., Atropine)	QUATERNARY (e.g., Ipratropium)
Respiratory tract	Bronchodilation	Bronchodilation
	Decreased mucociliary clearance	Little or no change in mucociliary clearance
	Blocks hypersecretion	Blocks nasal hypersecretion
Central nervous system	Altered CNS function (dose-related)	No effect
Eye	Mydriasis	Usually no effect*
	Cycloplegia	
	Increased intraocular pressure	
Cardiac	Minor slowing of heart rate (small dose); increased heart rate (larger dose)	No effect
Gastrointestinal	Dry mouth, dysphagia; dysphonia slows motility	Dry mouth
Genitourinary	Urinary retention	Usually no effect†

*Assumes aerosol is not sprayed into eye; use with caution in glaucoma.
†Use with caution in prostatic enlargement or urinary retention.
CNS, Central nervous system.

TERTIARY AMMONIUM COMPOUNDS

Tertiary compounds include *atropine sulfate, scopolamine,* and *homatropine.* They are well absorbed across mucosal surfaces and their effects increase with dose. Effects are summarized for these agents for the organ systems.

Respiratory Tract Effects. Atropine sulfate, a prototype tertiary compound, inhibits and reduces mucociliary clearance, as demonstrated by Groth and associates.[18] Atropine seems to block hypersecretion stimulated by cholinergic agonists in both the lower airway and the nose (upper airway) more than the basal secretion.[19] Atropine relaxes airway smooth muscle, the basis for its use in asthma.

Central Nervous System Effects. Tertiary compounds cross the blood-brain barrier and produce dose-related effects. Small doses of 0.5 of 1.0 mg can cause effects that include restlessness, irritability, drowsiness, fatigue or, alternatively, mild excitement. Increased doses can cause disorientation, hallucinations, or coma. Inhaled atropine has been reported to cause an acute psychotic reaction.[20-21]

Eye Effects. Tertiary anticholinergic compounds given by inhalation will distribute through the bloodstream and can affect vision. They block contraction of the iris to cause pupil dilation and paralyze the ciliary muscle of the lens to prevent thickening of the lens for near accommodation, causing blurred vision. These effects can raise intraocular pressure in glaucoma. Atropine-like agents are contraindicated in narrow-angle glaucoma.

Cardiac Effects. Atropine in small doses causes minor slowing of the heart rate; larger doses increase heart rate through vagal blockade.

Gastrointestinal Effects. Anticholinergic agents generally cause dryness of the mouth as a result of inhibition of salivary gland secretions, and atropine is used for this effect to reduce upper airway secretions before surgery and anesthesia or when reversing neuromuscular blockade (see Chapter 18). Larger doses can cause dysphagia and dysphonia. Gastrointestinal motility is slowed, an effect that is the basis for the inclusion of atropine in the brand Lomotil, an antidiarrheal. Inhibition of gastrointestinal motility and emptying has been noted with normal doses of atropine given by aerosol to asthmatics.[22]

Genitourinary Effects. Atropine-like agents can inhibit parasympathetic-controlled relaxation of the urinary sphincter. With prostate gland enlargement this can produce acute urinary retention. Atropine-like drugs can predispose to male impotency, because penile erection is also under parasympathetic control. Ejaculation is a sympathetic function.

QUATERNARY AMMONIUM COMPOUNDS

Quaternary compounds include the approved aerosol agent ipratropium, as well as tiotropium, glycopyrrolate, atropine methylnitrate, and oxitropium. The following effects are discussed primarily for ipratropium, which is well known as an inhaled bronchodilator. In general, quaternary ammonium compounds will not cross lipid membranes easily and therefore do not distribute throughout the body when inhaled. Agents such as ipratropium will produce an anticholinergic effect at the site of delivery. With inhalation this will be the nose or mouth and the upper and lower airway.

Respiratory Tract Effects. Ipratropium has minimal or no effect on mucociliary clearance or mucus viscosity, despite the fact that the aerosol is delivered topically to the airways. The drug does cause bronchodilation by blocking cholinergic contractile action. In the nasal passages, however, ipratropium does reduce hypersecretion, the basis for its use in rhinitis.

Central Nervous System Effects. Because quaternary compounds do not cross the blood-brain barrier, they do not cause CNS effects as the tertiary agents do.

Eye Effects. As long as ipratropium and other quaternary agents are not sprayed directly in the eye, there are no effects on intraocular pressure, pupil size, or lens accommodation when inhaled as an aerosol. Topical delivery to the eye can cause pupillary dilation (mydriasis) and lens paralysis (cycloplegia). Subjects using quaternary ammonium antimuscarinic bronchodilators must be cautioned to protect the eyes from aerosol drug.

Cardiac Effects. Ipratropium has minimal effects on heart rate or blood pressure when given by inhaled aerosol.

Gastrointestinal Effects. There is little effect on gastrointestinal motility with inhaled ipratropium in most patients. However, a portion of the aerosol dose is swallowed, thereby allowing exposure of the gastrointestinal tract to the drug. There has been a report of meconium ileus in an adult cystic fibrosis patient receiving nebulized ipratropium.[23] Use of a reservoir device with MDI administration can reduce oropharyngeal impaction and the amount of swallowed drug.

Genitourinary Effects. Ipratropium has no effect on urinary ability when tested in males 50 to 70 years of age.[24]

MODE OF ACTION

In Chapter 5 the autonomic innervation of the airway was outlined. This consists of the traditional sympathetic and the parasympathetic branches, as well as nonadrenergic, noncholinergic (NANC) inhibitory and excitatory branches.

The sympathetic branch does not actually extend its fibers beyond the peribronchial ganglia or plexa to the airway, although adrenergic receptors are present throughout the airway, especially in the periphery. Parasympathetic nerves do enter the lung at the hila, deriving from the vagus, and travel along the airways. Parasympathetic postganglionic fibers terminate on or near airway epithelium, submucosal mucous glands, smooth muscle, and probably mast cells. Parasympathetic innervation and muscarinic receptors are concentrated in the larger airways, although present from the trachea to the respiratory bronchioles.

In the normal airway a basal level of bronchomotor tone is caused by parasympathetic activity. This basal level of tone can be abolished by anticholinergic agents such as atropine, indicating it is mediated by acetylcholine. Administration of parasympathomimetic (cholinergic) agents such as methacholine (e.g., in bronchial provocation testing) can intensify the level of bronchial tone to the point of constriction in healthy subjects and more so in asthmatic patients.

Cholinergic stimulation of muscarinic receptors on airway smooth muscle and submucosal glands causes contraction and release of mucus. Anticholinergic agents such as atropine or ipratropium are antimuscarinic; they competitively block the action of acetylcholine at parasympathetic postganglionic effector cell receptors. Because of this action, anticholinergic agents block cholinergic-induced bronchoconstriction, as seen in Figure 7-2.

An important point to realize with use of a blocking agent, such as an anticholinergic bronchodilator, is that the effect seen will depend on the degree of tone present that can be blocked. In healthy subjects, there will be minimal airway dilation with an anticholinergic agent because there is only a basal or resting level of tone to be blocked. Variation in the clinical effect of such drugs will be partially due to variation in the degree of parasympathetic activity. One particular mechanism for parasympathetic activity in the lung is vagally mediated reflex bronchoconstriction, which is discussed next.

VAGALLY MEDIATED REFLEX BRONCHOCONSTRICTION

A portion of the bronchoconstriction seen in COPD may be due to a mechanism of vagally mediated reflex innervation of airway smooth muscle (Figure 7-3).

Sensory C-fiber nerves respond to a variety of stimuli, such as irritant aerosols (hypotonic or hypertonic),

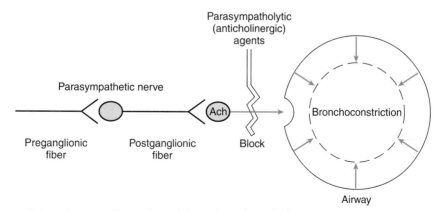

Figure 7-2 Conceptual overview of the action of anticholinergic (parasympatholytic) bronchodilating agents in preventing cholinergic-induced bronchoconstriction. *Ach,* Acetylcholine.

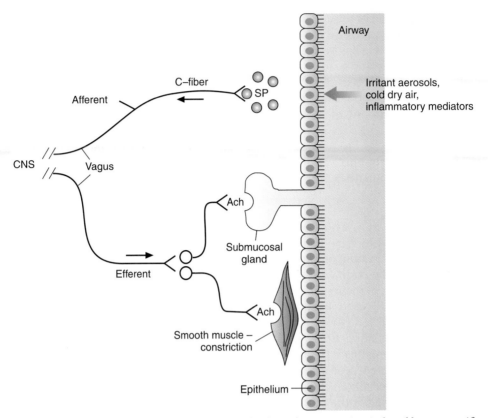

Figure 7-3   Mechanism of vagally mediated reflex bronchoconstriction induced by nonspecific stimuli on sensory C-fibers. *Ach,* Acetylcholine; *CNS,* central nervous system; *SP,* substance P.

cold air and high airflow rates, cigarette smoke, noxious fumes, and mediators of inflammation such as histamine. When activated, they produce an *afferent* nerve impulse to the central nervous system, which results in a reflex cholinergic *efferent* impulse, to cause constriction of airway smooth muscle and release of secretion from mucous glands, as well as cough.

Because atropine or its derivatives are competitive inhibitors of acetylcholine at the neuroeffector junction, such antagonists should block parasympathetic reflex bronchoconstriction. Atropine has been shown to inhibit exercise-induced asthma and psychogenic bronchospasm, as well as bronchoconstriction caused by β-blockade or cholinergic agents. Use of a topical anesthetic such as 4% lidocaine by aerosol to the large airways has also inhibited reflex bronchoconstriction, by blocking the sensory irritant receptors in the epithelial lining.

Changes in the airway may also sensitize the subepithelial cough receptors, making them more responsive to lower thresholds of stimulation. This is often seen during colds that involve lung congestion. Lung inflation during a deep breath stimulates the cough receptors, resulting not only in coughing but also increased bronchomotor tone. It has been suggested that greater bronchial reactivity in asthmatic patients or patients with COPD may be caused by mucosal edema and deformation of airway tissue, which increases the sensitivity of these receptors in response to irritants. Several reviews of cholinergic mechanisms of airway obstruction have been published.[25-29]

MUSCARINIC RECEPTOR SUBTYPES

Anticholinergic agents cause bronchodilation by blocking muscarinic receptor subtypes: M_1 receptors at the parasympathetic ganglia, which facilitate cholinergic neurotransmission and bronchoconstriction, and M_3 receptors on airway smooth muscle, which cause bronchoconstriction. Muscarinic receptor subtypes were reviewed in Chapter 5 and are illustrated for the lung in Figure 7-4. M_1 receptors on the postganglionic parasympathetic neuron facilitate cholinergic nerve transmission, leading to release of acetylcholine. Acetylcholine stimulates M_3 receptor

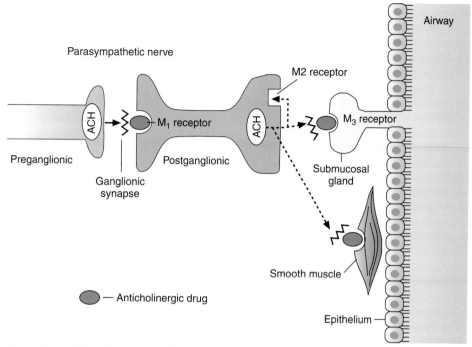

Figure 7-4 Identification and location of muscarinic receptor subtypes M_1, M_2, and M_3 in the vagal nerve, submucosal gland and bronchial smooth muscle in the airway, showing nonspecific blockade by anticholinergic drugs such as ipratropium. *Ach*, Acetylcholine.

subtypes on airway smooth muscle and submucosal glands, causing contraction of smooth muscle and exocytosis of secretion from the mucous gland. The M_2 receptor subtype at cholinergic nerve endings inhibits further acetylcholine release from the postganglionic neuron.

M_3 receptors are G protein–linked receptors, as introduced in Chapter 2 and again in Chapter 5. Table 7-4 lists the various muscarinic receptor subtypes and their G proteins, along with their effector enzymes. Stimulation of the M_3 receptor subtype activates a G_q protein that in turn activates phospholipase C (PLC). Phospholipase C causes the breakdown of phosphoinositides into inositol trisphosphate (IP_3) and diacylglycerol (DAG). This ultimately leads to an increase in the cytoplasmic concentration of free calcium and smooth muscle contraction or gland exocytosis. As shown in Figure 7-5 the competitive blockade of M_3 receptors by anticholinergic agents prevents this sequence. The blockade of M_1 receptor subtypes by anticholinergic agents also inhibits nerve transmission by acetylcholine at the ganglionic synapse. Both ipratropium and tiotropium also block the M_2 receptor. This receptor inhibits continued release of acetyl-

Table 7-4

Muscarinic receptor subtypes: Their G proteins and effector systems

RECEPTOR	G PROTEIN	EFFECTOR
M_1	G_q	Phospholipase C
M_2	G_i	Adenylyl cyclase (decreases)
M_3	G_q	Phospholipase C
M_4	G_i	Adenylyl cyclase (decreases)
M_5	G_q	Phospholipase C leads to an increase

choline. As a result, blockade of the M_2 receptor can enhance acetylcholine release, possibly counteracting the bronchodilator effect of M_3 receptor blockade. As noted in the discussion of ipratropium and tiotropium, tiotropium has selective affinity for M_1 and M_3 receptors because it dissociates much more rapidly from the M_2 receptor and remains bound to the M_1 and M_3 subtypes.

The use of agents such as ipratropium for allergic and nonallergic rhinitis is based on the parasympathetic control of submucosal glands in the nasal

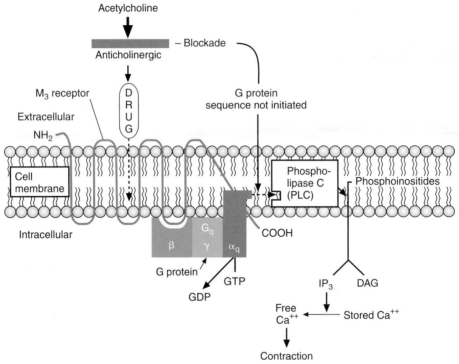

Figure 7-5   Illustration of the M_3 receptor as a G protein–linked receptor, showing the G_q protein; its effector system, phospholipase C; and the mechanism of smooth muscle constriction, which is blocked by an anticholinergic agent preventing stimulation of the M_3 receptor. *DAG*, Diacylglycerol; *IP_3*, inositol trisphosphate; *GDP*, guanosine diphosphate; *GTP*, guanosine triphosphate.

mucosa. Acetylcholine stimulates muscarinic receptors in the nose, where approximately 55% are M_3 and the rest are M_1.[30] M_2 receptors were not identified in human nasal mucosa with an autoradiographic study by Okayama and associates.[31] Blockade of muscarinic M_1 and M_3 receptors on submucosal nasal glands by ipratropium given as a nasal spray prevents gland secretion and rhinitis.

ADVERSE EFFECTS

It has been stated that the safety profile of quaternary ammonium antimuscarinic bronchodilators (e.g., ipratropium or tiotropium) is superior to that of β agonists, particularly with regard to cardiovascular effects.[14] Changes in electrocardiogram, blood pressure, or heart rate are not usually seen. There is no worsening of ventilation-perfusion abnormalities in COPD, which would otherwise cause an increase in hypoxemia. A tolerance to bronchodilation and loss of bronchoprotection have not been observed. The lack of these effects is due to the poor absorption and systemic distribution of quaternary compounds such as

ipratropium. A detailed review of the clinical pharmacology and toxicology of ipratropium is provided by Cugell and colleagues.[32]

The side effects seen with the MDI and SVN formulations of ipratropium, the agent with the most clinical experience, are primarily related to the local, topical delivery to the upper and lower airway with inhalation. Similar side effects would be expected with other antimuscarinic agents such as tiotropium or oxitropium. The most common side effect seen with this class of bronchodilator is dry mouth. Possible side effects are listed in Box 7-1. The SVN solution has also been associated with additional side effects in a few patients: pharyngitis, dyspnea, flulike symptoms, bronchitis, and upper respiratory infection. It should be noted that the amount of drug in the nebulizer dose is over 10 times greater than in the MDI dose (500 μg versus 40 μg). If the patient receives approximately 10% of an inhaled aerosol to the lung, a much larger dose is given with an SVN. The orally swallowed portion will be proportionately higher also. Systemic side effects such as tachycardia, palpitations, urinary hesitancy, constipation, blurred vision, or in-

Box 7-1 Side Effects Seen With Anticholinergic Aerosol Ipratropium*

MDI and SVN (common)
Dry mouth
Cough

MDI (occasional)
Nervousness
Irritation
Dizziness
Headache
Palpitation
Rash

SVN
Pharyngitis
Dyspnea
Flulike symptoms
Bronchitis
Upper respiratory infections
Nausea
Occasional bronchoconstriction
Eye pain
Urinary retention (<3%)

*Side effects were reported in a small percentage (<1% to 5%) of patients.
Precautions: Use with caution in patients with narrow-angle glaucoma, prostatic hypertrophy, bladder neck obstruction, constipation, bowel obstruction, or tachycardia.
MDI, Metered dose inhaler; *SVN,* small volume nebulizer.

Table 7-5

Comparison of effects for anticholinergic and β-adrenergic bronchodilators

	ANTICHOLINERGIC	β AGONIST
Onset	Slightly slower	Faster
Time to peak effect	Slower	Faster
Duration	Longer	Shorter
Tremor	None	Yes
Fall in Pao_2	None	Yes
Tolerance	None	Yes
Site of action	Larger, central airways	Central and peripheral airways

creased ocular pressure are less likely with quaternary agents such as ipratropium or tiotropium than with tertiary agents such as atropine. Although ipratropium is not contraindicated in subjects with prostatic hypertrophy, urinary retention, or glaucoma, the drug should be used with caution and adequate evaluation for possible systemic side effects in these subjects.

The eye must be protected from drug exposure with aerosol use resulting from accidental spraying or with nebulizer delivery. Blockade of muscarinic receptors causes mydriasis by blocking the sphincter muscle of the iris and inhibits the ciliary muscle of the lens preventing lens thickening (accommodation). As the iris dilates outward and the lens remains flattened, drainage of intraocular aqueous humor is reduced. In patients with narrow-angle glaucoma, intraocular pressure can rise. Because many COPD patients are older, the presence of narrow-angle glaucoma may be more common. Subjects using quaternary ammonium antimuscarinic bronchodilators must be in-

formed of this hazard and should use proper aerosol inhalation technique. A holding chamber should be used with MDI administration. With nebulizer delivery, the mouthpiece should be kept in the mouth and a reservoir tube attached to the expiratory side of the T to vent aerosol away from the face. The ideal nebulizer would be a dosimetric device with no ambient exposure from the device on exhalation. If the nebulizer solution is delivered by facemask (which is not recommended), the eyes should be closed or covered to prevent drug exposure. Because of the greater risk of eye exposure with a nebulizer, especially disposable, constant-output devices, an MDI with holding chamber is recommended for delivery of this class of bronchodilator.

CLINICAL APPLICATION

Anticholinergic (antimuscarinic) aerosols have been investigated for use with asthma and with COPD. Table 7-5 compares the general effects seen with anticholinergic bronchodilators and β-adrenergic bronchodilators.

USE IN CHRONIC OBSTRUCTIVE PULMONARY DISEASE

Antimuscarinic agents were found to be more potent bronchodilators than β-adrenergic agents in bronchitis-emphysema, and this is likely to be their primary clinical application. This difference is illustrated Figure 7-6 with data from Tashkin and colleagues.[33] In that 90-day, multicenter study, the investigation compared 40 µg of ipratropium with 1.5 mg of metaproterenol, both given by MDI, in a population of patients with COPD. Explanations for the superiority of

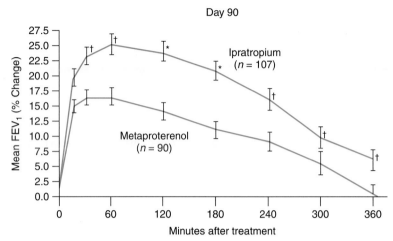

Figure 7-6   The effect of the β agonist metaproterenol and the anticholinergic ipratropium on FEV$_1$ in patients with COPD after 90 days of treatment (*, $P <0.01$; †, $P <0.05$). (From Tashkin and others: Comparison of the anticholinergic bronchodilator ipratropium with metaproterenol in chronic obstructive pulmonary disease, *Am J Med* 81[suppl 5A]:59, 1986. From Excerpta Medica, Inc.)

anticholinergic action in COPD are debated but may relate to the complicated, inflammatory, noncholinergic pathways seen in asthma, especially with antigen-antibody reactions mentioned previously in the section on the vagal reflex mechanism. Conversely, the pathology of COPD may reveal the reason for the superior effect of anticholinergic over β-adrenergic drugs. Ipratropium has been approved by the Food and Drug Administration (FDA) specifically for use in the treatment of COPD, although the drug is also prescribed for treatment of asthma.

An analysis of data from the clinical trials of ipratropium compared with a β agonist for FDA approval was conducted by Rennard and associates[34] and published in 1996. Their analysis showed that use of ipratropium over the 90-day interval tested was associated with improved baseline lung function and response to acute bronchodilator use. Subjects using β agonists over the same period had little change in baseline lung function and a small decrease in airway response to acute bronchodilator treatment.

Tiotropium, under investigation as an antimuscarinic bronchodilator, offers the possibility of a prolonged duration of action up to 24 hours with a single daily inhalation. In dose-ranging trials, an inhaled dose of 18 μg once a day has been found to give significant bronchodilation in patients with COPD, with few side effects.[14,16] Figure 7-7 illustrates the effect on FEV$_1$ with single inhaled doses of tiotropium of different strengths in comparison with placebo.[14] There is also prolonged

dose-dependent protection against inhaled methacholine challenge. Both the bronchodilating and the bronchoprotective effect can be compared with the 6-hour effect of ipratropium. Perhaps one of the more important effects of a long-acting drug such as tiotropium is the elevation in baseline, predose FEV$_1$. Unlike ipratropium, lung function is maintained more consistently at a higher level throughout the day with tiotropium. This may have a significant effect on quality of life and reduction of breathlessness in patients with COPD. The prolonged effect may also be useful in controlling nocturnal asthma symptoms, where cholinergic mechanisms appear to increase airway tone.[35]

USE IN ASTHMA

Anticholinergic (antimuscarinic) agents such as ipratropium do not have a labeled indication for asthma in the United States. Current asthma guidelines state that ipratropium may have some additive benefit when given with inhaled β agonsts.[36] Antimuscarinic bronchodilators are not clearly superior to β-adrenergic agents in treating asthma. Antimuscarinic and β-adrenergic agents have an approximately equal effect on flow rates in many patients. These agents may be especially useful in the following applications when prescribed for asthmatic patients[37]:

- Nocturnal asthma, in which the slightly longer duration of action may protect against nocturnal deterioration of flow rates[38]

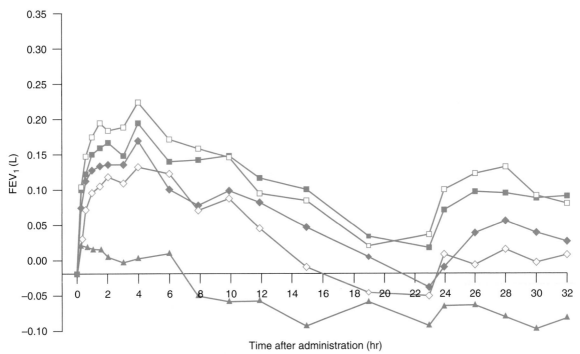

Figure 7-7 Bronchodilator responses measured with FEV_1 in patients with COPD given single doses of tiotropium, a long-acting antimuscarinic bronchodilator. Symbols: ■ 80 μg; □ 40 μg; ◆ 20 μg; ◇ 10 μg; ▲ placebo. (Data from Maesen FPV and others: Tiotropium, a new long-acting antimuscarinic bronchodilator: a pharmacodynamic study in patients with chronic obstructive pulmonary disease [COPD], *Eur Respir J* 8:1506, 1995.)

- Psychogenic asthma, which may be mediated through vagal parasympathetic fibers
- Asthmatic patients with glaucoma, angina, or hypertension who require treatment with β-blocking agents
- As an alternative to theophylline in patients with notable side effects from that drug
- Acute, severe episodes of asthma not responding well to β agonists

A large, randomized controlled study by Qureshi and colleagues[39] in 434 children 2 to 8 years of age with acute moderate to severe asthma found that the overall rate of hospitalization was lowered with addition of inhaled ipratropium to nebulized albuterol.[39] However, the most striking effect on admission was seen in children with severe asthma (peak expiratory flow <50% of predicted). A meta-analysis of the addition of anticholinergic bronchodilators to β agonists in children and adolescents, conducted by Plotnick and Ducharme,[40] concluded that adding multiple doses of anticholinergic (antimuscarinic) bronchodilators to $β_2$ agonists was safe, improved

lung function, and may avoid hospital admission in 1 of 11 treated patients. Multiple doses should be preferred to single doses of antimuscarinic agents.

COMBINATION THERAPY: β-ADRENERGIC AND ANTICHOLINERGIC AGENTS IN CHRONIC OBSTRUCTIVE PULMONARY DISEASE

Theoretically, a combination of β-adrenergic and anticholinergic agents should offer advantages in the treatment of COPD (or asthma as well), based on the following considerations:

- Complementarity of sites of action exists, with anticholinergic effect seen in the more central airways and β-agonist effect in the smaller, more peripheral airways.
- Mechanisms of action from anticholinergic and β-adrenergic agents are separate and complementary.

Pharmacokinetics of shorter-acting agents (albuterol or ipratropium) in the two classes of bronchodilator are somewhat complementary, with β agonists peaking sooner but also terminating sooner, while anticholinergics tend to peak more slowly and last longer. However, this consideration is not relevant with longer-acting agents in both classes, such as salmeterol and tiotropium.

ADDITIVE EFFECT OF β AGONISTS AND ANTICHOLINERGIC AGENTS

Conflicting results have been found on the question of whether the bronchodilator effect of β agonists is increased by adding an anticholinergic agent, in either COPD or asthma.[41-45] Many of the studies performed with combined anticholinergic and β-agonist bronchodilator therapy suffer from small sample sizes and poor statistical power. Before the approval of combined albuterol and ipratropium (Combivent) in late 1996, a large, well-controlled study was conducted over 85 days with 462 patients at 24 centers.[7] Patients represented stable COPD. The study showed superior efficacy of the combination therapy of ipratropium and albuterol compared with either agent alone. Figure 7-8 shows a comparison of ipratropium plus albuterol with albuterol or ipratropium alone on the percentage change in FEV_1, from this study. The mean *peak* increases in FEV_1 were 31% to 33% for combined drug therapy, compared with 24% to 25% for ipratropium alone and 24% to 27% for albuterol alone. Flow rates were significantly better on all test

days. Symptom scores did not differ among the three groups, however. As a large, well-designed study, these results support combination anticholinergic and β-agonist therapy in COPD.

SEQUENCE OF ADMINISTRATION

The order in which an MDI of β_2 agonist and an anticholinergic are administered has been debated. Because an anticholinergic bronchodilator acts in the central, larger airways, some practitioners argue that it should be given *before* the β_2 agonist. No data have been given to support this sequence, however. The β_2 agonist is often given first, and this can be rationalized for two reasons: (1) β_2 agonists have a more rapid onset of action than an anticholinergic bronchodilator and (2) β_2 receptors are distributed in large and small airways. The order of administration is probably not important. Combination products such as Combivent (ipratropium and albuterol) make order of administration a moot point.

RESPIRATORY CARE ASSESSMENT OF ANTICHOLINERGIC BRONCHODILATOR THERAPY

- Assess effectiveness of drug therapy based on the indication(s) for the aerosol agent: Presence of reversible airflow resulting from primary bronchospasm or obstruction secondary to an inflammatory response or secretions, either acute or chronic.
- Monitor flow rates using bedside peak flow meters, portable spirometry, or laboratory reports of pulmonary function. Before-and-after bronchodilator studies performed with a β agonist may not reliably predict response to an anticholinergic (antimuscarinic) agent such as ipratropium.
- Perform respiratory assessment: Breathing rate and pattern, and breath sounds by auscultation, before and after treatment.
- Assess pulse before, during, and after treatment.
- Assess patient's subjective reaction to treatment, for any change (positive or negative) in breathing effort or pattern.
- Assess arterial blood gases, or pulse oximeter saturation, as needed, for acute states with COPD or asthma, to monitor changes in ventilation and gas exchange (oxygenation).
- Long term: Monitor pulmonary function studies of lung volumes, capacities, and flows.
- Instruct and then verify correct use of aerosol delivery device (SVN, MDI, reservoir, DPI). Empha-

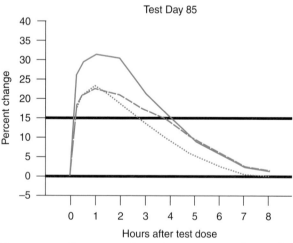

Figure 7-8   Percentage change in FEV_1 on test day 85, for combined ipratropium and albuterol compared with either drug alone, in patients with COPD. • • • = albuterol; - - - = ipratropium; — = ipratropium plus albuterol. (From COMBIVENT Inhalation Aerosol Study Group: In chronic obstructive pulmonary disease, a combination of ipratropium and albuterol is more effective than either agent alone: an 85-day multicenter trial, *Chest* 105:1411, 1994.)

size that the eye must be protected from aerosol sprays. Instruct patients in use, assembly, and especially cleaning of aerosol inhalation devices.

For long-acting antimuscarinic bronchodilators:

- Assess ongoing lung function, including predose FEV_1 over time.
- Assess amount of concomitant β agonist use and nocturnal symptoms.
- Assess number of exacerbations, unscheduled clinic visits, and hospitalizations.
- Assess days of absence because of symptoms.

SUMMARY KEY TERMS AND CONCEPTS

- *Anticholinergic* agents given by inhalation offer a second class of *bronchodilating agents.*
- The anticholinergic bronchodilators are specifically *parasympatholytic,* that is, *antimuscarinic* agents, blocking the effect of acetylcholine at the cholinergic (muscarinic) receptors on bronchial smooth muscle.
- The only approved anticholinergic agent for inhalation as an aerosol at this time is *ipratropium* (Atrovent), which is available as an MDI, an SVN solution, and an intranasal spray.
- Other anticholinergic agents used as bronchodilators include the long-acting agent tiotropium (investigational) and the drug oxitropium (available outside the United States).
- The anticholinergic agent ipratropium is *indicated* for treatment of airflow obstruction in COPD.
- At least a portion of the airflow obstruction in COPD may be due to *vagally mediated reflex bronchoconstriction* caused by stimulation of afferent sensory C-fibers, which trigger reflex, efferent vagal nerve activity, and constriction.
- The anticholinergic bronchodilators are *nonspecific blockers of muscarinic receptor* subtypes (M_1, M_2, and M_3) in the airway. Blockade of the M_3 receptor subtype on bronchial smooth muscle prevents activation of the linking G_q *protein,* its effector system phospholipase C (PLC), and subsequent increase in free calcium with bronchoconstriction or gland exocytosis.
- Blockade of M_1 and M_3 receptors in the nasal passages prevents gland secretion and rhinitis.
- *Quaternary compounds,* such as ipratropium, are fully ionized and less absorbed in body tissues than *tertiary compounds,* such as atropine sulfate. Consequently, side effects with quaternary compounds are localized to the site of drug exposure.
- The most common *side effect* with quaternary ammonium antimuscarinic bronchodilators such as ipratropium is a dry mouth and perhaps a cough caused by the aerosol particles.

- Direct spraying in the eye must be avoided to prevent ocular effects. Subjects with *COPD* can show a greater response in reversibility of airflow obstruction with an anticholinergic agent than a β agonist.
- Combined anticholinergic and β-agonist therapy may give additive bronchodilating results in COPD and in severe, acute asthma.

SELF-ASSESSMENT QUESTIONS

1. What is the first FDA-approved anticholinergic bronchodilator for aerosol inhalation?
2. What is the usual recommended dose of ipratropium by MDI and by SVN?
3. Identify a long-acting anticholinergic bronchodilator and give its duration of action.
4. What is the usual clinical indication for use of an anticholinergic bronchodilator such as ipratropium?
5. Which disease state, asthma or COPD, may show greater response to an anticholinergic bronchodilator rather than a β agonist?
6. With which type of anticholinergic agent are you more likely to observe systemic side effects: the tertiary ammonium or quaternary ammonium compounds?
7. What are the most common side effects seen with inhaled ipratropium?
8. Can ipratropium be used with subjects who have glaucoma?
9. Can ipratropium be alternated with or combined with a β agonist in the treatment of COPD and asthma?
10. What precautions should you observe if administering ipratropium by SVN?
11. What is the clinical indication for the use of an anticholinergic intranasal spray?

Answers to Self-Assessment Questions are found in Appendix A.

CLINICAL SCENARIO

Mr. James C. is a 66-year-old retired, well-educated middle level manager for a major film company. He is referred to a pulmonologist for his complaint of shortness of breath. On interview he states that he has increasingly noticed exertional dyspnea with mild physical activity over the past few months. With questioning, he admits to occasional social alcohol intake of either 1 or 2 beers or a couple of mixed drinks several times a week. He has been happily married to the same woman since he was 24. He also admits to regular cigarette smoking of around 1 pack/day since he was 20 years old. He leads a sedentary life with no physical exercise. He states that he does have a chronic cough, which is worse in the morning, although he denies much productivity. He appears to be well-nourished, is articulate, and his color is good. No cyanosis nor use of accessory muscles is noted at rest.

Physical examination reveals very mild digital clubbing, a slightly increased AP diameter, diminished and distant breath sounds bilaterally with some rhonchi, mildly hyperresonant percussion notes, no jugular venous distention upright or supine, and no peripheral edema. His vital signs are BP, 146/90, T, 37.2° C; P, 88 beats/min; RR, 16 breaths/min with no laboring. His arterial blood gas (room air) results are pH, 7.40; $PaCO_2$, 42.5 mm Hg; PaO_2, 62 mm Hg; base excess, 1.9 mEq/L; and Hgb, 14.5 g/dl.

His pulmonary function results are as follows:

Observed	% Predicted
FVC, 2.98 L	74
FEV_1, 1.94 L	60
FEV_1/FVC: 65%	83
RV/TLC: 42%	124
DLCO, 18.4	70
(ml/min/mm Hg)	

Mr. C's chest radiograph (PA, lateral) shows some loss of lung markings, mild flattening of the hemidiaphragms, and increased AP diameter. His electrolytes and white cell count are normal.

His chief complaint, smoking history, physical findings, and laboratory results all indicate early manifestations of COPD. He is mildly hypoxemic at rest (PaO_2, 62 mm Hg), but his acid-base status is normal. Moderate airflow obstruction is present as evidenced by the FEV_1 of 1.94 L, an FEV_1/FVC of 65%, and an increased RV/TLC ratio. Gas exchange is impaired, as seen in the below-normal DLCO. There is no evidence of cardiac failure or acute exacerbation at this time. His diagnosis is COPD with mixed bronchitis and emphysema.

Would you recommend a bronchodilator for Mr. C.?

What type of bronchodilator would you think best to start for Mr. C.?

If Mr. C. has trouble with MDI use, what actions could you take?

What lifestyle change(s) would you emphasize to Mr. C.?

Answers to Clinical Scenario Questions are found in Appendix A.

REFERENCES

1. Gandevia B: Historical review of the use of parasympatholytic agents in the treatment of respiratory disorders, *Postgrad Med J* 51(suppl 7):13, 1975.
2. Witek TJ Jr: Anticholinergic bronchodilators, *Respir Care Clinics North Am* 5:521, 1999.
3. Cavanaugh MJ, Cooper DM: Inhaled atropine sulfate: dose response characteristics, *Am Rev Respir Dis* 114:517, 1976.
4. Pak CCF and others: Inhaled atropine sulfate: dose-response characteristics in adult patients with chronic airflow obstruction, *Am Rev Respir Dis* 125:331, 1982.
5. Gross NJ: Anticholinergic agents: clinical application. In Leff AR, ed: *Pulmonary and critical care pharmacology and therapeutics*, New York, 1996, McGraw-Hill.
6. Meltzer EO: Intranasal anticholinergic therapy of rhinorrhea, *J Allergy Clin Immunol* 90:1055, 1992.
7. COMBIVENT Inhalation Aerosol Study Group: In chronic obstructive pulmonary disease, a combination of ipratropium and albuterol is more effective than either agent alone: an 85-day multicenter trial, *Chest* 105:1411, 1994.
8. Gal TJ, Suratt PM, Lu J: Glycopyrrolate and atropine inhalation: comparative effects on normal airway function, *Am Rev Respir Dis* 129:871, 1984.
9. Flohr E, Bischoff KO: Oxitropium bromide, a new anticholinergic drug, in a dose-response and placebo comparison in obstructive airway diseases, *Respiration* 38:98, 1979.
10. Frith PA and others: Oxitropium bromide: dose-response and time-response study of a new anticholinergic bronchodilator drug, *Chest* 89:249, 1986.
11. Skorodin MS and others: Oxitropium bromide: a new anticholinergic bronchodilator, *Ann Allergy* 56:229, 1986.
12. Nakano Y and others: Efficacy of adding multiple doses of oxitropium bromide to salbutamol delivered by means of a metered-dose inhaler with a spacer device in adults with acute severe asthma, *J Allergy Clin Immunol* 106:472, 2000.
13. Barnes PJ: The pharmacological properties of tiotropium, *Chest* 117:63S, 2000.
14. Maesen FPV and others: Tiotropium bromide, a new long-acting antimuscarinic bronchodilator: a pharmacodynamic study in patients with chronic obstructive pulmonary disease (COPD), *Eur Respir J* 8:1506, 1995.
15. Van Noord JA and others on behalf of the Dutch Tiotropium Study Group: A randomised controlled comparison of tiotropium and ipratropium in the treatment of chronic obstructive pulmonary disease, *Thorax* 55:289, 2000.
16. Littner MR and others: Long-acting bronchodilation with once-daily dosing of tiotropium (Spiriva) in stable chronic obstructive pulmonary disease, *Am J Respir Crit Care Med* 161:1136, 2000.
17. Chodosh S and others: Effective use of HandiHaler dry powder inhalation system over a broad range of COPD disease severity, *Am J Respir Crit Care Med* 159:A524, 1999.
18. Groth ML, Langenback EG, Foster WM: Influence of inhaled atropine on lung mucociliary function in humans, *Am Rev Respir Dis* 144:1042, 1991.
19. Wanner A: Effect of ipratropium bromide on airway mucociliary function, *Am J Med* 81(suppl 5A):32, 1986.

20. Bergman KR and others: Atropine-induced psychosis, an unusual complication of therapy with inhaled atropine sulfate, *Chest* 78:891, 1980.

21. Herschman ZL and others: Central nervous system toxicity from nebulized atropine sulfate, *J Toxicol Clin Toxicol* 29:273, 1991.

22. Botts LD and others: Prolongation of gastric emptying by aerosolized atropine, *Am Rev Respir Dis* 131:725, 1985.

23. Mulherin D, Fitzgerald MX: Meconium ileus equivalent in association with nebulized ipratropium bromide in cystic fibrosis, *Lancet* 335:552, 1990.

24. Molkenboer JFWM, Lardenoye JG: The effect of Atrovent on micturition function, double-blind cross-over study, *Scand J Respir Dis* 103(suppl):154, 1979.

25. Barnes PJ: Autonomic control of airway function in asthma, *Chest* 91(suppl):45S, 1987.

26. Bleecker ER: Cholinergic and neurogenic mechanisms in obstructive airways disease, *Am J Med* 81(suppl 5A):2, 1986.

27. Hogg JC: The pathophysiology of asthma, *Chest* 82(suppl):8S, 1982.

28. Leff A: Pathophysiology of asthmatic bronchoconstriction, *Chest* 82(suppl):13S, 1982.

29. Simonsson BG, Jacobs FM, Nadel JA: Role of autonomic nervous system and the cough reflex in the increased responsiveness of airways in patients with obstructive airway disease, *J Clin Invest* 46:1812, 1967.

30. Baraniuk JN: Muscarinic receptors. In Leff AR, ed: *Pulmonary and critical care pharmacology and therapeutics,* New York, 1996, McGraw-Hill.

31. Okayama M and others: Autoradiographic localization of muscarinic receptor subtypes in human nasal mucosa, *J Allergy Clin Immunol* 89:1144, 1992.

32. Cugell DW: Clinical pharmacology and toxicology of ipratropium bromide, *Am J Med* 81(suppl 5A):27, 1986.

33. Tashkin DP and others: Comparison of the anticholinergic bronchodilator ipratropium bromide with metaproterenol in chronic obstructive pulmonary disease: a 90-day multi-center study, *Am J Med* 81(suppl 5A):59, 1986.

34. Rennard SI and others: Extended therapy with ipratropium is associated with improved lung function in patients with COPD: a retrospective analysis of data from seven clinical trials, *Chest* 110:62, 1996.

35. Morrison JFJ, Pearson SB, Dean HG: Parasympathetic nervous system in nocturnal asthma, *Br Med J* 296:1427, 1988.

36. National Asthma Education and Prevention Program, Expert Panel Report II: *Guidelines for the diagnosis and management of asthma,* Bethesda, Md, 1997, National Institutes of Health.

37. Weber RW: Role of anticholinergics in asthma, *Ann Allergy* 65:348, 1990 (editorial).

38. Cox ID, Hughes DTD, McDonnell KA: Ipratropium bromide in patients with nocturnal asthma, *Postgrad Med J* 60:526, 1984.

39. Qureshi F and others: Effect of nebulized ipratropium on the hospitalization rates of children with asthma, *N Engl J Med* 339:1030, 1998.

40. Plotnick LH, Ducharme FM: Should inhaled anticholinergics be added to β_2 agonists for treating acute childhood and adolescent asthma? A systematic review, *Br Med J* 317:971, 1998.

41. Rebuck AS and others: Nebulized anticholinergic and sympathomimetic treatment of asthma and chronic obstructive airways disease in the emergency room, *Am J Med* 82:59, 1987.

42. Owens MW, George RB: Nebulized atropine sulfate in the treatment of acute asthma, *Chest* 99:1084, 1991.

43. Karpel JP: Bronchodilator responses to anticholinergic and β-adrenergic agents in acute and stable COPD, *Chest* 99:871, 1991.

44. Lightbody IM and others: Ipratropium bromide, salbutamol and prednisolone in bronchial asthma and chronic bronchitis, *Br J Dis Chest* 72:181, 1978.

45. Petrie GR, Palmer KNV: Comparison of aerosol ipratropium bromide and salbutamol in chronic bronchitis and asthma, *Br Med J* 1:430, 1975.

CHAPTER 8

Xanthines

Joseph L. Rau

CHAPTER OUTLINE

Chapter 8 reviews the pharmacology of the xanthine drugs, such as theophylline. Theophylline has been traditionally used to treat asthma and chronic obstructive pulmonary disease (COPD) patients in both stable and acute phases. The mechanism of action by xanthines is unclear, and their clinical use in asthma and COPD has been relegated to that of second- or third-line agents, although this remains an issue of some debate.

CLINICAL INDICATIONS FOR USE OF XANTHINES

Theophylline has traditionally been used in the management of asthma and COPD. Theophylline and caffeine have been used to treat apnea of prematurity. A now-obsolete use of theophylline was as a diuretic. Although theophylline is usually classified as a bronchodilator, it actually has a relatively weak bronchodilating effect compared with the β agonists. Its therapeutic action in asthma and COPD may occur by other means, such as stimulation of the ventilatory drive or direct strengthening of the diaphragm. Any of these actions could result in the clinical outcome of improved ventilatory flow rates. This is further discussed in the section on clinical application in this chapter.

USE IN ASTHMA

Sustained-release theophylline is indicated as a long-term controller drug, for maintenance therapy of mild, persistent (step 2) asthma or greater. Sustained-release theophylline is considered as a less-preferred alternative to low-dose inhaled corticosteroids or cromolyn-like agents as second-line maintenance drug therapy in stable asthma. The 1997 National Institutes of Health (NIH) guidelines on asthma do not clearly give a preference between theophylline and the anti-leukotriene agents (zafirlukast, montelukast), which were newly released at the time of the Expert Panel II recommendations.[1] Many clinicians believe that the antileukotrienes are preferable in terms of side effects and therapeutic margin to theophylline.

Methylxanthines are not generally recommended for acute exacerbations of asthma in the 1997 Expert Panel II report giving guidelines for managing asthma. Guidelines on drug therapy of asthma including the role of theophylline can be found in Appendix D.

USE IN CHRONIC OBSTRUCTIVE PULMONARY DISEASE

Current guidelines for treatment of stable COPD state that bronchodilators, including theophylline, are central to symptom management. Xanthines would be considered for moderate (Stage II) and severe (Stage III) COPD. The Global Initiative for Chronic Obstructive Lung Disease (GOLD) also states that inhaled bronchodilators are preferred when available. Theophylline is considered effective in COPD but, because of potential toxicity, is recommended as an alternative to the inhaled bronchodilators such as β_2 agonists or anticholinergic agents.[2-4]

The GOLD guidelines suggest use of intravenous theophylline in managing acute exacerbations of COPD if aggressive inhaled therapy with β agonists and anticholinergic bronchodilators is inadequate.

Guidelines on drug management of COPD from the National Heart, Lung, and Blood Institute (NHLBI)

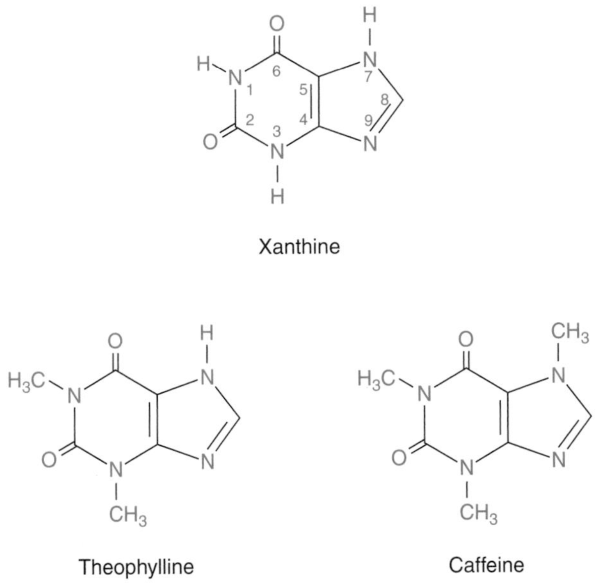

Figure 8-1 Chemical structure of xanthine and its methylated derivatives theophylline and caffeine.

and the World Health Organization (WHO) are given in Appendix D.

USE IN APNEA OF PREMATURITY

If pharmacological therapy is needed to stimulate breathing in apnea of prematurity (AOP), methylxanthines are considered as the first-line agents of choice. Theophylline has been most extensively used, but Bhatia[5] suggests that caffeine citrate may be the agent of choice. Caffeine citrate (Cafcit) has been approved for administration either intravenously or orally.

SPECIFIC XANTHINE AGENTS

Theophylline is related chemically to the natural metabolite xanthine, which is a precursor of uric acid. Figure 8-1 gives the general xanthine structure, along with that of theophylline (1,3-dimethylxanthine) and caffeine (1,3,7-trimethylxanthine). Because of their methyl attachments, these agents are often referred to as *methylxanthines*. Another xanthine is theobromine. All three agents are found as alkaloids in plant species. Caffeine is found in coffee beans and in kola nuts. Caffeine and theophylline are contained in tea leaves, and caffeine and theobromine are in cocoa seeds or beans. Historically, these natural plant substances have all been used as brews for their stimulant effect.

There are several synthetic modifications to the naturally occurring methylxanthines. These include dyphylline (7-[2,3-dihydroxypropyl theophylline]), proxyphylline (7-[2-hydroxypropyl]-theophylline), and enprofylline (3-propylxanthine). Table 8-1 lists xanthine derivatives, along with selected brand names and available formulations.

Theophylline is available in a variety of formulations, including sustained-release oral forms, as

Table 8-1

Xanthine derivatives used as bronchodilators in obstructive airways diseases, with selected brand names and available formulations

XANTHINE DERIVATIVE	SELECTED BRAND NAMES	FORMULATIONS
Theophylline	Slo-Phyllin, Theolair, Quibron-T, Dividose, Bronkodyl, Elixophyllin, Theo-Dur, Uni-Dur, Uniphyl	Tablets, capsules, syrup, elixir, extended-release tablets, capsules
Oxtriphylline	Choledyl SA	Tablets, syrup, elixir, stained-release tablets
Aminophylline	Aminophylline, Phyllocontin, Truphylline	Tablets, oral liquid, injection, suppositories
Dyphylline	Dilor, Lufyllin	Tablets, elixir, injection

Table 8-2

Differences in intensity of effects for caffeine and theophylline

EFFECT	CAFFEINE	THEOPHYLLINE
Central nervous system stimulation	+++	++
Cardiac stimulation	+	+++
Smooth muscle relaxation	+	+++
Skeletal muscle stimulation	+++	++
Diuresis	+	+++

aminophylline for oral or intravenous administration, and in rectal suppository forms. Aminophylline has been tried unsuccessfully by aerosol with asthmatic subjects.[6] The aerosol is irritating to the pharynx, has a bitter taste, and can cause coughing and wheezing.

GENERAL PHARMACOLOGICAL PROPERTIES

The xanthine group has the following general physiological effects in humans:

- Central nervous system stimulation
- Cardiac muscle stimulation
- Diuresis
- Bronchial, uterine, and vascular smooth muscle relaxation
- Peripheral and coronary vasodilation
- Cerebral vasoconstriction

Some of the effects seen with xanthines are well known to those who drink caffeinated beverages (e.g., coffee, colas, tea). Coffee in particular can be used for the central nervous system stimulatory effect to remain awake. The diuretic effect after drinking coffee or cola is also well known. Caffeine or theophylline can also cause tachycardia, and the cerebral vasoconstricting effect has been used to treat migraine headaches. A special agent intended for this use is Cafergot, which contains 100 mg of caffeine and 1 mg of ergotamine tartrate.

Caffeine and theophylline differ in the intensity of the effects listed previously. These differences are summarized in Table 8-2. Caffeine has more central nervous system stimulating effect than theophylline, and this includes ventilatory stimulation. In clinical use, theophylline is generally classified as a bronchodilator, because of the relaxing effect on bronchial smooth muscle.

MODE OF ACTION

STRUCTURE-ACTIVITY RELATIONS

Figure 8-2 illustrates the general xanthine structure and the effect of attachments at various sites on the molecule. Also, the chemical structure of theophylline is shown in comparison with that of the theophylline derivatives dyphylline and enprofylline. The methyl attachments at the nitrogen-1 and nitrogen-3 positions for theophylline enhance its bronchodilating effect, as well as its toxic side effects, which will be discussed later in this chapter. In contrast, the structure of caffeine (see Figure 8-1) has an additional methyl group at the nitrogen-7 position, thereby decreasing its bronchodilator effect in relation to theophylline. Dyphylline has the same methyl attachments at the nitrogen-1 and nitrogen-3 positions as theophylline but also has a large attachment at the nitrogen-7 position that decreases its bronchodilator potential. Enprofylline, which is not clinically available in the United States at this time, has potent bronchodilating effects, probably because of the large substitution at the nitrogen-3 position.

THEORIES OF ACTIVITY

The exact mechanism of action of the xanthines, and theophylline in particular, is not known.[7] It was originally thought that xanthines caused smooth muscle relaxation by inhibition of phosphodiesterase, leading to an increase in intracellular cyclic adenosine monophosphate (cyclic AMP, or cAMP). An increase in cAMP causes relaxation of bronchial smooth muscle. The effect of increased cAMP was described in Chapter 6 in the discussion of β-adrenergic agents. However, this explanation to account for therapeutic xanthine actions has been questioned.

Several alternative theories of action for xanthines have been proposed in addition to phosphodiesterase inhibition. Each of the modes of action proposed for xanthines is briefly described and commented on in the following sections.

INHIBITION OF PHOSPHODIESTERASE

Theophylline is a weak and nonselective inhibitor of cAMP-specific phosphodiesterase (PDE). The pathway by which this inhibition can lead to an increase in intracellular cAMP, with consequent bronchial relaxation or antiflammatory effects, is illustrated in Figure 8-3, *A*. However, at the dosage levels used clinically in humans, theophylline is a poor inhibitor of the enzyme.[8] As a result, this is not considered to be an acceptable explanation of how xanthines exert a therapeutic effect. *PDE is*

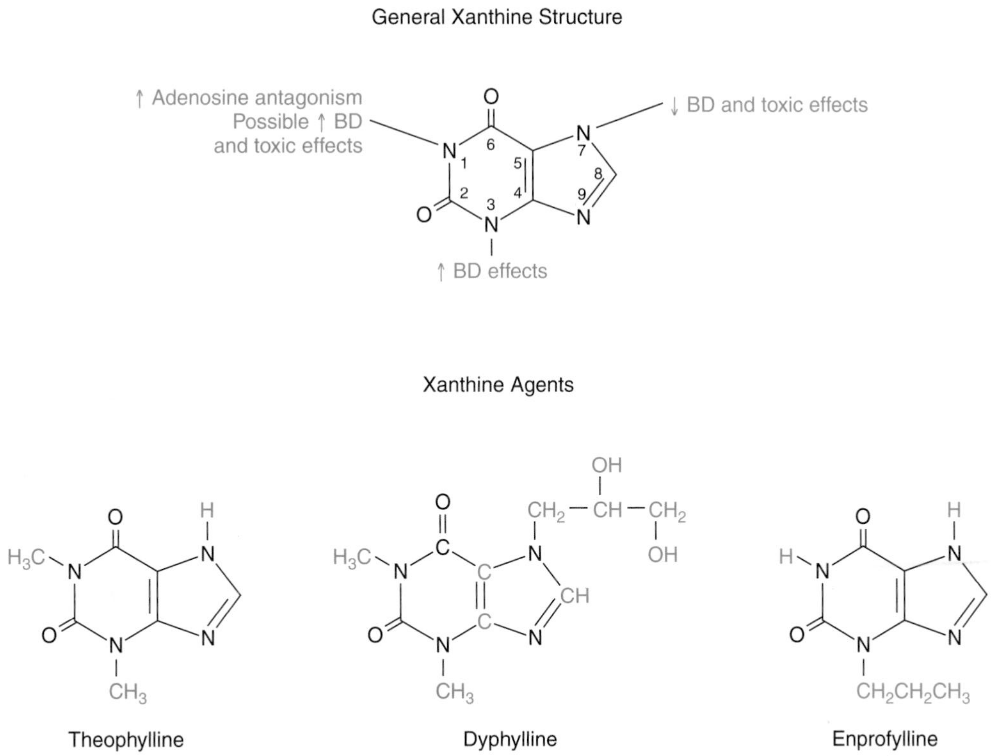

General Xanthine Structure

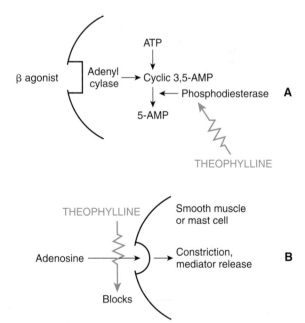

↑ Adenosine antagonism
Possible ↑ BD
and toxic effects

↓ BD and toxic effects

↑ BD effects

Xanthine Agents

Theophylline   Dyphylline   Enprofylline

Figure 8-2   Effect of attachments at different sites on the xanthine molecule and comparative illustration of the structures of theophylline, dyphylline, and enprofylline. *BD,* Bronchodilation.

a generic term referring to at least 11 distinct families that have been identified that hydrolyze cAMP or cyclic guanosine monophosphate (cyclic GMP, or cGMP) and have unique tissue and subcellular distributions. Various PDE families differ in substrate specificity, inhibitor sensitivity, and cofactor requirements.[7] There are two cAMP-hydrolyzing PDEs, referred to as *PDE3* and *PDE4*, which may play a role in asthma. PDE4 is expressed in airway smooth muscle, pulmonary nerves, and many proinflammatory and immune cells. PDE4 inhibitors suppress processes thought to contribute to asthma inflammation by blocking the degradation of cAMP in target cells and tissue. The antiinflammatory effect of theophylline and xanthines is reviewed in the discussion of the clinical application of these drugs in COPD and asthma.

ANTAGONISM OF ADENOSINE

An alternative explanation is that theophylline acts by blocking the action of adenosine. This mechanism is illustrated in Figure 8-3, *B*. Adenosine is a purine nucleoside that can stimulate A_1 and A_2 receptors. A_1-Receptor stimulation inhibits cAMP, whereas A_2-receptor stimulation increases cyclic AMP. Inhaled adenosine has

Figure 8-3   Two proposed mechanisms of action by which theophylline and xanthines reverse airway obstruction. **A,** Inhibition of phosphodiesterase. **B,** Blockade of adenosine receptors. *AMP,* Adenosine monophosphate; *ATP,* adenosine triphosphate.

produced bronchoconstriction in asthmatic patients. Theophylline is a potent inhibitor of both A_1 and A_2 receptors and could block smooth muscle contraction mediated by A_1 receptors.

This explanation is contradicted by the action of enprofylline, which is about five times more potent than theophylline for relaxing smooth muscle, yet lacks a sufficient attachment at the nitrogen-1 position to provide adenosine antagonism.[9] This can be seen in Figure 8-2 by comparing the structures of theophylline and enprofylline. In addition, A_1 receptors are sparse in smooth muscle, and isolated animal tissue preparations have actually shown smooth muscle relaxation through adenosine stimulation of the A_2 receptors.

CATECHOLAMINE RELEASE

A third explanation of xanthine action is that these agents cause the production and release of endogenous catecholamines, which in turn could cause muscle tremor, tachycardia, and bronchial relaxation. Studies on plasma levels of catecholamines such as epinephrine have reported conflicting results, with both an increase and no change reported.[10]

CONCLUSION

Other theories have been proposed for how xanthines exert their effects, in addition to those just described. Caffeine and theophylline may inhibit calcium uptake by the sarcoplasmic reticulum, thereby relaxing smooth muscle. Xanthines may also antagonize the effects of prostaglandins such as prostaglandin E_2 and prostaglandin $F_{2\alpha}$.

There is no accepted definitive explanation for the action of xanthines to date. It is possible that there are multiple mechanisms involved with the specific agents in this class. For example, theophylline may cause its effect on smooth muscle by antagonism of adenosine receptors (specifically A_1), whereas enprofylline does so by a different mechanism.

TITRATING THEOPHYLLINE DOSES

In the past, clinical use of the xanthine theophylline, in its many forms, was questioned because of wide variability in its therapeutic effect. It was subsequently found that individuals metabolize theophylline at differing rates, which makes it difficult to determine therapeutic doses. This is complicated further by the fact that different forms of the drug are not always equivalent.

EQUIVALENT DOSES OF THEOPHYLLINE SALTS

The standard with which salts of theophylline are compared is anhydrous theophylline. Anhydrous theophylline is 100% theophylline. By contrast, salts of theophylline such as oxtriphylline (Choledyl) are not pure theophylline by weight. A 200 mg dose of Choledyl (brand of theophylline) contains approximately 130 mg of theophylline, whereas Theo-Dur (brand of theophylline) is 100% anhydrous theophylline. A 200 mg dose of Choledyl will not give the same amount of theophylline as a 200 mg dose of Theo-Dur. Table 8-3 lists the equivalent dose of pure theophylline provided by the salts, such as oxtriphylline or aminophylline.

Because oxtriphylline is 64% theophylline, a dose equivalent to 100 mg of theophylline anhydrous would be 156 mg of oxtriphylline (100 mg/0.64 = 156 mg). Similarly, 127 mg of aminophylline dihydrate (theophylline ethylenediamine) would be required for equivalency to 100 mg of theophylline anhydrous. It should be noted that dyphylline is not a theophylline but a derivative of theophylline. It does not form theophylline in the body and is about one tenth as potent as theophylline. This is consistent with its structure-activity relation, described previously.

SERUM LEVELS OF THEOPHYLLINE

In 1972, Jenne and colleagues indicated that the optimum serum theophylline level for maximal bronchodilatation in adults was between 10 and 20 μg/ml.[11] The effects associated with a range of serum levels are as follows:

Table 8-3

Theophylline content of salts of theophylline, with amount needed for equivalence to 100% anhydrous theophylline

THEOPHYLLINE SALT	THEOPHYLLINE (%)	EQUIVALENT DOSE
Theophylline anhydrous	100	100 mg
Theophylline monohydrate	91	110 mg
Aminophylline anhydrous	86	116 mg
Aminophylline dihydrate	79	127 mg
Oxtriphylline	64	156 mg

<5 µg/ml: No effects seen
10 to 20 µg/ml: Therapeutic range
>20 µg/ml: Nausea
>30 µg/ml: Cardiac arrhythmias
40 to 45 µg/ml: Seizures

Since the originally proposed serum levels of 10 to 20 µg/ml, the recommended range has been changed to a somewhat more conservative 5 to 15 µg/ml for management of asthma.[12] ATS recommendations for use of theophylline in COPD suggest a target serum level of 10 to 12 µg/ml.[2] Both of these ranges seek maximal therapeutic effect with minimal toxicity and side effects. It is stressed that the ranges listed for toxic effects are general. It is possible for an individual to bypass the nauseous phase of toxicity and immediately enter the seizure phase.

Although there is a dose-related response to higher serum levels of the theophylline, there is evidence that the response does not continue at the same rate of increase as levels rise. This is illustrated in Figure 8-4. The improvement in forced expiratory volume in 1 second (FEV$_1$) tends to flatten above a serum level of 10 to 12 µg/ml, whereas the toxic effects of theophylline (to be discussed subsequently) tend to increase even within the therapeutic range of 10 to 20 µg/ml.[13]

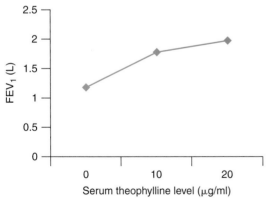

Figure 8-4   Conceptual illustration of the decreasing rate of improvement with theophylline levels above 10 µg/ml, even though levels may be in the therapeutic range of 10 to 20 µg/ml. (For illustration purposes only; not to be used to predict clinical response to serum levels.) *FEV$_1$,* Forced expiratory volume in 1 second. (Data from Tashkin DP: Measurement and significance of the bronchodilator response. In Jenne JW, Murphy S, eds: *Drug therapy for asthma: research and clinical practice,* New York, 1987, Marcel Dekker.)

Dosage Schedules

Because of the variability in the rate at which individuals metabolize theophylline and the other factors that affect theophylline metabolism and clearance rates, dosage schedules are used to titrate the drug. These schedules are found in the product literature, references such as *Facts and Comparisons, Physicians' Desk Reference,* and general pharmacology texts.

For rapid theophyllinization, the patient may be given an oral loading dose of 5 mg/kg, *provided* the patient was not previously receiving theophylline. This dose is based on anhydrous theophylline. Lean body weight should be used in calculating theophylline doses, because theophylline does not distribute into fatty tissue. In titrating the dose, each 0.5 mg/kg dose of theophylline given as a loading dose will result in a serum level of approximately 1 µg/ml. If theophylline was taken previously by the patient, a serum theophylline level should be measured if at all possible.

For chronic therapy, a slow titration is helpful, with an initial dose of 16 mg/kg/24 hr or 400 mg/24 hr, whichever is less. These dosages may need to be modified in the presence of factors such as age (younger children versus the elderly), congestive heart disease, or liver disease. The effect of these factors on serum theophylline levels and on dosage will be discussed subsequently. The dosage guidelines given are obtained from theophylline product information.

Dosage of theophylline can be guided by the clinical reaction of the patient or, better, by measurement of serum drug levels. Without a serum drug level, the dose of theophylline should be based on the benefit provided and should be reduced if the patient experiences toxic side effects.

When monitoring serum theophylline levels, take the sample at the time of peak absorption of the drug, that is, 1 to 2 hours after administration for immediate-release forms and 5 to 9 hours after the morning dose for sustained-release forms.

The previous examples of dosage schedules are by no means complete for all situations; they are intended only as an example of such schedules and of the complexity involved in treating patients with theophylline. Complete tables for different ages and clinical applications should be consulted when administering theophylline.

Theophylline Toxicity and Side Effects

An unfortunate and important problem with use of theophylline is its narrow therapeutic margin. This

| Box 8-1 | Adverse Reactions Seen With Theophylline Treatment, Organized by Organ System* |

Central Nervous System
Headache
Anxiety
Restlessness
Insomnia
Tremor
Convulsions

Gastrointestinal
Nausea
Vomiting
Anorexia
Abdominal pain
Diarrhea
Hematemesis
Gastroesophageal reflux

Respiratory
Tachypnea

Cardiovascular
Palpitations
Supraventricular tachycardia
Ventricular arrhythmias
Hypotension

Renal
Diuresis

*Effects are not listed in order of severity or progression.

refers to the fact that there is very little difference between the dose and serum level that give therapeutic benefit and those that cause toxic side effects. In fact, even within the therapeutic serum levels of 10 to 20 μg/ml, distressing side effects can be experienced. The most common adverse reactions usually seen with theophylline are listed in Box 8-1.

Gastric upset, headache, anxiety, and nervousness are not unusual as less toxic side effects of theophylline and can result in loss of school time or workdays. The diuretic effect should be noted in patients with excess airway secretions (e.g., patients with bronchitis or cystic fibrosis), with adequate fluid replacement when necessary to prevent dehydration and thickening of secretions.

Reactions to levels of theophylline also can be unpredictable from patient to patient. Studies are cited in which reported serum levels of 78.5 and 104.8 μg/ml caused only gastrointestinal symptoms, whereas mean levels of 35 μg/ml caused cardiac arrhythmias or seizures.[14] Also, there may be little warning from minor side effects before serious toxic effects such as arrhythmias or seizures occur.

FACTORS AFFECTING THEOPHYLLINE ACTIVITY

Theophylline is metabolized in the liver and eliminated by the kidneys. Any condition that affects these organs can affect theophylline levels in the body. Interactions between other drugs and theophylline can affect serum levels of the drug. Some of the common drugs and conditions that increase or decrease theophylline levels are listed in Box 8-2.

Viral hepatitis or left ventricular failure can cause elevated serum levels of theophylline for a given dose because of decreased liver metabolism of the drug. An opposite effect of decreased serum levels is caused by cigarette smoking, which stimulates the production of liver enzymes that inactivate the methylxanthines.[15] This necessitates higher theophylline doses. Some drugs used for treatment of tuberculosis, such as isoniazid, and the loop diuretics, such as furosemide (Lasix) or bumetanide (Bumex), are unpredictable in their effect and may either increase or decrease theophylline levels. Measurement of serum levels is extremely important when using these agents with theophylline.

The β agonists and theophylline have an additive effect and are often combined when treating patients with asthma or COPD. Theophylline may antagonize the sedative effect of the benzodiazepines (e.g., Valium). Theophylline can also reverse the paralyzing effect of the nondepolarizing neuromuscular blocking agents (pancuronium, atracurium) in a dose-dependent manner. This is important to realize when paralyzing patients with severe asthma to facilitate ventilatory support and when intravenous administration of aminophylline is used.

Box 8-2	Factors That Can Increase or Decrease Blood Levels of Theophylline, and Affect Dosage Requirements

Increase	Decrease
Alcohol (0.9 g/kg)	Barbiturates
β-Blocking agents	β Agonists
Calcium channel blockers	Aminoglutethimide
Cimetidine, ranitidine	Carbamazepine
Corticosteroids	Cigarette smoking
Disulfiram	Isoniazid (+ or −)*
Ephedrine	Isoproterenol (IV)
Estrogen	Ketoconazole
Influenza virus vaccine	Loop diuretics (+ or −)
Interferon	Moricizine
Mexlitine	Phenytoin
Macrolide antibiotics (e.g., clarithromycin)	Rifampin
Quinolones, oral contraceptives	Sulfinpyrazone
Methotrexate	
Pentoxifylline	
Tacrine	
Ticlopidine	
Troleandomycin	
Zileuton	
Hepatitis	
Cirrhosis	
Congestive heart failure	
Pneumonia	
Renal failure	

Data from Weinberger M, Hendeles L: Theophylline in asthma, *N Engl J Med* 334:1380, 1996; American Thoracic Society: Standards for the diagnosis and care of patients with chronic obstructive pulmonary disease, *Am J Respir Crit Care Med* 152:S77, 1995.

* +, Increase in theophylline level; −, decrease in theophylline level.

CLINICAL APPLICATION

Recent guidelines for the pharmacological management of asthma and COPD do not indicate theophylline as first-line therapy (see Appendix D). The disadvantages of theophylline are its narrow therapeutic margin, toxic effects, unpredictable blood levels and need for individual dosing, and numerous drug-drug and drug-condition interactions.

USE IN ASTHMA

The role of theophylline preparations in the management of acute and stable asthma and COPD has been debated.[16-17] In the treatment of asthma, theophylline is suggested after reliever agents, such as a β agonist, and other controller agents, such as inhaled steroids, or mediator antagonists (cromolyn-like drugs) targeting the underlying inflammation.[1]

USE IN CHRONIC OBSTRUCTIVE PULMONARY DISEASE

Use as a maintenance agent in COPD is indicated if ipratropium bromide and a β agonist fail to provide adequate control. Development of long-acting β agonists, such as salmeterol, offer an additional drug choice to preserve lung function in COPD before using theophylline, especially if theophylline was used to prevent nocturnal symptoms. The increased area under the FEV_1 curve (AUC) with salmeterol gives more consistent improvement in lung function on a 12-hour basis and maintains a higher baseline of lung function.[18] Theophylline or the intravenous salt aminophylline are listed as one of several bronchoactive agents for managing an acute exacerbation of COPD, in the GOLD guidelines.[2]

Because of side effects in the gastrointestinal system, xanthines are contraindicated in subjects with active peptic ulcer or acute gastritis. Suppositories should not be used if the rectum or lower colon is irritated. If stomach upset occurs with theophylline, the drug may be taken with food. Ingestion of large amounts of caffeine from other sources such as tea or coffee may precipitate side effects when taking theophylline.

NONBRONCHODILATING EFFECTS OF THEOPHYLLINE

Although theophylline is classified as a bronchodilator, it actually has a relatively weak bronchodilating action. The efficacy of theophylline in obstructive lung disease may be due to its nonbronchodilating effects on ventilation. This concept of the effectiveness of theophylline is consistent with the finding of significant clinical improvement despite little increase in expiratory flow rates in asthmatic patients.[19] Mahler and colleagues[20] documented the effect of theophylline in reducing dyspnea in COPD subjects when there was no reversibility of obstruction and no objective improvement in lung function, gas exchange, or exercise performance capability. The nonbronchodilating effects of theophylline are listed with a brief commentary.

RESPIRATORY MUSCLE STRENGTH

Theophylline can increase the force of respiratory muscle contractility, and this effect is thought to inhibit or even reverse muscle fatigue and subsequent ventilatory failure. Theophylline can have the same effect on limb skeletal muscle. Aubier and associates[21] demonstrated increased diaphragmatic strength and transdiaphragmatic pressure generation by using electromyographic stimuli before and after theophylline administration.

RESPIRATORY MUSCLE ENDURANCE

Methylxanthines also show evidence of increasing respiratory muscle endurance, as well as strength. This can prevent fatigue of the respiratory muscles, especially with an increased resistance. Xanthines have been shown to increase the time that an external inspiratory load could be sustained.[19]

CENTRAL VENTILATORY DRIVE

The methylxanthines have also been shown to increase ventilatory drive at the level of the central nervous system. In particular, theophylline can increase phrenic nerve activity for a given level of chemical stimulus.[21] This effect on ventilatory drive seems to occur at the level of the midbrain and may involve the neurotransmitter dopamine.

CARDIOVASCULAR EFFECTS

Theophylline use may have nonbronchodilating advantages in subjects with COPD who also have cardiac disease or cor pulmonale. Theophylline can increase cardiac output, decrease pulmonary vascular resistance, and improve myocardial muscle perfusion in ischemic regions.[22]

ANTIINFLAMMATORY EFFECTS

Theophylline also has some antiinflammatory effects, which may also explain its efficacy despite the fact the drug is a relatively weak bronchodilator.[16,23] Evidence indicates that theophylline can produce some degree of immunomodulation, and an antiinflammatory and bronchoprotective effect through inhibition of cAMP-specific phosphodiesterase enzymes, particularly PDE3 and PDE4, in proinflammatory cells and tissues. Theophylline has been shown to cause the following (see references for detailed antiinflammatory effects of theophylline[16,23-25]):

- Decreased migration of activated eosinophils into bronchial mucosa with allergen stimuli and reduced eosinophil survival
- Reduced T-cell proliferation and accumulation in atopic asthma with corresponding improvement in pulmonary function
- Inhibition of proinflammatory cytokines, such as IL-β, TNF-α, and IFN-γ, and increased production of the antiinflammatory cytokine IL-10
- Attenuation of the late-phase response to histamine in patients with allergic asthma
- Reduced airway responsiveness to stimuli such as histamine, methacholine, allergen, sulfur dioxide, distilled water, cyanates, and adenosine

The antiinflammatory and immunomodulating effects of theophylline occur at lower plasma concentrations such as 9 to 10 μg/ml, in contrast with those usually recommended for bronchodilation, and may result in a steroid-sparing effect.[24] Inhibitors of PDE4, with more selectivity than theophylline and reduced toxic effect profile, may offer a new class of antiinflammatory agents.[7]

USE IN APNEA OF PREMATURITY

When nonpharmacological methods are not successful in AOP, xanthines such as theophylline and caffeine are still considered a first-line choice of drug therapy, as stated in the indications for this class of drug. Theophylline is biotransformed to caffeine in neonates.[26] However, caffeine is preferred to theophylline for a variety of pharmacological reasons, as follows[5]:

- Caffeine penetrates more readily than theophylline into cerebrospinal fluid and can be effective in infants refractory to theophylline therapy.
- Caffeine is a more potent stimulant of the central nervous system and the respiratory system than theophylline.
- Dosing regimens are simpler and give more predictable results with caffeine than with theophylline, most likely because of smaller plasma fluctuations with caffeine.
- Caffeine has a wider therapeutic margin, with fewer side effects than theophylline.

A standard preparation of caffeine, caffeine citrate (Cafcit), is available, which can be administered either orally or intravenously. The recommended loading dose is 20 mg/kg of caffeine citrate (equivalent to 10 mg/kg of caffeine). This is followed 24 to 48 hours later by a single daily maintenance dose of 5 mg/kg of caffeine citrate (2.5 mg/kg of caffeine). Serum concentrations of 5 to 20 mg/L of caffeine have been found effective.[5]

CONCLUSION

The effects of respiratory muscle function and the ventilatory stimulus response could be as important or even more important than the bronchodilating action of xanthines. Such effects would be complementary to the bronchodilating action of β agonists and anticholinergic bronchodilators in managing COPD and asthma. As the structure-activity relations of the xanthines are better understood, it is hoped that new analogues may prove effective in preserving ventilatory function, while eliminating the troublesome side effects and the narrow therapeutic margin associated with current forms.

SUMMARY KEY TERMS AND CONCEPTS

- *Theophylline*, and its salt, *aminophylline*, are members of the *methylxanthine* group of drugs, which also includes *dyphylline* and *enprofylline*.

- Xanthines generally have *stimulant* properties, exemplified by the xanthine caffeine. Other effects of this class of drug include diuresis and smooth muscle relaxation (e.g., bronchodilation).
- The *clinical uses* of theophylline are management of asthma, COPD, and apnea of prematurity in neonates.
- The exact *mode of action* of xanthines is unclear; antagonism of adenosine receptors may occur, perhaps as a partial mechanism for the effects of drugs such as theophylline.
- Because individuals vary in the rate at which theophylline is metabolized, dosage must be titrated to clinical effect, avoidance of side effects, and, most precisely, a *therapeutic serum level* of 10 to 12 μg/ml in COPD and between 5 to 15 μg/ml in asthma management.
- Theophylline has a *narrow therapeutic margin,* and side effects such as gastric upset, headache, insomnia, nervousness, palpitations, and diuresis occur frequently, even within the therapeutic range of dosing. Blood levels of theophylline are affected by many factors, which can either increase or decrease the amount of the drug in the body.
- Theophylline has been relegated to the level of a second- or third-line drug in treating *asthma*, and is considered if β agonists and antiinflammatory therapy fail to control symptoms.
- In COPD the *nonbronchodilating effects* of theophylline, such as ventilatory drive stimulation, and enhanced respiratory muscle function are of value, although its use is debated.

SELF-ASSESSMENT QUESTIONS

1. What drug in the xanthine group is used most often therapeutically?
2. What is the difference between aminophylline and theophylline?
3. What is the recommended therapeutic plasma level for theophylline in asthma?
4. How do you know whether a given dose of theophylline will produce a satisfactory treatment effect in an asthmatic?
5. Identify at least three adverse side effects seen with theophylline.
6. What is meant by a "narrow therapeutic margin"?
7. Although theophylline is a weak bronchodilator, what other effects make it useful in treating chronic airflow obstruction?
8. True or False: theophylline causes bronchodilation and improved airflow solely by inhibiting phosphodiesterase, which breaks down cAMP.

Answers to Self-Assessment Questions are found in Appendix A.

CLINICAL SCENARIO

A 70-year-old white male brought himself to the hospital emergency department. He was severely short of breath (SOB) and could take only a few steps before complaining of dyspnea. He reported coughing up thick, greenish sputum, with some tinges of blood in the last few days. He appeared oriented, coherent, and somewhat malnourished, with thin arms. On interview he admitted to smoking two packs of cigarettes a day since age 18, stopping about 2 years ago. He has had six hospitalizations within the last 2 years. Current medications include ipratropium bromide by MDI, 2 puffs four times daily, with a β_2 agonist by MDI as needed, 1 to 3 puffs. He has been using the β_2 MDI regularly during the last month, at least four times daily.

On physical examination, he was very SOB, even at rest, and used accessory muscles with an RR of 22 breaths/min. There was little discernible chest expansion. His breath sounds were distant in all areas, with expiratory wheezes, and air movement appeared poor. He was afebrile; P, 120 beats/min; BP, 170/112 mm Hg. He was admitted with a diagnosis of acute exacerbation of COPD.

Laboratory values on admission showed normal electrolytes, but his WBC count was 15.2×10^3/cc and his hemoglobin was 10.6 g/dl. Arterial blood gas values on room air were as follows: pH, 7.40; $Paco_2$, 42.4 mm Hg; Pao_2, 64 mm Hg; base excess, +1.9 mEq/L; and Sao_2, 90%.

A chest radiograph (PA) shows hyperinflation of the lung fields, with flattened diaphragms.

What is the first drug that is indicated by this individual's blood sample values?

Would you continue his use of ipratropium bromide; if so, what dose would you suggest?

What additional bronchodilator therapy could you recommend?

What is the rationale for use of theophylline in this patient?

What would you check before initiating therapy with theophylline?

What serum theophylline level would you target, if the patient is started on theophylline?

Answers to Clinical Scenario Questions are found in Appendix A.

REFERENCES

1. National Asthma Education and Prevention Program, Expert Panel Report II: *Guidelines for the diagnosis and management of asthma*, Bethesda, 1997, National Institutes of Health.
2. Global Initiative for Chronic Obstructive Lung Disease (GOLD), Workshop Report: *Gold strategy for the diagnosis, management, and prevention of COPD*, National Heart, Lung, and Blood Institute, Bethesda, Md, World Health Organization, 2001.
3. Ferguson GT: Recommendations for the management of COPD, *Chest* 117:23S, 2000.
4. Pauwels RA: National and international guidelines for COPD: the need for evidence, *Chest* 117:20S, 2000
5. Bhatia J: Current options in the management of apnea of prematurity, *Clin Pediatr* 39:327, 2000.
6. Stewart BN, Block AJ: A trial of aerosolized theophylline in relieving bronchospasm, *Chest* 69:718, 1976.
7. Giembycz MA: Phosphodiesterase 4 inhibitors and the treatment of asthma, *Drugs* 59:193, 2000.
8. Persson CGA, Karlsson J: In vitro responses to bronchodilator drugs. In Jenne JW, Murphy S, eds: *Drug therapy for asthma: research and clinical practice*, New York, 1987, Marcel Dekker.
9. Jenne JW: Physiology and pharmacodynamics of the xanthines. In Jenne JW, Murphy S, eds: *Drug therapy for asthma: research and clinical practice*, New York, 1987, Marcel Dekker.
10. Svedmyr N: Theophylline, *Am Rev Respir Dis* 136(suppl):568, 1987.
11. Jenne JW and others: Pharmacokinetics of theophylline: application to adjustment of the clinical dose of aminophylline, *Clin Pharmacol Ther* 13:349, 1972.
12. Kaliner M: Goals of asthma therapy, *Ann Allergy Asthma Immunol* 75:169, 1995.
13. Tashkin DP: Measurement and significance of the bronchodilator response. In Jenne JW, Murphy S, eds: *Drug therapy for asthma: research and clinical practice*, New York, 1987, Marcel Dekker.
14. Kelly HW: Theophylline toxicity. In Jenne JW, Murphy S, eds: *Drug therapy for asthma: research and clinical practice*, New York, 1987, Marcel Dekker.
15. Powell JR and others: Theophylline disposition in acutely ill hospitalized patients: the effect of smoking, heart failure, severe airway obstruction and pneumonia, *Am Rev Respir Dis* 118:229, 1978.
16. Weinberger M, Hendeles L: Theophylline in asthma, *N Engl J Med* 334:1380, 1996.
17. Lam A, Newhouse MT: Management of asthma and chronic airflow limitation: are methylxanthines obsolete? *Chest* 98:44, 1990.
18. Mahler DA and others: Efficacy of salmeterol xinafoate in the treatment of COPD, *Chest* 115:957, 1999.
19. Supinski GS: Effects of methylxanthines on respiratory skeletal muscle and neural drive. In Jenne JW, Murphy S, eds: *Drug therapy for asthma: research and clinical practice*, New York, 1987, Marcel Dekker.
20. Mahler DA and others: Sustained-release theophylline reduces dyspnea in nonreversible obstructive airway disease, *Am Rev Respir Dis* 131:22, 1985.
21. Aubier M and others: Aminophylline improves diaphragmatic contractility, *N Engl J Med* 305:249, 1981.

22. Ziment I: Pharmacologic therapy of obstructive airway disease, *Clin Chest Med* 11:461, 1990.

23. Sullivan P and others: Antiinflammatory effects of low-dose oral theophylline in atopic asthma, *Lancet* 343:1006, 1994.

24. Page CP: Recent advances in our understanding of the use of theophylline in the treatment of asthma, *J Clin Pharmacol* 39:237, 1999.

25. Markham A, Faulds D: Theophylline: a review of its potential steroid sparing effects in asthma, *Drugs* 56:1081, 1998.

26. Yeh TF: *Drug therapy in the neonate and small infant,* St Louis, 1985, Mosby.

Mucus-Controlling Drug Therapy

Bruce K. Rubin • Mamta Fuloria • Joseph L. Rau

CHAPTER OUTLINE

Chapter 9 presents an in-depth review of the mucociliary system and the nature of mucus, as a basis for discussing pharmacological agents used in the treatment of respiratory secretions. The two drugs currently used in North America by aerosol administration, acetylcysteine and dornase alfa, are presented, along with several investigational agents. The effects of bland aerosols are considered, and possible future directions for mucoactive drug therapy are outlined.

DRUG CONTROL OF MUCUS: A PERSPECTIVE

One of the major defense mechanisms of the lung is the self-renewing, self-cleansing mucociliary escalator. Failure of this system results in mechanical obstruction of the airway, often with thickened, adhesive secretions. In many diseases associated with abnormal mucociliary function (e.g., bronchitis, asthma, and cystic fibrosis), a marked slowing of mucus transport is noted.[1,2] Whether such slowing is due to changes in the physical properties of mucus or to decreased cil-

Table 9-1

Mucoactive agents available for aerosol administration

DRUG	BRAND NAME	ADULT DOSAGE	USE
Acetylcysteine 10% Acetylcysteine 20% Mucosil-20	Mucomyst Mucosil-10 Mucomyst	SVN: 3-5 ml	Bronchitis; efficacy not proven
Dornase alfa	Pulmozyme	SVN: 2.5 mg/ampule one ampule daily*	Cystic fibrosis
Aqueous aerosols: water, saline (0.45%, 0.9%, 5%-10%)	N/A	SVN: 3-5 ml SVN: 3-5 ml, as ordered USN: 3-5 ml, as ordered	Sputum induction, secretion mobilization

*Use recommended nebulizer system (see package insert).
N/A, Not applicable; *SVN*, small volume nebulizer; *USN*, ultrasonic nebulizer.

iary activity, or both, is not always clear. Mucus is found in several areas of the body, including the airways, gastrointestinal tract, and genital tract. Regardless of its location, mucus seems to serve protective purposes, including lubrication, waterproofing, and protection against osmotic or inflammatory changes.

Historically in respiratory care, drug therapy for secretions has been aimed at liquefying thick mucus to a watery state. It is recognized that mucus is a gel with physical properties of viscosity *and* elasticity. Drug therapy for mucus secretions in acute and chronic bronchitis, asthma, respiratory infections, and cystic fibrosis should optimize the physical state of the mucous gel for efficient ciliary transport. As a result, the term *mucolytic*, indicating breakdown of mucus, is better replaced with *mucoactive agent*. A review of mucus physiology presents the concepts necessary for discussing the current and future pharmacological management of secretions. The amount of this chapter devoted to understanding the production, nature, and regulation of respiratory mucus reflects the current situation in which the knowledge of airway mucus has outstripped the development of therapies, including pharmacological, for control of secretion dysfunction.

CLINICAL INDICATION FOR USE

The general indication for mucoactive therapy is to reduce accumulation of airway secretions, with concomitant improvement in pulmonary function and gas exchange and the prevention of repeated infection and airway damage. Diseases in which mucoactive therapy is indicated are those with hypersecretion or poor clearance of airway secretions. These include cystic fibrosis, acute and chronic bronchitis, pneumonia,

diffuse panbronchiolitis, primary ciliary dyskinesia, and bronchiectasis. Not all subjects with mucus retention benefit from mucoactive drug therapy; those with adequately preserved expiratory airflow and cough have greater response. Specific indications for use of individual mucoactive agents are presented in more detail with each agent.

Use of mucoactive therapy to promote secretion clearance should be considered after therapy to decrease infection and inflammation and after minimizing or removing irritants to the airway, including environmental irritants (if possible) and tobacco smoke.[3]

IDENTIFICATION OF AGENTS

Table 9-1 lists general information on mucoactive agents that are approved, available, or commonly administered as inhaled aerosols. Greater detail will be given on indications, dosage and administration, hazards and side effects, and assessment of drug therapy in the discussion of each agent.

Mucoactive agents are intended to promote secretion clearance and differ in their mechanism of action. Secretion properties that impair airway clearance also differ among diseases and at different times in the course of a disease. The source and properties of airway secretions, as well as the mechanisms of action for the mucoactive agents, are the basis for clinical use of this class of drugs.

PHYSIOLOGY OF THE MUCOCILIARY SYSTEM

SOURCE OF AIRWAY SECRETIONS

The conducting airways in the lung and the nasal cavity to the oropharynx are lined by a mucociliary system (Figure 9-1). The secretion lining the surface of

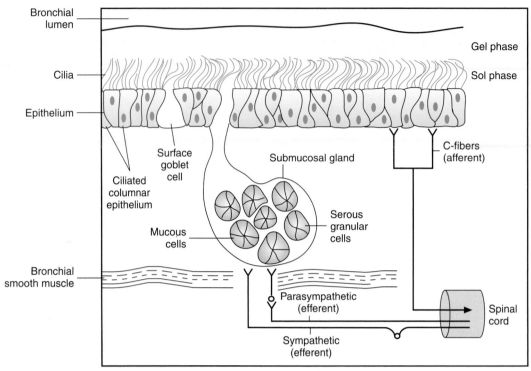

Figure 9-1   Principal components and innervation of the mucociliary system in the respiratory tract.

the airway is called *mucus;* it has been described as having two phases: a *gel* layer (0.5 to 20 μm) that is propelled toward the larynx by the cilia and floats on top of a watery *periciliary* layer (7 to 10 μm).[3] Cells responsible for secretion in the airway and the source of components found in respiratory mucus have been summarized by Basbaum and associates.[4] Although there are many cell types in the mammalian airway, the essential secretory structures of the mucociliary system are the following:

- Surface epithelial cells
- Pseudostratified, columnar, ciliated epithelial cells
- Surface goblet (or surface mucous) cells
- Clara cells in the distal airway
- Submucosal gland, with serous and mucous cells

Submucosal glands are found in cartilaginous airways. Beyond the distal airways, these mucus-producing cells are not found. Mucus secreted by surface epithelial cells and glands in the airway provide for basic protection of the respiratory tract, including humidification and warming of inspired gas, mucociliary

transport of debris, waterproofing and insulation, and antibacterial activity.[3]

TERMINOLOGY

Confusion has existed regarding the nomenclature used to classify mucoactive medications. Although some authors have used *mucolytic* as a generic term for these agents, it is clear that most of these medications are thought to mobilize secretions by mechanisms other than by the direct "thinning" of mucus. For example, although the mucociliary transportability of sputum is often improved by reducing sputum viscosity, the cough clearability of secretions is independent of sputum viscosity. Increased knowledge of the properties of mucus has given us tools to better understand the mechanisms of airway disease and mucoactive therapy.

Expectorants are thought to increase the volume or hydration of airway secretions. Systemic hydration and classic expectorants (guaifenesin, iodide) have not been demonstrated to be clinically effective. Modifiers of airway water transport including tricyclic nucleotides, hyperosmolar saline, or mannitol are being clinically investigated as expectorants.

Table 9-2

Terminology associated with secretions found in the airway and drug therapy of respiratory secretions*

TERM	DEFINITION
Mucus	Secretion from mucous membranes, including surface goblet cells and submucosal glands.[5] Purified glycoprotein from the secretion is termed *mucous glycoprotein* or *mucin*.[6]
Sputum	Expectorated secretions that contain respiratory tract, oropharyngeal, and nasopharyngeal secretions, as well as bacteria and products of inflammation.[5]
Gel	A macromolecular description of part of the respiratory secretion that has a structure determined by intermolecular attractions, along with properties of viscosity and elasticity.[5]
Sol	A macromolecular description of the respiratory secretion in true solution, with the physical property of viscosity (usually referred to as the *periciliary layer*)
Glycoprotein	A protein with covalently attached oligosaccharide units.[5] The principal constituent of mucus and a high-molecular-weight glycoprotein, it gives mucus its physical/chemical properties such as viscoelasticity.
Oligosaccharide	A sugar that is the individual carbohydrate unit of glycoproteins.[5]
Mucoactive	A general term connoting any agent that has an effect on mucus secretion; may include mucolytic, expectorant, mucospissic, mucoregulatory, or mucokinetic agents.[7]
Mucoregulatory	An agent that reduces mucus hypersecretion to normal levels.[7]
Mucolytic	Breaks down the structure of mucus, usually reducing viscosity and elasticity.[7]
Mucokinetic	An effect of improving the mobilization and clearance of respiratory mucus secretions.[7]
Mucospissic	An effect of increasing the viscosity and elasticity of mucus secretion.[7]
Expectorant	An agent improving expectoration of respiratory secretions, usually by stimulation of bronchial gland output.[7]

*Sources indicated in the numerical references.

Mucolytics degrade polymers in secretions. The *classic mucolytics* have free thiol groups to degrade mucin, and *peptide mucolytics* break pathological filaments of neutrophil-derived DNA or actin in sputum. These appear to be effective in chronic inflammatory airway diseases.

Mucokinetics are medications that increase mucociliary efficiency or cough efficiency. Cough flow can be increased by bronchodilators in patients with airway hyperreactivity. Abhesives such as surfactants decrease epithelial-mucus attachment augmenting both cough and mucociliary clearance.

Mucoregulatory agents reduce the volume of airway mucus secretion and appear to be especially effective in hypersecretory states such as bronchorrhea, diffuse panbronchiolitis, and some forms of asthma. These medications include antiinflammatory agents (indomethacin, glucocorticosteroids), anticholinergic agents, and some macrolide antibiotics. Table 9-2 lists terminology used with airway secretions.

SURFACE EPITHELIAL CELLS

The surface of the trachea and bronchi includes primarily ciliated cells and goblet cells, in a ratio of ap-proximately 5:1. Goblet cells contain granules of mucus that are electron-lucent and resemble the granules of the submucosal gland mucous cells. There are over 6000 goblet cells per square millimeter of normal airway mucosa. Goblet cells do not seem to be directly innervated in human lung, although they do respond to irritants by increasing the production of mucus, and they may respond to sympathomimetic agents. Figures 9-2 and 9-3 show scanning electron micrographs of the mucous lining (Figure 9-2) and of the bronchiolar surface with the mucus stripped away (Figure 9-3). In addition to ciliated and goblet cells, microvilli, which may have a reabsorptive function, can be seen in Figure 9-3.

SUBEPITHELIAL CELLS

Submucosal glands below the epithelial surface are thought to provide the majority of mucus secretion, having a total volume around 40 times greater than that of goblet cells in the proximal airways. The submucosal gland is under parasympathetic (vagal) control and responds to cholinergic stimulation by increasing the amount of mucus secreted. Evidence suggests that submucosal glands in the respiratory

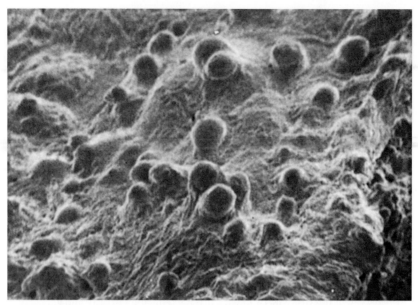

Figure 9-2   Scanning electron micrograph of the mucus blanket in a bronchiole, prepared from hamster lung. (From Nowell JA, Tyler WS: Scanning electron microscopy of the surface morphology of mammalian lungs, *Am Rev Respir Dis* 103:313, 1971.)

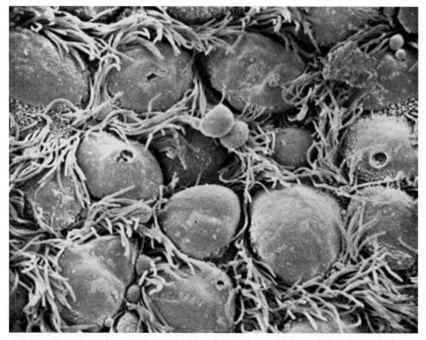

Figure 9-3   Scanning electron micrograph of the airway surface shows epithelial cells with cilia, possible surface goblet cells dehiscing, and some microvilli. (From Nowell JA, Tyler WS: Scanning electron microscopy of the surface morphology of mammalian lungs, *Am Rev Respir Dis* 103:313, 1971.)

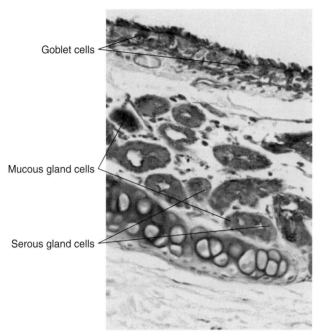

Goblet cells

Mucous gland cells

Serous gland cells

Figure 9-4   Light microscopy demonstrating immunohistochemical staining of the ferret airway using horseradish peroxidase conjugated DBA. The tracheal section shows the mucociliary apparatus, including surface mucous (goblet) cells, ciliated epithelial cells, and serous and mucous glands.

tract are innervated by sympathetic axons and the peptidergic nerve system described previously in Chapter 5.

Two types of cells, mucous and serous, are found in the gland. Figure 9-4 shows a section of the ferret airway stained for mucin with the surface mucous (goblet) cells and the submucosal gland serous and mucous cells identified. The secretions from the serous and mucous cells mix in the submucosal gland and are transported through a ciliated duct onto the airway lumen.

CILIARY SYSTEM

Droplets of mucus from the secretory cells form plaques or "flakes" in the distal, nonciliated airway and coalesce into clumps in the more proximal ciliated airway. It may be that the mucous flakes are stagnant for a short time before being propelled and that the watery periciliary layer separates from the upper viscoelastic layer. Mucociliary transport results from the movement of the mucous gel by the beating cilia. There are approximately 200 cilia on each cell. Cilia are approximately 7 μm in length in larger airways

and shorten to 5 μm or slightly less in smaller bronchioles. Luk and Dulfano[8] examined the frequency of ciliary beat on biopsy samples from various tracheobronchial regions and found rates of 8 to 18 Hz (Hz = 1 cycle/sec) at 37° C on epithelial fragments, which is 660 to 1080 beats/min. A ciliary beat is made up of an *effective* (power) stroke and a *recovery* stroke with about a 1:2 ratio. In the effective stroke the cilium moves in an upright position through a full forward arc, to contact the underside of the mucus layer and propel it forward. In the recovery stroke the cilium swings back around to the starting point near the cell surface, to avoid pulling secretions back. Cilia beat in a coordinated, metachronal wave of motion to propel airway secretions. A functional surfactant layer lies at the tips of the cilia and separates the periciliary fluid from the mucous gel. This layer allows the cilia to effectively transmit kinetic energy to the mucus without becoming entangled. This layer also facilitates mucus spreading as a continuous layer and prevents water loss from the periciliary fluid. The properties of cilia given here are described in detail in a 1988 review by Sleigh and colleagues, with a complete list of references.[9]

FACTORS AFFECTING MUCOCILIARY TRANSPORT

The rate of mucociliary transport varies in the normal lung and has been estimated at around 1.5 mm/min in peripheral airways and 21.5 mm/min in the trachea. Transport rates are slower in the presence of the following conditions or substances, many of which are associated with airway damage.

- Chronic obstructive pulmonary disease (COPD)
- Parasympatholytics (atropine)
- Narcotics
- Endotracheal suctioning and tracheostomy
- Cigarette smoke
- Atmospheric pollutants (SO_2 NO_2, ozone) may increase or decrease transport rates
- Hyperoxia and hypoxia

Table 9-3 summarizes the effects of drug groups commonly used in respiratory care, on ciliary beat, mucus output, and overall transport.

FOOD INTAKE AND MUCUS PRODUCTION

A common belief is that drinking dairy milk increases the production of mucus, or phlegm, and congestion in the respiratory tract. Respiratory care personnel may be asked for advice on withholding milk from children with colds, respiratory infections, or chronic

Table 9-3

Effects of various drug groups on mucociliary clearance

DRUG GROUP	CILIARY BEAT	MUCUS PRODUCTION	TRANSPORT
β Adrenergic	Increase	Increase*	±
Cholinergic	Increase	Increase	Increase
Methylxanthines	Increase	Increase	±
Cromolyn sodium	None	None	None
Corticosteroid (beclomethasone)	None	Decrease (if airway is inflamed)	None

*Data from Wanner A: Clinical aspects of mucociliary transport, *Am J Respir Dis* 116:73, 1977.

respiratory conditions such as cystic fibrosis. Pinnock and colleagues[10] inoculated 60 healthy subjects with rhinovirus 2 in a study designed to answer the question of whether milk causes increased mucus production. Milk intake ranged from 0 to 11 glasses a day. They reported no association between milk or dairy product intake and an increase in upper or lower respiratory tract symptoms of congestion or in nasal secretion weight. There was a trend for cough to be "loose" with increasing intake of milk, although this was not significant. None of the subjects were allergic to cow's milk. The authors concluded that the data do not support the withholding of milk or the belief that milk increases respiratory tract congestion.

NATURE OF MUCUS SECRETION

A healthy person is thought to produce around 100 ml of mucus per 24 hours, and the secretion is clear, viscoelastic, and adhesive. Apparently, most of this secretion is reabsorbed in the bronchial mucosa, with only 10 ml or so reaching the glottis. This amount is rarely noticed by the individual. During disease states, the volume of secretions can increase dramatically, and the secretions are expectorated or swallowed. One of the primary functions of respiratory tract mucus is thought to be transporting and removing trapped inhaled particles, cellular debris, or dead and aging cells.

STRUCTURE AND COMPOSITION OF MUCUS

The structure and major constituents of the mucus secreted by the submucosal glands and surface goblet cells are pictured in Figure 9-5 and have been reviewed by Basbaum.[6] Basbaum and colleagues[4] and Lundgren and Shelhamer[11] also provide summaries of the composition and structure of mucus.

Mucus is a complex, high-molecular-weight macromolecule consisting of a mucin protein backbone to which carbohydrate *(oligosaccharide)* side chains are attached. The carbohydrate content is 80% or more of the total weight of the macromolecule. This structure has been likened to a bottle brush in appearance. This general structure of protein and attached saccharide side chains is termed a *glycoprotein*. Mucus forms a flexible, threadlike strand from 200 nm up to 6 μm in length,[12] that is linearly cross-linked with disulfide (—S—S—) bonds. Strands may perhaps be further cross-linked with each other by disulfide and hydrogen bonding. The result is a gel that consists of a high water content (90% to 95%) organized around the structural elements; the gel is intensely hydrophilic and spongelike.[13,14] The final gelation of mucus is probably due to a combination of hydrogen, electrostatic and hydrophobic bonds, and the specific disulfide linkages.

Under normal circumstances, bonding within mucus produces low viscosity but moderate elasticity. Although mucous gel incorporates water during its formation, a gel is both a liquid and a solid, as will be discussed in a later section. A better analogy is Jell-O, which is mostly water but organizes into a semisolid by its chemical structure as the liquid "gels." It is important clinically to note that sufficient water must be available in the body to form mucus with normal physical properties, but once formed, mucus does not readily incorporate topically applied water, as shown by Dulfano and associates.[15]

Phospholipids are also present in the serous and mucous cell granules of the submucosal glands. When released onto the airway surface, they may serve as lubricants affecting the surface-active and adhesive properties of mucus, both of which can affect mucociliary transport function.[3]

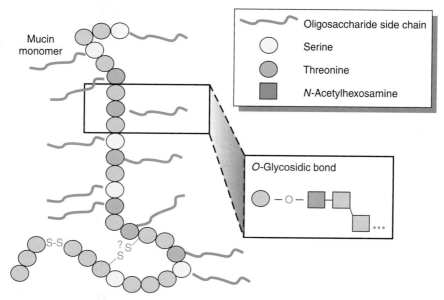

Figure 9-5   Basic structure and constituents of the mucus macromolecule.

In addition to the mucous gel secreted in the airway, bronchial secretions contain other substances such as serum proteins (albumin, secretory IgA and IgG immunoglobulins, α_1-antitrypsin, complement components), lysozyme, lactoferrin, and electrolytes (sodium, potassium, chloride, calcium). Antibacterial defense in the airway is provided by secretory IgA, IgG, lysozyme, lactoferrin, definsins, peroxidase, and serine proteases released by cells such as neutrophils. Bronchial secretions control the potentially destructive action of protease enzymes with two major antiproteases: α_1-protease inhibitor, or α_1AT, and secretory leukoprotease inhibitor (sLPI), a cationic protein found in serous secretory glandular cells.[3] In healthy airways, the antiproteases are present in higher quantities than the protease enzymes and provide a protease screen.[16]

EPITHELIAL ION TRANSPORT

The composition and amount of the periciliary fluid layer is regulated in part by ion transport across the epithelial cells lining the airway lumen. If the periciliary layer is not approximately the height of an extended cilium, effective mucus movement cannot occur.[17] Defective ion transport contributes to the cycle of retained secretions and infection seen in cystic fibrosis. Normal airway epithelial ion transport is illustrated in Figure 9-6.

In the basal, unstimulated state, sodium (Na^+) absorption into the epithelial cell is the dominant

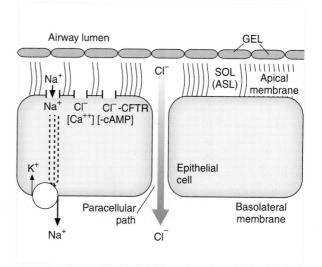

Figure 9-6   Illustration of ion exchange mechanisms across the normal airway epithelium controlling absorption/secretion for the periciliary airway surface liquid *(ASL)*, or *SOL*. Under basal conditions, sodium (Na^+) is absorbed along with liquid, with no net chloride (Cl^-) secretion from the cell into the liquid layer. *cAMP*, Cyclic adenosine monophosphate; *CFTR*, cystic fibrosis transmembrane regulator.

ion exchange that absorbs liquid from the airway periciliary layer. Sodium absorption occurs as an active transport process through sodium channels on the airway lumen side of the cell (apical cell membrane). The sodium in the epithelial cell is then pumped from the cell, driven by a sodium/potassium-ATPase pump on the basolateral membrane (blood vessel side) of the epithelial cell shown in Figure 9-6. When sodium is absorbed from the airway surface liquid, there is an accompanying absorption of chloride ions and water, which occurs through paracellular pathways.[18] Normally, there is no net chloride or liquid exchange into the airway fluid because this unbalances the electrochemical condition. Chloride secretion can occur through at least two different types of chloride channel in the cell apex. One channel is dependent on cyclic adenosine monophosphate (cAMP), also known as the *cystic fibrosis transmembrane regulator* (CFTR) channel; the other channel is calcium activated. The cAMP dependent channel is the channel that is dysfunctional as a result of the mutation in cystic fibrosis of the cystic fibrosis transmembrane regulator (CFTR) gene. The composition of human airway surface liquid reported in studies by Mentz and colleagues,[19] Joris and co-workers,[20] Jayaraman and colleagues,[21] and Baconnais and associates[22] is described in Table 9-4.

To summarize, under normal conditions, healthy airway epithelia can absorb salt and water driven by an active sodium (Na^+) transport; this is the usual basal condition. Normal epithelia can also secrete liquid into the periciliary fluid, driven by an active chloride (Cl^-) transport through ion channels.

MUCUS IN DISEASE STATES

The normal clearance of airway mucus can be altered by changes in the volume, hydration, or composition of the secretion (water, salts, protein, glycoconjugates). The volume is due to the production by surface goblet cells and submucosal gland cells. Water content is a function of transepithelial chloride secretion and osmosis. The composition of respiratory mucus is undergoing investigation by using molecular cloning techniques (Carlstadt)[22a,22b] that can reveal the structure of the varied mucin oligosaccharides, as well as the regulation of mucin synthesis and production[6] and by using structural analysis techniques.[23]

Knowledge of these features of respiratory mucus may lead to a better understanding of diseases characterized by an abnormal production of mucus such as chronic bronchitis, asthma, cystic fibrosis, and bronchiectasis. Acute bronchitis can be superimposed on any of the other diseases. Mucus hypersecretion and airway damage predisposes to bacterial infections in the respiratory tract in chronic bronchitis, asthma, or cystic fibrosis, probably because of impaired clearance of mucus. A green or yellow sputum is caused by the enzyme myeloperoxidase, seen with cellular breakdown, and indicates neutrophil activation.[24] In general, under pathological conditions, changes occur in the physical properties of mucus, including an increase in viscosity, slowed or stopped ciliary motion, and stasis, resulting in mucus impaction. Bronchial

Table 9-4

Composition of airway surface liquid (periciliary layer) in the human bronchi[19-22]

	HEALTHY	CYSTIC FIBROSIS	ASTHMA	ACUTE INFECTION
Sodium (Na^+) (mEq/L)[20]	82 ± 6	121 ± 3.5	27 ± 1.5	147 ± 5.2
Na^+ (mM/L)[21]	103 ± 3			
Na^+ (mM/L)[22]	63.9 ± 7.6	79.7 ± 11.6		
Potassium (K^+) (mEq/L)[20]	29 ± 5	23 ± 9.4	21 ± 5.1	
K^+ (mM/L)[22]	2.4 ± 0.5	3.2 ± 1.6		
Chloride (Cl^-) (mEq/L)[20]	84 ± 9	129 ± 5.3	37 ± 6.5	143 ± 2.9
Cl^- (mM/L)[21]	92 ± 4			
Cl^- (mM/L)[22]	64.9 ± 13.2	82.6 ± 15.7		
Magnesium (Mg^{2+}) (mM/L)[22]	1.9 ± 0.3	2.2 ± 0.4		
Sulfur (mM/L)[22]	4.9 ± 1.3	4.8 ± 0.5		
Osmolarity (mOsm/L)[19]	240			
Water, %[19]	87 ± 11			
pH[19]	7.0 ± 0.1			
pH[21]	6.78 ± 0.2			

See numerical references.

obstruction by secretions can increase airflow resistance and lead to complete airway obstruction and atelectasis.[11]

CHRONIC BRONCHITIS

Chronic bronchitis is defined clinically by the volume of sputum expectorated over time. Histological examination shows hyperplasia of submucosal glands and goblet cells. The number of goblet cells increases, and there is hypertrophy of the submucosal glands, as measured by the Reid index of gland to airway wall thickness ratio.[25] Submucosal glands from patients with chronic bronchitis produce excessive amounts of mucus when studied in vitro.[26] Tobacco smoke is considered the most important predisposing factor to airway irritation and mucus hypersecretion, but other factors include viral infections, pollutants, and genetic predisposition.[11,27]

ASTHMA

Mucus hypersecretion can occur during an acute asthmatic episode or can be a chronic feature of asthma accompanying airway inflammation. In acute episodes, an estimated 8% of patients will have bronchorrhea, discharging more than 100 ml of sputum per day.[28] Turner-Warwick and Openshaw[29] found that as many as 80% of patients with asthma report increased sputum expectoration.

BRONCHORRHEA

Bronchorrhea is the production of watery sputum of 100 ml or more per day.[30] Some of these patients respond well to antiinflammatory therapy such as corticosteroids,[31] H_1 but not H_2 antihistamines,[30] indomethacin by aerosol,[32] or macrolide antibiotics.[33] These are all considered mucoregulatory medications and are most effective when bronchorrhea is associated with airway inflammation. Patients with congenital fucosidosis also have a form of bronchorrhea resulting from the inability of mucins to polymerize. This form of bronchorrhea does not respond to mucoregulatory therapy.[34]

PLASTIC BRONCHITIS

Plastic bronchitis is an uncommon disease that occurs in children and adults. It is also known as fibrinous bronchitis or bronchitis fibroplastica, pseudomembranous bronchitis, or Hoffman's bronchitis. It denotes the formation of large branching mucoid bronchial casts that are expectorated, discovered at the time of bronchoscopy or at autopsy, or identified in a pneumonectomy specimen. The casts contain mainly mucin, and the branching pattern may match the bronchial distribution of an entire lobe or lung.[35] Most patients have underlying cardiac disease. Mucin casts can completely obstruct the airway and can lead to death. Urokinase has been reported to be effective in some patients.[36]

CYSTIC FIBROSIS

Cystic fibrosis is a chronic hereditary disease characterized by impaired function of the exocrine glands, including glands in the airway and the pancreas. Airway mucus hypersecretion results in bronchial obstruction and recurrent respiratory tract infections. The basic defect is a mutation of the cystic fibrosis transmembrane conductance regulator (CFTCR) gene, but it is unclear how abnormal CFTR function leads to abnormal mucus secretion. Airway epithelia in cystic fibrosis show excessive absorption of sodium (Na^+) compared with normal epithelia. There is a limited ability for the epithelial cells to secrete chloride (Cl^-) through the chloride CFTR channels (see Figure 9-6) stimulated by cAMP. The result of excessive Na^+ absorption and limited Cl^- secretion may lead to decreased water secretion and increased reabsorption of the periciliary fluid.[18] This causes impaired mucociliary clearance in patients with cystic fibrosis compared with normal subjects.[37] Abnormal phospholipid balance in cystic fibrosis secretions may also increase mucus adhesion and stickiness by altering surface properties of the secretion.[3] Retention of secretions leads to chronic bacterial infections with organisms such as *Staphylococcus aureus* and *Pseudomonas aeruginosa*.

PHYSICAL PROPERTIES OF MUCUS

As previously stated, the biochemical characteristics of mucus determine its physical properties, which influence the efficiency of the mucociliary interaction and resulting transport.

ADHESIVE FORCES

Adhesion refers to forces between *unlike molecules.* In the airway, adhesive forces refer to the attractive and frictional forces between the mucus and airway surface. Adhesion severely reduces the ability to clear secretions by airflow (cough).[38] Mucokinetic agents are either abhesives, such as surfactant, that reduce the adhesivity of secretions or agents that increase the power of expiratory airflow and cough. Mucolytics may work in part by severing the bonding of mucus to the epithelium, thus reducing inertial (frictional) adhesion.

COHESIVE FORCES

Cohesion refers to forces between *like molecules.* Cohesive forces result from the elongation of the mucus macromolecule. A property of spinnability has been described as a surrogate measure of cohesivity. These terms are defined as follows:

Rheology: Study of the deformation and flow of matter. The rheologic behavior of mucus is the way it responds to forces (stress) by *deforming* and/or *flowing* (strain).

Viscosity: Measure of the resistance of a fluid to flow. More specifically, viscosity is the proportionality constant (ratio) of applied force to rate of flow. The properties of an ideal or Newtonian liquid can be described by the loss modulus or viscosity.

Elasticity: Measure of the ability of a deformed material to return to its original shape. Ideal elastic solids store all of the energy or force during deformation, and this energy is available when the force is removed. The properties of an ideal or Hookian solid can be described by the storage modulus or elasticity.

Spinnability: The ability of mucus to be drawn into long threads by a standardized device and measured in millimeters of length.[39]

Figure 9-7 illustrates the concepts of viscosity (a property of fluids) and elasticity (a property of solids). King and Rubin give a clear discussion of such properties in their application to mucus.[40]

MUCUS AS A VISCOELASTIC MATERIAL

The mucous gel is a viscoelastic material and therefore behaves partially as a fluid and partially as a solid. As a solid, a gel has elastic deformation under applied force, and as a liquid, a gel flows under applied force. Cilia supply the force. As the tips of the cilia contact the gel during the forward power stroke, the gel is stretched and its elastic recovery causes it to snap forward. At the same time, the mucous gel flows forward as a liquid under the forward beat of the cilia.

This model of gel transport is seen in Figure 9-8, using unvulcanized rubber as an example of a viscoelastic substance. If such a rubber strip is loaded on one end with a weight and allowed to hang, it would stretch instantaneously as an elastic solid. If the

VISCOSITY AND ELASTICITY

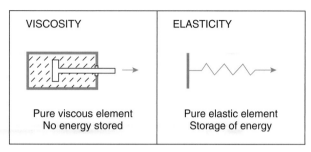

Viscosity: Resistance to <u>flow</u>.

Elasticity: Property of <u>deforming</u> under force, resuming shape.

Figure 9-7   Illustration of concepts of viscosity and elasticity.

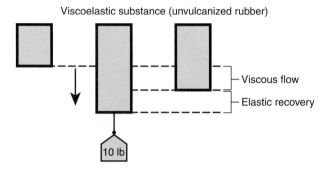

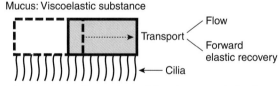

Figure 9-8   Illustration of the viscous and elastic properties affecting the movement of viscoelastic substances, such as unvulcanized rubber and mucus.

weight (applied force) remains, the strip will elongate very slowly because of its viscosity (i.e., the rubber would "flow"). After removing the weight, the rubber recovers the elastic elongation because of the stored energy, but will not recover the length caused by flow. Mucus behaves similarly. Mucociliary transport results from both flow and forward elastic recovery. For this reason, the physical properties of viscosity and elasticity are extremely important for efficient and adequate transport of respiratory secretions. In general, normal mucus has a relatively low viscosity, and its elasticity is high enough to provide forward propulsive energy.

SPINNABILITY (COHESIVITY) OF MUCUS

The ability of mucus to be drawn out into threads of varying length was initially identified for cervical mucus and termed *spinnability* by Reiner and Scott-Blair in 1966, although this was described much earlier in the German literature as *spinnbarkheit.* It was noted that this property was essential for the motility of sperm and female reproduction. The property of spinnability was subsequently studied by Puchelle and colleagues for respiratory mucus.[39] They used a device to draw mucus out vertically at a standardized constant rate, and measured the spinnability of mucus as the maximal length the thread can be drawn before breaking. Generally, a significant and positive correlation was demonstrated between the degree of spinnability of mucus and its mucociliary transport rate ($r = +0.61$). Spinnability also was found to decrease with increasing viscosity ($r = -0.50$) and to increase with increasing elasticity ($r = +0.54$). Spinnability varied widely, however, with low viscosities, and mucus with high spinnability showed a normal ciliary transport even though viscosity and elasticity were abnormally low. Spinnability, and therefore mucus transport, was also found to decrease as the purulence of sputum (quantified by the number of leukocytes present) from chronic bronchitic patients increased. The authors speculate that spinnability gives information about internal cohesion forces in mucus. Specifically, insufficiently polymerized mucus as in watery secretions will lower spinnability and therefore mucus transport. These results suggest that spinnability is a key physical factor for normal mucus transport and that it reflects cohesivity.

Cohesivity is defined as interfacial tension multiplied by the new area created after a test substance is pulled apart. For ideal or Newtonian fluids this equals twice the interfacial tension, γ. For a non-Newtonian gel, such as mucus, a distraction device (Filancemeter) is used to stretch the mucus until breaking. The measurement is performed with a 25-μl mucus sample at a distraction velocity of 10 mm/sec. An electric signal conducted through the sample is interrupted at the point where the stretched mucus thread is broken. Assuming a cone with a diameter of the base of the cone of 1 mm, at the point of breaking this would mean that cohesivity $= \gamma \times \pi \times$ length in mm/100.

NON-NEWTONIAN NATURE OF MUCUS

Evaluation of the properties of mucus is complicated by the fact that mucus exhibits non-Newtonian viscosity. In an ideal Newtonian liquid, the proportion of applied force to rate of flow remains constant with changing force. A non-Newtonian substance, such as mucus, has *varying* viscosity (defined as the proportionality constant of force to flow) with varying applied force (shear rate). As the force, or shear rate, increases, the apparent viscosity of mucus decreases. Mucus also exhibits a shear-thinning phenomenon: Viscosity decreases at a low shear rate *after* the mucus is subjected to a high shear rate.[41] Such changes in viscosity are consistent with the rupture or change in the macromolecular chains and cross-linking network of the gel. Because of its non-Newtonian behavior, evaluation of the properties of mucus and of the effect of drugs on those properties is complicated and must be performed under standardized conditions of shear rate. Otherwise, as pointed out by Dulfano and Adler,[42] interpretation of research findings on mucus viscosity is difficult.

Several review articles and compendia are devoted to the physiology of mucus secretion in the lung and the nature of mucus.[6,8,11,43-47]

MUCOACTIVE AGENTS

Two agents are approved, at the time of this edition, for administration as an aerosol to treat abnormal pulmonary secretions: acetylcysteine and dornase alfa. Both agents are mucolytic, disrupting the disulfide bond in mucus or enzymatically breaking down DNA material in airway secretions, respectively. Although not an approved agent, bicarbonate solutions of 2% concentration have been instilled in 2 to 5 ml amounts into the airway, to raise the topical pH and alter mucus bonding. Table 9-5 summarizes the spectrum of agents, both in current use and with the potential to improve mucus clearance.

MUCOLYSIS AND MUCOCILIARY CLEARANCE

Mucolytic agents decrease the elasticity and viscosity of mucus because the gel structure is broken down. Because elasticity is crucial for mucociliary transport, mucolytics have the potential for a negative effect on normal physiological mucus clearance. Reduction of mucous gel to a more liquid state *may* facilitate aspiration of secretions with use of suction catheters. However, it is undesirable to create the

Table 9-5

Drugs currently used or under investigation as mucus- and secretion-controlling agents in the respiratory tract for aerosolization

DRUG	DESCRIPTION
Acetylcysteine, nacystelyn	Classic mucolytics
Dornase alfa	Peptide mucolytic
P2Y2 agent (INS 365)	Increases epithelial mucus and chloride secretion
Hyperosmolar saline	Expectorant
Dry powder mannitol	Expectorant
Gelsolin, thymosin β4	Peptide mucolytics
Surfactants	Abhesive phospholipid, mucokinetic
β Agonists	Secretagogue and mucokinetic if increased airflow
Macrolide antibiotics	Mucoregulatory
Anticholinergic agents	Mucoregulatory
Corticosteroids	Mucoregulatory
Gene therapy	Normalize secretory cell function and mucociliary clearance.

need for tracheal suctioning, with its attendant trauma to the airway and risk of infection and hypoxemia, by liquefying secretions unless a person is unable to cough adequately. Ideally the goal should be to facilitate physiological clearance by optimizing the viscoelasticity of mucus. The status of mucolytic agents in pulmonary disease was well reviewed at the two conferences on the scientific basis of respiratory care.[48,49]

Until agents are developed to more specifically control the biochemical composition and viscoelastic properties of mucus, mucolytics such as acetylcysteine and dornase alfa form part of a program aimed at optimal clearance of the airway and at preventing the cycle of obstruction and infection that causes further hypersecretion. The therapeutic options for controlling mucus hypersecretion are outlined below:

1. **Remove causative factors where possible.**
   a. Treat infections
   b. Stop smoking
   c. Avoid pollution and allergens
2. **Optimize tracheobronchial clearance.**
   a. Use of bronchodilators only if there is an increase in expiratory airflow
   b. Bronchial hygiene measures
      (1). Cough, deep breathing
      (2). Postural drainage
   c. Improve airflow by exercise and nutrition rehabilitation

3. **Reduce inflammation.**
   a. Treat infection (antibiotics)
   b. Use of corticosteroids
4. **Use mucoactive agents as specifically indicated.**

N-ACETYL L-CYSTEINE (MUCOMYST)

Classic mucolytics reduce mucins by severing disulfide bonds or charge shielding.

INDICATION FOR USE

As a mucolytic, acetylcysteine has been used in the treatment of conditions associated with viscous mucus secretions. A second use of acetylcysteine is as an antidote (as an antioxidant) to reduce hepatic injury with acetaminophen overdose.[50] The drug is given orally, not by aerosol, for this use, and is designated an *orphan drug* for this application. Despite excellent in vitro mucolytic activity and a long history of use, no data clearly demonstrate that oral or aerosolized acetylcysteine is effective therapy for any lung disease. This may be due in part to acetylcysteine selectively depolymerizing the essential mucin polymer structure and leaving the pathologic polymers of DNA and F-actin intact.

DOSAGE AND ADMINISTRATION

Acetylcysteine is the *N*-acetyl derivative of the amino acid L-cysteine and is used as a solution for either aerosol administration or by direct instillation into the tracheobronchial tree. It is supplied in the following strengths:

    20% solution: 3 to 5 ml tid or qid
    10% solution: 6 to 10 ml tid or qid
    Direct instillation: 1 to 2 ml of 10% or 20% solution

It should be noted that the recommended amount of the 10% solution (6 to 10 ml) is not efficiently nebulized by the typical gas-powered, hand-held disposable nebulizer (see Chapter 3), which requires an optimal filling volume of 3.0 to 5.0 ml for mechanical efficiency and for reasonable times of administration.

MODE OF ACTION

Acetylcysteine disrupts the structure of the mucus molecule by substituting free thiol (sulfhydryl) groups for the disulfide bonds in the mucus. This action is illustrated in Figure 9-9, which also shows the molecular structure of acetylcysteine. The substituted sulfhydryl group in mucus does not provide a bond or cross-linking between strands, and as a result both the viscosity and the elasticity of the mucus are lowered. In physical contact with mucus, acetylcysteine begins to reduce viscosity immediately. Its mucolytic activity increases with higher pH and is optimal with a local pH of 7.0 to 9.0. The solution of acetylcysteine contains a chelating agent, ethylenediaminetetraacetic acid. A light-purple solution indicates metal ion removal and does not change the safety or efficacy of the drug. It is suggested that opened vials of the drug be stored in a refrigerator and discarded after 96 hours to prevent contamination. Additional details in the manufacturer's package insert should be reviewed.

HAZARDS

The most serious potential complication with acetylcysteine is bronchospasm. This is more likely with hyperreactive airways, such as in asthmatic patients, and can be lessened by using the 10% solution instead of the 20%, and by concomitant use of a bronchodilator. It is possible to use bronchodilators either mixed with acetylcysteine or administered previously by nebulizer or pressurized MDI (pMDI). If this is done, a bronchodilator with rapid onset and quick peak effect should be used. Noncatecholamine adrenergic bronchodilators (terbutaline, metaproterenol, albuterol) have a relatively slow time to peak effect and may not be as effective in preventing drug-induced bronchospasm.

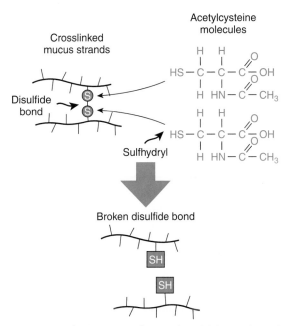

Figure 9-9   Mechanisms of action by which acetylcysteine reduces the viscosity of mucus. Acetylcysteine substitutes the sulfhydryl for the disulfide bonds.

Other complications can include stomatitis, nausea, and rhinorrhea. Mechanical obstruction of the airway can occur with liquefaction of copious secretions, and suction should be available with artificial airways. The disagreeable odor of acetylcysteine is due to the release of hydrogen sulfide, and this may provoke nausea or vomiting. In prolonged nebulization, the manufacturer suggests that after three fourths of the solution is nebulized, the remaining one fourth should be diluted with an equal volume of sterile water to prevent a highly concentrated residue, which could irritate the airway. An aerosol of acetylcysteine may leave a sticky film on hands or face. Overdosage with the drug is unlikely.

INCOMPATIBILITY WITH ANTIBIOTICS IN MIXTURE

Acetylcysteine is incompatible in mixture with the following major antibiotics and should not be combined in physical solution:

- Sodium ampicillin
- Amphotericin B
- Erythromycin lactobionate
- Tetracyclines (tetracycline, oxytetracycline)
- Aminoglycosides

Incompatibility is taken to mean the formation of a precipitate; a change in color, clarity, or odor; or other physical or chemical change. The topical use of acetylcysteine in the lung does not contraindicate the simultaneous use of antibiotics by *other* routes of administration.

Acetylcysteine is reactive with several substances, including rubber, copper, iron, and cork. Most conventional nebulizers made of plastic or glass are suitable for administering the drug. Aluminum, chromed metal, tantalum, sterling silver, or stainless steel are also safe to use, although silver may tarnish. A complete list of incompatibilities for acetylcysteine can be found in the manufacturer's literature.

ANTIOXIDANT PROPERTIES OF ACETYLCYSTEINE

Acetylcysteine has been investigated for use both in acute respiratory distress syndrome (ARDS) and for lung cancer prevention. Both uses are based on its antioxidant properties. Glutathione is a tripeptide antioxidant, and it antagonizes the effects of toxic radicals such as hydrogen peroxide (H_2O_2). Acetylcysteine is an aminothiol and is the precursor of intracellular cysteine and glutathione. When taken orally, acetylcysteine is rapidly absorbed, deacetylated, and incorporated in the intracellular and extracellular stores of glutathione.[51] The antioxidant properties of thiols such as acetylcysteine or glutathione may prevent pulmonary injury in patients with COPD, ARDS, or lung cancer. In ARDS, there is increased oxidant activity and a deficiency of glutathione. In a study of 61 adult patients with mild to moderate acute lung injury, Suter and colleagues[52] found that acetylcysteine, 40 mg/kg/day intravenously for 3 days, improved systemic oxygenation and reduced the need and length of ventilatory support compared with placebo. No adverse effects were observed in their study. Acetylcysteine may also provide a chemopreventive effect through multiple mechanisms and protect against a broad range of mutagens and carcinogens. A review by van Zandwijk[51] provides detailed references on the evidence for a chemopreventive effect with acetylcysteine.

DORNASE ALFA (PULMOZYME)

Peptide mucolytics reduce extracellular DNA or F-actin polymers. Dornase alfa is a clone of the natural human DNase I enzyme, which digests extracellular DNA material. The drug dornase alfa was produced by recombinant techniques and was initially referred to as rhDNase, for "recombinant human Dnase." In February, 1994, the FDA approved dornase alfa (Pulmozyme) for general use in treating the abnormally tenacious respiratory secretions seen in cystic fibrosis; it is designated as an *orphan drug.*

INDICATION AND USE IN CYSTIC FIBROSIS

Dornase alfa is indicated for the management of cystic fibrosis, to reduce the frequency of respiratory infections requiring parenteral antibiotics and to improve or preserve pulmonary function in these patients.

The bulk and surface properties of respiratory secretions in cystic fibrosis are due in part to the presence of DNA material from necrosing neutrophils present during chronic respiratory infections and to surfactant phospholipid hydrolysis by-products of inflammation. In the presence of infection, neutrophils are attracted to the airways, degenerate, and release DNA, which further increases the viscosity of secretions. DNA is an extremely viscous polyanion that is present in infected, but not in uninfected, respiratory secretions.[53,54] DNA in secretions may also contribute to reduced effectiveness of aminoglycoside antibiotics such as gentamicin. This could be caused by binding of the antibiotic to the polyvalent anions of the DNA and would tend to lessen the effectiveness of aerosolized antibiotics in cystic fibrosis.

MODE OF ACTION

The peptide mucolytic agent dornase alfa is similar in action to the proteolytic enzyme pancreatic dornase, which was approved for human use by inhalation in 1958 but is no longer available.[54]

Dornase alfa reduces the viscosity and adhesivity of infected respiratory secretions when given by aerosol (Figure 9-10). When mixed with purulent sputum from subjects with cystic fibrosis, dornase alfa lowered the viscosity and adhesivity of the sputum.[54] This was associated with a decrease in the size of the DNA in the sputum. The change in sputum viscosity with the addition of dornase alfa is dose dependent, with greater reduction occurring at higher concentrations of the drug.

Pancreatic dornase (Dornavac) (a product previously removed from the market), was a bovine pancreatic DNase. This product could cause serious bronchospasm when inhaled.[55] In addition, there was concern that the foreign protein might generate anti-DNase antibodies and cause allergic reactions. Differences between the human and bovine pancreatic

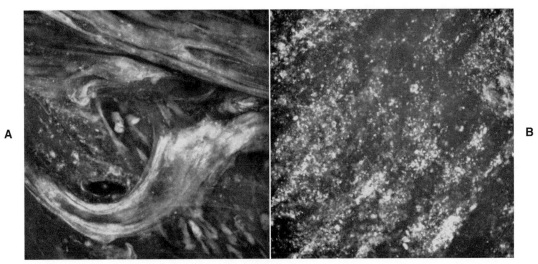

Figure 9-10   Illustration of the mode of action of dornase alfa in reducing DNA polymers in cystic fibrosis sputum. The figure is a confocal micrograph of cystic fibrosis sputum stained for DNA (with yoyo-1) before **(A)** and after **(B)** treatment with dornase alfa in vitro. The long DNA polymers are degraded into short units after dornase.

DNase I molecules in an immunogenic region imply that some of the adverse reactions to pancreatic dornase could have been caused by an immune response. Serum antibodies to DNase were found in some patients who were given multiple doses of bovine pancreatic DNase. Adverse effects with bovine DNase may also have been caused by the presence of contaminating proteinases, trypsin and chymotrypsin, in the drug.[54] On the other hand, studies revealed no allergic response or serum anti-DNase antibodies with inhaled dornase alfa in healthy subjects or in those with cystic fibrosis.[53]

DOSAGE AND ADMINISTRATION

The aerosol product dornase alfa is available as single use ampule, with 2.5 mg drug in 2.5 ml of clear, colorless solution. The solution should be refrigerated and protected from light. The usual dose is 2.5 mg daily, delivered by one of the following tested and approved nebulizers: Hudson T Updraft II or the Marquest Acorn II nebulizers with a Pulmo-Aide compressor, or the Pari LC Jet Plus nebulizer with the Pari Inhaler Boy compressor.[56] Although other nebulizer systems may perform suitably in nebulizing dornase alfa, this should not be assumed without testing. Optimal delivery of the enzyme requires a nebulizer system capable of suitable aerosol generation (i.e., particle size and quantity). This is especially important when administering very expensive drugs or aerosol medications with a narrow therapeutic index.

ADVERSE EFFECTS

Side effects with dornase alfa were little different from placebo in clinical trials, and the discontinuation rate was similar for dornase alfa (3%) and placebo (2%). Anti-DNase antibody production was not found with inhaled dornase alfa. Common side effects with use of the drug have included voice alteration, pharyngitis, laryngitis, rash, chest pain, and conjunctivitis. Other less common side effects reported include respiratory symptoms (increase in cough, dyspnea, pneumothorax, hemoptysis, rhinitis, sinusitis), flulike symptoms, malaise, gastrointestinal obstruction, hypoxia, and weight loss. Contraindications include hypersensitivity to dornase alfa.

CLINICAL APPLICATION AND EVALUATION

The intent of treatment with dornase alfa is to preserve or improve lung function in cystic fibrosis, while reducing the frequency and severity of respiratory infections by improving secretion clearance. A reduction in use of intravenous antibiotic therapy is also desired, as well as the need for hospitalizations. Institution of therapy is based on physician judgment of purulent sputum, infections, and need for antibiotic therapy. Evaluation of drug treatment is based not only on lung function, which may not improve appreciably, but also on a reduction in the number and severity of infections and corresponding need for antibiotics and hospitalization. In a study of aerosolized dornase alfa in *acute* pulmonary exacerbations requiring hospitalization, Wilmott and colleagues[57] found that rhDNase was safe and well tolerated, but there was no significant additional effect of the drug when given with the usual regimen of antibiotics and chest physical therapy. These findings reinforce the use of dornase alfa as maintenance therapy in cystic fibrosis when abnormal airway secretions lead to recurrent pulmonary infections. A Consensus Conference report on the application of dornase alfa in cystic fibrosis was published in *Pediatric Pulmonology* in 1994, and provides a useful reference.[58]

F-Actin Depolymerizing Drugs: Gelsolin and Thymosin β4

Chronic inflammation is characterized by inflammatory cell necrosis and release of undegraded DNA, filamentous actin (F-actin), and intracellular enzymes from neutrophils. These inflammatory products are present in the sputum from patients with cystic fibrosis. DNA and F-actin in the sputum copolymerize to form a rigid network that is entangled in the mucin gel. Peptide mucolytics degrade these filaments while leaving the glycoprotein network relatively intact. Gelsolin, an 85-kD actin-severing peptide, has been shown to significantly reduce the viscosity of cystic fibrosis sputum in a dose-dependent manner. Similarly, thymosin β4 decreases sputum cohesivity in a dose-dependent and time-dependent manner. In vitro studies have shown that F-actin depolymerizing agents along with dornase alfa result in greater reduction in sputum cohesivity and viscoelasticity than with either agent alone.[59,60] The actin depolymerizing agents both destabilize the actin-DNA filament network and increase the depolymerizing activity of dornase alfa on the DNA filaments.

Expectorants

Iodide-Containing Agents

Iodide-containing agents (e.g., SSKI [saturated solution potassium iodide]) are generally considered to be expectorants. They are thought to stimulate the secretion of airway fluid. Iodides have been shown in vitro to have a mucolytic effect on mucin networks. Iodopropylidene glycerol (IPG) may acutely increase tracheobronchial clearance as measured by radiola-

beled aerosol in patients with chronic bronchitis.[61] However, in a double-blind crossover study in 28 patients with stable bronchitis, therapy with IPG failed to demonstrate any changes in pulmonary function, gas trapping, or sputum properties.[62]

Sodium Bicarbonate

Sodium bicarbonate (2%) is a weak base that has occasionally been used for direct tracheal irrigation or as an aerosol. By increasing the local bronchial pH, sodium bicarbonate weakens the bonds between the saccharide side chains of the mucous molecule, resulting in lowering of the mucus viscosity and elasticity. Local bronchial irritation may occur with increase in the local bronchial pH to more than 8.0. Sodium bicarbonate has not been clinically demonstrated to improve airway mucus clearance. There is little to recommend its use.

Guaifenesin

Guaifenesin is usually considered an expectorant rather than a mucolytic. It may be ciliotoxic in vitro when applied directly to the respiratory epithelium.[63] It can stimulate the cholinergic pathway and induce increased mucus secretion from the airway submucosal glands, but neither guaifenesin nor glycerol guiacolate have been demonstrated to be clinically effective in randomized controlled trials.

Dissociating Solvents

Urea is a dissociating agent that can break ionic and hydrogen bonds. In mucin gels, urea disrupts the hydrogen bonds between the oligosaccharide side chains of the neighboring mucus molecules with subsequent decrease in the physical entanglements between the molecules and decreased viscosity of the mucus. Urea may also decrease the interaction between DNA molecules. Because the mucolytic action of urea occurs only at very high concentrations of urea (3 to 8 mol/L),[64,65] urea would not be considered appropriate for human usage.

Oligosaccharides

The oligosaccharide side chains make up about 80% of the mucin structure. These hydrogen bonds are weak and can be disrupted by agents such as dextran, mannitol, and lactose. The lower-molecular-weight fractions of dextran are primarily responsible for the mucoactive effects of dextran. Furthermore, an osmotic effect of dextran with increased hydration of the mucus could also result in improved clearance of secretions. Dextran administration via aerosol has been shown to improve tracheal mucus velocity in dogs.[66]

The charged oligosaccharide heparin has a greater mucolytic and mucokinetic capacity compared with the neutral oligosaccharide dextran. Heparin may cause both hydrogen bond disruption and improved ionic interactions. Aerosolized low-molecular-weight heparin shows promise in the treatment of asthma, presumably by interfering with antigen receptor binding.[67]

TYLOXAPOL

Tyloxapol is an alkylaryl polyether alcohol polymer, nonionic detergent, and antioxidant. Tyloxapol was used with a mixture of other mucolytic agents for the treatment of chronic bronchitis in the United States until 1981. It has recently been reported that tyloxapol inhibits the nuclear transcription factor, NF-κB, scavenges oxygen radicals, and reduces cystic fibrosis sputum viscosity in vitro.[68]

P2Y2 AGONISTS (ATP, UTP)

Chloride conductance through the Ca^{2+}-dependent chloride channels is preserved in the cystic fibrosis airway. The tricyclic nucleotides UTP and ATP regulate ion transport through P2Y2 purinergic receptors that increase intracellular calcium. UTP aerosol, alone or in combination with amiloride, increases transepithelial potential difference and the clearance of inhaled radioaerosol.[69] There is active development of novel P2Y2 purinergic receptor agonists for clinical use.

MUCOKINETIC AGENTS

Mucokinetic agents increase cough clearance by increasing expiratory airflow or by reducing sputum adhesivity and tenacity.

BRONCHODILATORS

The β agonists increase ciliary beat frequency, but this probably has little effect on mucus clearance. Of greater importance is that these medications can increase expiratory airflow in persons with an asthmatic component of airway disease.[70] However, airway muscle relaxation can also decease expiratory airflow by producing dynamic airway collapse in persons with "floppy airways," such as those with airway malacia or bronchiectasis. The β agonists are mucus secretagogues and therefore can potentially increase mucus

plugging if they increase dynamic collapse and decrease expiratory airflow.

SURFACE-ACTIVE PHOSPHOLIPIDS

Surfactant is produced in the conducting airways and alveolus and is essential for mucociliary and cough clearance. A thin surfactant layer between the periciliary fluid and the mucous gel prevents airway dehydration, permits mucus spreading upon extrusion from glands, and allows efficient ciliary coupling with mucus and, more importantly, ciliary release from mucus once kinetic energy is transmitted. With airway inflammation, surface active phospholipids such as surfactants are often consumed by secretory phospholipases and inflammatory peptides can further inhibit surfactant function. In the absence of surfactant, mucus sticks to the epithelium, rendering cough less effective.

Sputum adhesivity and cohesivity have a greater influence on the clearability of secretions than viscoelasticity. In chronic inflammatory airway diseases, including cystic fibrosis, inactivation of bronchial surfactant occurs and this increases secretion tenacity.[71] It has been reported in randomized, double-blind, placebo-controlled, multicenter studies that surfactant aerosol improves pulmonary function and sputum transportability in patients with chronic bronchitis or with cystic fibrosis and that this effect is dose dependent. No significant side effects were attributable to the surfactant therapy.[72] As a wetting and spreading agent, surfactant also has the ability to increase the lower airway deposition of other aerosol medications such as rhDNase or antibiotics.

ANTIPROTEASES

Persons with cystic fibrosis have increased activity of serine proteases on the respiratory epithelial surface. Neutrophils, when activated or degenerating, release proteases such as elastase that can directly damage epithelial cells and impair airway clearance. It has been shown that neutrophil proteases cause a secretory response from submucosal glands with very significant increase in mucus production.

Intravenous administration or inhalation of $α_1AT$ suppresses the activity of neutrophil elastase and restores the bacterial killing capacity of neutrophils. Recombinant secretory leukocyte protease inhibitor (rsLPI), given to a small number of cystic fibrosis patients at a dose of 100 mg twice daily for 2 weeks, decreased neutrophil elastase and IL-8 in airway fluid but was ineffective at a dose of 50 mg twice daily. No significant side effects were reported.[73]

Although this treatment is promising, several issues must be resolved before these or similar agents can be used to prevent damage resulting from unchecked protease activity in patients with cystic fibrosis. Airway-targeted antioxidant and antiprotease therapies, if effective, could decrease airway secretion volume and purulence.

GENE THERAPY

Gene therapy holds the promise of permanently correcting underlying abnormalities that predispose to mucus hypersecretion. Stable gene transfer into airway epithelia is limited by targeting the appropriate cells, achieving persistence of transfer or stable integration, evading the immune and inflammatory response, and activating the gene after transfer. Gene therapy was first attempted by inserting the normal CFTR gene into a replication defective (RD) adenovirus vector (E1 deleted adenovirus vectors). Transfected cells produced small amounts of normal CFTR, restoring the bioelectric properties of the cell.[74] However, in initial human trials, the RD-adenovirus induced a host inflammatory response that limited the usefulness of those vectors, especially for repeated administration. The host humoral immune response to the vector and genetically modified cells generates neutralizing antibodies that increase the risk of readministering the vector. If the RD-adenovirus vector could be made less immunogenic, it would probably be safer and have more stable expression once in the cell.

Adeno-associated virus (AAV) is a small single-stranded DNA parvovirus that is naturally replication defective and not pathogenic. When AAV infects a cell it usually requires coinfection with a helper virus to replicate and propagate. Infected with wild type AAV alone, the virus tends to become latent by stably integrating into a specific area on chromosome 19, thus minimizing the risk of insertional mutagenesis. AAV *rep* gene products appear to be needed for site-specific integration, meaning that AAV vectors without regulatory elements integrate at multiple sites and may not integrate at all unless the cell divides. Early trials using AAV vectors suggest that the CFTR gene package can be transferred successfully with safe, long-lasting, and stable vector expression.[75]

Cationic liposomes are lipid capsules with the ability to form complexes with DNA and then enter cells.

With the first generation of liposome vectors, the efficiency of gene transfer was poor, but this has improved with newer systems. Although progress has greatly increased uptake of liposomes into cells, transfer of DNA from the liposome into the cell nucleus is still relatively inefficient. Although most cationic lipids are toxic to cultured cells and can cause inflammation in animal systems, pilot studies have not shown cellular damage after exposure to liposome vectors. The duration of gene expression after liposome-mediated gene transfer has been transient, making frequent administration likely to be necessary.[76]

Lentiviruses are retroviruses with the ability to integrate into chromosomal DNA with stable and long-lasting expression. Because the integration site is random, insertional mutagenesis is possible. Although some lentiviruses are unable to infect postmitotic cells, others, including the human immunodeficiency virus (HIV), do not require cell division to insert their genome.[77]

OTHER MUCOACTIVE AGENTS

HYPEROSMOLAR SALINE

Sputum induction using hypertonic saline inhalation has been used to obtain specimens for diagnosing airway infection. In a recent study, 58 patients with cystic fibrosis were randomly assigned to receive 10 ml of either 0.9% saline or 6% saline twice daily by ultrasonic nebulization. Fifty-two patients completed the study. There was a significant increase in forced expiratory volume in 1 second (FEV_1) at 2 weeks in patients inhaling hypertonic saline, but FEV_1 returned to baseline by day 28. Despite pretreatment with 600 μg of inhaled albuterol, an acute decrease in FEV_1 was noted in several patients after inhaling hypertonic saline, and one patient in the saline group had to be withdrawn from the study because of acute hemoptysis.[78] Although hypertonic saline is inexpensive and readily available, making this a potentially attractive form of therapy, there is concern about the inactivation of definsins at the airway surface in the presence of high salt concentration and that this might increase the long-term risk of airway infection in these patients.[79]

FUTURE MUCUS-CONTROLLING AGENTS

To improve mucus transport, both elasticity and viscosity must be considered. Mucolytics have been targeted only at lowering the viscosity of mucus. Under the normal physiology of ciliary movement, logic dictates that thicker and denser strands of mucus would be moved more efficiently by ciliary contact and elastic recovery than would thin, low-viscosity solutions. The conceptual analogy is that of raking water—little transport will occur. This assumes mucus clearance is being optimized *physiologically.* Endotracheal aspiration of secretions using suction would be easier with low-viscosity mucus. Results of a study by Dulfano and Adler[42] and another by Gelman and Meyer[80] support the view that elasticity is extremely important for mucus transport. The former study found that high elastic recoil and low viscosity represent the best rheological combination for maximal velocity by the mucociliary type of system. Other studies have appeared to reach conflicting conclusions.[81]

It has been suggested that the treatment of bronchial hypersecretion would be better aimed at *normalizing* the rheological properties of mucus to optimize transport, rather than at simply lysing or liquefying bronchial secretions as traditionally done. It is suggested that the term *mucolytic* be replaced by *mucoactive* to connote such an approach to secretion clearance. In this view of mucus control, there is a an optimal range of elasticity and viscosity, as illustrated in Figure 9-11 using arbitrary units. Puchelle and colleagues[82] have distinguished possible states that would determine the treatment approach to be used.

Purulent sputum has high elasticity *and* viscosity, and mucolytic agents such as dornase alfa might restore normal transport properties by lowering tenacity (adhesivity), viscosity, and elasticity. With low viscoelasticity (e.g., bronchorrhea), restructuring or cross-linking agents would increase both viscosity and elasticity to improve transport. Such agents have been termed *mucospissic.*[8,83] Agents with mucospissic activity to cause improved gelation include sodium tetraborate, Congo red, and tetracycline.[80] The thickening effect of tetracycline can occur with oral and aerosol administration, although more so with direct aerosol. Tetracycline may bind to mucus proteins to increase viscosity and elasticity, although exact binding sites remain unclear.

With very adhesive sputum (cystic fibrosis, asthma, chronic bronchitis), mucokinetic agents that decrease tenacity while preserving viscoelasticity might be useful. Currently there are no drugs available as mucus-controlling agents in the United States that will selectively modify viscosity or elasticity. Proteolytic enzymes such as pancreatic dornase (Dornavac), chymin, or trypsin are also effective mucolytics but are hazardous because of their possible antigenic effect and lack of specificity. The new agent dornase alfa avoids this side effect but is still mucolytic in its effect.

Further investigation may produce clinically useful agents tailored to specific secretion problems. The first step has been to recognize the complex rheologic and tenacious nature of mucus and the necessity of cross-linking to provide adequate elasticity for efficient ciliary transport. A second step has been an increased understanding of the structure of mucus and regulation of its production. Finally, a better understanding of adhesivity and cohesivity, the components of tenacity, has focused attention on control of the abnormal surface properties of mucus and sputum and their role in cough clearance.

RESPIRATORY CARE ASSESSMENT OF MUCOACTIVE DRUG THERAPY

Assessment of drug therapy for respiratory secretions is difficult: FEV_1 is relatively insensitive to changes in mucociliary clearance. The rate of change in lung function over time is a better marker. In addition, during maintenance therapy, the volume of sputum expectorated is variable from day to day and does not reflect effective therapy. Therefore the following assessments should be performed.

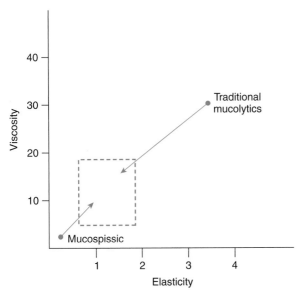

Figure 9-11 Conceptual representation of an optimal range of viscosity and elasticity of mucus for mucociliary transport.

Before Treatment

- Assess patient's adequacy of cough and level of consciousness to determine need for mechanical suctioning or need for adjunct bronchial hygiene (postural drainage or percussion, PEP therapy) to clear airway with treatment or if treatment is contraindicated.

During Treatment and Short Term

- Instruct and then verify correct use of aerosol nebulization system, including cleaning.
- Assess therapy based on indication for drug.
- Monitor airflow changes or adverse effects, such as fall in FEV_1 and gastroesophageal reflux.
- Assess breathing pattern and rate.
- Assess patient's subjective reaction to treatment (i.e., changes in breathing effort or pattern).
- Discontinue therapy if patient experiences adverse reactions.

Long Term

- Monitor number and severity of respiratory tract infections, need for antibiotic therapy, emergency visits, and hospitalizations.
- Monitor pulmonary function for improvement or slowing in the rate of deterioration.

General Contraindications

- Generally, if the FEV_1 is less than 25% of predicted, it becomes difficult to mobilize and expectorate secretions. Theoretically, with profound airflow compromise, secretion clearance could decline.
- Use mucoactive therapy with caution in patients with severely compromised vital capacity and expiratory flow, such as in the presence of end-stage pulmonary disease or neuromuscular disorders.
- Gastroesophageal reflux or inability of the patient to protect the airway are risk factors for postural drainage, if that is necessary with mucoactive therapy. Mucoactive agents should be discontinued if there is evidence of clinical deterioration.
- Patients with acute bronchitis or exacerbation of chronic disease (cystic fibrosis, COPD) may be less responsive to mucoactive therapy, possibly because of infection and muscular weakness, which can further reduce airflow-dependent mechanisms.

SUMMARY KEY TERMS AND CONCEPTS

- The physiology of *mucociliary function* in the airway involves secretory cells, including *surface goblet cells, submucosal glands,* and ciliated epithelium.
- The airway secretion consists of a *mucous layer,* where *mucus glycoprotein* is located, and a watery, *periciliary layer.*
- *Cilia* beat in a *metachronal* wave to escalate mucus and trapped particulates toward the upper airway.
- *Mucociliary clearance* is affected by numerous drug groups, including surfactants and anticholinergic agents.
- *Mucus* is 95% water by composition, with about 3% protein and carbohydrate, 1% lipids, and 1% miscellaneous.
- *Epithelial ion exchange,* particularly sodium and chloride reabsorption from the airway surface liquid, maintains normal periciliary fluid.
- Mucus or mucociliary clearance can be abnormal in pulmonary diseases such as chronic bronchitis, asthma, or cystic fibrosis.
- *Physical* properties of mucus include *viscosity, elasticity, cohesivity,* and *adhesivity;* normal ranges of these properties are needed for adequate mucus transport to occur.
- Currently two agents are administered by aerosol to modify airway secretions: *acetylcysteine* and *dornase alfa.* Both are *mucolytic* in action; dornase alfa is indicated for clearance of purulent secretions in *cystic fibrosis.* Acetylcysteine is used for lysis of excessive secretions, and is given orally for *acetaminophen overdose.* Other agents modifying airway secretions include inhaled anticholinergics such as atropine, tricyclic nucleotides, phospholipids, antiproteases, and gene therapy. Potassium iodide and glyceryl guaiacolate are considered *expectorants,* rather than mucolytics.
- Future mucus-controlling agents may be able to normalize and optimize physical properties of mucus to improve clearance.

SELF-ASSESSMENT QUESTIONS

1. Identify the two mucolytic agents approved for inhalation as an aerosol in the United States (give the generic and brand names).
2. What is the mode of action for acetylcysteine?
3. What is the mode of action for dornase alfa?
4. What is the clinical indication for use of dornase alfa?
5. What is the usual dose of acetylcysteine by nebulizer?
6. What is the recommended dose of dornase alfa?

7. How much active ingredient is contained in 4 cc of 10% acetylcysteine solution?
8. What is the percentage strength of the 1 mg/ml solution of dornase alfa available for nebulization?
9. What is a common side effect of acetylcysteine by nebulization? How is it detected?
10. What is a common side effect seen with aerosol administration of dornase alfa?

Answers to Self-Assessment Questions are found in Appendix A.

CLINICAL SCENARIO

A 17-year-old female with cystic fibrosis was admitted to a local children's hospital with an acute respiratory infection (pulmonary exacerbation). She is pleasant, mature, and extremely well informed concerning her disease. She complains of increased cough; increased sputum production, with some hemoptysis; and dyspnea with exertion over the past week.

She was diagnosed with cystic fibrosis at the age of 2 years and was asymptomatic until age 12. She has had a nasal polypectomy. A gastrostomy tube placed for night feeding several years ago resulted in a weight gain of 30 lb (13.6 kg). She has been admitted with exacerbations of her cystic fibrosis twice in the past year. She has been taking 300 mg of tobramycin (TOBI) by aerosol at home regularly this year, with courses of oral ciprofloxacin when symptoms of respiratory infection surfaced.

Her vital signs are T, 37.5° C; P, 116 beats/min and regular; RR, 36 breaths/min; BP, 110/60. Respiratory pattern exhibits mild effort while talking. Auscultation of the chest revealed crackles in all fields, with more in the right upper lobe. Extremities showed clubbing with no cyanosis. She has a cough productive of greenish, thick sputum.

Her electrolytes were normal; hemoglobin, 14.3 g/dl; hematocrit, 44%; and WBC count, 13.4×10^3 cells/mm³. Her SpO₂ is 91% in ambient air. Chest radiograph (PA and lateral) shows diffuse chronic changes with thick interstitial markings, no pneumothorax, no pleural fluid, and a normal cardiac silhouette. There is an infiltrate in the right upper lobe. Her pulmonary function test results show vital capacity, 82% predicted; FEV_1, 61% predicted; FEF_{25-75}, 45% predicted; and functional residual capacity, 121% predicted.

After her admission, she was treated for the next 14 days with a course of intravenous antibiotics in addition to her usual medications of pancreatic enzymes and vitamin supplements, albuterol by aerosol before chest physical therapy by autogenic drainage, nocturnal tube feedings, and oxygen 1 L/min at night. Chest percussion during postural drainage was withheld because of the hemoptysis. Her symptoms of dyspnea improved, along with her WBC count. She continues to have a productive cough with thick sputum, although the hemoptysis has disappeared. She is clinically stable, and is ready to be discharged.

What aerosol medications would be indicated for her?
What outcomes would you assess to determine the effectiveness of dornase alfa in her case?

Answers to Clinical Scenario Questions are found in Appendix A.

REFERENCES

1. Denton R and others: Viscoelasticity of mucus: its role in ciliary transport of pulmonary secretions, *Am Rev Respir Dis* 98:380, 1968.
2. Sackner MA: Effect of respiratory drugs on mucociliary clearance, *Chest* 73(suppl):958S, 1978.
3. Puchelle E, de Bentzmann S, Zahm JM: Physical and functional properties of airway secretions in cystic fibrosis: therapeutic approaches, *Respiration* 62(suppl 1):2, 1995.
4. Basbaum C and others: Cellular mechanisms of airway secretion, *Am Rev Respir Dis* 137:479, 1988.
5. Reid L, Clamp JR: Biochemical and histochemical nomenclature of mucus, *Br Med Bull* 34:5, 1978.
6. Basbaum CB: Airway mucin: chairman's summary, *Am Rev Respir Dis* 144(suppl):S2, 1991.
7. King M, Rubin BK: Mucus-controlling agent: past and present, *Respir Care Clin North Am* 5:575, 1999.
8. Luk CK, Dulfano MJ: Effect of pH, viscosity and ionic-strength changes on ciliary beating frequency of human bronchial explants, *Clin Sci* 64:449, 1983.
9. Sleigh MA, Blake JR, Liron N: The propulsion of mucus by cilia, *Am Rev Respir Dis* 137:726, 1988.
10. Pinnock CB and others: Relationship between milk intake and mucus production in adult volunteers challenged with rhinovirus-2, *Am Rev Respir Dis* 141:352, 1990.
11. Lundgren JD, Shelhamer JH: Pathogenesis of airway mucus hypersecretion, *J Allergy Clin Immunol* 85:399, 1990.
12. Rogers DF: Airway submucosal gland and goblet cell secretion. In Chung KF, Barnes PJ, eds: *Pharmacology of the respiratory tract*, New York, 1993, Marcel Dekker.
13. Lopez-Vidriero MT: Airway mucus: production and composition, *Chest* 80(suppl):799, 1981.
14. Matthews LW and others: Studies in pulmonary secretions. I, The overall composition of pulmonary secretions from patients with cystic fibrosis, bronchiectasis, and laryngectomy, *Am Rev Respir Dis* 88:199, 1963.

15. Dulfano JJ, Adler KB, Wooten O: Physical properties of sputum. IV, Effects of 100 percent humidity and water mist, *Am Rev Respir Dis* 107:130, 1973.

16. Birrer P: Proteases and antiproteases in cystic fibrosis: pathogenetic considerations and therapeutic strategies, *Respiration* 62(suppl 1):25, 1995.

17. Clarke LL, Boucher R: Ion and water transport across airway epithelia. In Chung KF, Barnes PJ, eds: *Pharmacology of the respiratory tract: experimental and clinical research,* New York, 1993, Marcel Dekker.

18. Knowles MR and others: Pharmacologic treatment of abnormal ion transport in the airway epithelium in cystic fibrosis, *Chest* 107(suppl, Feb):71S, 1995.

19. Mentz W and others: Measurement of airway surface liquid (ASL) composition of normal human subjects, *Am Rev Respir Dis* 129:315A, 1984 (abstract).

20. Joris L, Dab I, Quinton PM: Elemental composition of human airway surface fluid in health and diseased airways, *Am Rev Respir Dis* 148:1633, 1993.

21. Jayaraman S and others: Noninvasive in vivo fluorescence measurement of airway-surface liquid depth, salt concentration, and pH, *J Clin Invest* 107:317, 2001.

22. Baconnais S and others: Ion composition and rheology of airway liquid from cystic fibrosis fetal tracheal xenografts, *Am J Respir Cell Mol Biol* 20:605, 1999.

22a. Davies JR and others: Identification of MUC5B, MUC5AC and small amounts of MUC2 mucins in cystic fibrosis airway secretions, *Biochem J* 344(pt 2):321, 1999.

22b. Wickstrom C and others: MUC5B is a major gel-forming, oligomeric mucin from human salivary gland, respiratory tract and endocervix: identification of glycoforms and C-terminal cleavage, *Biochem J* 334:685, 1998.

23. Tomkiewicz RP and others: Effects of oscillating air flow on the rheological properties and clearability of mucous gel stimulants, *Biorheology* 31:511, 1994.

24. Hodgkin JE, ed: *Chronic obstructive pulmonary disease: current concepts in diagnosis and comprehensive care,* Park Ridge, Ill, 1979, American College of Chest Physicians.

25. Reid L: Measurement of the bronchial mucous gland layer, *Thorax* 15:132, 1960.

26. Sturgen J, Reid L: An organ culture study of the effects of drugs on secretory activity of human bronchial submucosal gland, *Clin Sci* 43:533, 1972.

27. Rubin BK and others: Mucus and mucoactive therapy in chronic bronchitis, *Clin Pulm Med* 5:1, 1998.

28. Shimura S and others: Bronchorrhea sputum in bronchial asthma, *Am Rev Respir Dis* 137:A14, 1988 (abstract).

29. Turner-Warwick M, Openshaw P: Sputum in asthma, *Postgrad Med J* 63(suppl 1):79, 1987.

30. Shimura S and others: Chemical properties of bronchorrhea sputum in bronchial asthma, *Chest* 94:1211, 1988

31. Marom Z and other: The effects of corticosteroids on mucous glycoprotein secretion from human airways in vitro, *Am Rev Respir Dis* 129:62, 1984.

32. Tamaoki J and others: Effect of indomethacin on bronchorrhea in patients with chronic bronchitis, diffuse panbronchiolitis, or bronchiectasis, *Am Rev Respir Dis* 145:548, 1992.

33. Marom ZM, Goswami SK: Respiratory mucus hypersecretion (bronchorrhea): a case discussion—possible mechanism(s) and treatment, *J Allergy Clin Immunol* 87:1050, 1991.

34. Rubin BK and others: Recurrent respiratory infections in a child with fucosidosis: is the mucus too thin for effective transport? *Ped Pulmonol* 10:304, 1991.

35. Seear M and others: Bronchial casts in children: a proposed classification based on nine cases and a review of the literature, *Am J Respir Crit Care Med* 155:364, 1997.

36. Quasney MW and others: Plastic bronchitis occurring late after the Fontan procedure: treatment with aerosolized urokinase, *Crit Care Med* 28:2107, 2000.

37. Regnis JA and others: Mucociliary clearance in patients with cystic fibrosis and in normal subjects, *Am J Respir Crit Care Med* 150:66, 1994.

38. Albers GM: Ring distraction technique for measuring surface tension of sputum: relationship to sputum clearability, *J Appl Physiol* 81:2690, 1996.

39. Puchelle E, Zahm JM, Duvivier C: Spinability of bronchial mucus: relationship with viscoelasticity and mucous transport properties, *Biorheology* 20:239, 1983.

40. King M, Rubin BK: Mucus rheology, relationship with transport. In Takishima T, ed: *Airway secretion: physiological bases for the control of mucus hypersecretion,* New York, 1994, Marcel Dekker.

41. Lourenco GV: Bronchial mucous secretions: introduction, *Chest* 63(suppl):55S, 1973.

42. Dulfano JJ, Adler KB: Physical properties of sputum. VII, Rheologic properties and mucociliary transport, *Am Rev Respir Dis* 112:341, 1975.

43. Hirsch SR: Airway mucus and the mucociliary system. In Middleton E Jr and others, eds: *Allergy: principles and practice,* ed 2, St Louis, 1983, Mosby.

44. Kaliner M and others: Human respiratory mucus, *J Allergy Clin Immunol* 73:318, 1984.

45. Kilburn K: A hypothesis for pulmonary clearance and its implications, *Am Rev Respir Dis* 98:449, 1968.

46. King M and others: On the transport of mucus and its rheologic stimulants in ciliated systems, *Am Rev Respir Dis* 110:740, 1974.

47. Marin MG: Pharmacology of airway secretion, *Pharmacol Rev* 38:273, 1986.

48. Barton AD: Aerosolized detergents and mucolytic agents in the treatment of stable chronic obstructive pulmonary disease, *Am Rev Respir Dis* 110:104S, 1974.

49. Wanner A, Rao A: Clinical indications for and effects of bland, mucolytic, and antimicrobial aerosols, *Am Rev Respir Dis* 122:79, 1980.

50. Macy AM: Preventing hepatotoxicity in acetaminophen overdose, *Am J Nurs* 79:301, 1979.

51. van Zandwijk N: *N*-Acetylcysteine for lung cancer prevention, *Chest* 107:1437, 1995.

52. Suter PM and others: *N*-Acetylcysteine enhances recovery from acute lung injury in man, *Chest* 105:190, 1994.

53. Aitken ML and others: Recombinant human DNase inhalation in normal subjects and patients with cystic fibrosis, *J Am Med Assoc* 267:1947, 1992.

54. Shak S and others: Recombinant human DNase I reduces the viscosity of cystic fibrosis sputum, *Proc Natl Acad Sci USA* 87:9188, 1990.

55. Raskin P: Bronchospasm after inhalation of pancreatic dornase, *Am Rev Respir Dis* 98:597, 1968.

56. Fiel SB and others: Comparison of three jet nebulizer aerosol delivery systems used to administer recombinant human DNase I to patients with cystic fibrosis, *Chest* 108:153, 1995.

57. Wilmott RW and others: Aerosolized recombinant human DNase in hospitalized cystic fibrosis patients with acute pulmonary exacerbations, *Am J Respir Crit Care Med* 153:1914, 1996.

58. Consensus Conference: Practical applications of Pulmozyme, *Ped Pulmonol* 17:404, 1994.

59. Vasconcellos CA and others: Reduction in viscosity of cystic fibrosis sputum in vitro by gelsolin, *Science* 263:969, 1994.

60. Dasgupta B and others: Rheological properties in cystic fibrosis and airway secretions with combined rhDNase and gelsolin treatment. In Singh M, Savena VP, eds: *Advances in physiological fluid dynamics*, New Delhi, 1996, Narosa.

61. Pavia and others: Effects of iodopropylidene glycerol on tracheobronchial clearance in stable, chronic bronchitis patients, *Eur J Respir Dis* 67:177, 1985.

62. Rubin BK and others: Iodinated glycerol has no effect on pulmonary function, symptom score, or sputum properties in patients with stable bronchitis, *Chest* 109:348, 1996.

63. Rubin BK: An in vitro comparison of the mucoactive properties of guaifenesin, iodinated glycerol, surfactant, and albuterol, *Chest* 116:195, 1999.

64. Waldron-Edward D, Skoryna SC: The mucolytic activity of amides: a new approach to mucus dispersion, *Can Med Assoc J* 94:1249, 1966.

65. Marriott C, Richards JH: The effects of storage and potassium iodide, urea, and *N*-acetyl-L-cysteine and Triton X-100 on the viscosity of bronchial mucus, *Br J Dis Chest* 68:171, 1974.

66. Feng W and others: Imroved clearability of cystic fibrosis sputum with dextran treatment in vitro, *Am J Respir Crit Care Med* 157(3 Pt 1):710, 1998.

67. Ahmed T and others: Preventing bronchoconstriction in exercise-induced asthma with inhaled heparin, *N Engl J Med* 329:90, 1993.

68. Ghio AJ and others: Tyloxapol inhibits NF-κB and cytokine release, scavenges HOCL, and reduces viscosity of cystic fibrosis sputum, *Am J Respir Crit Care Med* 154:783, 1996.

69. Stutts MJ and others: Multiple modes of regulation of airway epithelial chloride secretion by extracellular ATP, *Am J Physiol* 267:C1442, 1994.

70. Newhouse MT: Primary ciliary dyskinesia: what has it taught us about pulmonary disease? *Eur J Respir Dis* 64(suppl 127):151, 1983.

71. Girod S and others: Phospholipid composition and surface-active properties of tracheobronchial secretions from patients with cystic fibrosis and chronic obstructive pulmonary diseases, *Pediatr Pulmonol* 13:11, 1992.

72. Anzueto A and others: Effects of aerosolized surfactant in patients with stable chronic bronchitis: a prospective randomized controlled trial, *J Am Med Assoc* 278:1426, 1997.

73. McElvaney NG and others: Modulation of airway inflammation in cystic fibrosis: in vivo suppression of interleukin-8 levels on the respiratory epithelial surface by aerosolization of recombinant secretory leukoprotease inhibitor, *J Clin Invest* 90:1296, 1992.

74. Knowles MR and others: A controlled study of adenovirus-vector-mediated gene transfer in the nasal epithelium of patients with cystic fibrosis, *N Engl J Med* 333:823, 1995.

75. Flotte TR, Carter BJ: In vivo gene therapy with adeno-associated virus vectors for cystic fibrosis, *Advan Pharmacol* 40:85, 1997.

76. Gill DR and others: A placebo-controlled study of liposome-mediated gene transfer to the nasal epithelium of patients with cystic fibrosis, *Gene Ther* 4:199, 1997.

77. Naldini L and others: In vivo gene delivery and stable transduction of nondividing cells by a lentiviral vector, *Science* 272:2636, 1996.

78. Eng PA and others: Short term efficacy of ultrasonically nebulized hypertonic saline in cystic fibrosis, *Pediatr Pulmon* 21:77, 1996.

79. Smith JJ and others: Cystic fibrosis airway epithelia fail to kill bacteria because of abnormal airway surface fluid, *Cell* 85:229, 1996.

80. Gelman RA, Meyer FA: Mucociliary transference rate and mucus viscoelasticity: dependence on dynamic storage and loss modulus, *Am Rev Respir Dis* 120:553, 1979.

81. Giordano AM, Holsclaw D, Litt M: Mucus rheology and mucociliary clearance: normal physiologic state, *Am Rev Respir Dis* 118:245, 1978.

82. Puchelle E and others: Drug effects on viscoelasticity of mucus, *Eur J Respir Dis* 61(suppl 110):195, 1980.

83. Davis SS, Deverell LC: Rheological factors in mucociliary clearance. The assessment of mucotropic agents using an in vitro model, *Mod Probl Paediatr* 19:207, 1977.

CHAPTER 10

Surfactant Agents

Joseph L. Rau

*C*hapter 10 reviews pharmacological agents termed *surfactants,* which are intended to alter the surface tension of alveoli and the resulting pressures needed for alveolar inflation. The physical principles of surfactants and surface tension forces are reviewed as a basis for introducing agents that have been used or are currently used in respiratory care. The use of current exogenous surfactant agents in the treatment of respiratory distress syndrome of the newborn is presented.

PERSPECTIVE

PHYSICAL PRINCIPLES

Surface-active agents such as Alevaire or Tergemist (no longer available) have been used in the past to reduce the adhesiveness of mucus, and ethyl alcohol (ETOH) has been used to reduce the froth of pulmonary edema. Most recently, exogenous surfactants have been administered to replace missing pulmonary surfactant in respiratory distress syndrome (RDS) of the newborn. Surface-active agents act on liquids to affect surface tension. The following terms and concepts form the basis for an understanding of the application of surfactant preparations and their effects in the airway.

Surfactant: Surface-active agent that lowers surface tension. Examples include soap and various forms of detergent. Surfactants, or surface-active agents, have also been termed *detergents* for this reason.

Surface tension: Force caused by attraction between like molecules that occurs at liquid-gas interfaces and holds the liquid surface intact. The units of measure for surface tension are usually dynes per centimeter (dyn/cm), indicating the force required to cause a 1-cm rupture in the surface film. Because a liquid's molecules are more attracted to each other than to the surrounding gas, a droplet or spherical shape usually results (Figure 10-1, *A*).

LaPlace's Law: Physical principle describing and quantifying the relation between the internal pressure of a drop or bubble, the amount of surface tension, and the radius of the drop or bubble (Figure 10-1, *B*). For a bubble, which is a liquid film with gas inside and out, LaPlace's Law is as follows:

$$Pressure = (4 \times Surface\ tension)/Radius$$

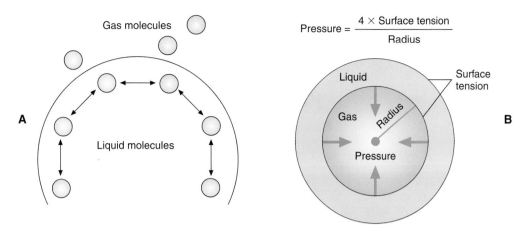

Figure 10-1 **A,** The concept of like liquid molecules producing the attractive force resulting in surface tension. **B,** LaPlace's Law illustrated for a bubble with two air-liquid interfaces. For alveoli, the relation is: Pressure = (2 × ST)/radius.

In alveoli there is only a single air-liquid interface, and LaPlace's Law is as follows:

$$\text{Pressure} = (2 \times \text{Surface tension})/\text{Radius}$$

APPLICATION TO THE LUNG

Because an alveolus has a liquid lining, surface tension forces apply. The higher the surface tension of the liquid, the greater is the compressing force inside the alveolus, which can cause collapse or difficulty in opening the alveolus. In foamy, bubbly pulmonary edema, the surface tension of the liquid allows the formation of the bubbly froth. In both cases, low compliance or pulmonary edema, lowering the surface tension will ease alveolar opening or cause the foam bubbles to collapse and liquefy.

CLINICAL INDICATIONS FOR EXOGENOUS SURFACTANTS

Exogenous surfactants are clinically indicated for the treatment or prevention of RDS in the newborn.

- *Prophylactic treatment:* Prevention of RDS in very-low-birth-weight infants and infants with higher birth weights who have evidence of immature lungs, at risk for developing RDS.
- *Rescue treatment:* Retroactive, or "rescue," treatment of infants who have developed RDS.

The basic problem in RDS is lack of pulmonary surfactant as a result of lung immaturity. This results in high surface tensions in the liquid-lined, gas-filled alveoli. Increased ventilating pressure is required to expand the alveoli during inspiration, which will lead to ventilatory and respiratory failure in the infant without ventilatory support. This concept, and the effect of exogenous surfactant, is shown in Figure 10-2. Exogenous surfactants are also being investigated for efficacy in the treatment of acute respiratory distress syndrome (ARDS), although this is not an approved clinical application at this time.

IDENTIFICATION OF SURFACTANT PREPARATIONS

Table 10-1 lists surfactant formulations that currently have Food and Drug Administration (FDA) approval for general clinical use in the United States, at the time of this edition. Detailed differences between these formulations and details of their dosing and administration are given subsequently for each agent in separate sections.

PREVIOUS SURFACTANT AGENTS IN RESPIRATORY CARE

The use of surfactant, or surface-active agents, in respiratory care predates the release of the exogenous surfactants currently applied in RDS of the newborn.

ETHYL ALCOHOL

Ethyl alcohol (ETOH) has been applied in acute fulminating pulmonary edema, in which the airway is obstructed with serous exudate. The exudate has

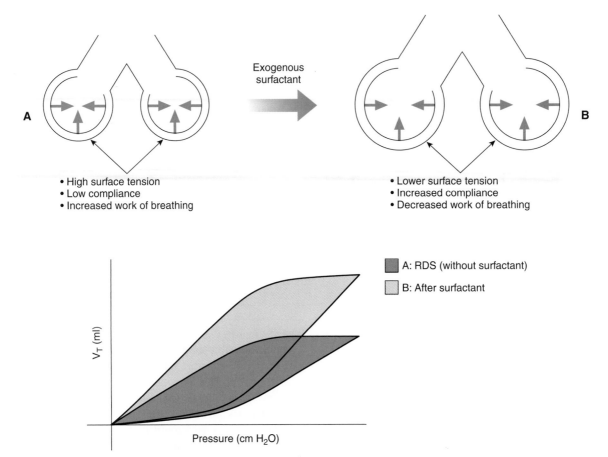

- High surface tension
- Low compliance
- Increased work of breathing

Exogenous surfactant

- Lower surface tension
- Increased compliance
- Decreased work of breathing

A: RDS (without surfactant)

B: After surfactant

V_T (ml)

Pressure (cm H_2O)

Figure 10-2   **A,** The lack of pulmonary surfactant in respiratory distress syndrome of the newborn results in high surface tension of the alveolar liquid lining and the need for high inspiratory pressures to expand alveoli. **B,** Exogenous surfactants reduce the high surface tension to reduce the pressures needed for alveolar expansion. A graph illustrates the change in the pressure-volume relation without pulmonary surfactant *(A)* and after exogenous surfactant therapy *(B)*.

Table 10-1

Exogenous surfactant preparations currently approved for use in the United States*

DRUG	BRAND NAME	FORMULATION AND INITIAL DOSE
Colfosceril palmitate	Exosurf Neonatal	10 ml vial, lyophilized powder, 108 mg colfosceril palmitate, 12 mg cetyl alcohol, and 9 mg tyloxapol, reconstituted in 8 ml sterile water *Dose:* 5 ml/kg, reconstituted suspension in two divided doses of 2.5 ml/kg by tracheal instillation
Beractant	Survanta	8 ml vial, 25 mg phospholipids/ml with 0.5-1.75 mg/ml triglycerides, 1.4-3.5 mg/ml free fatty acids, and <1 mg/ml protein *Dose:* 100 mg phospholipids/kg (4 ml/kg) in four divided doses by tracheal instillation
Calfactant	Infasurf	6 ml vial of 35 mg phospholipids/ml, 0.65 mg proteins *Dose:* 3 ml/kg in two divided doses of 1.5 ml/kg
Poractant alfa	Curosurf	1.5 ml (120 mg phospholipids) or 3 ml (240 mg phospholipids) vials *Dose:* 2.5 ml/kg (200 mg/kg) in two divided doses by tracheal instillation

*Individual agents are discussed subsequently in a separate section.
Detailed information on each should be obtained from manufacturer's drug insert.

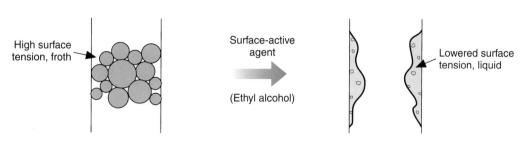

Effect of Surface-Active Agent
Pulmonary Edema

Figure 10-3   Illustration of the effect of alcohol on high surface tension foam to reduce the frothy bubbles to a liquid state.

sufficient surface tension to form a mass of bubbles, or foamy froth, that blocks gas exchange, precipitating acute hypoxemia. Ethyl alcohol has been given by nebulization or, more commonly, by direct tracheal instillation in a dilute strength of 30% to 50%, to lower the surface tension of the foam and reduce the froth to a liquid state that can be cleared by tracheobronchial aspiration (suctioning). This concept is illustrated in Figure 10-3.

MODE OF ACTION

Alcohol has the following surface tension at the concentrations given:

    100% strength: 22 dynes/cm
    50% strength: 28 dynes/cm
    30% strength: 32 dynes/cm

Frothy sputum is estimated to have a surface tension of approximately 60 dynes/cm. The addition of alcohol was thought to lower the surface tension of the foamy exudate, reducing it to a liquid, clearable state. Because alcohol can dissolve in water through hydrogen bonding, theoretically, physical mixing can occur between the alcohol and the aqueous exudate.

DISADVANTAGES

There is lack of an approved clinical use of alcohol in this application. Efficacy is not well established by controlled studies, which would be difficult to perform. Ethyl alcohol is toxic to membranes, and has been shown by Greiff and associates[1] to cause a bidirectional increase in permeability across the airway mucosal membrane. Exudation of plasma tracer substances onto the mucosal surface of the airway was significant. This is a process seen in airway inflammation, indicating that alcohol causes inflammatory

provocation of the airway. More sophisticated hemodynamic monitoring and the availability of improved diuretics and cardiotonics have replaced the use of topical ethyl alcohol in the airway.

MUCUS WETTING AGENTS (DETERGENTS)

Two agents were marketed, and subsequently removed, that were intended to alter the surface tension of mucus. The agents were prescribed for adhesive mucus, to improve water penetration and facilitate transport and expulsion.[2] Both agents were compounds with the following ingredients:

    Alevaire: Tyloxapol (Superinone), 0.125%
                Bicarbonate, 2.0%
                Glycerin, 5.0%
    Tergemist: Sodium ethasulfate, 0.125%
                Potassium iodide, 0.1%

The compounds were prescribed on a maintenance basis for chronic bronchitis. Of interest, alcohol in the form of vodka was also used by some physicians as a maintenance drug, given by nebulization, to reduce adhesiveness of mucus by its effect on surface tension. Perhaps the side effect of slight intoxication contributed to patient approval and compliance with this therapy.

MODE OF ACTION

In mucus, the attraction between water molecules is greater than the attraction between lipophilic groups of the macromolecule and water. Lipophilic groups tend to be pushed together to reduce the interfacial area of contact between lipophilic and water molecules. The resulting contacts of water and lipophilic groups are termed *hydrophobic bonds;* these provide junction points in the mucous gel.[3] It was thought that detergents may

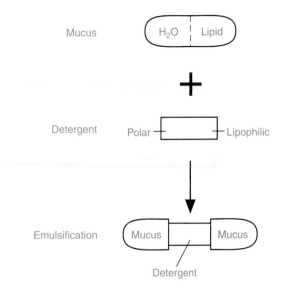

Mucus

Detergent

Emulsification

Detergent

Figure 10-4   Illustration of the theoretical effect of detergents, or "wetting agents," in emulsifying mucus to lower airway adhesion. Such agents have been withdrawn for lack of efficacy.

interact with mucus to produce emulsification, just as they do with grease and water. The lipophilic group on the detergent associates with that in the mucus, because the polar groups of the detergent orient to project into the aqueous phase and associate with the water molecules (Figure 10-4). Consequently the mucous gel will be "dissolved" or, better, dispersed into smaller particles. Sears and Stanitski[4] give a good illustration of this basic action of detergents in their discussion of solutions. The proposed mechanism of emulsification was described by Tainter and colleagues.[5]

EFFICACY OF DETERGENTS

Whether detergents actually have this emulsifying effect on mucus in vivo is questionable. The consensus ultimately was that clinical efficacy of surface-active agents with mucoid (as opposed to frothy edema) secretions could not be demonstrated and that some of the clinical effects seen could be due to the added ingredients, bicarbonate, glycerin, and potassium iodide, all of which have some mucolytic properties.[6,7] Tyloxapol *can* reduce surface tension and is an ingredient in one of the synthetic surfactant mixtures (Exosurf) discussed under exogenous surfactants.

USE OF PHOSPHOLIPIDS FOR MUCUS ADHESIVENESS

The influence of the physical properties of viscosity and elasticity, as well as spinnability, on mucociliary

clearance has been established, as reviewed in Chapter 9 (see Mucus-Controlling Agents). In addition, mucus adhesiveness may influence mucociliary clearance, as previously thought when surface active agents such as Alevaire, Tergemist, or vodka were prescribed to improve mucus transport. Phospholipids are present in the secretion of the mucous and serous cells in the submucosal glands.[8] Coating of the airway epithelium by phospholipids and mucin-like molecules may serve as a lubricant for mucus transport. Girod and associates[9] have shown that in cystic fibrosis, total phospholipids are increased in airway secretions compared with normals, and the *rigidifying* portions, such as sphingomyelin, are increased in comparison with the *surface-active* portions such as phosphatidylcholine and phosphatidylglycerol. This phospholipid imbalance may cause augmentation of mucus adhesion and stickiness in cystic fibrosis and chronic airway obstructive diseases. Treatment with surface-active phospholipids would therefore improve mucus clearance, and the in vitro data of Girod de Bentzmann and colleagues[10] support this theory. Transport of mucus by ciliary activity, as well as by cough, was significantly increased by coating mucus with liposomes of distearoyl phosphatidylglycerol (DSPG), with no toxicity to human airway epithelial cells. Therapeutic agents to act as lubricants and decrease mucus adhesivity would appear to offer another alternative to normalizing mucociliary transport and mucus clearance in disease states causing mucus hypersecretion or decreased clearance of secretions. There are no surfactant or phospholipid agents in general clinical use for mucus hypersecretion states at the time of this edition.

EXOGENOUS SURFACTANTS

The term *exogenous* used to describe this class of drugs refers to the fact that these are surfactant preparations from outside the patient's own body. These preparations may be obtained from other humans, from animals, or by laboratory synthesis. The clinical use of exogenous surfactants has been to replace the missing pulmonary surfactant of the premature or immature lung in RDS of the newborn. These agents have also been investigated for use in ARDS, and may prove to be beneficial, although results have not been entirely consistent.[11,12]

HISTORY AND DEVELOPMENT OF EXOGENOUS SURFACTANTS

Important events leading to the development and use of exogenous surfactant therapy in RDS of the new-

Box 10-1	Historical Events Leading to the Development of Exogenous Surfactants Used to Treat Respiratory Distress Syndrome (RDS)

1929	Von Meergaard showed that lungs were more difficult to inflate with air than with fluid.	1972	Enhorning and Robertson demonstrate the effectiveness of surfactant replacement in premature animals.
1956	Clements measured the surface tension of lung fluid extracts.	1980	Fujiwara and associates report success in exogenous surfactant therapy in infants, using a "lyophilised artificial surfactant" (bovine extract, Surfactant TA).
1958	Dipalmitoylphosphatidylcholine (DPPC) is identified by Clements and associates as the main surface-active component of pulmonary surfactant.	1990	Colfosceril palmitate (Exosurf Neonatal, Burroughs Wellcome) approved for general use.
1959	Avery and Mead showed that surface tension is higher in the lungs of infants with hyaline membrane disease than in the lungs of normal infants.	1991	Beractant (Survanta, Ross Laboratories) approved for general use.
		1998	Calfactant (Infasurf, Forest Pharamceuticals) approved for general use.
1964	Aerosols of synthetic DPPC are attempted in RDS, with little success.	1999	Poractant alfa (Curosurf, Dey) approved for general use.

born are listed in Box 10-1. Dipalmitoylphosphatidylcholine (DPPC) was not known to be the principal surface-active ingredient of normal pulmonary surfactant until 1958. In 1959, Avery and Mead[13] published their key paper describing the inability of lung extracts from infants who died of hyaline membrane disease to lower surface tension with deflation (film compression). Mary Ellen Avery gives a fascinating, first-hand description of how she was led to this discovery.[14] The understanding that surface tension is abnormally high in RDS and that this is caused by surfactant deficiency in immature lungs ultimately led to the development of exogenous surfactant products such as Exosurf, Survanta, and others and their application in RDS to normalize lung compliance. Although DPPC is the primary surface-active ingredient of natural surfactant, the use of DPPC alone was not successful in maintaining surface tension in the immature lung. Other components of pulmonary surfactant, described in the next section, were needed to reproduce the surface properties of natural surfactant.

COMPOSITION OF PULMONARY SURFACTANT

Pulmonary surfactant is a complex mixture of lipids and proteins (Box 10-2). The surfactant mixture is produced by alveolar type II cells, and its primary function, although not necessarily its only function, is to regulate the surface tension forces of the liquid alveolar lining. Surfactant regulates surface tension by forming a film at the air-liquid interface. Surfactant lowers surface tension as it is compressed during ex-

Box 10-2	Composition of Whole Surfactant From Bronchoalveolar Lavage Fluid (% by Weight)

Lipids (85%-90%)
Phospholipids (~90%)
   Phosphatidylcholine
     Half is dipalmitoylphosphatidylcholine, DPPC
   Phosphatidylglycerol
   Phosphatidylethanolamine
   Phosphatidylserine
   Phosphatidylinositol
   Sphingomyelin
Neutral lipids (10%)
   Cholesterol and others

Proteins (10%)
Surfactant protein A (SP-A)
Surfactant protein B (SP-B)
Surfactant protein C (SP-C)
Surfactant protein D (SP-D)

piration, thus reducing the amount of pressure and inspiratory effort required to reexpand the alveoli during a succeeding inspiration. The amount of extracellular (outside the type II cell) surfactant in animals is 10 to 15 mg/kg body weight in adults and 5 to 10 times that in mature newborns.[15] Figure 10-5 illustrates the source, basic composition, and regulation of pulmonary surfactant in the alveolus. Each of the major components is described.

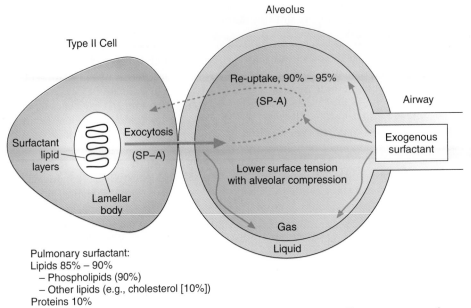

Figure 10-5   The production and reuptake of surfactant by type II cells. Exogenous surfactant is also taken up, to become part of the surfactant pool for alveoli.

LIPIDS

Lipids make up about 85% to 90% of surfactant by weight. The lipid component of surfactant is approximately 90% phospholipids, such as phosphatidylcholine, phosphatidylglycerol, sphingomyelin, and others, and 10% other lipids, most of which is cholesterol.[16] Phospholipids have both lipophilic and hydrophilic properties and are able to achieve low surface tensions at air-liquid interfaces. Phosphatidylcholine makes up about 75% to 80% of the phospholipids in surfactant, and about half of this is dipalmitoylphosphatidylcholine, or DPPC, which is also known as lecithin. DPPC is the surfactant component predominantly responsible for the reduction of alveolar surface tension. The hydrophilic choline residue of DPPC associates with the liquid phase in alveoli, while the hydrophobic palmitic acid residue projects into the air phase.[17]

PROTEINS

The total protein portion of surfactant is about 10% by weight. Approximately 80% of this portion is contaminating serum proteins and 20% is surfactant-specific proteins. There are currently four surfactant-specific proteins (SP) identified: SP-A, SP-B, SP-C, and SP-D.[14] Proteins of the surfactant mixture are reviewed by Johansson and associates.[18]

All of the components of surfactant are synthesized by the alveolar type II cell. The type I cell, which is the basic alveolar epithelial cell on 95% of the alveolar surface, has no known role in surfactant synthesis or metabolism. The type II cell also secretes other proteins, such as cytokines, growth factors, and antibacterial proteins into the alveolar space. The role of the surfactant-associated proteins is well-reviewed by Hawgood and Poulain[19] and Possmayer.[20]

Surfactant Protein A (SP-A). SP-A is a high-molecular-weight, water-soluble glycoprotein. This protein is specific to surfactant and has also been denoted by SP-35 and Apoprotein A or SAP-35.[15] SP-A seems to regulate both secretion and exocytosis of surfactant from the type II cell, as well as the reuptake of surfactant for recycling and reuse.

Surfactant Protein B and C (SP-B, SP-C). SP-B and SP-C are low-molecular-weight, hydrophobic proteins that improve the adsorption and spreading of the phospholipid throughout the air-liquid interface in the alveolus.

Surfactant Protein D (SP-D). SP-D is a fourth protein identified in natural endogenous surfactant. SP-D has similarities to SP-A as a large, water-soluble pro-

Table 10-2

Types of surfactant preparations and examples

CATEGORY	DESCRIPTION	EXAMPLES
Natural	Surfactant from natural sources (human or animal) with addition or removal of substances	Survanta (bovine) Surfactant TA (bovine) Curosurf (porcine) Infasurf (bovine) Alveofact (bovine)
Synthetic	Surfactant that is prepared by mixing in vitro synthesized substances that may or may not be in natural surfactant	Exosurf ALEC
Synthetic natural	Surfactant prepared in vitro with genetic engineering	None at present

tein, although differences exist in their molecular configuration.[19] There is no clear role for SP-D in surfactant function at this time, causing question as to whether SP-D is correctly designated as a surfactant-associated protein.

PRODUCTION AND REGULATION OF SURFACTANT SECRETION

The surfactant lipids are synthesized in the type II alveolar cells and stored in vesicles termed *lamellar bodies* (see Figure 10-5). The surfactant in the lamellar bodies is then secreted by exocytosis out of the type II cell and into the alveolus. The major stimulus for secretion of lamellar bodies into the alveolar space appears to be inflation of the lung, with a chemically coupled stretch response.[21] SP-A and SP-B facilitate the formation of an intermediate lattice form of surfactant termed tubular myelin, before it reaches the air-liquid interface. SP-C also helps to "break" the lipid layers of surfactant, so that adsorption and spreading of the compound as a monolayer will proceed quickly through the air-liquid interface. Surfactant is converted to small vesicles, which can be taken back into the type II cell or taken in alveolar macrophages. The two major alveolar forms of surfactant are large surfactant aggregates (lamellar bodies and tubular myelin-like structures) and small vesicles or aggregates.[22] The secretion of surfactant material from the type II cell is estimated at 10% of the intracellular pool every hour,[23] with an alveolar half-life between 15 and 30 hours.[16] The constant secretion of surfactant is balanced by two clearance mechanisms: endocytosis back into the type II cell, and clearance/degradation by alveolar macrophages.[19] In addition, clearance can occur by degradation within the alveoli, and by mucociliary removal and transport.[16]

A key feature of surfactant production which is the basis for the success of replacement therapy with ex-

ogenous compounds is the recycling activity in surfactant production. Most surfactant (90% to 95%) is taken back into the alveolar type II cell, reprocessed, and resecreted. It is for this reason that exogenously administered surfactant is successful in replacing missing surfactant, with one or two doses. The exogenous surfactant is taken into the type II cells and becomes the surfactant pool, through the reuptake and recycling mechanism. The reuptake is regulated, at least partly, by SP-A. It is clear the surfactant-specific proteins, or apoproteins, are critical for both the surface-active functioning of surfactant and the metabolic regulation of the surfactant pool. This process is well described by Wright and Clements[17] and Morton.[11] The normal function of endogenous surfactant also depends on the structural organization of the compound. Smaller surfactant aggregates have less SP-A and are less surface-active than larger aggregates.[15]

Pulmonary surfactant has also been found to contribute to host defense by increasing bacterial killing, modifying macrophage function and downregulating the inflammatory response through decreased mediator release from inflammatory cells.[24] Surfactant also enhances ciliary beat frequency and maintains patency of conducting airways.[22]

TYPES OF EXOGENOUS SURFACTANT PREPARATIONS

Exogenous surfactant preparations can be placed into three categories. These categories and examples of each are given in Table 10-2, and described in this section. A more complete technical description is given by Jobe and Ikegami.[15]

NATURAL/MODIFIED NATURAL SURFACTANT

Natural surfactant is an apt descriptive term for the category of surfactants obtained from animals or humans by alveolar wash or from amniotic fluid. The large surface-active aggregates of natural surfactant are recovered from the fluid by centrifugation or simple filtration. Because this is a natural surfactant, the ingredients necessary for effective function to regulate surface tension are present. Specifically this includes the surface proteins needed for adsorption and spreading. Depending on the source, natural surfactants can be expensive and time consuming to obtain and prepare. In addition, there is concern over contamination with viral infectious agents or immunological stimulation and antibody production from foreign proteins. Natural surfactant preparations are usually modified by the addition or removal of certain components. Examples of natural surfactants are given in Table 10-2. The natural surfactant Survanta, as an example, is obtained as an extract of minced cow lung, supplemented with other ingredients such as DPPC, palmitic acid, and tripalmitin. Usually, the modifications to the natural surfactant material are designed to improve functioning in the lung and to reduce protein contamination and provide sterility. Although Survanta contains the hydrophobic proteins SP-B and SP-C, the protein SP-A is missing, and this may shorten the duration of effect.

Other examples of a modified natural surfactant include *Surfactant TA*, prepared by the Tokyo-Akita Company in Japan and used by Fujiwara and colleagues in their 1980 work.[25] Surfactant TA is a reconstituted chloroform-methanol extract from minced bovine lungs, with DPPC and other lipids added. *Curosurf* is another modified natural surfactant, obtained as a porcine lung extract. *Infasurf* is a chloroform-methanol extract of fluid lavaged from calf lung and, like Survanta, contains only the surfactant proteins SP-B and SP-C, but not SP-A.[26] *Alveofact* is an organic solvent extract of cow lung lavage containing 99% phospholipids and neutral lipids and 1% surfactant proteins B and C (SP-B, SP-C).[27]

SYNTHETIC SURFACTANT

Synthetic surfactants are mixtures of synthetic components. An example is *Exosurf*, which is composed of DPPC, cetyl alcohol, and tyloxapol. The phospholipid DPPC can be synthesized in the laboratory. The characteristic feature of artificial surfactants is that none of the ingredients are obtained from natural sources, such as human or cow lung. Synthetic surfactants do not contain any of the surfactant proteins, including SP-B or SP-C, which are found in the natural preparations. A major advantage of this class of surfactant is its freedom from contaminating infectious agents and

additional foreign proteins that may be antigenic to the recipient. A possible disadvantage is the lack of equivalent performance between the organic chemicals substituted for the naturally occurring surfactant proteins, such as SP-A, B, or C.

ALEC is a preparation consisting of two phospholipids, DPPC and phosphatidylglycerol, in a 7:3 proportion by weight, which is available in Great Britain.[16]

SYNTHETIC NATURAL SURFACTANT

An ideal solution to the problems of concern in both natural and artificial surfactants would be genetically engineered surfactant using recombinant DNA technology. In such a preparation the phospholipid, lipid, and protein ingredients of the natural surfactant aggregate would be produced by characterizing with in vitro cloning the gene or genes responsible for human surfactant. There are no products available for general use at this time, but work progresses on their development. The genes and amino acid sequence for each of the surfactant proteins have been characterized.[28-30] A genetically engineered surfactant that closely resembles the structure and effect of natural human surfactant is the ideal preparation.

SPECIFIC EXOGENOUS SURFACTANT PREPARATIONS

Four exogenous surfactant preparations have been approved for general clinical use in the United States at the time of this edition. Each of these preparations is described in greater detail.

COLFOSCERIL PALMITATE (EXOSURF NEONATAL)

Colfosceril palmitate is a protein-free, synthetic lyophilised powder surfactant preparation (see Table 10-1). The powder preparation also contains sodium chloride to adjust osmolality, and its pH is adjusted with either sodium hydroxide (base) or hydrochloric acid. The powder form is reconstituted with 8 ml of preservative-free sterile water. The reconstituted suspension is milky white and has a pH in the range of 5 to 7; each milliliter of solution contains 13.5 mg of colfosceril palmitate, 1.5 mg of cetyl alcohol, and 1.0 mg of tyloxapol.

Colfosceril palmitate is another name used for dipalmitoylphosphatidylcholine, or DPPC. As a synthetic, or artificial mixture prepared in the laboratory, Exosurf does not contain any of the surfactant-associated proteins (SP-A, SP-B, or SP-C). Cetyl alcohol is a 16-carbon form of alcohol (hexadecanol) that acts as a spreading agent for DPPC at the liquid-air alveolar interface, because the proteins SP-B and SP-C are not contained in the artificial mixture. The tyloxapol additive (a polymeric long-chain alcohol) also acts to help disperse the DPPC and cetyl alcohol. A summary of prescribing information is given, with complete details on the Exosurf product found in the manufacturer's literature.

INDICATIONS FOR USE

Specific guidelines for use of colfosceril palmitate (Exosurf Neonatal) are the following:

1. Prophylactic therapy of infants weighing less than 1350 g birth weight
2. Prophylactic therapy of infants with birth weights greater than 1350 g with evidence of pulmonary immaturity and at risk for RDS
3. Rescue treatment of infants who have developed RDS

DOSAGE

The recommended dose of Exosurf is 5 ml/kg of the reconstituted suspension, given as two divided doses of 2.5 ml/kg, by direct tracheal administration.

Because the reconstituted suspension from a single vial of Exosurf has a volume of 8 ml, with 108 mg of colfosceril palmitate, a single vial can treat up to a 1600-g infant, based on a dose of 5 ml/kg, as follows:

$$5 \text{ ml/kg} \times 1.6 \text{ kg} = 8 \text{ ml}$$

With larger weight infants, additional vials are needed. A second dose of 5 ml/kg is administered 12 hours after the first, with a third dose if needed, 12 hours after the second.

ADMINISTRATION

Exosurf is instilled directly into the endotracheal tube (ETT) through a side-port adaptor that fits on the ETT and has a Luer-Lok. The first half of the dose is administered in bursts, timed to coincide with inspiration. The dose is given with the infant in midline position. The infant is then rotated to the right for half a minute and ventilated. The second half of the dose is then given, again in midline position, and the infant is rotated to the left.

Complete details of preparing the suspension, dosage, and administration are in the manufacturer's literature, which should be thoroughly read before using the drug.

BERACTANT (SURVANTA)

Beractant (Survanta) is considered a modified natural surfactant. It is a mixture with natural bovine lung extract, to which colfosceril palmitate (DPPC), palmitic acid, and tripalmitin are added. These last three ingredients are used to standardize the composition of the drug preparation, as well as to reproduce the surface-tension–lowering properties of natural surfactant. The colfosceril, or DPPC, is the same phospholipid contained in beractant. The ingredients are suspended in 0.9% saline. The composition of beractant, given in the product literature, is described in Table 10-1. The extract from minced bovine lung contains natural phospholipids; neutral lipids; fatty acids; and the low-molecular-weight, hydrophobic surfactant proteins SP-B and SP-C. The hydrophilic, large-molecular-weight protein SP-A is not contained in beractant. SP-A helps regulate surfactant reuptake and secretion by the type II cell. However, the addition of SP-A to beractant by Yamada and colleagues[31] did not improve the biophysical (spreading, absorption) *or* physiological (lung compliance change) activities of the mixture.

Beractant is available as Survanta from Ross Laboratories in a vial containing 8 ml of suspension, with a concentration of 25 mg per ml, in a 0.9% sodium chloride solution. The suspension does not require reconstitution. This gives a maximal total dose of 200 mg of phospholipids in a single vial of 8 ml of suspension.

INDICATIONS FOR USE

Specific guidelines for use of beractant are as follows:

1. Prophylactic therapy of premature infants less than 1250 g birth weight or with evidence of surfactant deficiency and risk of RDS
2. Rescue treatment of infants with evidence of RDS

DOSAGE

The recommended dose of beractant is 100 mg/kg of birth weight. Because there are 25 mg/ml in the beractant suspension, this is equivalent to a dose of 4 ml/kg of birth weight. For example, a 2000-g (2 kg) infant would require 8 ml, or the entire vial of suspension. Unlike Exosurf, Survanta does not require reconstitution because it is marketed as a suspension.

Repeat doses of beractant are given no sooner than 6 hours later if there is evidence of continuing respiratory distress. The manufacturer's literature recommends that manual hand-bag ventilation *not* be used for the repeat dose in place of mechanical ventilation. Ventilator adjustment may be necessary, however.

ADMINISTRATION

Beractant suspension is off-white to light brown in color. If settling has occurred in the suspension, the vial can be swirled gently but should not be shaken. The suspension is kept refrigerated and must be warmed by standing at room temperature for at least 20 minutes. Artificial warming methods should not be used.

The calculated dose is given in quarters from a syringe and instilled into the trachea through a 5-French catheter placed into the ETT. The catheter is removed and the infant manually ventilated or returned to the ventilator for at least 30 seconds or until stable, between doses. The remaining doses are given in similar fashion.

Unopened vials that have been warmed to room temperature may be returned for refrigerated storage within 8 hours. This should be done no more than once. Used vials should be discarded with residual drug. The preceding general description of beractant (Survanta) is intended to be instructional. Complete prescribing information from the manufacturer should be reviewed when using this product.

CALFACTANT (INFASURF)

Calfactant is another modified natural surfactant preparation from calf lung (bovine). It is an organic solvent extract of calf lung surfactant obtained by cell-free bronchoalveolar lavage. The extract contains phospholipids, neutral lipids, and hydrophobic proteins SP-B and SP-C. The preparation is a suspension, which does not require reconstitution. Its composition is given in Table 10-1. Each milliliter contains 35 mg total phospholipids, including 26 mg phosphatidylcholine, of which 16 mg is disaturated phosphatidylcholine, and 0.65 mg proteins, which includes 0.26 mg of SP-B. The protein SP-A is not contained in the preparation. The formulation is heat sterilized and contains no preservatives.

INDICATIONS FOR USE

Specific guidelines for use of calfactant (Infasurf) are as follows:

1. The prevention (prophylaxis) of RDS in premature infants less than 29 weeks of gestational age at high risk for RDS

2. The treatment (rescue) of premature infants less than or equal to 72 hours of age who develop RDS and require endotracheal intubation

It is noted in the drug insert that calfactant prophylaxis should be administered as soon as possible, preferably no more than 30 minutes after birth.

DOSAGE

The recommended dose of calfactant is 3 ml/kg body weight at birth. Each 6 ml of suspension contains enough preparation (210 mg of phospholipids) to treat a 2-kg infant.

Repeat doses, up to a total of three doses, can be given 12 hours apart. Repeat doses as early as 6 hours after the previous dose can be given if the infant is still intubated and requires 30% or greater oxygen for a PaO_2 of 80 mm Hg or less (manufacturer's literature).

ADMINISTRATION

Calfactant can be administered to an intubated infant either by side-port delivery or with a catheter. The preparation does not require reconstitution. Calfactant is an off-white suspension that requires gentle swirling or agitation, but not shaking, in the vial to ensure dispersion. Flecks may be visible in the suspension and foaming at the surface.

Side-port Adaptor. The dose is given in two aliquots of 1.5 ml/kg each. Position the infant with either the right or left side dependent for each aliquot. The suspension is instilled in small bursts timed to coincide with the inspiratory cycle, over 20 to 30 breaths. It is recommended that the infant be evaluated between repositioning for the second aliquot.

Catheter Administration. The dose is divided into four equal aliquots, with the catheter removed between each instillation, and mechanical ventilatory support for 0.5 to 2 minutes. Each aliquot is given with the infant in a different position (prone, supine, right lateral, and left lateral).

The preceding description of use of calfactant is for instructional purposes. Complete prescribing information from the manufacturer should be reviewed when using this product.

PORACTANT ALFA (CUROSURF)

Poractant alfa is a natural surfactant obtained as an extract of porcine lung. It is a suspension consisting of approximately 99% phospholipids (120 mg phospholipids in the 1.5-ml vial and 240 mg phospholipids in the 3-ml vial) and about 1% surfactant-associated proteins SP-B and SP-C. The preparation has been available in Europe since 1989 and was approved by the FDA for use in the United States on November 18, 1999.[32]

INDICATIONS FOR USE

Specific guidelines for use of poractant alfa (Curosurf) are as follows:

1. For the treatment or rescue of RDS in premature infants
2. Unlabeled uses: prophylaxis for RDS, ARDS resulting from viral pneumonia, human immunodeficiency virus (HIV)-infected infants with *Pneumocystis carinii* pneumonia, and treatment in ARDS after near drowning

DOSAGE

The initial dose of poractant is 2.5 ml/kg of birth weight. Subsequent doses of 1.25 ml/kg birth weight can be given twice in 12-hour intervals if needed. The maximum recommended total dose (initial plus repeat doses) is 5 ml/kg.

ADMINISTRATION

Before use, the vial should be slowly warmed to room temperature. The vial should be turned upside-down to uniformly disperse the suspension without shaking. Poractant does not need to be reconstituted. The dose is administered through a 5-French catheter positioned in the ETT, with the tip in the distal end of the ETT tube but not extended beyond the end of the ETT tube.

The dose is given in two divided aliquots. The infant is positioned with either the right or left side down for the first aliquot. The catheter is then removed and the infant is manually ventilated with 100% oxygen for 1 minute. When the infant is stable, the second aliquot is instilled with the alternate side dependent, after which the catheter is removed. The airway should not be suctioned for 1 hour unless significant airway obstruction is evident.

The preceding description of use of poractant alfa is for instructional purposes. Complete prescribing information from the manufacturer should be reviewed when using this product.

MODE OF ACTION

The mode of action of exogenous surfactants is to replace and replenish a deficient endogenous surfactant pool in neonatal RDS. As previously described, en-dogenous surfactant normally secreted by type II cells leaves the alveolar space and reenters the type II cell in the form of small vesicles. In the intracellular space, surfactant components are recycled. Exogenously administered surfactant that reaches the alveolar space can be recycled into the type II cells and form a surfactant pool to regulate surface tension.

There can be a dramatic improvement in oxygenation after surfactant administration, but Davis and associates[33] did not report a corresponding increase in compliance. Although exogenous surfactant should lower surface tension and thereby increase lung compliance, there is disagreement in the literature over whether the primary clinical effect of exogenous surfactant is one of increasing lung compliance.[34] Fujiwara and colleagues[25] noted that there was clearing of the chest radiograph associated with a good clinical response to surfactant, suggesting that surfactant treatment increased the functional residual capacity (FRC). A study by Goldsmith and associates[35] measured an increase in the FRC within 15 minutes of treatment with natural surfactant, correlating with the time of blood gas improvements. The surfactant stabilizes alveoli on expiration and prevents collapse, increasing residual volume and FRC. An increase in oxygenation would be seen with this effect.[34] An increase in lung volume resulting from improved residual volume and FRC shifts the tidal ventilation to a new pressure-volume curve. At higher lung volumes, chest wall elastic recoil is higher. A shift to the flatter part of the pressure-volume curve could give the same tidal volume for a given pressure change, masking the actual increase in static compliance.[30]

HAZARDS AND COMPLICATIONS OF SURFACTANT THERAPY

Some of the complications in exogenous surfactant therapy are due to the dosing procedure, and others can be caused by the therapeutic effect of the drug itself. In the dosing procedure, relatively large volumes of suspension are instilled in neonatal-size airways, and this can block gas exchange, causing desaturation and bradycardia.

The effect of the drug in improving pulmonary compliance can lead to overventilation, excessive volume delivery from pressure-limited ventilation, and overoxygenation with dangerously high PaO_2 levels. As a result, the following complications or hazards can occur with surfactant therapy. In general, complications of prematurity may affect the response to exogenous surfactant.

AIRWAY OCCLUSION, DESATURATION, AND BRADYCARDIA

Because the current method of administration is by direct tracheal instillation, a large volume of surfactant suspension may cause an acute obstruction of infant airways, with subsequent hypoxemia and bradycardia.[36] Repetitive small additions of the dose and a transient increase in ventilating pressure may help distribute the surfactant to the periphery.

HIGH ARTERIAL OXYGEN (Pao₂) VALUES

A good response to exogenous surfactant will result in better (higher) lung compliance, increased FRC, and concomitant improvement in oxygenation. Fractional inspired oxygen (FIO_2) settings must be lowered if Pao_2 improves, to prevent overoxygenation and the possibility of retrolental fibroplasia.

OVERVENTILATION AND HYPOCARBIA

As lung compliance improves, peak ventilating pressure, expiratory baseline pressures, and ventilatory rate must be adjusted, or overventilation and pneumothorax may occur.

APNEA

Apnea has been noted to occur with the intratracheal administration of surfactant.

PULMONARY HEMORRHAGE

In a study of infants weighing less than 700 g at birth, the incidence of pulmonary hemorrhage was 10% with Exosurf compared with 2% in the control group. This increase was not seen in infants greater than 700 g at birth. Pulmonary hemorrhage was more frequent in infants who were younger, smaller, male, and with a patent ductus arteriosus.*

FACTORS IN SURFACTANT SELECTION

There are differences between the two exogenous surfactant preparations, colfosceril palmitate and beractant, that form the basis for factors to be considered when selecting an agent. Several of these factors are summarized in Table 10-3. Despite the differences summarized in Table 10-3, both forms of exogenous surfactant have been effective in reducing overall infant mortality rates. Exogenous surfactants improve survival in RDS, improve oxygenation, and reduce days on ventilator support or with supplemental oxygen.[37] Comparisons between types of surfactant preparations are difficult because of variations in ventilator management, such as method of ventilation and weaning, and fluid management. In addition, results in studies of exogenous preparations are confounded by the associated risks of prematurity, including worsening of patent ductus arteriosus, increase in intraventricular hemorrhage, nosocomial-acquired infections, and pulmonary hemorrhage. Although natural biological surfactants give a more rapid response than a synthetic agent, it has not been shown that this changes overall mortality, morbidity, onset of bronchopulmonary dysplasia, or RDS-specific mortality.[38,39] As controlled comparative trials of synthetic versus natural products are performed, data may become available to guide a clinical choice of agent by

*From manufacturer's insert, Burroughs Wellcome.

Table 10-3

Summary of differences between the synthetic product colfosceril and a modified natural (biological) product, such as beractant

	SYNTHETIC (COLFOSCERIL)	NATURAL (BERACTANT)
Response time*	Slower in onset (several hours)	Rapid in onset (5-30 min)
Administration	During mechanical ventilator breath (ETT side-port adaptor)	Removed from ventilator
	Two divided doses, two positions	Four divided doses, four positions
Drug preparation	Must reconstitute before use	Refrigerated suspension; must warm to room temperature
Side effects	No proteins to stimulate immune response; no infectious agents present	Proteins may elicit immune response; concern over sterilization effectiveness
Cost	Similar (may change in future)	Similar

*Response = changes in oxygenation and lung mechanics.

supporting a net advantage or disadvantage with one type of product after all factors are considered.[37]

One such trial was conducted by Hudak and colleagues[40] as a large multicenter comparison of the natural surfactant Infasurf with the synthetic Exosurf, in 1033 infants. Assignment of treatment was random and masked, and the method of administration of both agents was the same. Infasurf (3 ml/kg) was found superior to the synthetic agent Exosurf (5 ml/kg) on the following variables: occurrence of pulmonary air leak (11% versus 21%), average oxygen concentration needed (0.39 versus 0.47), average mean airway pressure (7.2 versus 8.6 cm H_2O), and number of days of greater than 30% inspired oxygen and of assisted ventilation (both lower with Infasurf). Mortality, survival at 28 days without bronchopulmonary dysplasia, and duration of hospitalization did not differ between the two agents. The authors concluded that Infasurf was more effective as assessed by the severity of respiratory disease and the incidence of air leak complications.

Other questions in the use of exogenous surfactant continue to be investigated.

- When should surfactant be given for therapy in RDS? The advantage of rescue treatment is that there is no need to predict or anticipate the onset of RDS. The need for the treatment is clearly evident in the presence of RDS. However, does the delay with rescue treatment lead to increased risk and complications? With prophylactic therapy, there is the possibility of needless treatment, with possible adverse effects and unnecessary expense. The prophylactic approach administers surfactant as soon as possible after birth. There is discussion on waiting several hours after birth before giving surfactant, or even to withhold surfactant until and unless there is mild, or even moderate, RDS present.
- Are there other methods of administering surfactant preparations? An alternative to direct tracheal instillation is nebulization, and this is being investigated.[41] Other questions concern the use of high-frequency ventilation, ECMO, and even liquid ventilation for the administration of surfactant.

FUTURE DIRECTIONS IN SURFACTANT THERAPY

In addition to RDS of the newborn, surfactant replacement therapy has been considered for a variety of adult respiratory disorders. This topic is comprehensively reviewed by Hamm and colleagues.[16] Acute respiratory distress syndrome (ARDS) in the adult is a potential target for surfactant therapy. In RDS of the newborn, the primary abnormality of lung function is related to surfactant deficiency. In ARDS with adults, the surfactant deficiency is secondary to lung injury with complex inflammatory responses.[16] This would suggest a difference in clinical response to surfactant therapy between premature infants and adults with ARDS. In addition, dose amount and administration techniques may need to be modified for therapy in adults, who have large lung volumes compared with infants. If lung injury in ARDS is nonuniform in distribution, exogenous surfactant, especially if aerosolized, may distribute unevenly to more compliant lung areas instead of to areas needing surfactant the most.[22]

In one multicenter trial using the synthetic preparation Exosurf, surfactant was delivered for 5 days by continuous nebulization to over 200 patients with sepsis-induced ARDS. There was little physiological improvement and no difference in overall mortality compared with a conventionally treated control group.[42] Questions have been raised concerning the amount of aerosol deposited in the lungs in this study. A smaller clinical trial examined the use of the natural biological product, Survanta, in patients with ARDS.[43] The surfactant was instilled directly into the lungs, using up to four doses, with a dose of 100 mg/kg/dose. Mortality in the treated group was 17.8% compared with 43.8% in the control group. Similar favorable results were found in a study using Alveofact, which is also a natural preparation.[44] These results suggest a possible benefit to surfactant treatment in ARDS, as well as questions over the reasons for the difference in results. The availability of newer surfactant preparations, specifically human recombinant surfactants, may offer better results to improve outcomes in adults with ARDS.[30]

Other adult respiratory disorders in which either surfactant replacement therapy or abnormal surfactant regulation may occur include pneumonia, lung transplants, sarcoidosis, hypersensitivity pneumonitis, idiopathic pulmonary fibrosis, alveolar proteinosis, obstructive lung disease including asthma, radiation pneumonitis and drug-induced pulmonary disease.[14]

RESPIRATORY CARE ASSESSMENT OF SURFACTANT THERAPY

- Monitor pulse and cardiac rhythm during and after administration.
- Monitor the infant for signs of airway occlusion (desaturation and bradycardia) during and after

administration; if obstruction is evident, remove the infant from the ventilator and manually ventilate; in addition, saline lavage may be needed as well as aggressive suctioning to clear the airway.

- Monitor color and activity level of infant.
- Monitor chest rise for level of ventilation, or use electronic monitor if available.
- Monitor arterial oxygen saturation and adjust F_{IO_2} accordingly to prevent hyperoxia or hypoxia.
- Monitor transcutaneous P_{CO_2} if possible, and be prepared to adjust level of ventilation as needed to prevent hypercarbia or hypocarbia.
- Assess lung mechanics (exhaled volumes or peak inspiratory pressures) during mechanical ventilation to determine effectiveness of the exogenous agent in normalizing lung compliance. The instilled drug may cause changes within minutes in some cases.
- Consider the possible adverse effects if pulse, cardiac rhythm, or arterial/transcutanous blood gas values deteriorate.

SUMMARY KEY TERMS AND CONCEPTS

- *Surfactant agents* regulate *surface tension* in films at gas-liquid interfaces. The interrelation of surface tension, drop or bubble size, and pressure is described by *LaPlace's Law.*
- Previous use of surfactants included *ethyl alcohol* for *pulmonary edema*, and compounds such as *Alevaire* and *Tergemist* to decrease *mucus adhesiveness. Vodka* has also been nebulized for secretion clearance in chronic bronchitis.
- Four surfactant agents are currently used for treatment of *neonatal respiratory distress syndrome* (RDS). Colfosceril is a *synthetic* compound and beractant, calfactant, and poractant alfa are *modified natural* agents.
- Endogenous *pulmonary surfactant* is 90% lipids and 10% protein. The major phospholipid is *dipalmitoylphosphatidylcholine* (DPPC).
- *Surfactant-associated proteins*, such as SP-A, SP-B, or SP-C, regulate the function of endogenous pulmonary surfactant.
- Exogenous surfactant agents enter into the alveolar pool and replace deficient natural surfactant.
- Exogenous surfactants are given either *prophylactically* in RDS or as *rescue* treatment.
- There are possible *hazards* to use of exogenous surfactants, including airway occlusion, desaturation, bradycardia, overoxygenation and overventilation, apnea, and pulmonary hemorrhage.
- Differences between the two types of agents, synthetic and natural, should be considered by particular clinical sites when *selecting* an agent. Exogenous surfactants are being investigated for clinical use in disease states such as *ARDS* and *pneumonia.*

SELF-ASSESSMENT QUESTIONS

1. What is the definition of a surface-active substance?
2. What clinical problem was ethyl alcohol used for in the past?
3. In general, what is the clinical indication for use of exogenous surfactants?
4. What type (category) of exogenous surfactant is each of the following: colfosceril palmitate, beractant, calfactant, and poractant alfa?
5. What are the major ingredients of natural pulmonary surfactant?
6. Give the dosage schedule of each of the current exogenous surfactants.
7. What is the difference between "rescue" and "prophylaxis" treatment with these agents?
8. Identify at least three possible adverse effects with use of exogenous surfactant treatment.
9. Why does the improvement in lung mechanics last after only one or two administrations of exogenous surfactant?
10. How does the artificial surfactant colfosceril palmitate compensate for lack of the natural surfactant-associated proteins, such as SP-B or SP-C?
11. Which exogenous surfactants contain the proteins found in natural surfactant, such as SP-B?
12. How would you assess the effectiveness of exogenous surfactant treatment in a premature newborn with respiratory distress?

Answers to Self-Assessment Questions are found in Appendix A.

CLINICAL SCENARIO

Case courtesy **Robert Harwood, MSA, RRT, formerly of Georgia State University.**

A 16-year-old gravida 1000 female gave birth to a 25-week, 515-g baby girl by vaginal delivery. The mother had no prenatal care and she had premature rupture of the membranes 12 days before delivery. Immediately at birth the newborn was intubated with a 2.5-mm oral endotracheal tube. Apgar scores after intubation and application of positive-pressure ventilation with a bag and mask were 7 and 9 at 1 and 5 minutes, respectively. After transfer to the neonatal intensive care unit (NICU), umbilical venous and arterial catheters (UVC, UAC) were inserted and the infant placed on mechanical ventilation with PIP, 20 cm H_2O; PEEP, 5 cm H_2O; rate, 60/min; inspiratory time, 0.3 second; and F_{IO_2}, 1.0. Physical examination revealed P, 140 beats/min; BP, 34/22 mm Hg; T, 99.6° F; and Sp_{O_2}, 85% to 90%. Laboratory results revealed glucose, 39 mg/dl; WBC count of 11,900/mm³;

hematocrit, 47%; and platelets 297,000/mm³. Chest radiograph showed respiratory distress syndrome, stage II.

Is there an indication for administration of an exogenous surfactant in this case? Support your decision with the available data.
Would this administration of surfactant be a rescue or prophylactic treatment, if given immediately after placement on ventilatory support?

Twelve hours after the dose of surfactant was given, the infant exhibited signs of respiratory distress, with an RR increase from 46 breaths/min to 78 breaths/min, and a P increase from 140 beats/min to 185 beats/min. Periods of desaturation below 90% increased. Exhaled tidal volume decreased to 3 ml/kg body weight, and the FIO_2 was increased to 0.80. An arterial blood gas was obtained, with pH, 7.29; $PaCO_2$, 58 mm Hg; and PaO_2, 41 mm Hg.

What pharmacological treatment is now indicated?

Answers to Clinical Scenario Questions are found in Appendix A.

REFERENCES

1. Greiff L and others: Effects of histamine, ethanol, and a detergent on exudation and absorption across guinea pig airway mucosa in vivo, *Thorax* 46:700, 1991.
2. Miller JB and others: Alevaire inhalation for eliminating secretions in asthmatic sinusitis, bronchiectasis and bronchitis of adults, *Ann Allergy* 12:611, 1954.
3. Marriott C, Richards JH: The effects of storage and of potassium iodide, urea, N-acetyl-cysteine and triton X-100 on the viscosity of bronchial mucus, *Brit J Dis Chest* 68:171, 1974.
4. Sears CT Jr, Stanitski CL: *Chemistry for the health-related sciences: concepts and correlations*, ed 2, Englewood Cliffs, NJ, 1983, Prentice-Hall,.
5. Tainter ML and others: Alevaire as a mucolytic agent, *N Engl J Med* 253:764, 1955.
6. Paez PN, Miller WF: Surface active agents in sputum evacuation: a blind comparison with normal saline solution and distilled water, *Chest* 60:312, 1971.
7. Palmer KNV: Effect of an aerosol detergent in chronic bronchitis, *Lancet* 1:611, 1957.
8. Girod S and others: Identification of phospholipids in secretory granules of human submucosal gland respiratory cells, *J Histochem Cytochem* 39:193, 1991.
9. Girod S and others: Phospholipid composition and surface-active properties of tracheobronchial secretions from patients with cystic fibrosis and chronic obstructive pulmonary diseases, *Pediatr Pulmonol* 13:22, 1992.
10. Girod de Bentzmann S and others: Distearoyl phosphatidyl-glycerol liposomes improve surface and transport properties of CF mucus, *Eur Respir J* 6:1156, 1993.
11. Morton NS: Exogenous surfactant treatment for the adult respiratory distress syndrome? A historical perspective, *Thorax* 45:825, 1990 (editorial).
12. Holm BA, Matalon S: Role of pulmonary surfactant in the development and treatment of adult respiratory distress syndrome, *Anesth Analg* 69:805, 1989.
13. Avery ME, Mead J: Surface properties in relation to atelectasis and hyaline membrane disease, *Am J Dis Child* 97:517, 1959.
14. Avery ME: Surfactant deficiency in hyaline membrane disease: the story of discovery, *Am J Respir Crit Care Med* 161:1074, 2000.
15. Jobe A, Ikegami M: Surfactant for the treatment of respiratory distress syndrome, *Am Rev Respir Dis* 136:1256, 1987.
16. Hamm H, Kroegel C, Hohlfeld J: Surfactant: a review of its functions and relevance in adult respiratory disorders, *Respir Med* 90:251, 1996.
17. Wright JR, Clements JA: Metabolism and turnover of lung surfactant, *Am Rev Respir Dis* 135:427, 1987.
18. Johansson J, Curstedt T, Robertson B: The proteins of the surfactant system, *Eur Respir J* 7:372, 1994.
19. Hawgood S, Poulain FR: Functions of the surfactant proteins: a perspective, *Pediatr Pulmonol* 19:99, 1995.
20. Possmayer F: The role of surfactant-associated proteins (editorial), *Am Rev Respir Dis* 142:749, 1990.
21. Wirtz HR, Dobbs LG: Calcium mobilization and exocytosis after one mechanical stretch of lung epithelial cells, *Science* 250:1266, 1990.
22. Lewis J, Veldhuizen RAW: Surfactant: current and potential therapeutic application in infants and adults, *J Aerosol Med* 9:143, 1996.
23. Wright JR and others: Surfactant apoprotein Mr = 26,000-36,000 enhances uptake of liposomes by type II cells, *J Biol Chem* 262:2888, 1987.
24. Pison U and others: Host defence capacities of pulmonary surfactant: evidence for "non-surfactant" functions of the surfactant system, *Eur J Clin Invest* 24:586, 1994.
25. Fujiwara T and others: Artificial surfactant therapy in hyaline membrane disease, *Lancet* 1:55, 1980.
26. Notter RH and others: Lung surfactant replacement in premature lambs with extracted lipids from bovine lung lavage: effects of dose, dispersion techniques, and gestational age, *Pediatr Rev* 19:569, 1985.
27. Gortner L and others: Early treatment of respiratory distress syndrome with bovine surfactant in very preterm infants: a multicenter controlled clinical trial, *Pediatr Pulmonol* 14:4, 1992.
28. Floros J, Phelps DS, Taeusch HW: Biosynthesis and in vitro translation of the major surfactant-associated protein from human lung, *J Biol Chem* 260:495, 1985.
29. Avery ME, Merritt TA: Surfactant-replacement therapy, *N Engl J Med* 324:910, 1991.

30. Rodriguez RJ, Martin RJ: Exogenous surfactant therapy in newborns, *Respir Care Clin North Am* 5:595, 1999.

31. Yamada T and others: Effects of surfactant protein-A on surfactant function in preterm ventilated rabbits, *Am Rev Respir Dis* 142:754, 1990.

32. *The Medical Letter:* Curosurf, 42(Mar 20):27, 2000.

33. Davis J and others: Changes in pulmonary mechanics after the administration of surfactant to infants with respiratory distress syndrome, *N Engl J Med* 319:476, 1988.

34. Milner AD: How does exogenous surfactant work? *Arch Dis Childhood* 68:253, 1993.

35. Goldsmith LS and others: Immediate improvement in lung volume after exogenous surfactant: alveolar recruitment versus increased distention, *J Pediatr* 119:424, 1991.

36. Jobe AH: The role of surfactant therapy in neonatal respiratory distress, *Respir Care* 36:695, 1991.

37. Merritt TA: On exogenous surfactant therapy, *Pediatr Pulmonol* 14:1, 1992.

38. Merritt TA and others: Prophylactic treatment of very premature infants with human surfactant, *N Engl J Med* 315:785, 1986.

39. Bose C and others: Improved outcome at 28 days of age for very low birth weight infants treated with a single dose of a synthetic surfactant, *J Pediatr* 117:947, 1990.

40. Hudak ML and others: A multicenter randomized, masked comparison trial of natural versus synthetic surfactant for the treatment of respiratory distress syndrome, *J Pediatr* 128:396, 1996.

41. Lewis J and others: Nebulized vs. instilled exogenous surfactant in an adult lung injury model, *J Appl Physiol* 71:1270, 1991.

42. Anzueto A and others: An international, randomized, placebo-controlled trial evaluating the safety and efficacy of aerosolized surfactant in patients with sepsis-induced ARDS, *Am J Respir Crit Care Med* 149 (suppl, pt 2 of 2): A567, 1994.

43. Gregory TJ and others: Survanta supplementation in patients with acute respiratory distress syndrome (ARDS), *Am J Respir Crit Care Med* 149(suppl, pt 2 of 2):A567, 1994.

44. Walmrath D and others: Bronchoscopic surfactant administration in patients with severe ARDS and sepsis, *Am J Respir Crit Care Med* 154:57, 1995.

CHAPTER 11

Corticosteroids in Respiratory Care

Joseph L. Rau

CHAPTER OUTLINE

*C*hapter 11 presents the use of corticosteroids in respiratory care and provides a brief review of the physiology of endogenous corticosteroid hormones in the body. A summary description of inflammation, and specifically of airway inflammation in asthma, forms the basis for a discussion of the pharmacology of corticosteroids as antiinflammatory drugs. Aerosolized glucocorticoids are presented, along with their uses and side effects. The chapter concludes with a brief review of androgenic (anabolic) corticosteroids.

CLINICAL INDICATIONS FOR USE OF INHALED CORTICOSTEROIDS

Inhaled corticosteroids are available in formulations for oral inhalation (lung delivery) and intranasal delivery. Specific clinical applications are discussed more fully at the end of this chapter. General clinical indications for use of inhaled corticosteroids are as follows:

- Orally inhaled agents: Maintenance, control therapy of chronic asthma, identified as Step 2

or greater by the National Asthma Education and Prevention Program Expert Panel Report 2 (NAEPP EPR-II).[1]
- *Step 2 asthma:* Greater than 2 days/week of symptoms, greater than 2 nights/mo with symptoms, FEV_1 or peak expiratory flow (PEF) 80% or greater, but PEF variability is 20% to 30% (see Appendix D).
- Inhaled agents can be used together with systemic corticosteroids in severe asthma, and may allow systemic dose reduction or elimination for asthma control.
- Inhaled corticosteroids are not recommended by the American Thoracic Society (ATS) for chronic obstructive pulmonary disease (COPD) at this time and their use is debated, although they can be considered if oral corticosteroid therapy is found helpful. In steroid responders with COPD, inhaled steroids may reduce or replace oral corticosteroids.[2,3]
  - ○ Oral corticosteroids are indicated for management of acute exacerbations of COPD, by ATS guidelines.

- Intranasal aerosol agents: Management of seasonal and perennial allergic and nonallergic rhinitis.

IDENTIFICATION OF AEROSOLIZED CORTICOSTEROIDS

An increasing number of aerosolized corticosteroid preparations are becoming available for both oral inhalation and intransal delivery. Table 11-1 lists the currently available aerosol formulations of corticosteroids for oral inhalation, and Table 11-2 gives intranasal formulations. Discussion of the rationale for inhaled aerosol agents and a description of the properties of corticosteroids required for success as topical agents are given subsequently, along with additional detail on individual agents.

PHYSIOLOGY OF CORTICOSTEROIDS

IDENTIFICATION AND SOURCE

Corticosteroids are a group of chemicals secreted by the adrenal cortex, and are referred to as *adrenal cortical hormones*. The adrenal or suprarenal gland is composed of two portions (Figure 11-1). The inner zone is the adrenal medulla, and produces epinephrine. The outer zone is the cortex, the source of corticosteroids. Three types of corticosteroid hormone are produced by the adrenal cortex: the glucocorticoids (e.g., cortisol), the mineralocorticoids (e.g., aldosterone), and the sex hormones (e.g., androgens and estrogens). The mineralocorticoid aldosterone regulates body water by increasing the amount of sodium reabsorption in the renal tubules. Androgenic corticosteroids, such as testosterone, the male sex hormone, cause secondary sex characteristics to appear and will be discussed briefly in the section on androgenic corticosteroids. The corticosteroids used in pulmonary disease are all analogs of cortisol, or *hydrocortisone* as it is also termed. Box 11-1 lists the major developments in the introduction of corticosteroids, specifically the glucocorticoids, for treatment of asthma. Cortisone was isolated in 1935 by Kendall as compound E and later synthesized in 1948. Its antiinflammatory action was reported in rheumatoid arthritis by Hench and colleagues[4] in 1949. It was found to be effective in asthma in the early 1950s, and since the 1970s there has been increasing development and introduction of aerosolized glucocorticoids for maintenance therapy of asthma.[5-10] Glucocorticoid agents are referred to as

glucocorticosteroids, by the more general term *corticosteroid,* or simply as *steroids.*

THE HYPOTHALAMIC-PITUITARY-ADRENAL AXIS

The side effects of corticosteroids and the rationale for aerosol or alternate-day therapy can be understood if the production and control of endogenous (the body's own) corticosteroids are grasped. The pathway for release and control of corticosteroids is the hypothalamic-pituitary-adrenal (HPA) axis (Figure 11-2). Stimulation of the hypothalamus causes impulses to be sent to the area known as the median eminence, where corticotropin releasing factor (CRF) is released. CRF circulates through the portal vessel to the anterior pituitary gland, which then releases adrenocorticotropic hormone (ACTH) into the bloodstream. ACTH in turn stimulates the adrenal cortex to secrete glucocorticoids, such as cortisol. Cortisol and glucocorticoids in general regulate the metabolism of carbohydrates, fats, and proteins, generally to increase levels of glucose for body energy. This is the reason cortisol and its analogues are called glucocorticoids. They can also cause lipolysis, redistribution of fat stores, and breakdown of tissue protein stores. These actions are the basis for many of the side effects seen with glucocorticoid drugs. The breakdown of proteins for use of the amino acids (gluconeogenesis) is responsible for muscle wasting, and the effects on glucose metabolism can increase plasma glucose levels. This last is sometimes referred to as *steroid diabetes.*[11]

HYPOTHALAMIC-PITUITARY-ADRENAL SUPPRESSION WITH STEROID USE

One of the most significant side effects of treating with glucocorticoid drugs (exogenous corticosteroids) is adrenal suppression or, more generally, HPA suppression. When the body produces *endogenous* glucocorticoids, there is a normal feedback mechanism within the HPA axis to limit production. As glucocorticoid levels rise, release of CRF and ACTH is inhibited, and further adrenal production of glucocorticoids is stopped. This feedback inhibition of the hypothalamus and the pituitary can be seen in Figure 11-2, and is analogous to the servo mechanism by which a thermostat regulates furnace production of heat by monitoring temperature levels. Unfortunately, the body cannot distinguish between its own *endogenous* glucocorticoids and *exogenous* glucocorticoid drugs. Administration of glucocorticoid drugs raises the body's level of these hormones, and this

Table 11-1

Corticosteroids available by aerosol for oral inhalation*

DRUG	BRAND NAME	FORMULATION AND DOSAGE
Beclomethasone dipropionate	Beclovent, Vanceril	MDI: 42 µg/puff Adults: 2 puffs tid or qid Children: 1-2 puffs tid or qid
	Vanceril 84 µg Double Strength	MDI: 84 µg/puff Adults and children ≥6 yr: 2 inhalations bid
Beclomethasone dipropionate HFA	QVAR	MDI: 40 µg/puff and 80 µg/puff Adults ≥12 yr: 40 to 80 µg twice daily,† or 40 to 160 µg twice daily‡
Triamcinolone acetonide	Azmacort	MDI: 100 µg/puff Adults: 2 puffs tid or qid Children: 1-2 puffs tid or qid
Flunisolide	AeroBid, AeroBid-M	MDI: 250 µg/puff Adults: 2 puffs bid Children: 2 puffs bid
Fluticasone propionate	Flovent	MDI: 44 µg/puff, 110 µg/puff, 220 µg/puff Adults ≥12 yr: 88 µg bid,† 88-220 µg bid,‡ or 880 µg bid¶
	Flovent Rotadisk	DPI: 50 µg, 100 µg, 250 µg Adults: 100 µg bid,† 100-250 µg bid,‡ 1000 µg bid¶ Children 4-11 yr: 50 µg twice daily
Budesonide	Pulmicort Turbuhaler	DPI: 200 µg/actuation Adults: 200-400 µg bid,† 200-400 µg bid,‡ 400-800 µg bid¶ Children ≥6 yr: 200 µg bid
	Pulmicort Respules	SVN: 0.25 mg/2 ml, 0.5 mg/2 ml Children 1 to 8 yr: 0.5 mg total dose given once daily, or twice daily in divided doses†,‡; 1 mg given as 0.5 mg bid or once daily¶
Fluticasone propionate/ salmeterol	Advair Diskus	DPI: 100 µg fluticasone/50 µg salmeterol, 250 µg fluticasone/50 µg salmeterol, or 500 µg fluticasone/50 µg salmeterol Adults and children ≥12 yr: 100 µg fluticasone/50 µg salmeterol, 1 inhalation twice daily, about 12 hours apart (starting dose if not currently on inhaled corticosteroids) Maximum recommended dose is 500 µg fluticasone/50 µg salmeterol twice daily

*Individual agents are discussed subsequently in a separate section. Detailed information on each agent should be obtained from manufacturers' drug insert.
†Recommended starting dose if on bronchodilators alone.
‡Recommended starting dose if on inhaled corticosteroids previously.
¶Recommended starting dose if on oral corticosteroids previously.

Table 11-2

Aerosol corticosteroid preparations available for intranasal delivery*

DRUG	BRAND NAME	FORMULATION AND DOSAGE
Beclomethasone	Beconase, Vancenase, Vancenase Pockethaler Beconase AQ	MDI: 42 µg/actuation Adults ≥12 yr: 1 inhalation each nostril, 2 to 4 times daily Children 6-12 yr: 1 inhalation each nostril 3 times daily Spray: 0.042%
	Vancenase AQ 84 µg	Adults ≥12 yr: 1-2 inhalations each nostril, twice daily Children 6-12 yr: 1 inhalation each nostril twice daily Spray: 0.084% Adults and children ≥6 yr: 1-2 inhalations each nostril once daily
Triamcinolone acetonide	Nasacort	MDI: 55 µg/actuation Adults and children ≥12 yr: 2 sprays each nostril once daily (starting dose)
	Nasacort AQ	Children 6-12 yr: 2 sprays each nostril once daily (starting dose) Spray: 55 µg/actuation Adults and children ≥12 yr: 2 sprays each nostril once daily (starting dose) Children 6-12 yr: 1 spray each nostril once daily (starting dose)
Flunisolide	Nasalide, Nasarel	Spray: 0.025%/actuation Adults: 2 sprays each nostril 2 times daily (starting dose) Children 6-14 yr: 1 spray each nostril 3 times daily or 2 sprays each nostril 2 times daily (starting dose)
Budesonide	Rhinocort	MDI: 32 µg/actuation Adults and children ≥6 yr: 2 sprays each nostril morning and evening or 4 sprays each nostril in the morning (starting dose)
Fluticasone	Flonase	Spray: 0.05% Adults: 2 sprays each nostril once daily (starting dose) Adolescents ≥4 yr: 1 spray each nostril once daily (starting dose)
Mometasone furoate monohydrate	Nasonex	Spray: 50 µg/actuation Adults and children ≥12 yr: 2 sprays each nostril once daily (starting dose)

*Detailed information on each agent should be obtained from manufacturers' drug insert.

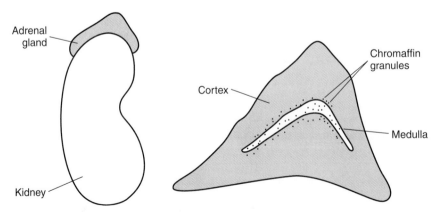

Figure 11-1   Location and cross-section of the adrenal, or suprarenal, gland. The outer portion, or cortex, of the adrenal gland is the source of corticosteroid hormones.

Box 11-1	Significant Events in the Development and Clinical Application of Aerosolized Inhaled Corticosteroids

1949	Hench and others report the antiinflammatory activity of compound E (cortisone) in rheumatoid arthritis.	1972	Topically active aerosolized steroids become available to treat asthma in the United Kingdom.
1950	Cortisone is reported to be effective in asthma.	1976	The topically active aerosol beclomethasone dipropionate is available in the United States.
1951	Cortisone is reported given by aerosol.	1984	Triamcinolone acetonide and flunisolide are approved for oral inhalation in the United States.
1956	Treatment of asthma with aerosolized hydrocortisone is reported.	1996	Fluticasone propionate approved for oral inhalation in the United States.
1957-1958	The use of aerosolized prednisolone in asthma is reported.	1997	Budesonide designated "approvable" as an orally inhaled aerosol in the United States.
1962	The aerosolized form of dexamethasone is reported.		

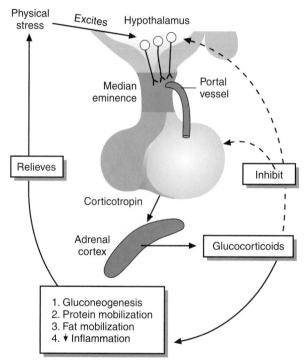

Figure 11-2   Hypothalamic-pituitary-adrenal (HPA) axis regulation of corticosteroid secretion (see text for complete description of function).

inhibits the hypothalamus and pituitary glands, which in turn decreases adrenal production. This is referred to as *HPA suppression* or, specifically, *adrenal suppression*. It is seen with systemic administration of corticosteroids, begins after a single day, and is significant after a week of oral therapy at usual doses. One of the primary reasons for using aerosolized glucocorticoids is to minimize adrenal, or HPA, suppression by both minimizing the dosage and localizing the site of treatment.

If a patient has received oral corticosteroids and adrenal suppression has occurred, weaning from the exogenous corticosteroids through use of tapered dose therapy allows time for recovery of the body's own adrenal secretion. It should be noted that aerosolized corticosteroids do not deposit sufficient amounts of drug to replace the missing output of a suppressed adrenal gland. Therefore a patient with adrenal suppression cannot be abruptly withdrawn from oral corticosteroids and placed on an aerosol dosage. The aerosol should be started, and the oral agent tapered off slowly at the same time.

THE DIURNAL STEROID CYCLE

The production of the body's own glucocorticoids also follows a rhythmical cycle, termed a *diurnal* or *circadian rhythm*. This daily rise and fall of glucocorticoid levels in the body is shown in Figure 11-3. On a daily schedule of daytime work and nighttime sleep, cortisol levels are highest in the morning around 8 AM. These high plasma levels inhibit further production and release of glucocorticoids and ACTH by the HPA axis because of the feedback mechanism previously presented. The high levels mobilize the body's energy resources in response to the anticipated stress and challenge of earning a living! During the day, plasma levels of both ACTH *(dotted line)* and cortisol *(solid line)* gradually fall. As the glucocorticoid level falls, the anterior pituitary is reactivated to begin releasing ACTH, which in turn stimulates production of cortisol by the adrenal cortex. This lag between the increased ACTH and cortisol levels is illustrated in Figure 11-3. One of the reasons for jet lag and the delay in adjusting to night shift from day shift is that this diurnal

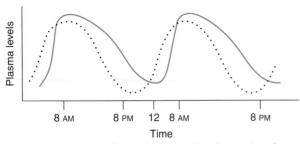

Figure 11-3   Diurnal variations in ACTH (·········) and cortisol (———) (see text for detailed description).

and regular rhythm of corticosteroid levels becomes out of synchronization with the time zone and the work time. Although the worker needs to sleep at 8 AM after working all night, the body is wide awake, with energy stores being released.

ALTERNATE-DAY STEROID THERAPY

Alternate-day therapy mimics the natural diurnal rhythm by giving a steroid drug early in the morning, when normal tissue levels are high. Thus suppression of the hypothalamic-pituitary system occurs at the same time it normally would with the body's own steroid, and on the alternate day the regular diurnal secretion in the hypothalamic-pituitary-adrenal (HPA) system can resume. Tissue side effects are minimized because the drug is administered at the time when tissues are normally exposed to high corticosteroid levels by the body's rhythm. Use of an intermediate-acting corticosteroid drug, with a duration of 12 to 36 hours, allows drug therapy to be restricted to alternate days.

NATURE OF THE INFLAMMATORY RESPONSE

One of the major therapeutic effects seen with analogs of the natural (endogenous) adrenal cortical hormone hydrocortisone is an antiinflammatory action. Glucocorticoid analogs of natural (endogenous) hydrocortisone are used for this effect in treating asthma, which is an inflammatory process in the lungs. To understand the antiinflammatory activity of the glucocorticoid drugs used in asthma, the nature of inflammation in general, and airway inflammation in particular will be reviewed briefly.

INFLAMMATION

A general definition of inflammation is the response of vascularized tissue to injury. An excellent and still-

applicable description of inflammation was given in the first century AD by Celsus: *"rubor et tumor cum calore et dolore."* This is translated as "redness and swelling with heat and pain." This is the most general description of an inflammatory reaction to injury, such as a cut, wound infection, splinter, burn, scrape, or bee sting.

An update of Celsus' description occurred in the 1920s with Lewis Thomas' characterization known as the *triple response:*

Redness: The local dilation of blood vessels, occurring in seconds
Flare: A reddish color several centimeters from the site, occurring 15 to 30 seconds after injury
Wheal: Local swelling, occurring in minutes

The process of inflammation producing the visible results described by Celsus, Thomas, and others is caused by the following four major categories of activity:

Increased vascular permeability: Produces an exudate into surrounding tissues.
Leukocytic infiltration: The emigration of white cells through capillary walls (diapedesis) in response to attractant chemicals (chemotaxis).
Phagocytosis: White cells and macrophages (in the lungs) ingest and process foreign material such as bacteria.
Mediator cascade: Histamine and chemoattractant factors are released at the site of injury, and various inflammatory mediators such as complement and arachidonic acid products are generated.

INFLAMMATION IN THE AIRWAY

Inflammation can occur in the lungs in response to a variety of causes. These include direct trauma (gunshot wound, stabbing), indirect trauma (blunt chest injury), inhalation of noxious or toxic substances (chlorine gas, smoke), respiratory infections and systemic infections producing septicemia and septic shock with acute respiratory distress syndrome (ARDS), and allergenic or nonallergenic stimulation in asthma. The two most common inflammatory diseases of the airway seen in respiratory care are chronic bronchitis, usually caused by tobacco smoking, and asthma, which can be caused by a range of triggers and involves a complex pathophysiology.

Because glucocorticoids are a mainstay for treating asthma, a brief description of the multiple pathways and mediators for the genesis of airway inflammation seen in asthma is given. Asthma is currently un-

Box 11-2   Operational Definition of Asthma

Asthma is a chronic inflammatory disorder of the airways in which many cells and cellular elements play a role, in particular, mast cells, eosinophils, T lymphocytes, macrophages, neutrophils, and epithelial cells. In susceptible individuals, this inflammation causes recurrent episodes of wheezing, breathlessness, chest tightness, and coughing, particularly at night or in the early morning. These episodes are usually associated with widespread but variable airflow obstruction that is often reversible either spontaneously or with treatment. The inflammation also causes an associated increase in the existing bronchial hyperresponsiveness to a variety of stimuli.

National Asthma Education and Prevention Program, Expert Panel II: *Guidelines for the diagnosis and management of asthma*, Bethesda, Md, 1997, National Institutes of Health.

derstood as a disease in which there is chronic inflammation of the airway wall, causing airflow limitation and a hyperresponsiveness to a variety of stimuli (Box 11-2).[11,12] The airway inflammation is mediated by inflammatory cells such as the mast cell, eosinophils, T lymphocytes, and macrophages. The mast cell and the eosinophil are considered to be the major effector cells of the inflammatory response, regardless of whether the asthma is allergic or nonallergic.[12] T lymphocytes may be pivotal in coordinating the inflammatory response by release of numerous proinflammatory cytokines (proteins that regulate immune/inflammatory responses), which in turn act on basophils, epithelial cells, and endothelial cells in the airway to further the inflammatory process. The potent mediators released during an asthmatic reaction cause airway smooth muscle contraction (bronchospasm), increased microvascular leakage and airway wall swelling, mucus secretion, and over the longer term remodeling of the airway wall. In an acute state, asthmatic individuals exhibit wheezing, breathlessness, chest tightness, and cough, especially at night or early morning. The acute symptoms produced by the airway inflammation are at least partly reversible either spontaneously or with pharmacological treatment. Treatment with antiinflammatory agents such as glucocorticoids are important to reduce the basal level of airway inflammation and thereby reduce airway hyperresponsiveness and the predisposition to acute episodes of obstruction.

Asthmatic reactions are distinguished into an early-phase and a late-phase reaction. A conceptual representation of the overall process is given in Figure 11-4. After an insult to the asthmatic airway by an allergen, cold air, viral infection, or noxious gas, there is evidence that the early asthmatic response is caused by immunoglobulin E (IgE)-dependent activation of airway mast cells, which can release inflammatory mediators such as histamine, prostaglandin D_2 (PGD_2), and leukotriene C_4.[12] The immediate response of the airway to chemicals such as histamine is bronchospasm. This response peaks at around 15 minutes and then declines over the next hour. This produces the early-phase decrease in expiratory flow rates illustrated in Figure 11-4. Although the early bronchoconstriction of smooth muscle may self-limit or respond to β agonists (described Chapter 6), the progression of cellular events can continue. Mast cell mediators and the release of cytokines recruit other inflammatory cells (eosinophils, basophils, monocytes/macrophages, lymphocytes), by activating epithelial cells and endothelial cells to release adhesion molecules (e.g., intercellular adhesion molecule [ICAM]) and other cytokines to cause the late-phase reaction. During the late-phase response, mast cells and recruited eosinophils, lymphocytes, or macrophages that have infiltrated the airway release a range of inflammatory mediators. Neutrophils are not generally associated with asthma and allergic reactions in the absence of infection. The late asthmatic response occurs 6 to 8 hours after a challenge, and it may last for up to 24 hours. The late-phase reaction is thought to be reflective of the chronic inflammation characterizing asthma between acute episodes.[13]

Phospholipids in the cell membrane of mast cells and other cells are converted by phospholipase A_2 to arachidonic acid and then to a variety of bronchoactive and vasoactive substances by the two metabolic paths shown: the cyclooxygenase and lipoxygenase pathways. The term *eicosanoid* is used to refer to the products of the two pathways. The migration of eosinophils and lymphocytes and further development of inflammation-producing chemicals such as the arachidonic acid metabolites and cytokines all contribute to build an inflammatory response in the lung.[14] In addition to smooth muscle spasm, mucus secretion occurs, along with mucosal swelling resulting from increased vascular permeability. Shedding of airway cells (desquamation) and goblet cell hyperplasia are seen. The result is mucus plugging of the airway, complicated by the cellular debris in

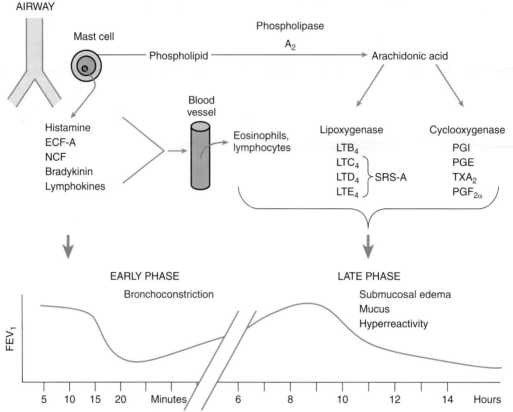

Figure 11-4   Conceptual illustration of the inflammatory asthmatic response in the airway, producing a biphasic deterioration in expiratory flow rates described as an early-phase and late-phase response to triggering stimuli. *ECF-A*, Eosinophilic chemotactic factor; *FEV$_1$*, forced expiratory volume in 1 second; *LTB$_4$*, leukotriene B$_4$; *LTC$_4$*, leukotriene C$_4$; *LTD$_4$*, leukotriene D$_4$; *LTE$_4$*, leukotriene E$_4$; *NCF*, neutrophil chemotactic factor; *PGI*, prostaglandin I; *PGE*, prostaglandin E; *PGF$_{2\alpha}$*, prostaglandin F$_2$-alpha; *SRS-A*, slow-reacting substance of anaphylaxis; *TXA$_2$*, thromboxane A$_2$.

the bronchial lumen. The pathology of bronchial asthma has been described as "chronic desquamating eosinophilic bronchitis."[15] These airway changes lead to further bronchial hyperreactivity seen in asthma. There is evidence of airway remodeling, with increased tenascin (an extracellular matrix protein for cell development), collagens, and fibronectin, all of which can cause thickening of the basement membrane in the airway wall. This deregulates communication between cells, promoting epithelial damage and enhancing the inflammatory response.[16]

AEROSOLIZED CORTICOSTEROIDS

Several corticosteroid preparations are available, such as hydrocortisone, cortisone, prednisone, prednisolone, and methylprednisolone, all of which have antiinflammatory activity. However, they produce undesirable systemic side effects when used to treat asthma, an inflammation of the lung.

EARLY TRIALS OF AEROSOL STEROIDS

The attempt to introduce aerosolized corticosteroids directly into the lung to avoid systemic side effects began in 1951, shortly after the identification of steroids. The development of this effort, resulting in the currently available aerosolized steroid agents, is highlighted in Box 11-1.

Glucocorticoid receptors are similar throughout the body, and therefore it has not been feasible to develop a steroid that would control bronchial inflammation without causing systemic side effects when given orally or intravenously. These side effects include adrenal suppression and Cushingoid symptoms such as moon face, edema, and central fat deposition ("hump" back). The alternative is to target the lung locally with an aerosol formulation. Direct application of steroids to inflamed tissue, as in the treatment of dermatitis, maximizes local concentration while minimizing systemic concentrations of the drug.

Cortisone, hydrocortisone, prednisone, and finally dexamethasone were all tried by aerosol between 1951 and 1963; although all produced the desired therapeutic effect of reduced airway inflammation, each unfortunately caused hypercortical effects and adrenal suppression. In each agent, the therapeutic dose was large enough to lead to systemic absorption, with the resulting side effects. Because of this, the aerosol route was not especially beneficial compared with the oral route for long-term administration. Until 1976, dexamethasone, in its metered spray formulation, remained the aerosolizable steroid of choice despite this fact. However, the introduction of the newer synthetic analogues of hydrocortisone, which have a high topical antiinflammatory activity, paved the way for effective use of aerosolized steroids with few systemic side effects. These agents include beclomethasone, triamcinolone, flunisolide, budesonide, and fluticasone.

TOPICAL TO SYSTEMIC ACTIVITY RATIOS

The agents cited have a high ratio of topical to systemic activity. Check and Kaliner review[17] the chemical principles involved in the development of these steroid analogues to achieve local effect in the lungs with less potential for systemic absorption and side effects. The high topical/systemic activity ratios of aerosolized corticosteroids are facilitated by the following combination of factors:

- Direct introduction into the airway by aerosol
- Rapid inactivation of drug absorbed into the plasma
- An intrinsic topical antiinflammatory effect

The topical potency of a steroid is measured by the vasoconstriction assay, devised by McKenzie and Stoughton.[18,19] In this method, test doses of the steroid are applied to the skin of the inner forearm and the blanching resulting from vasoconstriction is assessed visually in comparison with a standard agent such as dexamethasone or fluocinolone acetonide. The topical potency of aerosolized agents given by inhalation are listed in Table 11-3, which indicates binding affinity and blanching activity in relation to a dexamethasone standard of 1.0.

Table 11-3

Relative binding affinity and topical activity of inhaled glucocorticoids

	BINDING AFFINITY	BLANCHING POTENCY
Dexamethasone	1.0	1.0
Beclomethasone dipropionate	0.4	600
Beclomethasone monopropionate*	13.5	450
Triamcinolone-16,17-acetonide	3.6	330
Flunisolide	1.8	330
Budesonide	9.4	980
Fluticasone	18.0	1200†

Data from Barnes PJ: Inhaled glucocorticoids for asthma, *N Engl J Med* 332:868, 1995; and Barnes PJ, Pedersen S: Efficacy and safety of inhaled corticosteroids in asthma, *Am Rev Respir Dis* 148(Oct suppl):S1, 1993.
*Beclomethasone dipropionate (beclomethasone-17,21-dipropionate) is metabolized to the active product, beclomethasone monopropionate (beclomethasone-17-propionate), in the airway and liver when inhaled.
†Fluticasone was allotted a relative potency of 945 in reference to fluocinolone acetonide.[22]

Although differences are seen in binding affinity and relative topical potency of aerosolized glucocorticoids, as indicated in Table 11-3, very few studies compare the efficacy of these different compounds in the same individuals and with the same aerosol delivery systems. Usually comparisons are confounded by differences in severity of asthma, selection of patients, and aerosol generator systems.[20]

AEROSOLIZED CORTICOSTEROID AGENTS

Several aerosol steroid agents, all of which are glucocorticoids, are available for inhalational use in the United States at the time of this edition. These were previously identified in Table 11-1, which summarized steroids used for oral inhalation, and Table 11-2, which listed agents for intranasal delivery, giving strengths and recommended doses. Originally, in the United States, all of the orally inhaled corticosteroids were available as MDI formulations. More recently, two powder inhalers, the Diskhaler (fluticasone) and the Turbuhaler (budesonide) have been introduced, along with the first approved nebulizer formulation (budesonide [Pulmicort Respules]).

These agents possess the high topical to systemic potency ratio described, to make them suitable for control of asthma with minimal systemic side effects. The chemical structures of the aerosol agents available for oral and nasal inhalation are shown in Figure 11-5. A brief description of each of the aerosol agents is given. A more detailed review of the structure-activity relations of these agents has been published by Check and Kaliner[17] and Johnson.[21]

Beclomethasone dipropionate (Vanceril, Beclovent, QVAR) was the second inhaled aerosol corticosteroid available in the United States. Dexamethasone sodium phosphate (Decadron Respihaler), which is no longer available, was the first inhaled aerosol for general clinical use. Beclomethasone is an effective antiinflammatory aerosol for use in controlling asthma that requires steroid therapy. The drug's success as an aerosol in reducing or replacing the use of systemic steroids is due to its high topical to systemic activity ratio, as previously discussed. With the transition from chlorofluorocarbon (CFC)-propelled MDI formulations, beclomethasone dipropionate has been reformulated with an HFA propellant, in a 40 μg and 80 μg MDI strength as QVAR (see Table 11-1). Along with the change in propellant, many components of the MDI system were reengineered, significantly increasing the efficiency of this drug-delivery system. Lung deposition with QVAR has been measured at 50% to 60% of the emitted dose (see discussion of MDIs in Chapter 3). As seen in Table 11-1, the usual starting dose of QVAR is 40 to 80 μg twice daily; beclomethasone in the CFC formulation is 84 μg three or four times a day. The lower dosing with the HFA formulation is possible because of the increased efficiency in lung deposition.

An aerosol dose of 400 μg is approximately equivalent to 5 to 10 mg of oral prednisone. It has a topical to systemic potency ratio approximately 500 times that of dexamethasone. When inhaled by aerosol, the swallowed drug is slowly absorbed from the gastrointestinal tract, and most of what is absorbed is quickly (half-life in the liver = 10 minutes) broken down in its first passage through the liver, preventing high plasma levels.

Absorption of the drug across the pulmonary epithelium is good, but rapid inactivation prevents systemic accumulation. After inhalation of a 2 mg dose, plasma levels of beclomethasone dipropionate are very low, but the active metabolite, beclomethasone monopropionate (often designated 17-BMP), reached significant plasma levels of 1.8 to 2.5 ng/ml.[21]

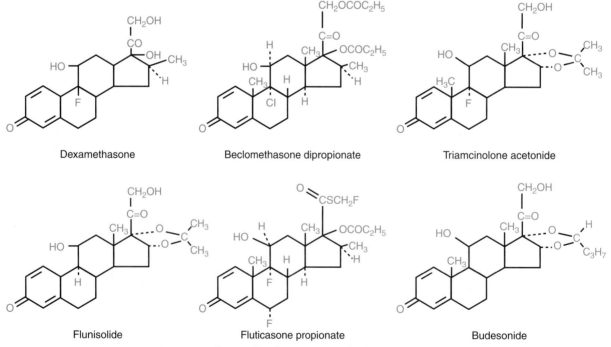

Figure 11-5   Structures of aerosolized corticosteroids, showing a common steroid nucleus, and modifications to enhance topical antiinflammatory action.

Triamcinolone acetonide (Azmacort) is also topically active and was available as Aristocort and Kenalog before its release as an aerosol. Triamcinolone acetonide is nonpolar and water insoluble, resulting in a lower potential for systemic absorption. This drug is slightly less topically active than beclomethasone dipropionate.[17] High initial doses of 12 to 16 inhalations/day may be needed in severe asthma. This agent is marketed with a built-in spacer device.

Flunisolide (AeroBid) is another topically active aerosol preparation, similar in potency to triamcinolone, and is said to have a longer duration of action. The name indicates the dosing schedule, which is twice daily. Flunisolide shows a peak plasma level after inhalation between 2 and 60 minutes, indicating good absorption from the lungs, as with beclomethasone. The half-life in plasma with inhalation is approximately 1.8 hours and similar to that with oral or intravenous dosing, indicating a rapid first-pass metabolism. The pharmacokinetics of flunisolide have been studied by Chaplin and associates.[22]

Fluticasone propionate (Flovent, Flonase) is a synthetic, trifluorinated glucocorticoid with high topical antiinflammatory potency and is available in MDI form, with three different strengths: 44 μg, 110 μg, and 220 μg. Each actuation of the MDI gives 50 μg, 125 μg, or 250 μg of fluticasone propionate from the valve, and 44 μg, 110 μg, or 220 μg from the actuator mouthpiece. The drug is a further analogue of previous agents with high topical potency, synthesized in an attempt to avoid systemic side effects. Fluticasone is derived from the 17β-carbothioate series of androstane analogues, a group that has very weak HPA inhibitory activity but high antiinflammatory effect.[23] Using fluocinolone acetonide as a reference standard, fluticasone propionate was found to have an antiinflammatory potency of 91 in mice, with an HPA inhibitory activity of only 1, giving a therapeutic index (antiinflammatory potency/HPA potency) of 91. By comparison, beclomethasone dipropionate has an antiinflammatory potency of 21, with an HPA inhibitory potency of 49 in mice.[24] If given by subcutaneous injection to mice, fluticasone propionate does exhibit HPA inhibition; however, the oral route gives only weak HPA suppression. This is useful with inhaled aerosols, because a portion of the aerosol may be swallowed and contribute to systemic activity of a drug (see Chapter 2, pharmacokinetics of inhaled drugs). An explanation for the weak HPA suppression when given orally may be its high first-pass effect, resulting in less than 1% of active drug in the circulation, because fluticasone is rapidly metabolized in the liver to the inactive product, 17β-carboxylic acid.[24]

Budesonide (Pulmicort, Rhinocort) is a topically active inhaled corticosteroid with a potency greater than that of beclomethasone dipropionate or monopropionate, triamcinolone, or flunisolide, but less potent than fluticasone, as estimated by skin vasoconstriction assay. With oral administration, only 10% of budesonide enters the systemic circulation because of a high (approximately 89%) first-pass metabolism in the liver. After inhalation with a spacer device, peak plasma concentrations occur between 15 and 45 minutes. The plasma half-life is 2 hours. There appears to be minimal metabolism in the lung, with approximately 70% of the inhaled dose reaching the circulation.[20] Budesonide was found to exhibit about half the adrenal suppression of fluticasone, on a microgram equivalent basis in asthmatic patients, by Clark and associates.[25]

Fluticasone propionate/salmeterol (Advair) is a combination product of the corticosteroid fluticasone, with the long-acting β₂-agonist bronchodilator, salmeterol (see Chapter 6 for a discussion of salmeterol). The combination of inhaled steroid and long-acting β₂ agonist in a convenient dose package would be useful in patients in Step 3 asthma, requiring both types of drug. In a large multicenter clinical study by Shapiro and colleagues,[26] patients with asthma who were on medium doses of inhaled corticosteroids were treated with 250 μg fluticasone in combination with 50 μg salmeterol from the DPI Diskus device for 12 weeks. Patients in the treatment group had significantly better FEV_1 profiles over 12 hours, a significantly greater probability of remaining in the study and not withdrawing because of worsening symptoms, a significantly increased morning peak flow (PEF), reduced asthma symptom scores, reduced rescue albuterol use, and significantly fewer nights with no awakenings, compared with salmeterol or fluticasone alone or placebo.

Although combination products have the disadvantage of not allowing changes in dose for each drug separately and have been discouraged, there is evidence of a beneficial, complementary interaction between glucocorticoids and β-adrenergic agonists. The addition of long-acting bronchodilators to inhaled corticosteroids has no negative effect and shows improvements in lung function and symptom control, as demonstrated in the clinical trial by Shapiro and associates[26] and Chung for Advair.[26,27] The interaction results from the following known or investigational actions of steroids and β agonists:

- Steroids increase β_2-adrenergic receptor transcription (upregulation of β receptors).[27,28]
- Inhaled corticosteroid therapy can provide partial protection against development of tolerance to β_2 adrenergic agonists.[27]
- Salmeterol has been shown to promote binding of the glucocorticoid receptor to the response element of the cell's nuclear DNA, *without the glucocorticoid present*, in vascular cells, thus initiating the antiinflammatory effect at least partially.[28]

If management of asthma requires both a long-acting β agonist and an inhaled corticosteroid, the combination product of fluticasone propionate/salmeterol offers the advantage of more-convenient, single-formulation dosing.

INTRANASAL CORTICOSTEROIDS

Many of the steroids available as orally inhaled agents are also available in an intranasal formulation. Exact indications for the intranasal preparations vary by specific agent, but generally, intranasal steroids are used for treatment of allergic or inflammatory nasal conditions and seasonal or perennial allergic or non-allergic rhinitis and to prevent reoccurrence of nasal polyps. Available preparations are listed in Table 11-2, with strengths and recommended doses. Other agents that are used to treat seasonal allergic rhinitis include H_1-receptor antagonists (e.g., loratidine), cromolyn sodium (see Chapter 12), topical vasoconstrictors (see Chapter 15) such as oxymetazoline or ephedrine, and anticholinergics such as ipratropium bromide (see Chapter 7).[29]

PHARMACOLOGY OF CORTICOSTEROIDS

The inflammatory process can be reduced or blocked by the antiinflammatory effects of glucocorticoids. The beneficial effect of glucocorticoids in asthma and other diseases of inflammation, is due to their ability to inhibit the activity of inflammatory cells and mediators of inflammation.

MODE OF ACTION

Glucocorticoids are highly lipophilic and enter airway cells to bind to intracellular receptors.[30] This mechanism of drug signaling action was described briefly in Chapter 2 in the discussion of the pharmacodynamics of lipid-soluble drugs that interact with intracellular

receptors. Originally, investigators thought that corticosteroids or, more simply, steroids, exerted antiinflammatory activity by stabilizing lysosomes within neutrophils. This prevented degranulation and an inflammatory response. In the mid-1960s, steroid receptors were discovered, and the realization developed that steroids modify the inflammatory response by inducing gene expression within the cell. By the 1980s, it was demonstrated that glucocorticoids induce gene expression for the antiinflammatory protein lipocortin, which inhibits the enzyme phospholipase A_2 (PLA$_2$), preventing the arachidonic acid cascade, which leads to prostaglandin synthesis and lipoxygenase products. However, now it is understood that PLA$_2$ inhibition is only one of multiple mechanisms by which steroids attenuate the inflammatory response.[13,31,32]

Steroids suppress a local or systemic inflammatory response by at least three general actions. These actions are illustrated in Figure 11-6. In general, steroids

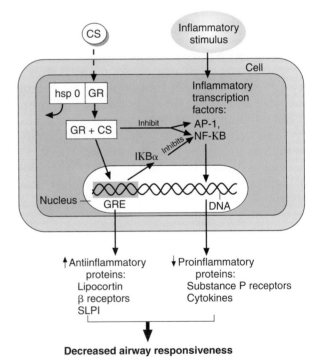

Decreased airway responsiveness

Figure 11-6   Proposed mechanism of action by which glucocorticoids exert an antiinflammatory effect. *AP-1*, Activator protein 1; *CS*, corticosteroid; *DNA*, deoxyribonucleic acid; *GR*, glucocorticoid receptor; *GRE*, glucocorticoid response element; *hsp 90*, heat shock protein 90; IκBα inhibitor of nuclear factor-κBα; *NF-κB*, nuclear factor-κB; *SLPI*, secretory leukocyte protease inhibitor.

diffuse into the cell and bind to a glucocorticoid receptor. Before binding by a steroid, the glucocorticoid receptor is in an inactive state and is bound to a protein complex termed *heat shock protein 90* (hsp 90), which prevents the unoccupied receptor from translocating to the nucleus of the cell. When the steroid binds to the receptor, the hsp 90 dissociates, and the steroid-receptor complex then translocates to the cell nucleus. One general action (not necessarily the first temporally) of a glucocorticoid is to upregulate the transcription of antiinflammatory genes for substances such as lipocortin, previously described.[31,32] In the nucleus the steroid produces this part of its effect on the cell by binding to portions of the nuclear DNA termed *glucocorticoid response elements.* Binding of the drug-receptor complex to glucocorticoid response elements upregulates, or induces, transcription of antiinflammatory substances such as lipocortin, neutral endopeptidase, secretory leukocyte protease inhibitor (SLPI), or inhibitors of plasminogen activator.[13] These are all antiinflammatory substances. A second general action of glucocorticoids is suppression of factors such as activator protein 1 (AP-1) and nuclear factor-kappa B (NF-κB), which cause transcription of genes involved in inflammation. This may be by means of a direct interaction with these transcription factors, by which the transcription factor is inactivated before it induces gene expression in the nucleus.[31] Direct inactivation of AP-1 and NF-κB leads to downregulation of gene expression for proinflammatory mediators such as cytokines. NF-κB regulates genes that have an increased expression in asthma for cytokines such as interleukins (IL-1, IL-3, etc.); chemokines; tumor necrosis factor-α (TNF-α); nitric oxide synthase, which produces nitric oxide in the airway; and adhesion molecules, which promote recruitment and attachment of leukocytes (eosinophils, basophils) from the circulation to the airway endothelium.[13,31,32] A direct inactivation of inflammatory transcription factors such as AP-1 or NF-κB may account for the rapidity with which some cellular effects of steroids are seen and that are not well explained by the time needed for modification of gene expression within a cell. A third action of glucocorticoids is to upregulate the expression of inhibitors of NF-κB, such as the inhibitor protein IκBα. This inhibitor of nuclear factor-κB further suppresses gene expression for proinflammatory proteins, such as cytokines.[32,33]

The general result of these actions is to *induce* gene expression for *antiinflammatory* proteins and receptors and to *suppress* gene expression for *proinflammatory*

proteins. Overall, glucocorticoids inhibit the cytokine production responsible for recruitment and migration of inflammatory cells such as eosinophils and lymphocytes into the airway. Examples of cytokines that are suppressed through gene suppression activity of steroids are listed in Box 11-3.

Glucocorticoids inhibit many of the cells involved in airway inflammation, including macrophages, T lymphocytes, eosinophils, and mast cells in the bronchial airway epithelium and submucosa and reverse the shedding of epithelial cells and goblet cell hyperplasia seen in asthma.[30] By decreasing cytokine-mediated survival of eosinophils, apoptosis of eosinophils occurs, reducing the number of eosinophils in the circulation and in the airway of subjects with asthma. Glucocorticoids also reduce the number of mast cells within the airways, which are sources of histamine and other mediators of inflammation, and inhibit plasma exudation, as well as mucus secretion in inflamed airways.[30]

Box 11-3 **Cytokines* Involved in Airway Inflammation That Are Suppressed by Glucocorticoids**

Tumor Necrosis Factor-α (TNF-α) and Interleukin-1 (IL-1)
Released from macrophages, monocytes, and other cells to activate endothelial cells to recruit neutrophils, eosinophils, basophils from the circulation.

Interleukin-4 (IL-4), Interleukin-13 (IL-13)
Released from lymphocytes and basophils and associated with allergic diseases; cause endothelium to bind basophils, eosinophils, monocytes, lymphocytes.

Interleukin-3 (IL-3), Interleukin-5 (IL-5), Granulocyte-macrophage colony-stimulating factor (GM-CSF), Interferon-γ (IFN-γ)
Cause eosinophil priming, resulting in prolonged eosinophil survival and potentiated degranulation to release inflammatory substances.

Chemokines
A family of small cytokines (molecules with weights of 8 to 10 kD) having many chemotactic properties to attract cells to a site. Example: Regulated on activation normal T-cell expressed and secreted (RANTES), one of the most potent chemokines, which induces eosinophil and lymphocyte migration and attraction.

---

*Cytokines are proteins secreted by a variety of cells, such as lymphocytes, that regulate local and systemic inflammatory responses.

EFFECT ON WHITE BLOOD CELL COUNT

Leukocytes, such as monocytes, macrophages, neutrophils, and basophils, are also essential to the inflammatory response and are attracted to an area of injury by the chemotactic factors identified among the mediators of inflammation. Neutrophils usually adhere ("marginate") to the capillary endothelium of storage sites in the lung. Glucocorticoids cause depletion of these stores and reduce their accumulation at inflammatory sites and in exudates. This is termed *demargination,* and can increase the number of neutrophils in circulation as the cells leave their storage sites. An overall increase in the white cell count can then be seen in patients on glucocorticoids. Glucocorticoids affect other leukocytes by inhibiting the number of monocytes, basophils, and eosinophils. This can also be seen in the differential count of these cells. An allergic asthmatic who would otherwise have a higher than normal eosinophil count will show a low count after initiation of drug therapy. Finally, glucocorticoids constrict the microvasculature to reduce leakage of the above cells and fluids into inflammatory sites.

EFFECT ON β RECEPTORS

β-Adrenergic agents are among the most potent inhibitors of mast cell release, yet the asthmatic in an acute episode may be unresponsive to these drugs. A very beneficial effect of glucocorticoids is their ability to restore responsiveness to β-adrenergic stimulation.[28,34] This effect can be seen within 1 to 4 hours after intravenous administration of glucocorticoids and is the rationale for administering a bolus of steroid in status asthmaticus as part of acute treatment. Even though steroid action is slow, the sooner they are given, the sooner the asthmatic will begin to respond to β-adrenergic drugs, and supported ventilation may be avoided. Glucocorticoids enhance β-receptor stimulation by increasing the number and availability of β receptors on the cell surfaces and by increasing affinity of the receptor for β agonists. There is also evidence that glucocorticoids prolong endogenous circulatory catecholamine action by inhibiting the uptake-2 mechanism (extraneuronal uptake), as discussed in Chapter 5. The mechanisms for a positive interaction between β_2 agonists and corticosteroids were described in the discussion of the compound fluticasone propionate/salmeterol in the section on aerosolized corticosteroids.

HAZARDS AND SIDE EFFECTS OF STEROIDS

SYSTEMIC ADMINISTRATION OF STEROIDS

The complicating side effects of systemic steroid treatment are well known and provide the motivation to switch to aerosolized, inhaled steroids when possible. These complications arise from the physiological effects of steroids on the body. These physiological effects are often exaggerated with systemic drug therapy, because potency and plasma levels are higher than with the body's own steroids. Complications of systemic therapy are reviewed by Truhan and Ahmed.[35] These complications are summarized in Box 11-4 and briefly described below.

- Suppression of the HPA axis by exogenous steroids may occur, causing inhibition of ACTH release and cortisol secretion from the adrenal gland. The length of time to recover from this suppression varies with patient, dose, and duration of treatment.
- With sufficient dose and duration, immunosuppression can be caused by systemic use of steroids. This can lead to increased susceptibility to infection by bacterial, viral, or fungal agents.
- Psychiatric reactions can occur, including insomnia, mood changes, and manic-depressive or schizophrenic psychoses.
- Cataract formation has been noted, and, rarely, intraocular pressure may increase with systemic steroid therapy.

Box 11-4   Side Effects Seen With Systemic Administration of Corticosteroids

Hypothalamic-pituitary-adrenal suppression
Immunosuppression
Psychiatric reactions
Cataract formation
Myopathy of skeletal muscle
Osteoporosis
Peptic ulcer (?)
Fluid retention
Hypertension
Increased white blood cell count
Dermatological changes
Growth restriction
Increased glucose levels

- Myopathy of striated skeletal muscle can occur.
- Steroid-induced osteoporosis is debated, but is thought to be a limitation of extended steroid therapy. Aseptic necrosis of the bone is also caused by steroid therapy.
- Peptic ulcer is thought to be a complication of steroid therapy, but evidence for this is debated. Patients may often be receiving other ulcerogenic medications such as aspirin or nonsteroidal anti-inflammatory drugs (NSAIDs).
- Fluid retention can occur as a result of the sodium-sparing effects of glucocorticoids, giving a puffy appearance.
- Hypertension may accompany the fluid retention or be aggravated by it.
- Corticosteroids given systemically can increase the white blood cell count, with an increase in neutrophils and a decrease in lymphocytes and eosinophils.
- Dermatological changes can occur with steroid therapy, including a redistribution of subcutaneous fat causing the cushingoid appearance of central obesity, hump back, and moon face.
- Growth of children can be slowed by prolonged systemic therapy, because corticosteroids retard bone growth and epiphyseal maturation.
- Corticosteroids lead to gluconeogenesis and antagonize glucose uptake, causing hyperglycemia. This can lead to a reversible steroid-induced diabetes.

SYSTEMIC SIDE EFFECTS WITH AEROSOL ADMINISTRATION

The rationale for the introduction of inhaled aerosol steroids was to eliminate or reduce the side effects seen with systemic therapy. Although the aerosol steroids introduced since dexamethasone are administered in low doses because of their high topical activity, local side effects may occur and certain systemic side effects, listed in Box 11-5, are also a concern. Some side effects may occur with transfer from oral therapy to the inhaled route. Three systemic effects of concern with inhaled steroids have been HPA suppression, loss of bone density, and growth restriction in children. A review and brief comment on possible systemic side effects with inhaled steroids is summarized below.

- Adrenal insufficiency may occur after transfer from systemic to aerosol inhaled steroids. Weaning from systemic steroids to allow recovery of adrenal cortex and HPA function and careful monitoring of pulmonary function can help control this problem.

- There may be a recurrence of allergic inflammation in other organs, such as nasal polyps or atopic dermatitis, after cessation of systemic steroids.
- Acute severe episodes of asthma may occur after withdrawal from oral steroids and transfer to inhaled forms. Aerosolized steroids may not be adequate to control asthma, especially during periods of stress, and short courses of oral drug may be necessary ("burst" therapy).
- Suppression of HPA function is nonexistent or small at low doses of inhaled aerosol steroids and increases with higher doses. Clinically significant suppression is rare at inhaled doses below 800 µg/day in adults and below 400 µg/day in children.[36] Goldberg and associates[37] investigated MDI beclomethasone administration in children with and without a reservoir.[37] They found that 7 of 15 subjects using the MDI alone (average dose = 474 ± 220 µg/day) showed adrenal suppression as measured by 24-hour urinary free cortisol excretion. Only 2 of 24 subjects using an MDI-reservoir system (average dose = 563 ± 249 µg/day) showed such suppression. Their results indicated that inhalation of low to moderate doses can cause some adrenal suppression and that use of a reservoir can reduce this, probably by reducing the swallowed amount of drug. Although higher inhaled doses of steroid have a greater risk of adrenal suppression, the dose at which the risk for toxicity outweighs the beneficial effect of an inhaled steroid is not known.[36]

Box 11-5	Potential Hazards and Side Effects with Inhaled Aerosol Corticosteroids	
Systemic		**Local (Topical)**
Adrenal insufficiency*		Oropharyngeal fungal
Extrapulmonary allergy*		infections
Acute asthma*		Dysphonia
HPA suppression (minimal, dose dependent)		Cough, broncho-constriction
Growth restriction (?) (dose-dependent)		Incorrect use of MDI (inadequate dose)

*After transfer from systemic corticosteroid therapy.

- Questions have been raised about the effect of inhaled steroids on growth when used in prepubertal children. A study by Wolthers and Pedersen[38] found a reduction in rate of lower leg growth with inhaled budesonide compared with placebo. Growth restriction was seen in some studies with beclomethasone dipropionate, yet other studies have found no effect on growth with the same drug by inhalation. Results may be confounded by the moderate growth restriction and delay in puberty seen as a result of asthma.[38] The authors cite a meta-analysis that found no association between growth impairment and inhaled beclomethasone dipropionate, even at higher doses.[39]
- No data have demonstrated clearly the effect of inhaled glucocorticoids on bone density and osteoporosis in asthma. Studies investigating the long-term effects of inhaled steroids on bone density and risk of fracture are needed.[36]

In summary, it is logical that the risks of steroid-induced adverse effects are lower with the relatively low doses of inhaled steroids compared with systemic administration. However, the threshold doses by inhalation causing adrenal suppression or other effects are not known. Generally these effects are rare with doses of 800 μg/day or less in adults and 400 μg/day or less in children. Absorption of inhaled steroid leads to systemic bioavailability, from both the swallowed portion and the inhaled portion reaching the lung. Table 11-4 summarizes data on the bioavailability of four agents. When administered orally, bioavailability ranges from less than 1% to over 20% of the total dose. This is due to the high first-pass metabolism of the swallowed drug. In contrast, all of the inhaled dose reaching the lung is absorbed and enters the systemic circulation, where it is ultimately metabolized in the liver or extrapulmonary tissues.[21,40] The efficiency of the delivery device in depositing drug in the lungs will therefore determine the amount of drug entering the systemic circulation from the airway. Thorsson and colleagues[41] reported that an MDI of budesonide delivered 18% of the dose to the lungs, whereas a DPI preparation (Turbuhaler) delivered nearly twice as much (32%). Unless a lower dose is used with the DPI, greater systemic drug levels will result compared with those with an equal dose from an MDI. Total bioavailability, and thus the amount of drug that can cause systemic side effects such as HPA suppression, is a function of both the swallowed amount, with its bioavailability, and the inhaled amount, all of which is absorbed into the circulation. Use of a reservoir device and mouth rinsing can minimize the oropharyngeal loss and amount of swallowed drug contributing to systemic bioavailability and potential side effects. It will be necessary to adjust doses based on efficiency of the delivery system and the amount reaching the airway.

TOPICAL (LOCAL) SIDE EFFECTS WITH AEROSOL ADMINISTRATION

Two of the most common side effects caused by topical application of inhaled steroids in the respiratory tract are oropharyngeal candidiasis (oral thrush) and dysphonia. Several other complications and precautions with the inhaled route are summarized below.

- *Orophyaryngeal fungal infections:* Infections with *Candida albicans* or *Aspergillus niger* may occur in the mouth, pharynx, or larynx with aerosolized steroid treatment. Some form of this may be seen in up to one third of patients on the aerosol formulations, but such an infection responds to topical antifungal agents and seems to diminish with continued aerosol steroid use.[15] Occurrence and severity are dose related and are more likely in patients who are also taking oral steroids. The use of a spacer device and gargling after treatment can reduce oropharyngeal deposition of the steroid and the incidence or severity of such infections.
- *Dysphonia:* Hoarseness and changes in voice quality also may occur with inhaled steroids in a third

Table 11-4

Bioavailability of oral and inhaled corticosteroid agents

	ORAL (%)*	INHALED (%)†
Beclomethasone dipropionate	<20	≈20
Triamcinolone acetonide	22.5	21.5
Budesonide	11.0	25.0
Fluticasone propionate	<1	20.0

Modified from Johnson M: Pharmacodynamics and pharmacokinetics of inhaled glucocorticoids, *J Allergy Clin Immunol* 97(Jan suppl):169, 1996.
*Figures represent percentages of a 100% oral dose.
†Figures represent the 20% of an inhaled dose that reaches the lungs and indicate complete absorption of that fraction.

of patients. This can be minimized with use of a spacer and by gargling. The effect is primarily caused by adductor vocal cord paresis, which is thought to be a local steroid-induced myopathy.[42]

- *Cough and bronchoconstriction:* Occasionally, cough or bronchoconstriction may occur after inhalation of an aerosol steroid.[15]
- *Incorrect use:* Incorrect use of the metered dose inhaler delivery vehicle also represents a possible risk factor, because inadequate amounts of the topical inhaled steroid will be delivered.

With inhaled steroids the following can minimize risk of adverse effects, both local and systemic:

- Use of minimal doses (400 μg/day or 800 μg/day) in children and adults, or the lowest effective dose
- Use of a reservoir device
- Mouth-rinsing after treatments

CLINICAL APPLICATION OF AEROSOL STEROIDS

Corticosteroids are used for a wide variety of conditions, with the therapeutic goal of reducing inflammation. These applications include clinical conditions such as contact dermatitis, rheumatoid arthritis, and systemic lupus erythematosus (SLE), as well as asthma and COPD and include topical cream application, oral, parenteral, and inhaled formulations.

USE IN ASTHMA

The 1995 *Global Initiative for Asthma* and the 1997 Expert Panel Report II of the National Asthma Education and Prevention Program (NAEPP)'s *Guidelines for the Diagnosis and Management of Asthma* identify corticosteroids as long-term-control agents rather than quick-relief agents.[1,11]

Corticosteroids have traditionally been used in asthma by the oral route for maintenance therapy of severe asthma and by oral or intravenous routes for treatment of status asthmaticus, as well as by inhalation for maintenance of asthma control. However, the increased emphasis on asthma as a disease of inflammation leading to bronchial hyperresponsiveness has shifted the use of inhaled aerosol steroids from second-line or third-line therapy to first-line, primary therapy. Appendix D offers a summary of the pharmacological management of asthma based on the NAEPP EPR-II. The following summarizes the princi-

ples of corticosteroid use in asthma, based on those guidelines.

- Bronchial hyperresponsiveness is characteristic of asthma and is related to the degree of airway inflammation.
- The basic pathology of asthma, previously emphasizing bronchospasm, is now understood to be a chronic inflammatory disorder of the airways resulting from a complex interaction among inflammatory cells, mediators, and airway tissue.[1] The phrase "chronic desquamating eosinophilic bronchitis" has been used to describe asthma.[15]
- Inhaled corticosteroids are considered to be the most effective long-term therapy for mild, moderate, or severe persistent asthma, and they are well tolerated and safe at recommended dosages.[1,11] Several points are related to the use of inhaled steroids.
  - Barnes suggests starting inhaled steroids at a high enough dose to be effective and then reducing the dose.[43] Alternatively, a short course of systemic corticosteroids can be used to gain control of symptoms followed by a step-down in therapy.[1] Loss of patient confidence and compliance with prescribed use of inhaled corticosteroids may be avoided in this way, especially because steroids do not give an immediate effect as a bronchodilator does. Any reduction in pharmacological management should be monitored by symptoms, concomitant need for β_2 agonists, and peak flow rates.
  - An increase in dose of inhaled steroids, such as doubling of the current dose, if peak expiratory flow rates decline 25% to 30%, may avoid the need for oral steroids. However, controlled studies are needed to confirm the effectiveness of such practice.[43]
  - If asthma is not controlled by inhaled steroids and other types of drug therapy, a short burst of oral steroids may be required to regain control of the asthma and help clear the airways.[1,15]

EARLY USE OF CORTICOSTEROIDS IN ASTHMA

There is evidence that the addition of an inhaled corticosteroid to first-line β agonist maintenance treatment of asthma reduces morbidity and airway hyperresponsiveness.[44] Haahtela and associates[45] demonstrated that subjects with mild asthma maintained on inhaled budesonide (1200 μg/day for 2 years, then 400 μg/day) had decreased bronchial response to histamine challenge compared with subjects on inhaled terbutaline (375 μg twice daily), over a 2-year period. Perhaps the most significant finding was that the later addition of inhaled budesonide after use of a β_2 agonist was not able to give as high a level of bronchoprotection as achieved by subjects who had started with and stayed on the inhaled steroid. This suggests that irreversible changes had occurred during the 2 years of β_2-agonist therapy and supports earlier use of inhaled steroids.

Although inhaled corticosteroids are first-line anti-inflammatory agents and acceptable for primary therapy of moderate asthma in children, the anti-asthmatic prophylactic agents cromolyn sodium or nedocromil sodium may be used as an initial choice for long-term control therapy in mild persistent asthma (Step 2 therapy) with children, because these medications have excellent safety profiles.[1]

INHALED CORTICOSTEROIDS FOR ACUTE SEVERE ASTHMA

Inhaled corticosteroids have not been considered useful for treatment of acute, severe asthma episodes, and in fact drug labeling contraindicates this use, because there is no bronchodilator effect. In addition, the dose of inhaled steroids is low compared with oral administration. However a study by Rodrigo and Rodrigo examined the addition of high, cumulative doses of inhaled flunisolide added to albuterol in emergency room treatment of acute adult asthma.[46] Both drugs were given by MDI with a spacer. Flunisolide was given as 4 puffs (250 μg per actuation) every 10 minutes. Their protocol allowed 3 hours of this treatment, with a cumulative dose of 6 mg flunisolide each hour, and equally aggressive albuterol dosing. The use of flunisolide resulted in better lung function at 90 minutes and following, compared with use of albuterol alone. Although preliminary, these results suggest that the contraindication to use of inhaled corticosteroids for treating acute severe asthma may need to be reconsidered.

CLINICAL USE OF INHALED CORTICOSTEROIDS

Other considerations in the clinical application of inhaled corticosteroids are as follows:

- High-dose inhaled steroids can be tried in cases of severe, persistent asthma to replace or reduce oral corticosteroid dependence. High doses of inhaled steroids are two to four times the usual recommended dose. Oral steroid therapy can be reduced slowly while monitoring the patient's pulmonary function.[1] (Note that relative inhaled doses considered low, medium, and high are given in the NAEPP EPR-II guidelines.)

- Although more control may be achieved with high doses of inhaled steroids, side effects, including systemic ones, are also likely to increase with inhaled doses above 1 mg per day. However, if oral steroids can be replaced or even reduced, this can be an overall improvement in the risk to benefit ratio.[47]

- Aerosol treatment is more effective when administered in several doses throughout the day in severe asthma.[15,48]

- All aerosolized corticosteroids should be administered for oral inhalation using a reservoir device (preferably a holding chamber rather than a spacer) and mouth rinsing, to reduce the risk of oropharyngeal candidiasis or other fungal infections and to reduce systemic absorption from swallowed drug.

- Use of a long-acting β_2 agonist such as salmeterol in subjects with inadequate symptom control, who are already receiving low to moderate doses of inhaled corticosteroids, may prevent the need to increase the inhaled corticosteroid dose.[1]

- Compliance with prescribed steroid therapy by inhalation appears to be poor and can be a complicating factor in the management of asthma. One study noted that overall compliance with two controller agents (a steroid, and a cromolyn-like agent) was approximately 37% and involved both overuse and underuse of drug.[49] Compliance has also been found to be worse with four-times-daily dosing compared with twice-daily dosing. Unfortunately, evidence indicates that symptoms and peak flow rates may be better in some cases with the four-times-daily rather than the two-times-daily schedule.[43] Wasserfallen and Baraniuk[49] note that the absence of immediate effect with inhaled steroids compared with bronchodilators may explain the lack of compliance.

USE IN CHRONIC OBSTRUCTIVE PULMONARY DISEASE

The use of steroids in COPD is debated, and, additionally, the 1995 ATS recommendations on drug management of COPD are in revision. Guidelines on managing COPD and potential changes are reviewed in the February, 2000 supplement of *Chest*.[3,50] COPD is characterized by a different pattern of inflammatory cells than athma.[51] Whereas eosinophils predominate in asthma, neutrophils are mostly seen in COPD. Oral and inhaled corticosteroids do not influence the inflammatory changes driven by neutrophils.[32,51]

With stable COPD, especially severe disease, corticosteroids may be helpful in improving lung function if treatment with other inhaled therapy, including bronchodilators, is suboptimal. However, a study by Eliasson and others[52] estimated that the proportion of stable COPD patients showing improvement with corticosteroids is small.[44] Therefore pulmonary function results, symptoms, and change in response to β agonists ought to be evaluated when determining whether corticosteroids will benefit a patient with COPD. If patients do not show a response to systemic corticosteroid therapy, inhaled steroids have a minimal effect in COPD. If there is objective improvement with systemic steroid treatment, the oral corticosteroid should be reduced to the minimum dosage possible, with attempted conversion to inhaled steroid agents.[53]

In acute exacerbations of COPD, oral or parenteral steroids are often given. Short-term corticosteroid therapy has shown benefit in hospitalized patients.[53-55] Systemic steroid therapy is indicated in patients who are on chronic corticosteroids who have a documented response to corticosteroids previously and in those who do not respond to the usual bronchodilator and antibiotic therapy.[53]

ANDROGENIC (ANABOLIC) CORTICOSTEROIDS

Testosterone is a hormone, generally referred to as the male sex hormone, and is the third type of steroid secreted by the adrenal cortex. This hormone is androgenic and is responsible for secondary male sex characteristics; it is present in both men and women, although to a lesser degree in women. The hormone also causes anabolic effects such as an increase in muscle and lean body mass (*ana* means "building up"). Derivatives of testosterone have been developed in an effort to minimize the androgenic, or masculinizing, effects and still maintain the anabolic effects. Medical uses of these derivatives, which are termed *anabolic steroids,* include stimulation of red blood cells in certain forms of anemia and stimulation of sexual development in hypogonadal males.

The structure of testosterone, cortisol, and anabolic steroid derivatives are illustrated in Figure 11-7. The common steroid nucleus is clearly seen in all of these

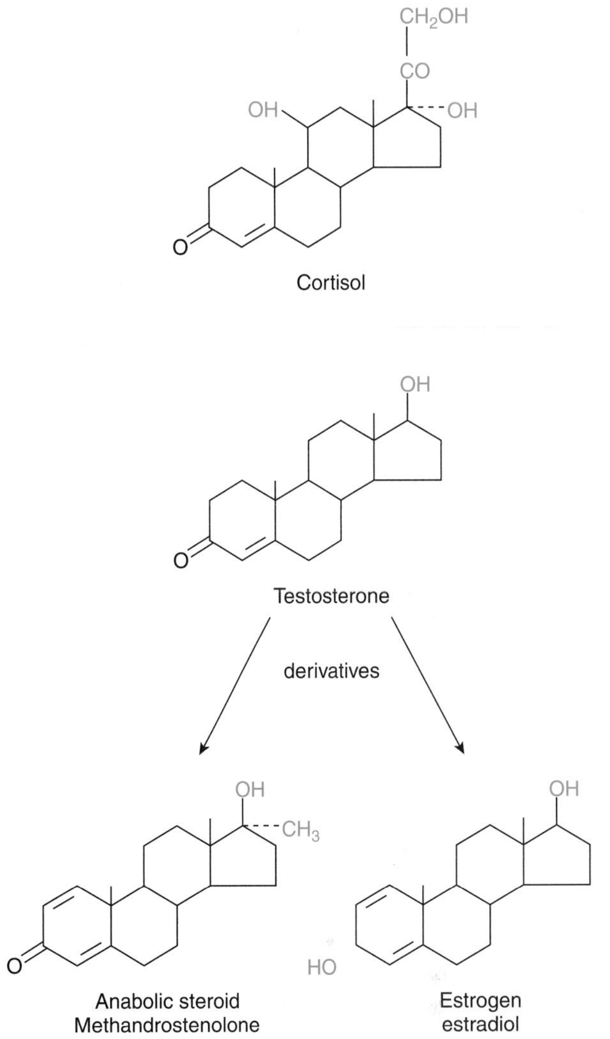

Figure 11-7 The structural similarity of cortisol, testosterone, and the testosterone derivatives, methandrostenolone and estradiol.

agents. Testosterone can also be converted by the body to estradiol, which is an estrogenic, or feminizing, hormone (Figure 11-7). One of the side effects of anabolic steroids is gynecomastia, which implies that these testosterone derivatives can also be converted to estrogens. Generally, testosterone and its derivatives bind with an androgen receptor in the cytoplasm of skeletal muscles, the prostate gland, and other organs. The steroid-receptor complex then causes the cell nucleus to increase ribonucleic acid synthesis and in turn protein synthesis in cell ribosomes. There is no question that the anabolic steroids increase nitrogen retention and body mass and enhance muscle growth in castrated male animals and normal female

Box 11-6	Selected Anabolic Steroids Used Therapeutically

Nandrolone phenpropionate (Durabolin)
Nandrolone decanoate (Deca-Durabolin)
Oxandrolone (Oxandrin)
Oxymetholone (Anadrol-50)
Stanozolol (Winstrol)

animals. Anabolic steroid therapy is effective in stimulating muscular development in castrated human males or those otherwise deficient in natural androgens. A partial list of therapeutic androgenic steroids is given in Box 11-6. Greater detail on the pharmacology of these agents and their clinical application can be found in standard texts of clinical pharmacology.[56]

RESPIRATORY CARE ASSESSMENT OF INHALED CORTICOSTEROID THERAPY

- Instruct and then verify correct use of aerosol delivery system (MDI, holding chamber, SVN, or DPI).
- Assess breathing rate and pattern.
- Assess breath sounds by auscultation, before and after treatment.
- Assess pulse before and after treatment.
- Assess patient's subjective reaction to treatment, for any change in breathing effort or pattern.
- Verify that patient understands that a corticosteroid is a controller agent and is aware of its difference from a rescue bronchodilator (relieving agent); assess patient's understanding of the need for consistent use of an inhaled corticosteroid (compliance with therapy).
- Instruct subject in use of a peak flow meter, to monitor baseline PEF and changes. Verify that there is a specific action plan, based on symptoms and peak flow results. Subject should be clear on when to contact a physician with deterioration in PEF or exacerbation of symptoms.
- Long-term: Assess severity of symptoms (coughing, wheezing, nocturnal awakenings), symptoms during exertion; use of rescue bronchodilator; and number of exacerbations, missed work/school days, and pulmonary function and modify level of asthma therapy (up or down, as described in NAEPP EPR-II guidelines for step therapy).
- Assess for presence of side effects with inhaled steroid therapy (oral thrush, hoarseness or voice changes, cough/wheezing with MDI use); have patient use a reservoir (preferably a holding chamber) with MDI use and verify correct use.

SUMMARY KEY TERMS AND CONCEPTS

- The *physiology* of *endogenous corticosteroids* involves a sequence of stimulation of the adrenal cortex through the *hypothalamic-pituitary-adrenal* (HPA) axis, in which increased blood levels of corticosteroid inhibit the HPA and adrenal cortex from further secretion.
- Levels of endogenous corticosteroids follow a daily, or *diurnal, rhythm.*
- *Exogenous* corticosteroid agents can *suppress the HPA axis* and the adrenal gland.
- Corticosteroids secreted by the adrenal cortex include the *glucocorticoids* (e.g., cortisol), the *mineralocorticoids* (e.g., aldosterone) and the *androgen/estrogen* hormones.
- Glucocorticoids, often referred to simply as *steroids,* exert an *antiinflammatory effect* in the body.
- *Inflammation* produces general symptoms of redness, swelling, heat, and pain.
- In the airway, inflammation is mediated by various cells, such as *eosinophils, basophils, macrophages, mast cells, T lymphocytes,* and *epithelial* or *endothelial* cells in response to the release of *mediators of inflammation.* This process is complex and involves several mediators, including the *arachidonic acid cascade* (prostaglandins, leukotrienes), *histamine,* and a variety of *cytokines,* such as interleukins. These mediators further amplify the inflammatory response by attracting the cells mentioned previously to the airway and inducing the release of *adhesion* factors (intercellular adhesion molecule [ICAM]) to bind inflammatory cells to the airway surface.
- Glucocorticoids are lipid soluble and act on intracellular receptors to produce their antiinflammatory effects.
- The *mode of action* of glucocorticoids is through the *up-regulation* of antiinflammatory proteins (e.g., β receptors, lipocortin), and the *downregulation* of proinflammatory proteins (e.g., cytokines, substance P).
- *Aerosolized glucocorticoids* are all topically active drugs and include beclomethasone dipropionate, triamcinolone acetonide, flunisolide, budesonide, and fluticasone propionate, as well as the older agent dexamethasone. Aerosol agents are available for both *oral inhalation* in control of *asthma* and *intranasal* administration for *rhinitis.*
- *Hazards* to *systemically* administered steroids include HPA suppression, immunosuppression, fluid retention, muscle wasting, and others.
- Inhaled agents may cause local *oral candidiasis, hoarseness, cough,* or even bronchoconstriction in some cases.

- HPA suppression is minimal or absent with inhaled agents, although high doses can cause adrenal suppression in a dose-dependent fashion.
- Side effects with inhaled steroids can be *minimized* by use of a reservoir device, rinsing of the mouth after treatments, and use of minimal doses.
- Inhaled steroids are used in asthma as a *first-line therapy* for mild to moderate asthma.
- Glucocorticoids may be of use in COPD and are often administered systemically.
- *Androgenic*, or *anabolic*, steroids can increase muscle mass, but have significant side effects.

SELF-ASSESSMENT QUESTIONS

1. Identify five corticosteroids approved for clinical use by oral inhalation in the United States, using generic names.
2. What is the major therapeutic effect of corticosteroids?
3. Identify two common respiratory diseases in which inhaled corticosteroids are prescribed.
4. What is the rationale for use of inhaled corticosteroids instead of oral routes in asthma?
5. Contrast the effects of β agonists with those of corticosteroids on the early phase and late phase of asthma.
6. What is the effect of orally administered corticosteroids on growth, bone density, and adrenal function?
7. What is the purpose of alternate-day steroid therapy?
8. Can you transfer an asthmatic patient from oral steroid use to inhaled steroid use? Explain the precautions or reasons, as appropriate.
9. Identify a common side effect with inhaled steroids.
10. Identify two methods of minimizing the side effect identified in question 9.
11. Have inhaled corticosteroids traditionally been used with an asthmatic during an acute episode?

Answers to Self-Assessment Questions are found in Appendix A.

CLINICAL SCENARIO

A 55-year-old white female presents to the emergency department (ED) with a chief complaint of cough, wheezing, shortness of breath, and chest pain. She is well nourished and educated. She is a known asthmatic, with one hospitalization in the previous year for asthma exacerbation. Two days earlier, she reported rhinorrhea, sore throat, sinus congestion, and subsequent increase in dyspnea and wheeze.

Physical examination on admission to the ED exhibited wheezing on auscultation, use of accessory muscles, no cyanosis or diaphoresis, and mild respiratory distress. Vital signs were T, 98.4° F; P, 96 beats/min and regular; RR, 22 breaths/min; and BP, 92/68 mm Hg.

Chest radiograph showed hyperinflation, but no infiltrates or other abnormalities. Electrocardiogram revealed sinus tachycardia. An arterial blood gas on room air indicated pH, 7.44; $Paco_2$, 38 mm Hg; Pao_2, 54 mm Hg; base excess (BE), 2.2; HCO_3^-, 25.9 mEq/L; and Sao_2, 89.4%. Hemoglobin was 13.3 g/dl, and WBC count, 8.8 × 10³/mm³. Administration of MDI albuterol by reservoir showed little improvement in her peak flow rates.

She was subsequently admitted to the hospital after failing to improve in her flow rates, blood gas values, or symptoms of dyspnea, and albuterol 0.5 cc of a 0.5% solution was administered by SVN, with 3 L/min of oxygen by nasal cannula. She was placed on theophylline orally, given intravenous methylprednisolone 40 mg and a brand of phenylephrine for nasal decongestion and sinus clearance, and ipratropium bromide by MDI was added to her inhaled albuterol. Over a 5-day course in the hospital, her peak flow rates improved to within 80% of her predicted and her chest sounds were clear to auscultation. A throat culture returned normal flora, and follow-up theophylline levels showed 10 to 12 μg/ml. An arterial sample on day 5 gave the following: pH, 7.45; $Paco_2$, 37 mm Hg; Pao_2, 68 mm HGO_3^-, 26.2 mEq/L; BE, 2.7; and Sao2, 94% on room air. Hemoglobin was 12.9 g/dl. In preparation for discharge, respiratory care was consulted for appropriate inhaled medications.

What inhaled aerosol agents would you recommend as appropriate at this time for discharge?

What precautions and recommendations would you make with this subject?

Answers to Clinical Scenario Questions are found in Appendix A.

REFERENCES

1. National Asthma Education and Prevention Program, Expert Panel II: *Guidelines for the diagnosis and management of asthma*, Bethesda, Md, 1997, National Institutes of Health.
2. American Thoracic Society: Standards for the diagnosis and care of patients with chronic obstructive pulmonary disease, *Am J Respir Crit Care Med* 152 (suppl):S77, 1995.
3. Ferguson GT: Recommendations for the management of COPD, *Chest* 117:23S, 2000.

4. Hench PS and others: The effect of a hormone of the adrenal cortex (17-hydroxy-11-dehydrocortisone, compound E) and of pituitary adrenocorticotropic hormone on rheumatoid arthritis, *Mayo Clin Proc* 24:181, 1949.

5. Carryer HM and others: The effect of cortisone on bronchial asthma and hay fever occurring in subjects sensitive to ragweed pollen, *J Allergy* 21:282, 1950.

6. Gelfand ML: Administration of cortisone by the aerosol method in the treatment of bronchial asthma, *N Engl J Med* 245:203, 1951.

7. Brockbank W, Brebner H, Pengelly CDR: Chronic asthma treated with aerosol hydrocortisone, *Lancet* ii:807, 1956.

8. Peters GA, Henderson LL: Prednisolone aerosol in asthmatic bronchitis: a preliminary report, *Proc Staff Meet Mayo Clinic* 33:57, 1958.

9. Fisch BR, Grater WC: Dexamethasone aerosol in respiratory tract disease, *J New Drugs* 2:298, 1962.

10. Morrow-Brown H, Storey G, George WHS: Beclomethasone dipropionate: a new steroid aerosol for the treatment of allergic asthma, *Br Med J* 1:585, 1972.

11. National Institutes of Health: Global initiative for asthma: global strategy for asthma management and prevention, NHLBI/WHO workshop report, Bethesda, Md, National Institutes of Health, January, 1995.

12. Holgate ST: The immunopharmacology of mild asthma, *J Allergy Clin Immunol* 98:S7, 1996.

13. Schwiebert LA and others: Glucocorticosteroid inhibition of cytokine production: Relevance to antiallergic actions, *J Allergy Clin Immunol* 97(Jan suppl):143, 1996.

14. Kay AB: Mediators and inflammatory cells in allergic disease, *Ann Allergy* 59:35, 1987.

15. Reed CE: Aerosol glucocorticoid treatment of asthma: adults, *Am Rev Respir Dis* 141(suppl):S82, Feb 1990.

16. Laitinen LA, Laitinen A: Remodeling of asthmatic airways by glucocorticosteroids, *J Allergy Clin Immunol* 97:153, 1996.

17. Check WA, Kaliner, MA: Pharmacology and pharmacokinetics of topical corticosteroid derivatives used for asthma therapy, *Am Rev Respir Dis* 141(suppl):S44, 1990.

18. McKenzie AW: Percutaneous absorption of steroids, *Arch Dermatol* 86:611, 1962.

19. McKenzie AW, Stoughton RB: Method for comparing percutaneous absorption of steroids, *Arch Dermatol* 86:608, 1962.

20. Barnes PJ, Pedersen S: Efficacy and safety of inhaled corticosteroids in asthma, *Am Rev Respir Dis* 148(Oct. suppl):S1, 1993.

21. Johnson M: Pharmacodynamics and pharmacokinetics of inhaled glucocorticoids, *J Allergy Clin Immunol* 97(Jan suppl): 169, 1996.

22. Chaplin MD and others: Flunisolide metabolism and dynamics of a metabolite, *Clin Pharmacol Ther* 27:402, 1980.

23. Holliday SM, Faulds D, Sorkin EM: Inhaled fluticasone propionate: a review of its pharmacodynamic and pharmacokinetic properties, and therapeutic use in asthma, *Drugs* 47:318, 1994.

24. Phillipps GH: Structure-activity relationships of topically active steroids: the selection of fluticasone propionate, *Respir Med* 84(suppl A):19, 1990.

25. Clark DJ and others: Comparative adrenal suppression with inhaled budesonide and fluticasone propionate in adult asthmatic patients, *Thorax* 51:262, 1996.

26. Shapiro G and others: Combined salmeterol 50 µg and fluticasone propionate 250 µg in the Diskus device for the treatment of asthma, *Am J Respir Crit Care Med* 161:527, 2000.

27. Chung KF: The complementary role of glucocorticosteroids and long-acting β-adrenergic agonists, *Allergy* 53:7, 1998.

28. Anderson GP: Interactions between corticosteroids and β-adrenergic agonists in asthma disease induction, progression, and exacerbation, *Am J Respir Crit Care Med* 161:S188, 2000.

29. Bousquet J, Chanez P, Michel FB: Pathophysiology and treatment of seasonal allergic rhinitis, *Respir Med* 84 (suppl A):11, 1990.

30. Barnes PJ: Inhaled glucocorticoids for asthma, *N Engl J Med* 332:868, 1995.

31. Barnes PJ: Molecular mechanisms of steroid action in asthma, *J Allergy Clin Imuununol* 97(Jan suppl):159, 1996.

32. Barnes PJ, Pedersen S, Busse WW: Efficacy and safety of inhaled corticosteroids: new developments, *Am J Respir Crit Care Med* 157:S1, 1998.

33. Baraniuk JN: Molecular actions of glucocorticoids: an introduction, *J Allergy Clin Immunol* 97:141, 1996.

34. Svedmyr N: Action of corticosteroids on beta-adrenergic receptors, clinical aspects, *Am Rev Respir Dis* 141(suppl):S31, Feb 1990.

35. Truhan AP, Ahmed AR: Corticosteroids: a review with emphasis on complications of prolonged systemic therapy, *Ann Allergy* 62:375, 1989.

36. Kamada AK and others: Issues in the use of inhaled glucocorticoids, *Am J Respir Crit Care Med* 153:1739, 1996.

37. Goldberg S and others: Adrenal suppression among asthmatic children receiving chronic therapy with inhaled corticosteroid with and without spacer device, *Ann Allergy Asthma Immunol* 76:234, 1996.

38. Wolthers OD, Pedersen S: Controlled study of linear growth in asthmatic children during treatment with inhaled glucocorticoids, *Pediatrics* 89:839, 1992.

39. Allen DB, Mullen M, Mullen B: A meta-analysis of the effect of oral and inhaled corticosteroids on growth, *J Allergy Clin Immunol* 93:967, 1994.

40. Brattsand R, Selroos O: Current drugs for respiratory diseases. In Page CP, Metzger WJ, eds: *Drugs and the lung*, New York, 1994, Raven Press.

41. Thorsson L, Edsbacker S, Conradson T-B: Lung deposition of budesonide from Turbuhaler is twice that from a pressurized metered-dose inhaler P-MDI, *Eur Respir J* 7:1839, 1994.

42. Williams AJ and others: Dysphonia caused by inhaled steroids: recognition of a characteristic laryngeal abnormality, *Thorax* 38:813, 1983.

43. Barnes PJ: Inhaled glucocorticoids: new developments relevant to updating of the Asthma Management Guidelines, *Respir Med* 90:379, 1996.

44. Kerstjens HAM and others: A comparison of bronchodilator therapy with or without inhaled corticosteroid therapy for obstructive airways disease, *N Engl J Med* 327:1413, 1992.

45. Haahtela T and others: Effects of reducing or discontinuing inhaled budesonide in patients with mild asthma, *N Engl J Med* 331:700, 1994.

46. Rodrigo G, Rodrigo C: Inhaled flunisolide for acute severe asthma, *Am J Respir Crit Care Med* 157:698, 1998.

47. Geddes DM: Inhaled corticosteroids: benefits and risks, *Thorax* 47:404, 1992 (editorial).

48. Malo JL and others: Four-times-a-day dosing frequency is better than twice-a-day regimen in subjects requiring a high-dose inhaled steroid, budesonide, to control moderate to severe asthma, *Am Rev Respir Dis* 140:624, 1989.

49. Wasserfallen J, Baraniuk JN: Clinical use of inhaled corticosteroids in asthma, *J Allergy Clin Immunol* 97:177, 1996.

50. Pauwels RA: National and international guidelines for COPD: the need for evidence, *Chest* 117:20S, 2000.

51. Barnes PJ: Mechanisms in COPD. Differences from asthma, *Chest* 117:10S, 2000.

52. Eliasson O and others: Corticosteroids in COPD: a clinical trial and reassessment of the literature, *Chest* 89:484, 1986.

53. National COPD Awareness Panel: Early detection and management of COPD, *J Respir Dis* 21:9(suppl), 2000.

54. Davies L, Angus RM, Calverley PM: Oral corticosteroids in patients admitted to hospital with exacerbations of chronic obstructive pulmonary disease: a prospective randomised controlled trial, *Lancet* 354:456, 1999.

55. Niewoehner DE and others: Effect of systemic glucocorticoids on exacerbations of chronic obstructive pulmonary disease, *N Engl J Med* 340:1941, 1999.

56. Goldfien A: The gonadal hormones & inhibitors. In Katzung BG, ed: *Basic & clinical pharmacology*, ed 7, New York, 1998, Appleton & Lange.

Nonsteroidal Antiasthma Agents

Joseph L. Rau

*I*n Chapter 11 the concept of airway inflammation was introduced and some of the numerous cells and chemicals involved in an inflammatory response were described, in order to discuss the antiinflammatory actions of glucocorticoids. Chapter 12 presents drug groups that also have an antiinflammatory effect through mechanisms different from those of the corticosteroids. Two subgroups of agents are included in the nonsteroidal antiasthma group: cromolyn-like drugs (mast cell stabilizers) and the antileukotrienes (anti-LTs). A brief summary of the immune mechanisms involved in allergic responses is given as an introduction to the specific mechanisms of action for the drug groups discussed in this chapter.

CLINICAL INDICATION FOR NONSTEROIDAL ANTIASTHMA AGENTS

The general indication for clinical use of nonsteroidal antiasthma agents described in this chapter is *prophylactic* management (control) of mild persistent asthma (Step 2 asthma, using the classification in the 1997 National Asthma Education and Prevention Program guidelines[1]).

Step 2 asthma: Greater than 2 days/wk of symptoms, greater than 2 nights/mo with symptoms; forced expiratory volume in 1 second (FEV_1) or peak expiratory flow (PEF) 80% or greater; PEF but variability is 20% to 30% (see Appendix D).

The following are qualifications to the general indication for use of these agents:

- Cromolyn-like drugs and the antileukotrienes (anti-LTs) are typically recommended as alternatives to inhaled corticosteroids in Step 2 asthma.
- Cromolyn and nedocromil in particular are often used with infants and young children as alternatives to inhaled corticosteroids in Step 2 asthma because of their safety profiles.
- The anti-LT agents can be useful in combination with inhaled steroids to reduce the dose of the steroid.

All of the nonsteroidal antiasthma drugs described in this chapter are controllers, not relievers, and are used in asthma requiring antiinflammatory drug therapy. A summary of agents used in drug therapy for asthma, both relievers and controllers, is presented in Box 12-1 and lists both cromolyn-like agents and antileukotrienes as controllers. Use of rescue β_2-agonist agents more than twice a week (i.e., Step 2 asthma) is an indicator of the need for initiation of controller drug therapy.

IDENTIFICATION OF NONSTEROIDAL ANTIASTHMA AGENTS

Individual agents in the cromolyn-like group and in the antileukotriene group are identified in Table 12-1, with generic and brand names, formulations and strengths, and usual recommended dosages.

Box 12-1	Drug Groups Used in the Pharmacological Management of Asthma (Categorized as Controllers or Relievers)

Controllers
Inhaled corticosteroids
Oral corticosteroids
Cromolyn sodium and nedocromil
Long-acting inhaled β_2 agonists
Long-acting oral β_2 agonists
Leukotriene modifiers
Sustained-release theophylline

Relievers
Short-acting inhaled β_2 agonists
Systemic corticosteroids (oral burst therapy, intravenous)
Inhaled anticholinergic bronchodilators

Table 12-1

Nonsteroidal antiasthma medications, with brand and generic names, formulations, and usual recommended dosages*

DRUG	BRAND NAME	FORMULATION AND DOSAGE
CROMOLYN-LIKE (MAST CELL STABILIZERS)		
Cromolyn sodium†	Intal	MDI: 800 µg/actuation Adults and children ≥5 yr: 2 inhalations 4 times daily SVN: 20 mg/amp or 20 mg/vial Adults and children ≥2 yr: 20 mg inhaled 4 times daily
	Nasalcrom	Spray: 40 mg/ml (4%) Adults and children ≥6 yr: 1 spray each nostril, 3-6 times daily every 4-6 hr
Nedocromil sodium	Tilade	MDI: 1.75 mg/actuation Adults and children ≥12 yr: 2 inhalations 4 times daily
ANTI-LEUKOTRIENES		
Zafirlukast	Accolate	Tablets: 20 mg Adults and children ≥12 yr: 20 mg (1 tab) twice daily, without food
Montelukast	Singulair	Tablets: 10 mg, 4 mg, and 5 mg cherry-flavored chewable Adults and children ≥15 yr: one 10 mg tab each evening Children 6-14 yr: one 5 mg chewable tablet each evening Children 2-5 years: one 4 mg chewable tablet each evening
Zileuton	Zyflo	Tablets: 600 mg Adults and children ≥12 yr: one 600 mg tablet 4 times a day

*Detailed prescribing information should be obtained from the manufacturer's package insert.
†NOTE: Cromolyn sodium is also available in an oral concentrate giving 100 mg in 5 ml (Gastrocrom), for treatment of systemic mastocytosis, and as an ophthalmic 4% solution (Opticrom, 40 mg/ml) for treatment of vernal keratoconjunctivitis.

MECHANISMS OF INFLAMMATION IN ASTHMA

Asthma was previously defined in Chapter 11 as a chronic inflammatory disorder of the airways.[1] Asthma has been distinguished into extrinsic and intrinsic forms on the basis of the triggers for asthma. *Extrinsic* asthma is dependent on allergy, or atopy, whereas the *intrinsic* form shows no evidence of sensitization to common inhaled allergens.[2] The allergic, or extrinsic, form of asthma, which is immunoglobu-lin E (IgE) mediated, is associated with younger subjects, and the intrinsic, or nonallergic, form is associated with adults and later onset in which childhood asthma may not have been present. Holgate[3] describes asthma as an "evolving" disease in early childhood, when viruses are an important trigger, whereas in school and teen years, allergens stimulate an immune response. As asthma progresses, and in adults, the disease becomes intrinsic and may be driven by T cells (lymphocytes) that release various cytokines, as described in Chapter 11. The asthma is chronic and persistent, with continual inflammation and episodes of acute obstruction. Three components of asthma are described by Drazen and Turino[4] as follows:

1. The acute asthma attack, which resolves spontaneously or with treatment
2. A hyperresponsiveness of the airways to various stimuli
3. Persistent inflammation that is now appreciated

In both forms of asthma, intrinsic and extrinsic, mediators and enzymes are released to act on target tissues in the airway and cells involved in inflammation are recruited and activated in the airway. Airway inflammation is manifested in the responses of bronchoconstriction, airway swelling, mucus secretion and obstruction, and subsequent airway wall remodeling that furthers the responsiveness of the airway.[5]

THE IMMUNOLOGICAL (ALLERGIC) RESPONSE

The majority of asthma is primarily an allergic response, which involves mast cells and immunoglobulin E (IgE).[1] An overview of the immunological response is outlined in Box 12-2. An understanding of the immune response is fundamental to discussing both asthma and the mediator antagonists presented in this chapter, because allergy is essentially a mistaken immune response. Generation of an immune response, and specifically an allergic asthmatic response, is considered to be *initiated* by the interaction of T lymphocytes with an antigen presented by other cells, such as macrophages or B lymphocytes.[4] Activation of T lymphocytes results in production of IgE by B lymphocytes. Antigen-specific IgE binds to effector cells such as mast cells and is termed a *cytophilic* antibody because of this. When activated by subsequent exposure to an antigen or allergen, mast cells release physiologically active mediators of inflammation such as prostaglandins, leukotrienes and proteases, histamine, platelet-activating factor (PAF), and certain cytokines.[4] The cytokines released, which include tumor necrosis factor-α (TNF-α) and interleukin-4 (IL-4), can upregulate endothelial adhesion molecules.[3] This cascade of mediators causes an inflammatory response manifested by vascular leakage, bronchoconstriction, mucus secretion, and mucosal swelling, all of which obstruct airflow in the bronchi-

---

Box 12-2   **An Overview of the Immune Mechanisms Involved in Allergy and Inflammation**

Cell Mediated

T lymphocytes (from bone marrow stem cells, processed in the thymus) mediate by several mechanisms, including cytotoxicity and secretion of cytokines. The family of T lymphocytes outlined below are the basis of cellular immunity.

Helper/T4 (CD4+) cells, which are subdivided into the following:

*   **Type 1 (Th1):** Regulate classic delayed hypersensitivity reactions and other actions related to macrophage activation and T-cell mediated immunity by the production of interferon-γ and interleukin-2 (IL-2).
*   **Type 2 (Th2):** Translate mRNA for interleukin-4 (IL-4) and interleukin-5 (IL-5) and are involved in atopic allergy. IL-4 is essential for production of IgE (see below) by B cells; IL-5 and granulocyte-macrophage colony-stimulating factor (GM-CSF) and interleukin-3 (IL-3) promote eosinophil maturation, activation, and survival.

Suppressor/T8 (CD8+): Inhibit the immune response to an antigen after the immune response has begun.

Cytotoxic T cells: Bind to viral antigen on the surface of infected cells, to destroy the cell.

Natural killer cells: Lymphocyte related to the cytotoxic T cell, whose targets are thought to be tumor cells or cells infected by organisms other than viruses.

Antibody Mediated

Antibodies are serum globulins (proteins) modified to specifically combine and react with an antigen (substance capable of provoking antibodies or cellular immunity).

B lymphocytes: Antibody-producing plasma cells; memory cells for later antibody production.

Classes of antibody: The classes of immunoglobulins are as follows:

*   Immunoglobulin G (IgG)
*   Immunoglobulin A (IgA)
*   Immunoglobulin M (IgM)
*   Immunoglobulin D (IgD)
*   Immunoglobulin E (IgE): Cytophilic antibody (binds to effector cells such as mast cells); termed *reaginic antibody*; involved in allergic responses, atopy

oles. T lymphocytes also release cytokines (such as interleukins), causing accumulation and activation of eosinophils, which also release chemicals to damage the airway. The process of initiating the inflammatory response and continuing it through amplification, as discussed next, is illustrated in Figure 12-1.

Once initiated by exposure to antigen, the inflammatory response in the airway is *amplified* by chemoattraction of more lymphocytes, eosinophils, basophils, and neutrophils and an increase in mast cells. Adhesion molecules increase after stimulation of lymphocytes and mast cells by antigen or allergen. These molecules, found in epithelial (intercellular adhesion molecule-1 [ICAM-1]) and vascular endothelial cells (vascular cell adhesion molecule-1 [VCAM-1]) in the airway, are responsible for eosinophil, neutrophil, and lymphocyte recruitment from the microvascular circulation into the airways. The adhesion molecules enable leukocytes to marginate, cross the

blood vessel wall, and migrate to the airway mucosa, continuing and further amplifying the inflammation begun.[5] The increase and activation of eosinophils is associated with increased inflammation and severity in asthma.[3]

Nonspecific stimuli such as fog, sulfur dioxide, dust, and cold air can stimulate sensory receptors and cause reflex bronchoconstriction (see Chapter 7).[5] Asthmatic subjects are more sensitive to such stimuli, reflecting either altered neural control or the result of chronic inflammation sensitizing the airway, or both. Nerve fibers of the noncholinergic nonadrenergic excitatory system, containing potent peptide mediators, contribute to local effects on smooth muscle and mucous glands and reflexly stimulate cholinergic activity. Some of these peptides include substance P (SP), neurokinin A (NKA), and neurokinin B (NKB); they are released from sensory C-fiber nerve endings. These neuropeptides can also contribute to inflammation

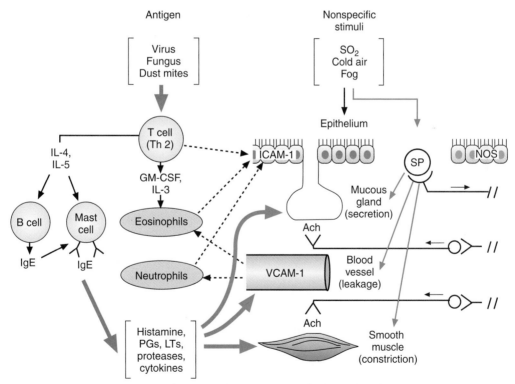

Figure 12-1   Illustration of the complex interaction of cells and mediators that are thought to initiate and amplify the inflammation of the airway in asthma, resulting in acute episodes of bronchoconstriction and persistent airway damage. *Ach,* Acetylcholine; *GM-CSF,* granulocyte-macrophage colony-stimulating factor; *ICAM-1,* intercellular adhesion molecule-1; *IgE,* immunoglobulin E; *IL-3, 4, 5,* interleukin-3, 4, 5; *LTs,* leukotrienes; *NOS,* nitric oxide synthase; *PGs,* prostaglandins; *SP,* substance P; *VCAM-1,* vascular cell adhesion molecule-1.

and the features of asthma previously described, such as mucus hypersecretion, smooth muscle contraction, plasma leakage, inflammatory cell activation, and adhesion. Neutral endopeptidase (NEP) is an enzyme that inactivates neuropeptides to limit their activity; NEP is found on the surface of cells that contain receptors for neuropeptides (smooth muscle, airway epithelium, vascular endothelium). An increased release of excitatory neuropeptides may be involved in asthma.[5]

Nitric oxide is formed in airway tissue through the action of the enzyme nitric oxide synthase (NOS). There is evidence that in asthma this enzyme is upregulated in airway epithelium.[5] Nitric oxide, a potent vasodilator and bronchodilator, may be the neurotransmitter for the nonadrenergic noncholinergic inhibitory nervous system (see Chapter 5). It is possible that nitric oxide, which can damage cells, is induced by proinflammatory cytokines in asthma and contributes to the observed epithelial damage seen in Figure 12-1.[6,7]

A better understanding of the inflammatory process just described has spurred the development of drugs targeted at interrupting the inflammatory processes, thereby blocking the asthmatic response. These drugs include mast cell stabilizers, such as cromolyn sodium and nedocromil sodium, as well as a newer group of antileukotriene drugs such as montelukast, zafirlukast, and zileuton.

CROMOLYN-LIKE (MAST CELL STABILIZING) AGENTS

Both cromolyn sodium, or *disodium cromoglycate*, as it is also termed, and nedocromil sodium are used as inhaled prophylactic aerosol drugs to prevent the inflammatory response in asthma. These drugs differ in structure and activity from the drug groups considered in previous chapters. Their chemical structures are illustrated in Figure 12-2. The basic catecholamine xanthine and steroid structures are given for comparison. Neither cromolyn nor nedocromil is related to the

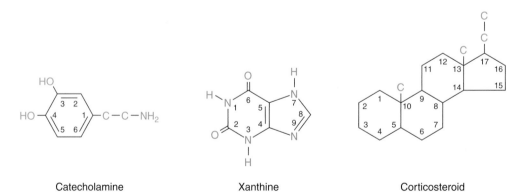

Figure 12-2   Chemical structures of cromolyn sodium (disodium cromoglycate) and nedocromil sodium, in comparison with the basic catecholamine, xanthine, and corticosteroid structures.

β agonists, xanthines, theophylline, or antiinflammatory glucocorticoids. These drugs have no intrinsic bronchodilating capability.

CROMOLYN SODIUM (DISODIUM CROMOGLYCATE)

In January 1965 a bischromone, later known as cromolyn sodium, was synthesized in the laboratory of the Fisons Corporation (Bedford, Mass.). Dr. Roger Altounyan, an investigator of the drug who himself has asthma, found that prior inhalation of cromolyn sodium inhibited and reduced his symptoms.[8] This drug, a synthetic derivative of khellin, the active ingredient found in the Mediterranean plant *Ammi visnaga,* was first introduced for clinical use in 1967 and became available for use in the United States in 1973.

The antiinflammatory, mast cell stabilizing effect of cromolyn has led to uses other than asthma prophylaxis, including the following:

- Allergic rhinitis (nasal solution)
- Mastocytosis, to improve diarrhea, abdominal pain, headaches, nausea, and itching (oral)
- Vernal keratoconjunctivitis (eye drops)

Administration and dosage for these alternative applications are listed briefly in the next section, along with inhaled formulations for asthma and allergic rhinitis.

DOSAGE AND ADMINISTRATION

Table 12-1 lists the inhaled oral and nasal formulations of cromolyn sodium, along with recommended doses. A stronger formulation for MDI use that delivers 5 mg per actuation is available in Great Britain. The original formulation of the drug was 20 mg of dry powder contained in a gelatin capsule. The capsule was placed in a specially designed inhaler apparatus, the Spinhaler, which was the first breath-actuated dry powder inhaler (DPI) and was introduced in 1971.

Ampule/Vial for Nebulization. The ampule or vial contains 20 mg in 2 ml of aqueous solution (a 1% strength). This solution can be nebulized in any small reservoir device powered by compressed air that will produce suitably small particles of 3 to 5 μm. Additional diluent will be needed for most nebulizers to function well. Slow tidal breathing reduces the need for inspiratory maneuvers as seen with the MDI, although longer administration times and lack of portability become a disadvantage.

Metered Dose Inhaler. The MDI is the most easily carried device and employs lower doses than the nebulized solution—only 2 mg per dose (approximately) rather than 20 mg per dose. This is typical of the dose ratio of MDIs versus nebulizers, as discussed in Chapter 3.

Nasal Solution (Nasalcrom). Cromolyn is available as a 4% solution for treatment of seasonal and perennial allergic rhinitis. As with the inhaled solution, protection requires prior administration, although the drug does not need to be taken outside of seasonal exposure to allergens. The solution is delivered by using a metered pump spray device.

Ophthalmic Solution (Opticrom). A 4% solution of cromolyn is available as Opticrom for use in treating ocular symptoms of allergic conjunctivitis. This drug is effective within 7 days and is poorly absorbed from the eye into the body, giving a localized effect. After initiation of the eye solution at regular intervals as prescribed, there is a decrease in the allergic symptoms of itching, tearing, redness, or discharge. This formulation has been given an orphan drug designation.

Oral Solution (Gastrocrom). A 100 mg capsule of cromolyn sodium has been released for oral use and is indicated for the management of systemic mastocytosis.

Mastocytosis: Condition involving the formation of clumps of mast cells in the skin. These may appear as brown areas that itch. Other organs may be involved. Symptoms include diarrhea, vomiting, and abdominal pain, as well as itching of the skin (urticaria).

In this use of cromolyn, the powder contents of the capsule are dissolved in one-half glass of hot water to which cold water is added. Usual starting dosage is 200 mg four times daily, one-half hour before meals and at bedtime.

MODE OF ACTION

Cromolyn sodium is considered an antiasthmatic, an antiallergic, and a mast cell stabilizer. Pretreatment with inhaled cromolyn sodium results in inhibition of mast cell degranulation, thereby blocking release of the chemical mediators of inflammation (Figure 12-3). By its action, cromolyn is effective in blocking the late-phase reaction in asthma. (The late-phase reaction in asthma was discussed in the review of corticosteroids in Chapter 11.)

CROMOLYN SODIUM (INTAL)

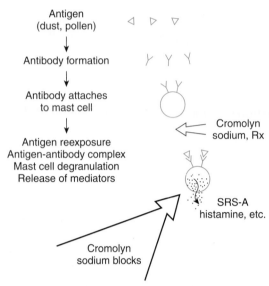

Figure 12-3   Mode of action of cromolyn sodium in preventing mast cell degranulation. *SRS-A,* Slow-reacting substance of anaphylaxis.

Cromolyn prevents the extrusion of the granules containing the mediators of inflammation to the cell exterior. For this reason, cromolyn is often classified as a "mast cell stabilizer." The exact mechanism by which this inhibition is accomplished is not completely understood, but the following details of cromolyn activity and mast cell function are known.

- The mode of action of cromolyn sodium is *prophylactic;* pretreatment is necessary for inhibition of mast cell degranulation.
- Cromolyn sodium may inhibit mediator release by preventing calcium influx necessary for microfilament contraction and extrusion of mast cell granules.[9,10]
- Cromolyn sodium does not have an antagonist effect on any of the chemical mediators themselves.
- Cromolyn sodium does not operate through the cyclic adenosine monophosphate (cAMP) system and does not affect α or β receptors.
- Antibody formation, attachment of antibody (IgE) to the mast cell, and antigen-antibody union are *not* prevented by cromolyn; cromolyn does prevent release of mediators.

- Cromolyn sodium can prevent or attenuate the late-phase response in an asthmatic episode, which can otherwise cause more severe airway obstruction 6 to 8 hours after initial bronchoconstriction.[11,12]

The protective effect of cromolyn in inhibiting mast cell degranulation has been captured using scanning electron microscopy and is shown in the sequence in Figure 12-4. Initial understanding of cromolyn's activity focused on allergy-triggered mast cell release of mediators, and therefore the drug came to be considered useful primarily in allergic asthma. There is evidence that the activity of cromolyn is not limited to preventing allergen-stimulated asthma. Cromolyn inhibits mast cell mediator release caused by nonallergic stimuli and may even reduce reflex-induced asthma. The latter requires about twice the usual dose of cromolyn. Understanding of the broader protection given by cromolyn has supported its successful use in allergic and nonallergic asthma and specifically with exercise-induced asthma. This view of the broader pharmacological activity of cromolyn is discussed by Bernstein.[13,14]

PHARMACOKINETICS

As with other inhaled aerosols, cromolyn sodium is distributed to the airway and to the stomach via a swallowed portion. Distribution to the stomach (swallowed portion) can be modified by use of reservoir devices with the MDI formulation. The dose reaching the airway is absorbed from the lung and quickly excreted unchanged in the bile and urine. The lung portion does not appear to be metabolized in the airway. The swallowed portion is largely unabsorbed from the gastrointestinal tract (less than 1%) and excreted in the feces.

SIDE EFFECTS

Cromolyn sodium is a safe drug. It has an effectiveness similar to theophylline in controlling asthma, with a better therapeutic margin than theophylline.[11] In studies comparing the two agents, subjects using theophylline reported more side effects, including nervousness, nausea, school behavioral problems, and more office visits. The overall incidence of adverse effects with cromolyn has been reported at 2%.[15] Nasal congestion may be seen after beginning cromolyn sodium use. Dermatitis, myositis (muscle tissue inflammation), and gastroenteritis occurred in a very few patients.

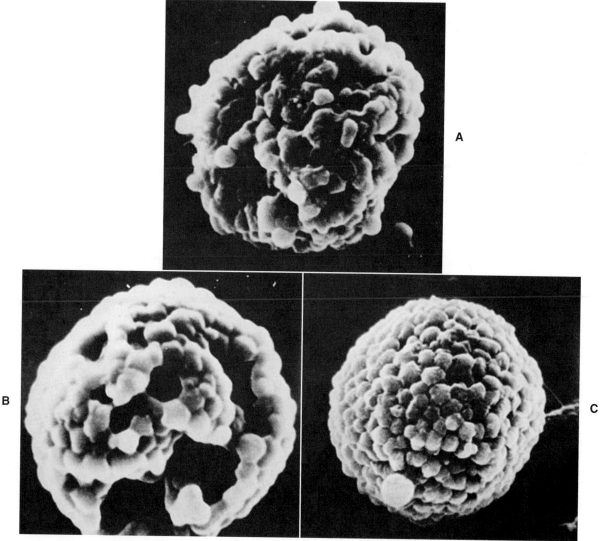

Figure 12-4   Degranulation of a mast cell. **A,** Mast cell undergoing gross degranulation shows free granules. **B,** The pores now occupy a large area of the cytoplasm. **C,** A sensitized mast cell fails to degranulate after challenge when pretreated with cromolyn sodium. (Courtesy Rhone-Poulenc Rorer Pharmaceuticals, Inc., Collegeville, Pa.)

Use of the *nebulizer solution* has been associated with cough, nasal congestion, wheezing, sneezing, nasal itching, epistaxis, or nose burning. Use of the *nasal solution* has most commonly been associated with sneezing (approximately 10% of patients), as well as nasal stinging or burning (5%), nasal irritation (2.5%), and a bad taste (2%). Side effects with the *oral capsules* for mastocytosis are difficult to differentiate from effects of the disease itself. Adverse events with this use of cromolyn sodium were transient and included headache and diarrhea.

CLINICAL EFFICACY OF CROMOLYN SODIUM

The original trials of cromolyn sodium as a prophylactic agent in asthma were performed with the 20 mg Spinhaler formulation. Studies were conducted in both adult and pediatric subjects and included both intrinsic and extrinsic forms of asthma. The conclusion of these early studies was that inhaled cromolyn sodium is effective as a treatment for approximately 70% of patients.[16] Edwards gives a review of data supporting the use of cromolyn sodium in chronic asthma.[17] In a long-term study by Konig and Shaffer,[18] 175 children were followed for an average of 8.4 years (2.2 to 16.8 years). Their results showed that pulmonary function improved to normal values in both the group treated with corticosteroids and the group on cromolyn sodium. Cockcroft and Murdock[19] found evidence of protection against antigen challenge, with attenuation of both the early and the late phase asthmatic response with cromolyn sodium.

MDI Strength. As seen in Table 12-1, the difference between the nebulizer dose (20 mg) and the MDI dose (approximately 1.0 mg/actuation) of cromolyn sodium is 10-fold. If we assume that approximately 10% of an inhaled dose reaches the airway, as seen previously with adrenergic bronchodilators (see Chapter 6), equivalent doses are not available with the usual dose from the nebulizer and the MDI. Although not available in the United States, a 5 mg per actuation MDI strength is used in Great Britain. Holgate[16] cites several studies that have demonstrated that increased doses using the 5 mg MDI with two actuations give better protection against exercise challenge, with a longer duration of protection in more subjects.

Use in Angiotensin-Converting–Enzyme (ACE) Inhibitor Cough. Hargreaves and Benson[20] reported that cromolyn sodium two actuations, four times daily of the 5 mg MDI formulation, provided protection against the cough often seen as a side effect with use of angiotensin-converting–enzyme (ACE) inhibitors.[20] Cromolyn sodium significantly improved cough scores (frequency and severity) in 9 of the 10 patients in the study after 2 weeks. Cough was not completely suppressed in any of the 10 patients.

Anti–Sickle Cell Effects. Both the 4% intranasal solution and the 20 mg inhaled powder capsule of cromolyn given as a single dose were observed to cause a striking decrease in sickle cell percentage in nine African children with severe sickle cell disease. Improvement was seen 24 hours after administration of the single dose. The reduction in sickling is hypothesized to be due to the blocking of calcium-activated potassium channels, which play a major part in water loss and erythrocyte dehydration.[21]

CLINICAL APPLICATION OF CROMOLYN SODIUM

Three points should be emphasized concerning the clinical application of cromolyn sodium with asthma and hyperreactive airway states.

1. First, the drug is only prophylactic and should not be used during acute bronchospasm. This is based on its mode of action, because the drug must already be present to prevent mast cell degranulation. *It has no bronchodilating action* and in fact may cause further bronchial irritation as an aerosol.
2. Second, abrupt withdrawal of oral corticosteroids and substitution of cromolyn sodium in asthmatic patients can result in inadequate adrenal function. Cromolyn has no effect on the adrenal system, and tapered withdrawal of corticosteroids is necessary while beginning cromolyn use with patients.
3. Third, it may take from 2 to 4 weeks for improvement in the patient's symptoms, enabling a decrease in concomitant therapy such as bronchodilator or steroid use.

Guidelines for the management of asthma indicate that cromolyn sodium is used in subjects requiring regular use of β agonists for control of symptoms. It is considered an alternative to the use of inhaled corticosteroids, especially in children (see Appendix D).[1]

Dosage Regulation. The protective effect of cromolyn in allergic, nonallergic, or reflex-induced asthma is dose dependent. The usual dosage of 20 mg four times daily (80 mg/day) with the nebulized solution in some cases can be reduced to a maintenance dosage of 40 to 60 mg/day after the patient is stabilized for 1 or 2 months. Likewise, if stimuli for asthma increase in severity (e.g., heavy exercise in cold weather [skiing] as opposed to walking in warm weather), higher dosages or addition of a β agonist may be required. For seasonal allergy, cromolyn should be started at least 1 week before allergen exposure. The drug will protect if given 30 minutes before a specific allergen exposure (e.g., cat fur), and a single dose 15 minutes before exercise on an occasional instead of continuous basis is effective. As stated previously, the degree of exercise and the conditions must be considered in estimating the protection required. Long-term continual maintenance with cromolyn may be needed for patients with reflex-induced asthma or for those with late-phase reactions or severe bronchial reactivity and lability.[13,14]

NEDOCROMIL SODIUM (TILADE)

Nedocromil sodium was approved for general clinical use by the Food and Drug Administration (FDA) on December 30, 1992. The drug is an inhaled prophylactic antiasthmatic agent and is extensively reviewed by Gonzalez and Brogden.[22] Nedocromil is marketed as Tilade in an MDI formulation. Nedocromil is considered a second-generation antiasthmatic agent and is a cromolyn-like drug in its action and clinical use. The structure of nedocromil is illustrated in Figure 12-2. The drug is a disodium salt of a pyranoquinolone dicarboxylic acid.

As with cromolyn sodium, nedocromil sodium is indicated as prophylactic therapy in the management of mild to moderate asthma. The drug is a controller, not a reliever, has no bronchodilator properties, and is not indicated for use in the reversal of acute bronchospasm. Optimum control of asthma symptoms depends on regular use of the drug, even if symptoms of airway obstruction are not apparent.

DOSAGE AND ADMINISTRATION

Nedocromil is available as an MDI, with 1.75 mg per actuation, with at least 104 metered inhalations per canister. The recommended dosage by MDI for maintenance therapy in asthma is two inhalations four times a day.

MODE OF ACTION

Nedocromil sodium exerts its antiinflammatory and antiasthmatic effect by inhibiting the activation and activity of multiple inflammatory cells, including mast cells, eosinophils, airway epithelial cells, and sensory neurons.[23] Specific activities of nedocromil sodium are listed and illustrated in Figure 12-5.

- Nedocromil sodium inhibits mast cell cytokine release, such as release of histamine, tryptase, and tumor necrosis factor-α (TNF-α).
- Nedocromil sodium modulates the synthesis and release of proinflammatory cytokines such as IL-1β, IL-6, IL-8, granulocyte macrophage colony-stimulating factor (GM-CSF), tumor necrosis factor-α (TFN-α), and "regulated on activation, normal T cell expressed and secreted" (RANTES, an eosinophil-attracting chemokine), and adhesion molecules from airway epithelial cells.[23]
- Nedocromil sodium can inhibit eosinophil chemotaxis and adhesion in culture media containing the chemoattractive factors released from airway epithelial cells and can block the release of eosinophil cationic protein, which is involved in epithelial cell damage in the airway.[3]

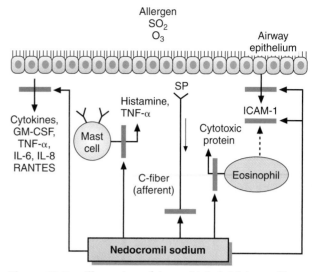

Figure 12-5   Illustration of the multiple inhibitory effects by which nedocromil sodium attenuates and prevents inflammation in the airway. *GM-CSF*, Granulocyte-macrophage colony-stimulating factor; *ICAM-1*, intercellular adhesion molecule-1; *IL-6, 8*, interleukin-6, 8; *RANTES*, regulated on activation, normal T cell expressed and secreted; *SP*, substance P; *TNF-α*, tumor necrosis factor-α.

- Nedocromil sodium can prevent neuronally mediated bronchoconstriction by inhibiting afferent sensory nerve impulses.[3] Nedocromil sodium can also inhibit the cytokines that lead to increased synthesis of neuropeptides, such as substance P, or other tachykinins.

It has been suggested that the activity of nedocromil sodium, as well as cromolyn sodium, in inhibiting activation and activity of inflammatory cells may be through a common pathway of chloride ion transport blockade. An influx of chloride ions is thought to be responsible for some of the high intracellular calcium concentration in *mast cells,* needed for degranulation. An efflux of chloride mediates in part the regulation of airway *epithelial cell size* and volume decrease with hypotonic induced swelling. Exercise probably causes a hypertonic airway surface fluid. By preventing chloride-regulated cell volume decrease in this instance, nedocromil sodium may alter the availability of afferent sensory nerves in the airways to mechanical or chemical irritants.[24] Finally, chloride efflux from *sensory nerves* produces depolarization and the action potential needed for nerve signal propagation. Evidence suggests that nedocromil sodium inhibits the chloride channels and the transport needed for each of these cell functions. This nonspecific chloride-channel blocking activity may protect the airway from nerve stimulation, which produces bronchospasm and cough, and inhibit the activity of mast cells and eosinophils in releasing mediators.

In summary, nedocromil sodium can inhibit mast cells, eosinophils, and airway epithelial cells, which taken together can release a wide range of mediators, inflammatory cytokines, and enzymes, all of which would otherwise produce airway inflammation in asthma. Unlike corticosteroids, which downregulate cytokine production to reverse inflammation in the airway, nedocromil sodium blocks further inflammation by blocking the activation of inflammatory cells.[23]

PHARMACOKINETICS

In asthmatic subjects given nedocromil sodium by inhalation, the peak plasma concentration varied between 5 and 90 minutes, with a terminal half-life of 1.5 hours. The drug is not metabolized and is excreted unchanged in humans. It is confined to the extravascular space and does not penetrate the central nervous system well. There is reversible binding to plasma protein (approximately 89% of the drug), and systemic bioavailability is low, although there is good absorption from the airway. Plasma clearance is more rapid than the absorption, at 10 ml/min/kg in humans, with urinary excretion.[25]

SIDE EFFECTS

Nedrocromil was well tolerated in both healthy volunteers and asthmatic subjects. The most commonly reported side effects are as follows[22]:

Unpleasant taste (13.6%)
Headache (4.8%)
Nausea (4.0%)
Vomiting (1.8%)
Dizziness (1% to 2%)

CLINICAL EFFICACY

Holgate[26] has reviewed the literature addressing the efficacy of nedocromil sodium in adults and in children ages 3 to 19 years.

Efficacy in Adults. In adults a dose of 2 MDI actuations two or four times daily has been shown to provide equal or better control of mild to moderate asthma compared with theophylline, based on daytime and nighttime asthma symptoms, need for inhaled bronchodilator, cough, and morning tightness. Nedocromil sodium has also been shown to be of potential use in reducing high-dose inhaled steroid use. Patients using 2000 µg of inhaled steroid were able to reduce their daily usage by 31% after using 4 mg (approximately two MDI actuations) four times daily. In a large meta-analysis of double-blind, placebo-controlled clinical trials of nedocromil sodium, nedocromil sodium demonstrated a significant effect compared with placebo on outcome variables of daytime and nighttime asthma symptoms, cough, peak expiratory flow rate, FEV_1, inhaled bronchodilator use, and patient report of control.[27] Doses included both twice-daily and four-times-daily schedules of two actuations. Clinical improvement was greatest in mild to moderate asthma and with continued bronchodilator treatment.

Efficacy in Children. When nedocromil sodium in a four-times-daily dose was added to current therapy in stable mild asthmatic children in placebo comparisons, there was significant improvement in daily peak expiratory flow and a reduction in daily bronchodilator use.[28] Nedocromil sodium 4 mg given twice daily has also been found to be equally effective compared with cromolyn sodium 5 mg four times daily in controlling asthma in children, offering a compliance advantage in the reduced dosing frequency. A long-term safety study in 65 chronic asthmatic children receiving nedocromil sodium 4 mg four times daily for 1 year showed excellent acceptability and only minor expected side effects of headache, cough, or pharyngitis.[29]

ANTILEUKOTRIENE AGENTS

The availability of the antileukotriene drugs represents the first new drug class in the treatment of asthma since the cromolyn-like agents became available in the early 1970s. These drugs are the culmination of chemical research that can be dated to the identification of the leukotrienes in 1979 and 1980 and the elucidation of their biochemical pathways and effects. Box 12-3 lists some of the notable events associated with the development of this class. The name *leukotriene* is based on the fact that these molecules were originally isolated from leukocytes and the carbon backbone has three double bonds in series, termed a *triene*. Chemical structures of the three antileukotriene drugs currently available in the United States are given in Figure 12-6. Two of these agents

Box 12-3	Historical Events Leading to the Development of the Antileukotriene Drugs for Asthma

1938	The laboratory of Feldberg and Kellaway named a material released from guinea pig lungs perfused with cobra venom and that caused smooth muscle contraction "slow-reacting muscle-stimulant substance" because the contraction was slower to develop than with histamine.	1979-1980	Identification of leukotriene A_4 (LTA_4); identification of the leukotrienes C_4, D_4, and E_4 (LTC_4, LTD_4, LTE_4) as the active components of SRS-A.
1960	The substance of Feldberg and Kellaway is subsequently named "slow-reacting substance of anaphylaxis" (SRS-A) by Brocklehurst and colleagues, based on its role in anaphylaxis-induced bronchoconstriction.	1996	Zafirlukast (Accolate) is approved by the FDA in late 1996.
		1997	Zileuton (Zyflo) is approved by the FDA.
		1998	Montelukast (Singulair) is approved by the FDA.
		1999	Cloning and characterization of the human cysteinyl leukotriene receptor $CysLT_1$ is reported.

FDA, Food and Drug Administration.

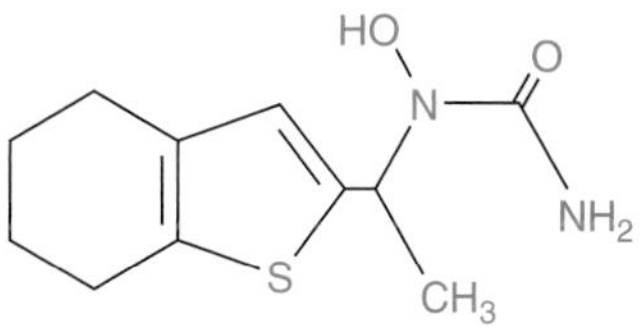

Zileuton

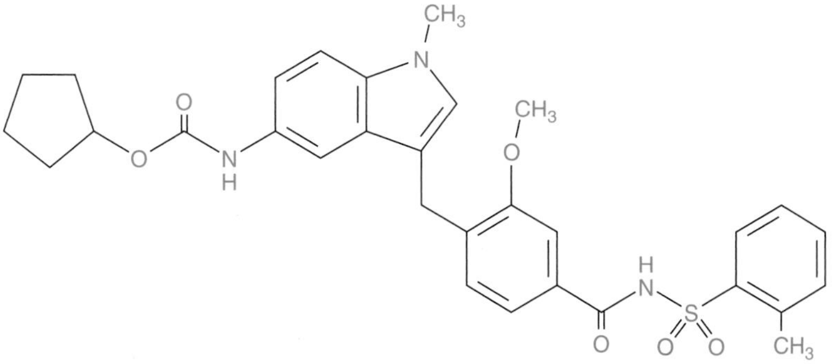

Zafirlukast

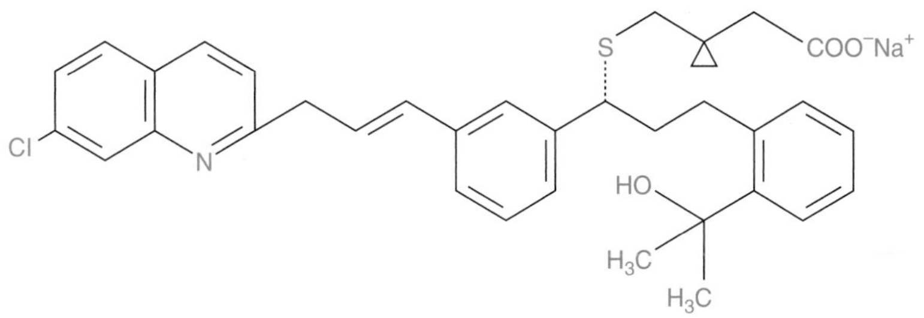

Montelukast

Figure 12-6 Chemical structures of the three antileukotriene agents (zileuton, zafirlukast, and montelukast).

(zafirlukast and montelukast) attach to and block the receptor for leukotrienes, and a third agent (zileuton) inhibits synthesis of leukotrienes.

LEUKOTRIENES AND INFLAMMATION

The following summary of the source, synthesis, and effects of leukotrienes is based on several sources, which offer more detailed information on these interesting mediators.[30-35]

The leukotrienes are members of a group of biologically active fatty acids including prostaglandins, thromboxanes, and lipoxins that are known as *eicosanoids*. These molecules are lipid mediators of inflammation that are synthesized from the fatty acid precursor arachidonic acid (5,8,11,14-eicosatetraenoic acid). Arachidonic acid is found in cell nuclear membrane phospholipids. The leukotrienes mediate directly or indirectly at least some of the inflammatory process seen in asthma. They are potent bronchoconstrictors and stimulate other cells to cause airway edema, mucus secretion, ciliary beat inhibition, and recruitment of other inflammatory cells into the airway.

CELL SOURCES OF LEUKOTRIENES

The leukotrienes and other lipid mediators are not preformed and stored in cells, but rather are synthesized after a mechanical, chemical, or physical stimulus that activates phospholipase A_2, an enzyme. These stimuli include antigen challenge of sensitized tissues and exposure to platelet activating factor (PAF) or other cytokines. Certain cells have the necessary enzymes to synthesize leukotrienes and other mediators. These include eosinophils, mast cells, monocytes, macrophages, basophils, neutrophils, and B lymphocytes.[31] Eosinophils, mast cells, and macrophages are present and recruited to the lung in asthma.[32]

BIOCHEMICAL PATHWAYS

A simplified diagrammatic view of the arachidonic acid cascade, which results in the various lipid mediators, is given in Figure 12-7. Essentially, free arachidonic acid is converted to various lipid mediators through two pathways: the cyclooxygenase and the 5-lipoxygenase. The cyclooxygenase pathway results in the prostaglandins (PGs) and thromboxane, and the 5-lipoxygenase (5-LO) pathway results in the

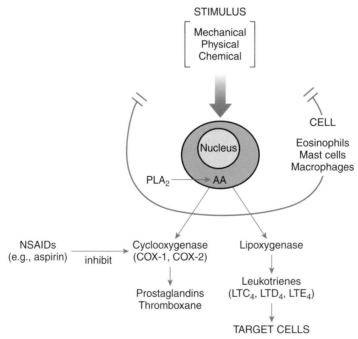

Figure 12-7   A simplified diagrammatic overview of stimuli and cell types involved in the arachidonic acid cascade and resulting in the cyclooxygenase products such as prostaglandins and the lipoxygenase pathway that produces leukotrienes. *AA*, Arachidonic acid; *COX-1*, *COX-2*, isoenzyme forms of cyclooxygenase; *LTC$_4$*, *LTD$_4$*, *LTE$_4$*, leukotrienes C$_4$, D$_4$, and E$_4$. *NSAIDs*, nonsteroidal antiinflammatory drugs; *PLA$_2$*, phospholipase A$_2$.

leukotrienes. Aspirin and other nonsteroidal antiinflammatory drugs (NSAIDs, e.g., ibuprofen) inhibit the cyclooxygenase enzyme to block prostaglandin and thromboxane production. There are two forms of the cyclooxygenase (COX) enzyme: COX-1 and COX-2. Many NSAIDs are mainly COX-1 selective, such as aspirin, ketoprofen, and indomethacin; some are slightly COX-1 selective, such as ibuprofen and naproxen. Other agents such as celecoxib and rofecoxib, used to treat arthritis, have primarily selective inhibition of COX-2. The 5-LO pathway results in the synthesis of the leukotrienes; this pathway is the target for drugs in the antileukotriene group.

Leukotriene Production

The lipoxygenase pathway resulting in leukotriene production is illustrated in Figure 12-8. After stimulation of an appropriate cell, the enzyme phospholi-

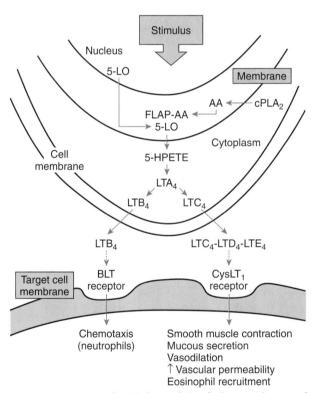

Figure 12-8 A detailed model of the synthesis of leukotrienes through the 5-lipoxygenase (5-LO) pathway and their effects on target cells. See text for a detailed description. *AA*, Arachidonic acid; *BLT*, B leukotriene (LTB_4) receptor; *cPLA₂*, cytosolic phospholipase A_2; *CysLT₁*, cysteinyl leukotriene receptor; *FLAP*, 5-lipoxygenase–activating protein; *5-HPETE*, 5-hydroperoxyeicosatetraenoic acid; *LTA₄*, *LTB₄*, *LTC₄*, *LTD₄*, *LTE₄*, leukotrienes A_4, B_4, C_4, D_4, and E_4.

pase A_2 (PLA_2), which is located in the cell cytoplasm, moves to the cell nuclear membrane. In the nuclear membrane, PLA_2 hydrolyzes phospholipids to liberate free arachidonic acid. Arachidonic acid (AA) binds to 5-LO activating protein (FLAP) (AA-FLAP). Another enzyme, 5-LO, moves from both the nucleus and the cell cytoplasm to the nuclear membrane and interacts with the AA-FLAP complex to oxygenate the arachidonic acid. This results in 5-hydroperoxyeicosatetraenoic acid (HPETE), which is then converted to the unstable intermediate, leukotriene A_4 (LTA_4). Leukotriene A_4 is the source of all the other leukotrienes. LTA_4 is converted either into leukotriene B_4 (LTB_4) or the cysteinyl leukotriene C_4 (LTC_4). Both LTB_4 and LTC_4 are exported from the cell to the extracellular space; LTC_4 is converted to leukotrienes D_4 and E_4 (LTD_4 and LTE_4). These three LTs are termed *cysteinyl LTs* because they each have the amino acid cysteine in their chemical structure. This is abbreviated to *CysLTs*. The three CysLTs, LTC_4, LTD_4, and LTE_4, have been identified as the components of the previously termed SRS-A (see Box 12-3).

CysLT Receptors and Effects of Leukotrienes

Leukotrienes bind to leukotriene receptors to exert their inflammatory effects. There are several different receptor types identified to date. LTB_4 binds to a seven-transmembrane spanning receptor, termed the *B leukotriene receptor* (BLT). The BLT receptor is involved in cellular recruitment (chemotaxis), probably of neutrophils, and may be involved in acute respiratory distress syndrome (ARDS). The cysteinyl LTs (CysLTs) attach to two subtypes of receptors: *CysLT₁* and *CysLT₂*. The proasthmatic actions of the cysteinyl LTs are mediated by the CysLT₁ receptor, which is located on smooth muscle cells in the airway and other cell types. The human CysLT₁ receptor has been cloned and characterized.[36] Stimulation of the CysLT₁ receptor causes bronchoconstriction, and the cysteinyl LTs are more potent airway constrictors than histamine.[32] In addition to direct bronchoconstriction, there is also an increase in bronchial hyperresponsiveness to other irritants such as histamine. Other effects include mucus secretion in the airway, increased vascular permeability causing airway wall edema, and plasma exudation into the airway lumen. The resulting protein and cellular debris in the airway, together with the mucous secretion, increases secretion viscosity and may lead to airway occlusion such as that seen in asthma. The cysLTs may also have an eosinophilic chemoattractant effect. Drugs that block the binding of leukotrienes to $CysLT_1$ receptors are named with the generic suffix -*lukast* (e.g., zafirlukast, montelukast, pranlukast). The $CysLT_2$ receptor subtype mediates constriction of pulmonary vascular smooth muscle.[37]

The CysLTs are produced largely by eosinophils, mast cells, and macrophages, all of which are cell types seen in the airways of asthmatics. Elevated levels of CysLTs may be markers of asthma. Leukocytes of asthmatics release more CysLTs than nonasthmatics. Plasma levels of LTE_4 correlate with asthma severity and are elevated in the urine of patients during an asthma attack, during exercise-induced asthma, and in the presence of nocturnal asthma symptoms.[32] Urinary LTE_4 is also elevated after challenge with allergen in atopic asthma or with aspirin in aspirin-sensitive asthmatics.[30]

ZILEUTON (ZYFLO)

Zileuton was approved for use in early 1997 as Zyflo, as an orally active inhibitor of 5-LO. Its structure is shown in Figure 12-6. This drug is indicated for the prophylaxis and chronic treatment of asthma and is approved for use in adults and children 12 years of age or older. It is considered as a controller agent rather than a reliever and has no indication for use in an acute asthma episode.

DOSAGE AND ADMINISTRATION

Zileuton is available in a single tablet strength of 600 mg. The recommended dosage for asthma is one 600 mg tablet, four times daily, for a total daily dose of 2400 mg. Zileuton is taken at meals and at bedtime. Hepatic transaminase enzymes should be measured and evaluated before initiation of treatment, once a month for the first 3 months, and every 2 to 3 months thereafter for the first year, with periodic monitoring for longer-term therapy. If clinical signs of liver injury (right upper quadrant pain, nausea, fatigue, lethargy, pruritus, jaundice, or flulike symptoms) develop, the drug should be discontinued.

MODE OF ACTION

Taken orally, zileuton inhibits the 5-LO enzyme, which would otherwise catalyze the formation of leukotrienes from arachidonic acid. Specifically, 5-LO in the presence of FLAP catalyzes the conversion of arachidonic acid to the intermediate 5-HPETE, which is converted to LTA_4 and ultimately the other leukotrienes. By interrupting the synthesis of these

biologically active leukotrienes, their contribution to the inflammatory responses in asthma is effectively blocked. Both the R- and the S-enantiomers are active as 5-LO inhibitors. The mode of action of zileuton is illustrated along with that of the other antileukotrienes in Figure 12-9.

PHARMACOKINETICS

Zileuton is rapidly absorbed when taken orally, with an apparent volume of distribution of 1.2 L/kg. The drug is about 93% bound to plasma proteins, including albumin. The drug has a half-life of 2.5 hours, is metabolized to glucuronide conjugates and an *N*-dehydroxylated metabolite in the liver by cytochrome P450 enzymes, and is eliminated in the urine and feces.

HAZARDS AND SIDE EFFECTS

Side effects with oral zileuton that are greater than those with placebo include headache, general pain,

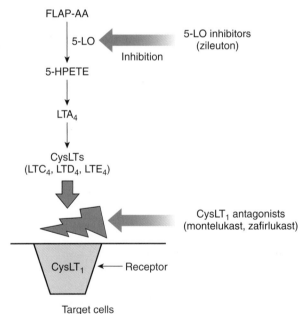

Figure 12-9   Illustration of the mode and site of action of the antileukotriene agents, zileuton, zafirlukast, and montelukast. Zileuton inhibits the 5-lipoxygenase (5-LO) enzyme to prevent leukotriene production, and zafirlukast and montelukast antagonize the action of the cysteinyl leukotrienes (*CysLTs*) at the leukotriene receptor, $CysLT_1$. *FLAP-AA*, 5-Lipoxygenase–activating protein, arachidonic acid; *5-HPETE*, 5-hydroperoxyeicosatetraenoic acid; LTA_4, C_4, D_4, E_4, leukotrienes A_4, C_4, D_4, E_4.

abdominal pain, loss of strength, and dyspepsia. Elevations of one or more liver function test values have occurred with zileuton, and it is recommended that hepatic transaminases be monitored before and during treatment. Liver enzyme levels may decrease or return to normal either during therapy or after discontinuation. Serum alanine aminotransferase (ALT, also known as SGPT) is a good indicator of liver injury. Zileuton is contraindicated in subjects with acute liver disease or transaminase elevations greater than three times the upper limit of normal.

Zileuton interacts with two important drugs in respiratory care: theophylline and warfarin. Zileuton can increase serum theophylline concentrations and can increase prothrombin time when given concomitantly with warfarin. Dose adjustments of theophylline and oral warfarin may be needed.

ZAFIRLUKAST (ACCOLATE)

Zafirlukast is a synthetic asthma prophylactic agent (a controller) approved for use in the United States in late 1996 as Accolate (its structure is illustrated in Figure 12-6). It is indicated for the prophylaxis and chronic treatment of asthma and has been approved for use in those 12 years of age or older. Zafirlukast was previously referred to by the code name ICI 204,219 in the literature. This drug inhibits asthma reactions induced by exercise, cold air, allergen, and aspirin. Oral forms of the drug inhibit both the early and late phase of asthma, but an inhaled formulation inhibits only the early response. The oral form of zafirlukast also causes modest bronchodilation, which is not produced by the inhaled form.[38,39]

DOSAGE AND ADMINISTRATION

Zafirlukast is taken as an oral tablet, 20 mg, twice daily in adults and children 12 years and older. Food reduces the bioavailability of the drug, and it should be taken at least 1 hour before or 2 hours after eating.

MODE OF ACTION

Zafirlukast, along with montelukast, are both leukotriene receptor antagonists and thereby block the inflammatory effects of leukotrienes (see Figure 12-9). Specifically, zafirlukast binds to the $CysLT_1$ receptors, with no agonist effect. This causes competitive inhibition of the leukotrienes LTC_4, LTD_4, and LTE_4 and subsequent blockade of the inflammatory effects described previously (in the discussion of leukotrienes and inflammation).

PHARMACOKINETICS

Zafirlukast is rapidly absorbed when taken orally. Peak plasma levels are reached 3 hours after dosing, with an elimination half-life of approximately 10 hours. Zafirlukast is metabolized in the liver, with 10% excreted in the urine and the remainder in the feces. Administration of zafirlukast with food reduces mean bioavailability by about 40%.

HAZARDS AND SIDE EFFECTS

The most common side effects reported in healthy volunteers and patients were headache, infection, nausea, diarrhea, and generalized and abdominal pain. Infections were predominantly respiratory. Because zafirlukast is metabolized by liver enzymes, hepatic impairment (e.g., in cirrhosis) will increase drug plasma levels. Although not noted in 6-month trials of zafirlukast, postmarketing surveillance indicated that doses higher than the 40 mg daily dose can cause elevations in serum aminotransferase concentrations.[37] A case of hepatitis and hyperbilirubinemia with no other attributable cause has been reported in a patient receiving 40 mg a day for 100 days, indicating the possibility of liver enzyme dysfunction with the drug (this case was reported in the manufacturer's drug literature).

MONTELUKAST (SINGULAIR)

In February, 1998, montelukast (Singulair) was approved by the FDA for general clinical use. The drug is an orally active leukotriene receptor antagonist (its structure is illustrated in Figure 12-6). Montelukast was previously referred to by its code name, MK-0476, in the literature. It is indicated for the prophylaxis and chronic treatment of asthma (a controller) and has no bronchodilating effect for use in acute asthma treatment. Montelukast is the only one of the three currently available antileukotriene agents that is approved for used in pediatrics (children 2 years or older). Montelukast has been shown to have clinical efficacy in treating mild to moderate asthma and exercise-induced bronchoconstriction. Compared with placebo, montelukast significantly improved asthma control in both children 6 to 14 years of age and adults over 15 years of age.[40-42] To date, no safety issues have appeared with pediatric use.

DOSAGE AND ADMINISTRATION

Montelukast is available as a 10 mg tablet and as a 4 mg and 5 mg chewable cherry-flavored tablet.

Adults and adolescents ≥15 years: One 10 mg tablet daily, taken in the evening

Pediatric patients 6 to 14 years: One 5 mg chewable tablet daily, taken in the evening

Pediatric patients 2 to 5 years: One 4 mg chewable tablet daily, taken in the evening

The drug can be taken with or without meals. Bioavailability when taken orally was not altered by a standard meal.

MODE OF ACTION

Like zafirlukast, montelukast is a competitive antagonist for the cysteinyl leukotrienes LTC_4, LTD_4, and LTE_4. It binds with high affinity and selectivity to the $CysLT_1$ receptor subtype (see Figure 12-9). Blockade of the $CysLT_1$ receptor prevents leukotriene stimulation of the receptor on target cells such as airway smooth muscle and secretory glands. Montelukast has been shown to inhibit both early- and late-phase bronchoconstriction caused by antigen challenge.

PHARMACOKINETICS

Montelukast is rapidly absorbed after oral administration. With a 10 mg dose, peak plasma concentration occurred in 3 to 4 hours, with a mean oral bioavailability of 64%. This bioavailability was not influenced by a standard meal in the morning. Concentration levels were slightly higher with the 5 mg chewable tablet taken while fasting in adults. For the 4 mg chewable tablet, the peak plasma concentration was reached in 2 hours. The drug is metabolized extensively in the liver and excreted via the bile, with little urinary excretion. Mean plasma half-life in adults ranged from 2.7 to 5.5 hours. Mild to moderate hepatic insufficiency will increase plasma levels, but no dosage adjustment is required. Severe hepatic impairment was not evaluated.

HAZARDS AND SIDE EFFECTS

The safety profile of montelukast is similar to placebo in drug testing. Adverse events that occurred in 2% or more of cases included diarrhea, laryngitis, pharyngitis, nausea, otitis, sinusitis, and viral infection. Hypersensitivity reactions were reported. Liver enzymes were not altered compared with placebo. Phenobarbital decreases the plasma level of montelukast, but the manufacturer suggests no dosage adjustment. If potent cytochrome P450 enzyme inducers such as phenobarbital or rifampin are used, appropriate clinical monitoring is suggested.

ROLE OF ANTILEUKOTRIENE DRUGS IN ASTHMA MANAGEMENT

The antileukotriene drugs, or leukotriene modifiers as they are also termed, are the first new drugs introduced for managing asthma since cromolyn sodium defined a new group in the early 1970s. Clinical experience is accumulating and helping to define the use of antileukotrienes in asthma. A summary of comparative features for the three currently available antileukotriene agents is given in Table 12-2. An excellent review of asthma management with these agents is given by Drazen and colleagues.[37]

PROTECTION AGAINST SPECIFIC ASTHMA TRIGGERS

Antileukotrienes are particularly useful in controlling asthma resulting from certain triggers, including exercise-induced asthma, aspirin-induced asthma, and, to a lesser extent, allergen-induced asthma.[37]

- *Exercise-induced asthma:* In exercise-induced asthma, cooling and drying of the airway promotes generation of leukotrienes, resulting in bronchoconstriction. Although protection varies from complete to very little, the antileukotrienes develop no tolerance and may benefit those who want to exercise or whose jobs require exercise under cold, dry conditions, without use of short-acting rescue β agonists.
- *Aspirin-induced asthma:* In 3% to 8% of asthma cases, aspirin or NSAIDs can cause bronchoconstriction as a result of an increase in leukotriene C_4 synthase activity. Based on such a pathophysiology, which involves leukotriene production, leukotriene modifiers are the treatment of choice of patients with aspirin-induced asthma.
- *Allergen-induced asthma:* Antileukotrienes also block the early asthma response to allergen challenge and attenuate airway obstruction in the late-phase response. They are not completely effective in abolishing the late response that is also due to histamine release.

CHRONIC PERSISTENT ASTHMA

The evidence to date supports the use of antileukotriene agents in the management of chronic asthma, including mild, moderate, or severe.[37,43,44] In mild to moderate asthma, antileukotrienes improve lung function, reduce the need for rescue β agonist use, and decrease asthma symptoms, including nocturnal symptoms. In moderate to severe asthma, the additive effect between antileukotrienes and inhaled

Table 12-2

Summary of comparative features of the three currently available antileukotriene agents

	ZILEUTON (ZYFLO)	ZAFIRLUKAST (ACCOLATE)	MONTELUKAST (SINGULAIR)
Action	5-LO inhibitor	$CysLT_1$ receptor block	$CysLT_1$ receptor block
Age range	≥12 yr	≥12 yr	≥2 yr
Dose	600 mg tab qid	20 mg tab bid	Adult: 10 mg tab q evening Children 6-14 yr: 5 mg tab q evening Children 2-5 yr: 4 mg tab q evening
Administration	Can be taken with food	1 hr before or 2 hr after meal	Taken with or without food
Drug interactions	Yes (theophylline, warfarin, propranolol)	Yes (warfarin, theophylline, aspirin)	No
Side effects (common)	Headache, dyspepsia, unspecified pain, liver enzyme elevations	Headache, infection, nausea, possible liver enzyme changes	Headache, influenza, abdominal pain
Contraindications	Active liver disease or elevated liver enzymes; hypersensitivity to components	Hypersensitivity to components	Hypersensitivity to components

$CysLT_1$, Cysteinyl leukotriene type 1; *5-LO*, lipoxygenase.

Box 12-4   Advantages and Disadvantages of Antileukotriene Drug Therapy in Managing Asthma

Advantages

- Oral administration, possible once-daily dosing
- Safe, with few side effects to date
- Effective in aspirin-sensitivity and often in exercise-induced asthma
- Systemic distribution reaches entire lung through the circulation
- Additive effect with inhaled steroids
- May reduce steroid dose, or prevent an increase in steroid dose
- A formulation approved for pediatric dosing (montelukast)

Disadvantages

- Relatively limited antiinflammatory action limited to one mediator pathway
- Unknown long-term toxicity
- Variable response—effective in about 50%-70% of patients
- No predictor of patients who will respond
- Systemic drug exposure, not limited to lung
- Generally not useful as monotherapy

---

corticosteroids is the basis for asthma control with lower steroid doses or without an increase in steroid dosing (inhaled or oral). There are advantages and disadvantages to antileukotriene drug therapy in asthma, which are summarized in Box 12-4.

Antileukotriene drug therapy is effective in approximately 50% of patients (although this proportion is higher in aspirin-sensitive individuals), but there is no method to predict which patients will be responders.[45,46] Considerable intersubject variability in re-

sponse has been seen. In a study of exercise challenge, 20 mg of zafirlukast gave complete protection in three subjects, partial protection in four subjects and no protection in one subject.[47]

ANTILEUKOTRIENES IN RELATION TO CORTICOSTEROIDS

Asthma guidelines agree that corticosteroids are the most effective antiinflammatory drugs for use in asthma, and they have a broader antiinflammatory activity than the more limited effect of the antileukotrienes. Leukotriene modifiers affect only one biochemical pathway—the lipoxygenase path and resulting leukotriene effects. Two aspects of antileukotriene therapy should be considered in relation to use of corticosteroids in asthma.

- Choosing between an inhaled steroid and an antileukotriene in mild persistent asthma is based on offsetting advantages: the superior efficacy of inhaled steroids with possibly poor compliance versus the anticipated superior compliance of the orally administered antileukotrienes with their more limited antiinflammatory action.[37]
- There is an additive effect between antileukotriene and inhaled corticosteroid therapy in mild to moderate asthma. A study by Laviolette and colleagues[48] showed a greater response to inhaled beclomethasone alone compared with oral montelukast alone. However, the combination of the two treatments resulted in the greatest improvement in lung function, as seen in Figure 12-10. In

another study, use of montelukast in adult asthmatics on chronic inhaled steroids resulted in a 47% reduction in steroid dose, compared with a 30% reduction in the placebo group.[49]

CHURG-STRAUSS SYNDROME

Churg-Strauss syndrome has been reported in a few patients treated with zafirlukast[50] or montelukast (postmarketing letter).[51] Churg-Strauss syndrome is a vasculitis of unknown etiology, usually occurring in adults between 20 and 40 years of age, marked by peripheral eosinophilia, eosinophilic infiltration of tissues, and necrotizing vasculitis that can result in major organ damage and death if left untreated. The syndrome is rare, with a prevalence of about 1 case per 15,000 to 20,000 patient-years of treatment. Cases to date who developed this syndrome have had difficult to control asthma and have been on oral or high doses of inhaled corticosteroids. It is not completely clear whether this is an effect of antileukotriene treatment or the syndrome is unmasked by a reduction in corticosteroid therapy allowed by the antileukotriene therapy.[37] A review by Wechsler and associates[51] of eight patients concluded that the occurrence of Churg-Strauss syndrome in asthmatic patients receiving antileukotriene treatment appeared to be due to unmasking of an underlying vasculitic syndrome diagnosed as moderate to severe asthma and treated with corticosteroids. Nevertheless, experience in humans with antileukotriene drugs, specifically $CysLT_1$ receptor antagonists, is still new, and all of the processes associated with 5-LO products are not completely understood. For example, a type 2 leukotriene receptor ($CysLT_2$), which is *not* blocked by the $CysLT_1$ antagonists such as zafirlukast or montelukast, has been identified on human pulmonary vasculature.[32] The effect of introducing a potential imbalance with $CysLT_1$ antileukotriene therapy is not well understood. Although antileukotriene drugs appear safe and effective, additional clinical experience is needed.

SUMMARY OF CLINICAL USE OF ANTILEUKOTRIENE THERAPY

The following points attempt to summarize current understanding of the role of antileukotriene drug therapy for asthma:

- Antileukotriene agents are prophylactic controller drugs used in persistent asthma, including mild, moderate, and severe states; they are not indicated for acute relief or rescue therapy.

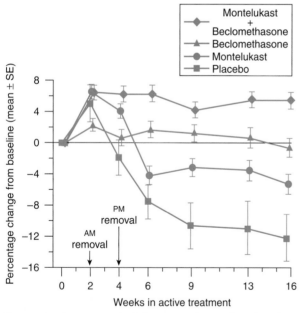

Figure 12-10   Mean (±SE) percent change from baseline in four treatment groups receiving combined inhaled beclomethasone and oral montelukast, beclomethasone alone, montelukast alone, or placebo. The AM and PM beclomethasone inhalers were replaced with placebo in the montelukast and placebo groups during the run-in period. (From Laviolette M and others: Montelukast added to inhaled beclomethasone in treatment of asthma, *Am J Respir Crit Care Med* 160:1862-1868, 1999.)

- Antileukotrienes can be tried as an alternative to inhaled corticosteroids or cromolyn-like agents in mild persistent asthma requiring more than as-needed β_2 agonists.
- Antileukotrienes may not be optimal as monotherapy in persistent asthma.
- Antileukotrienes may allow reduction of high-dose inhaled corticosteroids or prevent an increase in the dose of inhaled corticosteroids, and they reduce or prevent the need for oral corticosteroids.
- Evidence to date shows these agents as safe and often effective choices in managing a wide range of asthma severity.

FUTURE DIRECTIONS FOR ASTHMA THERAPY

Although questions exist concerning the usefulness of blocking the synthesis or activity of a single family of mediators such as leukotrienes, there is an unexpectedly high efficacy in clinical trials of these drugs that supports further development. This has fueled an interest in pursuing other mediator targets for treating allergic airway disease. These include new types of antileukotriene agents, as well as a variety of antagonists that can inhibit T cell–mediated inflammation. A review by Coyle and colleagues[52] gives more information on these biotherapeutic targets for treating allergic airway disease.

- *Additional antileukotriene agents:* There are two other potential points to interrupt the 5-LO pathway, which produces leukotrienes. These are (1) FLAP inhibitors, which prevent the protein (FLAP) from providing arachidonic acid as a substrate for LT synthesis by 5-LO and (2) competitive antagonists at the LTB_4 receptor. Agents acting at these points in the lipoxygenase pathway have been under investigation.
- *Cytokine receptor blockers:* Cytokines such as interleukin-5 (IL-5) and interleukin-4 (IL-4) attach to IL receptors and mediate some of the lymphocyte processes in allergic airway diseases. Humanized monclonal antibodies (MAbs) such as IL-5 MAb has been shown to provide protection in primate studies of allergic airway disease. Nebulized IL-4 receptor α subunit (IL-4rα), to which IL-4 binds, improved FEV_1 in patients with moderate asthma.
- *Anti-IgE monoclonal antibodies:* A recombinant antihuman IgE MAb designated as E25 has been shown to inhibit IgE-mediated bronchoconstrictor response to inhaled antigen, as well as the late-phase response associated with eosinophil infiltration into the airway.
- *Chemokine receptor antagonists:* The chemokines play an important role in the migration of leukocytes from blood vessels into the extracellular site of inflammation. The effects of chemokines are mediated by a family of transmembrane G protein–linked receptors. Selectively targeting these receptors may allow modification of the effector functions of T and B lymphocytes.
- *IL-1 receptor antagonists:* The IL-1 receptor superfamily is found on both Th1 and Th2 lymphocytes. Activation of both types of lymphocytes by interleukins leads to inflammation, including the Th2-driven eosinophilic inflammation of the airways.

As understanding of the mechanisms for immune reactions and allergy at the cellular level continue to increase, it is hoped that new and effective, safe, and nontoxic drug treatment will follow.

RESPIRATORY CARE ASSESSMENT OF NONSTEROIDAL ANTIASTHMA AGENTS

- Evaluate patient for optimal aerosol delivery formulation for inhaled medications, if more than one delivery system is available (e.g., SVN, MDI). Note age, ability to understand instructions, and need for reservoir with MDI.
- Initially for aerosol medications: Instruct patient in use of aerosol delivery system selected (MDI, reservoir, SVN) and then verify correct use.
  - Assess breathing rate and pattern.
  - Assess breath sounds by auscultation, before and after treatment.
  - Assess pulse before and after treatment.
  - Assess patient's subjective reaction to treatment, for any change in breathing effort or pattern.
- Verify that patient understands that nonsteroidal antiasthma agents are controller drugs and understands their difference from a rescue bronchodilator (relieving agent); assess patient's understanding of the need for consistent use of these agents (compliance with therapy).
- Instruct patient in use of a peak flow meter, to monitor baseline PEF and changes. Verify that there is a specific action plan based on symptoms and peak flow results. The patient should be clear

on when to contact a physician with deterioration in PEF or exacerbation of symptoms.

- Long term: Assess severity of symptoms (coughing, wheezing, nocturnal awakenings, symptoms during exertion); use of rescue medication; number of exacerbations, missed work/school days, and pulmonary function. Modify level of asthma therapy (up or down, as described in NAEPP EPR-II guidelines for step therapy).
- Assess for presence of side effects with nonsteroidal antiasthma agents (refer to particular agent and its side effects, as listed previously).

SUMMARY KEY TERMS AND CONCEPTS

- *Asthma* is an inflammatory disorder of the airways in which *allergic stimuli* often trigger *IgE-mediated mast cell* release of mediators of inflammation. Airway reactivity can be triggered by *nonspecific stimuli* such as cold air or dust as well.
- Allergic inflammation of the airway is a product of an *immune* response, and the *T lymphocyte* plays a central role in attracting mast cells and *eosinophils,* which in turn release mediators that attract other cells and damage epithelial cells.
- The *clinical result* of asthma is chronic persistent airway inflammation and occasional acute episodes of wheezing and airway obstruction caused by *bronchoconstriction, mucosal swelling,* and *mucus secretion.*
- Drugs that act to *inhibit the mediators* of inflammation include *cromolyn sodium, nedocromil sodium, zafirlukast, montelukast,* and *zileuton.* These agents are *prophylactic* and intended for the management of chronic asthma rather than for relief of acute airway obstruction. They do not provide bronchodilation in an acute asthma episode. *Cromolyn* is available as a DPI, a nebulizer solution and an MDI, and acts as a mast cell stabilizer. *Nedocromil sodium* is available as an MDI, and acts on multiple cells (mast cells, eosinophils, airway epithelium), sensory neurons and mediators to inhibit the inflammatory response. These agents are indicated in the management of *mild to moderate asthma,* when more than occasional β agonist use is needed. *Zafirlukast* and *montelukast* are available as oral agents, and act by competitive antagonism of the leukotriene receptor CysLT$_1$, to prevent bronchoconstriction, vascular permeability and mucus secretion. *Zileuton* is another oral agent, and acts by inhibiting the 5-lipoxygenase enzyme, to prevent generation of leukotrienes.

SELF-ASSESSMENT QUESTIONS

1. Identify five nonsteroidal antiasthma drugs used in the management of chronic asthma; give both generic and brand names.
2. Which immunoglobulin is implicated in allergy and is termed cytophilic?
3. Which type of asthma involves allergic reaction to an antigenic stimulus?
4. Which type of helper T cell, Th1 or Th2, is involved primarily in the atopic allergic response?
5. A resident wishes to order nebulized cromolyn sodium for a young asthmatic patient in the emergency department who is wheezing and in moderate distress. Would you agree?
6. Which of the following could be recommended as possible choices for the asthmatic patient in question 5: inhaled albuterol, inhaled salmeterol, inhaled ipratropium bromide, theophylline either orally or intravenously?
7. What is the usual dose of nedocromil sodium by inhalation in adults?
8. An asthmatic patient has been on 40 mg of oral prednisone for a week after an acute asthma attack and an emergency department visit. His physician now wants to switch him to inhaled nedocromil and discontinue the oral prednisone. What is the risk in doing this and what would you recommend?
9. Briefly compare and distinguish the mode of action of nedocromil sodium versus cromolyn sodium.
10. How does the mode of action of zafirlukast and montelukast differ from that of zileuton?
11. What is the recommended dose and route of administration for zafirlukast, montelukast, and zileuton?
12. Which of the three antileukotriene agents in question 11 offers the most convenient dosing and the fewest drug interactions?

Answers to Self-Assessment Questions are found in Appendix A.

CLINICAL SCENARIO

A 45-year-old white female calls her pulmonologist and is seen in the emergency department with a complaint of chest tightness, shortness of breath, and wheezing for the past 1.5 days. She also complains of a cough, with only occasional thin whitish sputum during that period. She denies any fever or chills. She has been diagnosed with adult-onset asthma for the past 3 years and is aspirin-sensitive. She has no history of tobacco use. She had a nasal polypectomy two years ago. Since that time she has been maintained on pirbuterol breath-actuated inhaler as needed and since about 4 months ago on oral theophylline 300 mg twice daily. She is alert but mildly anxious.

Her vital signs are T, 97° F; P, 92 beats/min and regular; BP, 90/60 mm Hg; and RR, 22 breaths/min with no laboring. Expiration is slightly prolonged, but there is no use of accessory muscles. No cyanosis is evident. Auscultation reveals diffuse wheezes, greater on expiration than inspiration, and rhonchi bilaterally. Routine blood work later showed hemoglobin, 13.5 g/dl and WBC count, $6.1 \times 10^3/mm^3$ with 13% eosinophils. Electrolytes were also found to be within normal limits, except for a plasma glucose of 281 mg/dl. A chest radiograph showed some hyperinflation bilaterally, with no infiltrates, no pneumothorax, and normal heart size. An arterial blood gas on room air revealed pH, 7.38; $Paco_2$, 42 mm Hg; Pao_2, 72 mm Hg; base excess, +0.3 mEq/L; and Sao_2, 96%.

On questioning, she states that she has been using her as-needed pirbuterol, two inhalations, almost every 4 hours over the past 24 hours, with little improvement. She has found it necessary to use her inhaler most days of the week. She also states that she has been experiencing many headaches, upset stomach, some lack of appetite, and insomnia often during the week. It has been 2 to 3 hours since she last used her pirbuterol inhaler.

How would you treat her asthma attack at this point?
What medications would you consider for maintenance of her asthma, given her recent history and prior medications?

Answers to Clinical Scenario Questions are found in Appendix A.

REFERENCES

1. National Asthma Education and Prevention Program, Expert Panel Report II: *Guidelines for the diagnosis and management of asthma*, Bethesda, Md, 1997, National Institutes of Health.
2. Platts-Mills TAE and others: Changing concepts of allergic disease: the attempt to keep up with real changes in lifestyles, *J Allergy Clin Immunol* 98:S297, 1996.
3. Holgate ST: A rationale for the use of nedocromil sodium in the treatment of asthma, *J Allergy Clin Immunol* 98:S157, 1996.
4. Drazen JM, Turino GM: Progress at the interface of inflammation and asthma: report of an ATS-sponsored workshop November, 1993, *Am J Respir Crit Care Med* 152:386, 1995.
5. National Institutes of Health: *Global initiative for asthma, Global strategy for asthma management and prevention*, NHLBI/WHO workshop report, Bethesda, Md, 1995, National Institutes of Health.
6. Flak TA, Goldman WE: Autotoxicity of nitric oxide in airway disease, *Am J Respir Crit Care Med* 154:S202, 1996.
7. Liggett SB, Levi R, Metzger H: G-protein coupled receptors, nitric oxide, and the IgE receptor in asthma, *Am J Respir Crit Care Med* 152:394, 1995.
8. Altounyan REC: Inhibition of experimental asthma by a new compound: disodium cromoglycate (Intal), *Allergy* 22:487, 1967.
9. Orr TSC: Mast cells and allergic asthma, *Br J Dis Chest* 67:87, 1973.
10. Orr TSC, Hall DE, Allison AC: Role of contractile microfilaments in the release of histamine from mast cells, *Nature* 236:350, 1972.
11. McFadden ER Jr: Cromolyn: first-line therapy for chronic asthma? *J Respir Dis* 8:39, 1987.
12. O'Byrne PM, Dolovich J, Hargeave FE: Late asthmatic responses, *Am Rev Respir Dis* 136:740, 1987.
13. Bernstein IL: Cromolyn sodium, *Chest* 87(suppl):68S, 1985.
14. Bernstein IL: Cromolyn sodium in the treatment of asthma: coming of age in the United States, *J Allergy Clin Immunol* 76:381, 1985.
15. Settipane GA, Klein DE, Boyd GK: Adverse reactions to cromolyn, *J Am Med Assoc* 241:811, 1979.
16. Holgate ST: Inhaled sodium cromoglycate, *Respir Med* 90:387, 1996.
17. Edwards AM: Sodium cromoglycate (Intal) as an anti-inflammatory agent for the treatment of chronic asthma, *Clin Exp Allergy* 24:612, 1994.
18. Konig P, Shaffer J: Long-term (3-14 years) outcome in children with asthma treated with cromolyn sodium, *Am J Respir Crit Care Med* 149:A210, 1994.
19. Cockcroft DW, Murdock KY: Comparative effects of inhaled salbutamol, sodium cromoglycate, and beclomethasone dipropionate on allergen-induced early asthmatic responses, late asthmatic responses, and increased bronchial responsiveness to histamine, *J Allergy Clin Immunol* 79:734, 1987.
20. Hargreaves MR, Benson MK: Inhaled sodium cromoglycate in angiotensin-converting- enzyme inhibitor cough, *Lancet* 345:13, 1995.
21. Toppet M and others: Antisickling activity of sodium cromoglycate in sickle-cell disease *Lancet* 356:309, 2000 (research letter).
22. Gonzalez JP, Brogden RN: Nedocromil sodium: a preliminary review of its pharmacodynamic and pharmacokinetic properties, and therapeutic efficacy in the treatment of reversible obstructive airways disease, *Drugs* 34:560, 1987.
23. Devalia JL and others: Nedocromil sodium and airway inflammation in vivo and in vitro, *J Allergy Clin Immunol* 98:S51, 1996.

24. Alton EWFW, Norris AA: Chloride transport and the actions of nedocromil sodium and cromolyn sodium in asthma, *J Allergy Clin Immunol* 98:S102, 1996.

25. Clark B: General pharmacology, pharmacokinetics, and toxicology of nedocromil sodium, *J Allergy Clin Immunol* 92:200, 1993.

26. Holgate ST: The efficacy and therapeutic position of nedocromil sodium, *Respir Med* 90:391, 1996.

27. Edwards AM, Stevens MT: The clinical efficacy of inhaled nedocromil sodium (Tilade) in the treatment of asthma, *Eur Respir J* 6:35, 1993.

28. Armenio L and others: Double blind, placebo controlled study of nedocromil sodium in asthma, *Arch Dis Child* 68:193, 1993.

29. Shields M and others: One year of treatment with flavoured nedocromil sodium in young children, *Eur Respir J* 7(suppl 18):139S, 1994.

30. Busse W: The role and contribution of leukotrienes in asthma, *Ann Allergy Asthma Immunol* 81:17, 1998.

31. Busse W: Leukotrienes and inflammation, *Am J Respir Crit Care Med* 157(June suppl):S210, 1998.

32. Bisgaard H: Role of leukotrienes in asthma pathophysiology, *Pediatr Pulmonol* 30:166, 2000.

33. Samuelsson B: The discovery of the leukotrienes, *Am J Respir Crit Care Med* 161(Feb suppl):S2, 2000.

34. Peters-Golden M, Brock TG: Intracellular compartmentalization of leukotriene biosynthesis, *Am J Respir Crit Care Med* 161(Feb suppl):S36, 2000.

35. Peters-Golden M: Cell biology of the 5-lipoxygenase pathway, *Am J Respir Crit Care Med* 157(June suppl):S227, 1998.

36. Lynch KR and others: Characterization of the human cysteinyl leukotriene CysLT$_1$ receptor, *Nature* 399:789, 1999.

37. Drazen JM, Israel E, O'Byrne PM: Treatment of asthma with drugs modifying the leukotriene pathway, *N Engl J Med* 340:197, 1999.

38. Holgate ST, Bradding P, Sampson AP: Leukotriene antagonists and synthesis inhibitors: new directions in asthma therapy, *J Allergy Clin Immunol* 98:1, 1996.

39. Dahlen B and others: The leukotriene-antagonist ICI-204,219 inhibits the early airway reaction to cumulative bronchial challenge with allergen in atopic asthmatics, *Eur Respir J* 7:324, 1994.

40. Knorr B and others: Montelukast for chronic asthma in 6- to 14-year-old children: a randomized, double-blind trial, *J Am Med Assoc* 279:1181, 1998.

41. Reiss TF and others: Montelukast, a once-daily leukotriene receptor antagonist, in the treatment of chronic asthma: a multicenter, randomized, double-blind trial, *Arch Intern Med* 158:1213, 1998.

42. Leff JA and others: Montelukast, a leukotriene-receptor antagonist, for the treatment of mild asthma and exercise-induced bronchoconstriction, *N Engl J Med* 339:147, 1998.

43. Becker A: Leukotriene receptor antagonists: efficacy and safety in children with asthma, *Pediatr Pulmonol* 30:183, 2000.

44. Kemp J: Role of leukotriene receptor antagonists in pediatric asthma, *Pediatr Pulmonol* 30:177, 2000.

45. Ind PW: Anti-leukotriene intervention: is there adequate information for clinical use in asthma? *Respir Med* 90:575, 1996.

46. Smith LJ: Newer asthma therapies, *Ann Internal Med* 130:531, 1999.

47. Finnerty JP and others: Role of leukotrienes in exercise-induced asthma, *Am Rev Respir Dis* 145:746, 1992.

48. Laviolette M and others: Montelukast added to inhaled beclomethasone in treatment of asthma, *Am J Respir Crit Care Med* 160:1862, 1999.

49. Löfdahl C and others: Randomised, placebo controlled trial of effect of a leukotriene receptor antagonists, montelukast, on tapering inhaled corticosteroids in asthmatic patients, *Br Med J* 319:87, 1999.

50. Wechsler ME and others: Pulmonary infiltrates, eosinophilia, and cardiomyopathy following corticosteroid withdrawal in patients with asthma receiving zafirlukast, *J Am Med Assoc* 279:455, 1998.

51. Wechsler ME and others: Churg-Strauss syndrome in patients receiving montelukast as treatment for asthma, *Chest* 117:708, 2000.

52. Coyle AJ, Lloyd CM, Gutierrez-Ramos J: Biotherapeutic targets for the treatment of allergic airway disease, *Am J Respir Crit Care Med* 162:S179, 2000.

CHAPTER 13

Aerosolized Antiinfective Agents

Joseph L. Rau

*C*hapter 13 discusses antiinfective agents currently approved for administration as inhaled aerosols: pentamidine isethionate (NebuPent), ribavirin (Virazole), tobramycin (TOBI), and zanamivir (Relenza). Pentamidine is used to prevent and treat *Pneumocystis carinii* pneumonia (PCP) in patients with acquired immunodeficiency syndrome (AIDS), and ribavirin is used for treating respiratory syncytial virus (RSV) infection. A formulation of prepared antibody to RSV, termed *respiratory syncytial virus immune globulin intravenous (RSV-IGIV)*, offers prophylaxis; a monoclonal antibody, palivizumab (Synagis), offers prophylaxis and treatment for RSV infection. Inhaled tobramycin is available for management of *Pseudomonas aeruginosa* infections in patients with cystic fibrosis.

Zanamivir is an inhaled antiviral agent used to treat influenza.

CLINICAL INDICATIONS FOR AEROSOLIZED ANTIINFECTIVE AGENTS

Clinical indications for each of the aerosolized antiinfective agents available at the time of this edition are given. Each agent is discussed separately in detail.

INDICATION FOR AEROSOLIZED PENTAMIDINE

Pentamidine by inhalation is indicated as second-line therapy for the *prevention* of PCP in high-risk human immunodeficiency virus (HIV)-infected patients who have a history of one or more episodes of PCP or a

Table 13-1

Currently available inhaled antiinfective agents, listed by generic and brand name, along with formulations, usual recommended dosage, and clinical use*

DRUG	BRAND NAME	FORMULATION AND DOSAGE	CLINICAL USE
Pentamidine isethionate	NebuPent	300 mg powder in 6 ml sterile water; 300 mg once every 4 wk	PCP prophylaxis
Ribavirin	Virazole	6 g powder in 300 ml sterile water (20 mg/ml solution); given 12-18 hr/day for 3-7 days by SPAG nebulizer	RSV
Tobramycin	TOBI	300 mg/5 ml ampule Adults and children ≥6 yr: 300 mg bid, 28 days on/28 days off the drug	*Pseudomonas* aeruginosa in CF
Zanamivir	Relenza	DPI: 5 mg/inhalation Adults ≥12 yr: 2 inhalations (one 5 mg blister per inhalation) bid ≈12 hr apart for 5 days	Influenza

*Details on use and administration should be obtained from manufacturer's drug insert material before use.
CF, Cystic fibrosis; *PCP, Pneumocystis carinii* pneumonia; *RSV,* respiratory syncytial virus; *SPAG,* small particle aerosol generator.

peripheral CD4+ (T4 helper cell) lymphocyte count of 200/mm^3 or less.

INDICATION FOR AEROSOLIZED RIBAVIRIN

Aerosolized ribavirin is indicated for the *treatment* of hospitalized infants with severe lower respiratory tract infection caused by RSV.

INDICATION FOR AEROSOLIZED TOBRAMYCIN

Aerosolized tobramycin is indicated for the *management* (control) of chronic *P. aeruginosa* infection in cystic fibrosis.

INDICATION FOR INHALED ZANAMIVIR

Inhaled zanamivir is indicated for the *treatment* of uncomplicated acute illness caused by influenza virus in adults and adolescents age 12 years or over who have been symptomatic for no more than 2 days.

IDENTIFICATION OF AEROSOLIZED ANTIINFECTIVE AGENTS

Each of the antiinfective agents available for inhalation is listed in Table 13-1, along with details of formulation, usual recommended dosage, and clinical use. These agents are each discussed in more detail.

AEROSOLIZED PENTAMIDINE

Pentamidine isethionate is an antiprotozoal agent that is active against *P. carinii,* the causative organism for

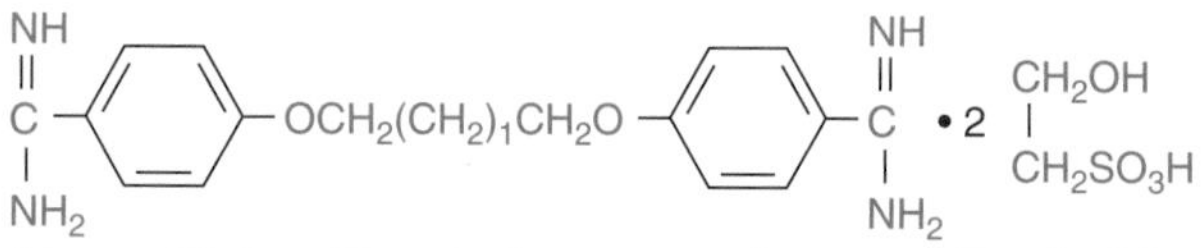

Figure 13-1 Chemical structure of pentamidine isethionate (NebuPent).

PCP. Chemically, it is an aromatic diamidine, whose structure is seen in Figure 13-1. Pentamidine is an old agent and has been used for years to treat protozoal infections. The drug was first synthesized in 1937, and it has been used since the 1940s to treat African sleeping sickness (trypanosomiasis). Pentamidine is also effective against other protozoal infections, including leishmaniasis, pneumocystosis, and babesiosis (a disease caused by an erythrocytic protozoan parasite).[1] Pentamidine can be given either parenterally or as an inhaled aerosol, but it is not absorbed with oral administration. When given parenterally, either intravenously or intramuscularly, the drug distributes quickly to the major organs (liver, kidneys, lung, pancreas). There it binds to tissues and is stored for months. After a single intramuscular dose, the drug can be detected in the urine 270 days later.

INTRODUCTION OF AEROSOLIZED PENTAMIDINE (NEBUPENT)

Both systemic and aerosol administration of pentamidine have been used for the treatment of PCP, which occurs as a common opportunistic respiratory infection in individuals with AIDS. In addition to the prophylactic use of aerosolized pentamidine, the aerosol form has also been used for treatment of acute episodes. The first report by Montgomery and associates in 1987 was for therapy of acute episodes of PCP.[2]

The rationale for aerosol administration of pentamidine to treat or prevent PCP is based on the same rationale as for other inhaled aerosol drugs used to treat the pulmonary system: local targeted lung delivery, with fewer or less severe side effects compared with systemic administration. Aerosolized pentamidine produces significantly higher lung concentrations than intravenous administration.[3] The San Francisco prophylaxis trial, published in 1990, showed that 300 mg of aerosol pentamidine every 4 weeks was effective in preventing PCP in patients with HIV infection.[4] Unfortunately, subsequent clinical experience with aerosolized pentamidine did not show improved clinical efficacy compared with oral drugs such as trimethoprim-sulfamethoxazole (TMP-SMX), and toxic side effects still occurred.

DESCRIPTION OF PNEUMOCYSTIS CARINII PNEUMONIA

The organism *P. carinii* was first noted in the lungs of guinea pigs by Chagas in 1909 and Carinii in 1910. It was named as a new organism by Delanöe and Delanöe in 1912, as *Pneumocystis carinii*, to describe the cystic form in the lungs and its earlier discoverer. Mammals are commonly infected with the organism at an early age, probably through an airborne vector. Disease occurs when there is suppression of the immune system. Before the AIDS pandemic, PCP was reported in malnourished infants in the 1940s and 1950s and in the 1970s in premature infants able to survive.[5] When not contained by a competent immune system, *P. carinii* causes the pneumonia termed *PCP*. This produces a foamy intraalveolar exudate, which contains cysts of *P. carinii*. The life cycle of *P. carinii* and the resulting pneumonia is illustrated in Figure 13-2. Both pentamidine and TMP-SMX are effective against PCP and are usually given parenterally to treat an acute episode.

DOSAGE AND ADMINISTRATION

Details of dose and administration of NebuPent, the aerosolized brand of pentamidine, can be found in manufacturer's literature. The following summary is not intended to replace the more detailed instructions that accompany the drug.

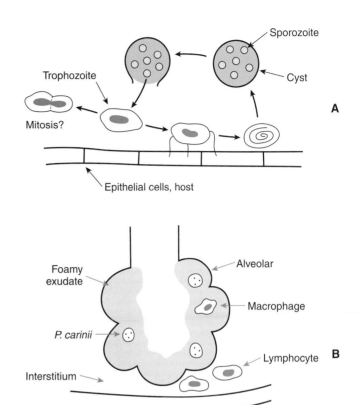

Figure 13-2   Pathogenesis of *Pneumocystis carinii* pneumonia (PCP). **A,** Life cycle of *P. carinii.* **B,** *P. carinii.* pneumonia pathology.

DOSAGE

The approved dose of aerosolized pentamidine for prophylaxis of PCP in AIDS subjects is 300 mg, given by inhalation once every 4 weeks. This dose may be altered by physicians in treating individual patients.

NebuPent, the brand of pentamidine approved for inhalation as an aerosol, is supplied as a dry powder, with 300 mg in a single vial. This must be reconstituted with 6 ml of sterile water for injection, USP (not saline, which can cause precipitation), added to the vial. The entire 6 ml of reconstituted solution is placed into the nebulizer.

ADMINISTRATION

Approval of aerosolized pentamidine by the Food and Drug Administration (FDA) was for administration with the Respirgard II nebulizer. This is a small

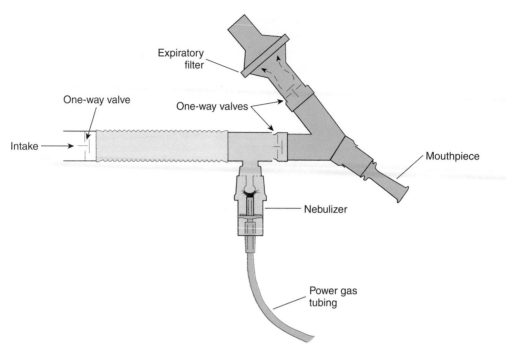

Figure 13-3   Diagrammatic illustration of the Respirgard II nebulizer system, showing one-way valves and expiratory filter to scavenge exhaust aerosol.

volume nebulizer (SVN) system, powered by compressed gas, fitted with a series of one-way valves and an expiratory filter (Figure 13-3). This nebulizer system has been described by Montgomery and associates.[3] The Respirgard II should be powered with a flow rate of 5 to 7 L/min from a 50-psi source or, alternatively, by controlling the flow with a 22- to 25-psi pressure source connected to the small-bore tubing of the nebulizer. Pressures below 20 psi are not sufficient to produce the desired particle size necessary for peripheral delivery of the drug. These requirements with the Respirgard II are found in the manufacturer's literature and further discussed in Corkery.[6]

NEBULIZER PERFORMANCE

Although nebulized pentamidine was approved for general clinical use with the Respirgard II nebulizer system, other nebulizers are used to administer the drug. Table 13-2 summarizes various reports in the literature on the particle sizes produced by different nebulizers with pentamidine.

The general requirement for effective nebulization of pentamidine is a particle size or distribution of sizes with a mass median diameter (MMD) of 1 to 2 microns. This is needed for the following two reasons[6]:

1. To achieve peripheral intraalveolar deposition targeted at the location of the microorganism
2. To reduce or prevent airway irritation seen with larger particle sizes, which will deposit more in larger airways

Studies by Vinciguerra and Smaldone[10] and Smaldone and associates[7] have examined nebulizer performance and compared treatment time and patient tolerance of aerosolized pentamidine with the Respirgard II versus other nebulizers. Both treatment times and efficiency in drug availability was actually greater with the AeroTech II than the approved Respirgard II.

MODE OF ACTION

The exact mode of action of pentamidine is not known. The drug's toxic effect on *P. carinii* may be due to multiple actions. Pentamidine blocks RNA and DNA synthesis, inhibits oxidative phosphorylation, and interferes with folate transformation.[1,5,11] Resistance to pentamidine by *P. carinii* has not been shown, and this may be due to the multiple effects of the drug on the organism's metabolism.[1]

Table 13-2

Particle size production of nebulizing systems used to deliver pentamidine by aerosol for inhalation*

NEBULIZER	MMD (MICRONS)	REFERENCE
AeroTech II	1.0 (at 10 L/min)	Smaldone, 1988[7]
	2.0 (at 7 L/min)	Corkery, 1988[8]
Respirgard II	0.76 (at 6 L/min)	Smaldone, 1988[7]
	0.93 (at 7 L/min)	Corkery, 1988[8]
	1.24 (at 6 L/min)	Dolovich, 1990[9]
Fisoneb USN	2.5 (on minimum)	Smaldone, 1988[7]
	5.0 (at 7 L/min)†	Corkery, 1988[8]
	2.6 (on minimum)	Dolovich, 1990[9]
Pulmosonic USN	4.2 (at 7 L/min)	Corkery, 1988[8]
Porta-sonic USN	1.6 (at 7 L/min)	Corkery, 1988[8]
	1.95 (at 6 L/min)	Dolovich, 1990[9]
Fan Jet	4.3 (at 7 L/min)	Corkery, 1988[8]

*As reported in the literature. First authors of each study are given, with the complete citation provided in the reference list.
†Use of auxiliary gas flow to drive aerosol from chamber.

When given by inhaled aerosol, pentamidine reaches significantly higher concentrations in the lung than when given intravenously.[3] The inhaled drug first binds to lung tissue. Although plasma levels are much less than with parenteral administration, the drug is slowly absorbed into the circulation and distributed to body tissues, as with parenteral administration. As a result, prolonged aerosol administration can result in systemic accumulation. Approximately 75% of the drug is excreted in urine and 25% in feces over the months after administration.

SIDE EFFECTS

The side effects seen with systemic therapy of PCP using either pentamidine or TMP-SMX provided part of the rationale for aerosol administration of pentamidine. Although both of these drugs are effective in a majority of patients with PCP when given systemically, over 50% of patients experience adverse effects.

SIDE EFFECTS WITH PARENTERAL PENTAMIDINE

Side effects with *parenteral* administration of pentamidine have been summarized in several reviews, with numerous references.[1,6] Parenteral use of pentamidine has resulted in the following:

- Pain, swelling, and abscess formation at the site of injection, with intramuscular administration
- Thrombophlebitis and urticarial eruptions, with intravenous administration

- Hypoglycemia (up to 62% of patients), with a cumulative cytotoxic effect on pancreatic β cells
- Impaired renal function and azotemia
- Hypotension
- Leukopenia
- Hepatic dysfunction

SIDE EFFECTS WITH AEROSOL ADMINISTRATION

Side effects with aerosol administration can be differentiated into local airway effects and systemic effects. *Local airway effects* with aerosol administration have included the following:

- Cough and bronchial irritation in 36% of patients in one study[4]
- Shortness of breath
- Bad taste (bitter or burning) of the aerosol impacting in the oropharynx
- Bronchospasm and wheezing in 11% of patients[4]
- Spontaneous pneumothoraces[12]

In addition, the following *systemic reactions* have occurred with aerosolized pentamidine:

- Conjunctivitis
- Rash
- Neutropenia
- Pancreatitis[13]
- Renal insufficiency
- Dysglycemia (hypoglycemia and diabetes)

- Digital necrosis in both feet[14]
- Appearance of extrapulmonary *P. carinii* infection.

Because of the pharmacokinetics of pentamidine, chronic treatment with the aerosol can lead to tissue accumulation in the body, causing some of the same side effects as with parenteral administration. Suppression of *P. carinii* with local targeting of the lung has resulted in the appearance of infection elsewhere in the body.

PREVENTING AIRWAY EFFECTS

Use of a β-adrenergic bronchodilator before inhaling aerosolized pentamidine can reduce or prevent local airway reaction, including reduction of coughing or wheezing. Ipratropium has also been shown to prevent bronchoconstriction by Quieffin and colleagues.[15] The airway reaction may be caused by the sulfite moiety in isethionate, which is known to cause airway irritation or by the drug itself.[16,17] This effect can be reduced by use of a nebulizing system producing very small particle sizes, which will lessen airway deposition and increase alveolar targeting.[6]

ENVIRONMENTAL CONTAMINATION BY NEBULIZED PENTAMIDINE

The following concerns exist regarding environmental contamination from nebulized pentamidine:

1. Exposure to the drug itself from the exhaust aerosol
2. Risk of infection with tuberculosis (TB), a disease associated with AIDS, from patients being treated with aerosolized pentamidine

Pentamidine is not known to be teratogenic, based on its use in pregnant women with African sleeping sickness (trypanosomiasis), although detailed clinical data were not kept. The drug is not mutagenic and its carcinogenic potential is considered minimal.[1] Studies have shown that low levels of pentamidine can be detected in healthcare workers exposed to the drug during treatments.[18,19] The investigators concluded that exposure probably occurred during treatment interruptions, usually caused by coughing episodes. Healthcare workers have also complained of conjunctivitis and bronchospasm when aerosolizing the drug.[1] Based on these reports and the long tissue half-life of pentamidine, contact with the drug should be held to a minimum or prevented if possible.

The risk of TB when treating AIDS patients with nebulized pentamidine is based on an association of TB and AIDS, the airborne mode of transmission of TB, and the fact that pentamidine aerosol can cause coughing and expulsion of droplet nuclei containing tuberculosis bacilli during aerosol treatments.

ENVIRONMENTAL PRECAUTIONS

The following precautionary measures are suggested in administering the drug, to reduce the risk of both drug exposure and TB infection with aerosolized pentamidine.[20-23]

- Use a nebulizer system with one-way valves and expiratory filter.
- Stop nebulization if the patient takes the mouthpiece out of the mouth (a thumb control on the power gas tubing gives more control).
- Use nebulizers producing an MMD of 1 to 2 microns, to increase alveolar targeting and lessen large airway deposition and cough production.
- Always use a suitable expiratory filter and one-way valves with the nebulizer. Instruct patients to turn off the nebulizer when talking or when taking it out of the mouth.
- Screen patients for cough history and pretreat with a β agonist, with sufficient lead time for effect in reducing the bronchial reactivity.
- Administer aerosol in a negative-pressure room, with six air changes per hour, or consider using an isolation booth/hood assembly with an exhaust fan and air directed through a high-efficiency filter.
- Use barrier protection (gloves, mask, eyewear) for healthcare workers.
- Screen patients with HIV infection for TB, and treat where evidence of infection exists.
- Do not allow treatment patients to mix with others until coughing subsides.
- Healthcare workers should periodically screen themselves for TB.
- Pregnant women and nursing mothers should avoid exposure to the drug, and all practitioners should limit exposure to the extent possible.

Although measures exist to radically limit environmental contamination with aerosolized pentamidine, many of these are expensive, such as negative-pressure rooms and improved ventilation exchange in older buildings. Others are difficult, such as the wearing of effective high-efficiency masks in a busy clinical setting for a prolonged period. The use of room disinfection with ultraviolet light has been reviewed[24] but is debated.[21]

AEROSOL THERAPY FOR PROPHYLAXIS OF PNEUMOCYSTIS CARINII PNEUMONIA: CLINICAL APPLICATION

Comparisons between the efficacy of aerosolized pentamidine with oral TMP-SMX, together with reports of serious adverse effects with aerosolized pentamidine, caused a reevaluation of aerosol therapy with pentamidine for prophylaxis of PCP. General recommendations for prophylaxis of PCP have been published by the Centers for Disease Control (CDC) in *Morbidity and Mortality Weekly Report* (MMWR) for HIV-positive adults[26] and for children.[25] In the 1992 CDC recommendations, oral TMP-SMX was preferred over aerosol pentamidine for prophylaxis of PCP, as long as adverse side effects from TMP-SMX were absent or acceptable.[26] Aerosolized pentamidine is now recommended as a second-line therapy for prophylaxis of PCP.

AEROSOL THERAPY OF ACUTE PNEUMOCYSTIS CARINII PNEUMONIA

It is important to note the difference between the acute use of aerosolized pentamidine and the prophylactic use. The use reported by Montgomery and associates[2] in 1987 was an acute use. In that report, aerosolized pentamidine was given to 15 patients with AIDS who were experiencing a first episode of pneumonia caused by *P. carinii*. Patients received 600 mg of aerosolized pentamidine once a day for 21 days. Of the 15 patients, 13 responded to therapy.

A study by Conte and colleagues[27] compared aerosol pentamidine, 600 mg with intravenous pentamidine, 3 mg/kg, in 45 patients with mild to mod-erate first episodes of PCP. Their conclusion was that the reduced-dose intravenous pentamidine was more effective than aerosolized pentamidine for treating mild to moderate PCP. The study enrollment was in fact halted because of relapse, none-response, or early recurrence of symptoms in the aerosol group.

RIBAVIRIN

Ribavirin (Virazole) is classified as an antiviral drug; it is active against respiratory syncytial virus (RSV), influenza viruses, and herpes simplex virus. Chemically, it is a nucleoside analogue and resembles guanosine and inosine; it was first synthesized in 1972.[28] Ribavirin is virostatic, not viricidal, and inhibits both DNA and RNA (retrovirus) viruses.

Ribavirin has been used throughout the world for a variety of viral infections, including RSV, influenza types A and B, and Lassa fever. Clinical trials of aerosolized ribavirin for severe RSV infection were conducted by Caroline Hall and associates[29,30] and showed significant improvement with ribavirin treatment compared with placebo. Ribavirin was approved as an antiviral agent by the FDA in 1986 for aerosol treatment of serious RSV infections in hospitalized patients.

CLINICAL USE

Infection with RSV in children results in either bronchiolitis or pneumonia. Guidelines concerning use of ribavirin were published by the Committee on Infectious Diseases of the American Academy of Pediatrics in 1987, and the recommendations were updated in 1993.[31,32] Box 13-1 summarizes the recommendations from the 1993 committee report. In general, the drug

---

Box 13-1	**American Academy of Pediatrics Recommendations for Use of Ribavirin in Treatment of Respiratory Syncytial Virus (RSV) Infection**

Patients hospitalized with RSV lower respiratory tract disease, at high risk for severe/complicated RSV infection secondary to other conditions, such as the following:

- Complicated congenital heart disease
- Bronchopulmonary dysplasia, cystic fibrosis, or other chronic lung conditions
- Premature infants
- Immunodeficiency
- Recent transplant recipients

- Those on chemotherapy for malignancy
- Infants who are severely ill (Pao_2, 65 torr; Sao_2, <90%, increasing $Paco_2$)
- Patients on mechanical ventilation for RSV infection
- Hospitalized infants at increased risk of progressing from mild to complicated course because of young age (<6 weeks) or underlying condition (multiple congenital anomalies, certain neurological or metabolic diseases [e.g., severe cerebral palsy, myasthenia])

From American Academy of Pediatrics, Committee on Infectious Disease: Uses of ribavirin in the treatment of respiratory syncytial virus infection, *Pediatrics* 92:501, 1993.

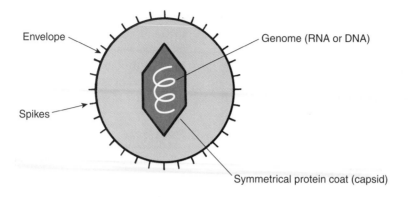

Virion: extracellular virus particle

Figure 13-4   Structure of a virus, showing nuclear material (DNA, RNA), protein coat, and an envelope.

is recommended primarily for infants and children at increased risk for severe lower respiratory tract disease and for those severely ill with RSV, including all patients on mechanical ventilation for RSV infection.[32]

The clinical use of ribavirin to treat RSV infection in infants and children remains the subject of debate, and the 1993 recommendations of the American Academy of Pediatrics have been questioned.[33] Ribavirin treatment by aerosol is expensive and risks environmental exposure to the drug by personnel. Studies have given conflicting results on whether use of ribavirin significantly reduces outcomes such as ventilator days, oxygen needs, intensive care unit days, hospital days, or mortality.[34,35]

NATURE OF VIRAL INFECTION

A short summary of viruses and viral infection is presented to establish key principles and concepts needed for understanding the difficulties in treating viral diseases, as well as the mode of action of ribavirin.

Virus: A virus can be defined as an obligate intracellular parasite, containing either DNA or RNA, that reproduces by synthesis of subunits within the host cell and causes disease as a consequence of this replication.

Figure 13-4 illustrates the simple structure of a virus. These are primitive members of the animal kingdom, submicronic in size, that consist of a strand of DNA or RNA that is surrounded by a protein coat. A virus may or may not be surrounded by an envelope, whose glycoprotein spikes are partially obtained from the host cell.

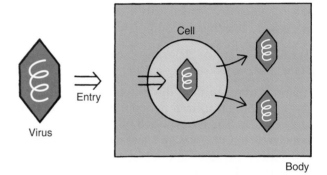

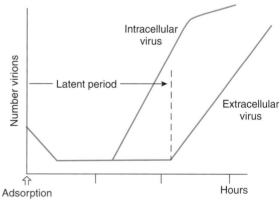

Figure 13-5   Sequence of viral infection, illustrating intracellular replication before dissemination in the body.

The concept and sequence of a viral infection is shown in Figure 13-5. A virus enters the body through a variety of routes (oral, inhaled, mucous membranes) and then invades a host cell. This is a multistep process consisting of phases in which the virus adsorbs to the cell, penetrates the cell, uncoats itself, goes through a process of recoding cell DNA (transcription, translation, synthesis), assembles itself, and sheds from the cell. The host cell usually dies in the process. Clinically, signs of a viral infection do not occur until after the initial latent period, when the virus leaves the cell, as illustrated in Figure 13-5. At this point, infection is well-established. The diagnosis of viral illness is usually based on clinical signs, including the symptoms, age of the patient, and time of year. Definitive diagnosis requires isolating the virus or demonstrating an antibody titer increase. Diseases produced by viruses include chickenpox, smallpox, fever blisters (herpes simplex virus), genital herpes, poliomyelitis, the common cold, AIDS, influenza, mumps, and measles.

Because of the nature of viral infection, as just outlined, antiviral drug treatment, whether for the common cold or for HIV infection, is difficult. In particular, there are three complications in treating viral disease with drugs, as follows:

1. Attacking the intracellular virus may harm the host cell.
2. Viral replication is maximal before the appearance of symptoms.
3. Viruses have the property of antigenic mutability; that is, they change their appearance to the immune system.

RESPIRATORY SYNCYTIAL VIRUS INFECTION

Respiratory syncytial virus (RSV), isolated in 1956, can cause bronchiolitis and pneumonia. Almost all children are exposed to the virus by their second year of life, and in most the infection is mild and self-limiting. Outbreaks of RSV pneumonia are seasonal and peak during winter months (November to March), with some variation according to geographical region.

The name of the virus reflects its effects on cells, which is to cause the formation of large, multinucleated cells, or a syncytium. The virus spreads easily by personal contact or hand contamination from surfaces. No effective vaccine exists to prevent RSV respiratory disease. Prepared antibody to RSV is available and is discussed below (RSV Immune Globulin).

DOSAGE AND ADMINISTRATION

The following is a descriptive summary of ribavirin dosage and administration. It is not intended to replace detailed instructions contained in manufac-

turer's literature, which should be reviewed before administering this drug. This includes the operating manual for the small particle aerosol generator (SPAG) nebulizing system.

DOSAGE

Ribavirin is given in a 20 mg/ml solution, which is administered by nebulizer (SPAG-2) for 12 to 18 hours per day, for a minimum of 3 days and not more than 7 days. The drug is supplied as 6 g of powder in a 100-ml vial. The powder is reconstituted first in the vial with sterile United States Pharmacopeia (USP) water for injection/inhalation, transferred to the large volume (500 ml) reservoir of the nebulizer, and further diluted to a total volume of 300 ml with sterile water. This gives a concentration of 6 g/300 ml, or 20 mg/ml, a 2% strength solution.

ADMINISTRATION

Clinical trials of ribavirin aerosol were carried out using a large volume nebulizing system, known as a small particle aerosol generator (SPAG). The drug was approved for general use with this aerosol generator. A diagram of the SPAG unit is shown in Figure 13-6. It is a large volume, pneumatically powered nebulizer operating on a jet shearing principle, with baffling of aerosol particles and with a drying chamber to further reduce particle size to a level of approximately 1.3 microns, MMD. Solutions in the SPAG reservoir should be replaced after 24 hours. Residual solution in the reservoir should be discarded before adding newly reconstituted solution. The drug solution should always be visually inspected for particulate matter or discoloration before use.

The nebulizer is connected to a hood as the patient interface. The manufacturer specifically warns against administration of the drug to infants requiring mechanical ventilation, because of the risk of drug precipitation occluding expiratory valves and sensors or even the endotracheal tube. However, the sickest infants with RSV are likely to need ventilatory support, and there are reports of drug use with mechanical ventilation. Detailed information concerning precautions with ventilator use during administration of the drug have been described by Demers and colleagues.[36] A clinical study of aerosol administration with mechanical ventilation of infants with severe RSV infection was reported by Smith and associates,[34] who showed that treatment reduced duration of ventilation, oxygen support, and hospital stay. Although labor-intensive,

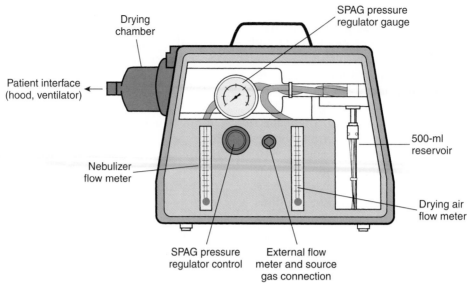

Figure 13-6   Diagrammatic illustration of the small particle aerosol generator (SPAG) unit used for nebulizing ribavirin.

mechanical ventilatory administration of ribavirin actually simplifies environmental control.

MODE OF ACTION

The mechanism of action by which ribavirin exerts its virostatic effect is not completely understood. Its viral inhibition is probably based on its structural resemblance to the nucleosides used to construct the DNA chain.[28] Figure 13-7 shows the structures of the natural nucleoside guanosine together with that of ribavirin, which is a synthetic nucleoside analogue. During the formation and assembly of new viral protein within the cell, ribavirin is most likely taken up instead of the natural nucleoside to form the DNA chain. This prevents construction of viable viral particles and subsequent shedding of virus into the bloodstream. A conceptual illustration of the process is shown in Figure 13-8. Ribavirin does not prevent the attachment or the penetration of respiratory syncytial virus into the cell and does not induce interferon.[28]

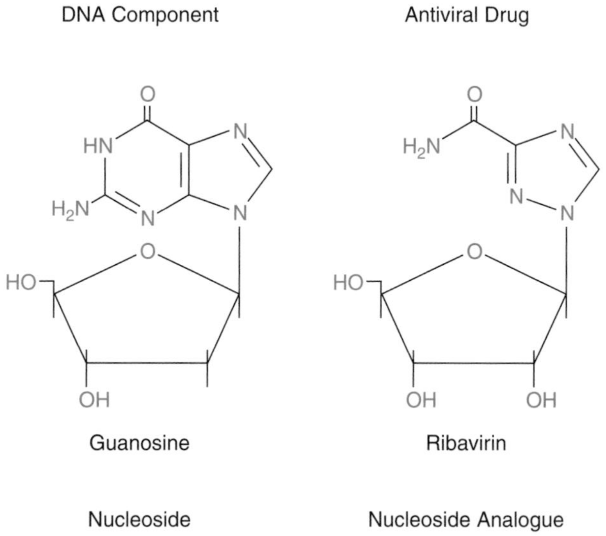

When given by inhaled aerosol, ribavirin levels are much greater in respiratory secretions than in the bloodstream. Waskin[1] gives a referenced summary of ribavirin kinetics. With 8 to 20 hours of aerosol treatment, peak plasma levels are 1 to 3 μg/ml, and respiratory secretion levels are greater than 1000 μg/ml. The minimal inhibitory concentration (MIC) for RSV is in the range of 4 to 16 μg/ml. The half-life of rib-

Figure 13-7   The similarity of the ribavirin molecule to the DNA precursor component, guanosine, may be the basis for the drug's virostatic effect.

avirin is about 9 hours in plasma and about 1 to 2 hours in respiratory secretions, which is the rationale for the almost continuous administration by aerosol.

SIDE EFFECTS

Side effects seen with aerosolized ribavirin are listed in product literature and have been reviewed by Waskin,[1] who gives detailed references. The following

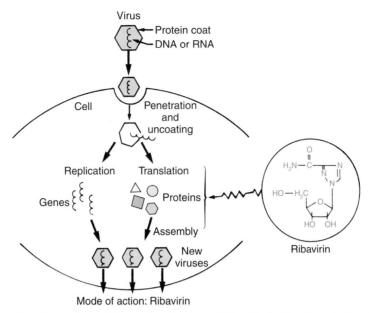

Mode of action: Ribavirin

Figure 13-8   Illustration of the mode of action of ribavirin in blocking viral replication.

list summarizes adverse effects reported, including those seen with adults receiving the drug.

Pulmonary: Deterioration of pulmonary function and worsening of asthma or chronic obstructive disease; pneumothorax, apnea, and bacterial pneumonia.

Cardiovascular: Cardiovascular instability, including hypotension, cardiac arrest, and digitalis toxicity.

Hematological: Effects on blood cells have been reported with oral or parenteral administration but not with aerosol use. Reticulocytosis (excess of young erythrocytes in the circulation) has been reported, however, with aerosol use.

Dermatological/Topical: Rash, eyelid erythema, and conjunctivitis have also been noted.

Equipment related: Equipment-related adverse effects with ribavirin treatment include occlusion and impairment of expiratory valves and sensors with ventilator use and endotracheal tube blockage from drug precipitate.

Although the above effects have been reported, common effects clinically are pulmonary function deterioration, equipment malfunction from drug precipitate, and skin irritation from excess drug precipitation.

ENVIRONMENTAL CONTAMINATION WITH AEROSOLIZED RIBAVIRIN

There is concern among healthcare workers over exposure to ribavirin. The drug has potential for mutagenic and carcinogenic effects, based on in vitro and

animal studies.[1] The effect on fertility is uncertain, but the drug has caused testicular lesions in rats. The effect on pregnancy is of particular concern because the drug is teratogenic or embryocidal in animal species. Acute effects from aerosolized ribavirin reported by healthcare workers have included precipitation on contact lens and conjunctivitis, headache (51%), rhinitis, nausea, rash, dizziness, pharyngitis, and lacrimation (10% to 20%). Several cases of bronchospasm or chest pain have been reported by individuals with reactive airway disease. The symptoms noted have resolved within hours after discontinuing exposure to the drug.[37]

Minimal levels of ribavirin exposure are difficult to specify because of lack of dose-response data for humans.[38] Corkery and others[39] state that the California Department of Health Services recommended an acceptable occupational airborne concentration for 8 hours of limited exposure to be $1/1000$th of the lowest no-observed effect level, which would be 2.5 $\mu g/m^3$.

Although there are no reports to date of serious effects from drug exposure by aerosol, precautions to limit or avoid exposure to the drug are well indicated, as advocated by Kacmarek.[40] Pregnant females, or those wishing to become pregnant, should avoid exposure to the drug if at all possible. In addition, environmental containment is superior to personnel barrier protection alone. Standard surgical masks do not prevent inhalation of 1- to 2-μm particles. Dermal absorption of ribavirin appears to be negligible.[32] ICN Pharmaceuticals makes available a containment system for use when the drug is aerosolized to an oxyhood, and several similar systems have been proposed in the literature.[41-43] All have common features of enclosure around the hood, with vacuum extraction and filtering of gas from the enclosure. Details needed for use can be found in the references given. It is recommended that the drug be administered in well-ventilated areas, that is, six or more air changes per hour.

RESPIRATORY SYNCYTIAL VIRUS IMMUNE GLOBULIN INTRAVENOUS (HUMAN)

Respiratory syncytial virus immune globulin intravenous (RSV-IGIV) is a sterile liquid formulation of immunoglobulin G (IgG) containing neutralizing antibody to RSV. The immunoglobulin is prepared from pooled human plasma containing high titers of neutralizing antibody against RSV. RSV-IGIV is available as RespiGam, and each milliliter contains 50 mg immunoglobulin, primarily IgG, and trace amounts of IgA and IgM. A vaccine against RSV, which has not been successfully developed yet, would stimulate active immunity against RSV. RSV-IGIV, as prepared antibody against RSV, confers passive immunity. The product was approved by the FDA on January 18, 1996. The drug is used on a prophylactic basis against RSV.

INDICATION FOR USE

RSV-IGIV is indicated for the prevention of serious lower respiratory tract infection with RSV in children younger than 24 months with bronchopulmonary dysplasia (BPD) or history of premature birth (less than 35 weeks of gestation).

DOSAGE AND ADMINISTRATION

The drug is available in 50-ml vials, containing 2500 mg of RSV immunoglobulin. It is administered as a monthly intravenous infusion of 750 mg/kg. The solution is infused at 1.5 ml/kg/hr for 15 minutes and then increased to 3 ml/kg/hr for 15 minutes if no adverse clinical effects occur. The dose is increased to a maximum rate of 6 ml/kg/hr, which should not be exceeded. Slower infusion rates may be needed in very ill children.

Infusion should begin within 6 hours and be completed by 12 hours after beginning to use the vial. Infuse children at risk (as indicated) each month during RSV season (usually November through April in the Northern Hemisphere).

MODE OF ACTION

RSV-IGIV is prepared immunoglobulin specific to RSV. As such, it is the antibody to RSV. When given intravenously, the product places antibody to RSV in the bloodstream of the patient, and the patient achieves a level of immunity to RSV. Because the recipient did not develop the antibody in response to RSV infection (which would be active immunity), this is a passive immunity. Upon exposure to RSV, the subject's immune system is prepared to neutralize the infecting agent.

ADVERSE REACTIONS

Side effects with infusion of RSV-IGIV can include fluid volume overload. Fever/pyrexia has also occurred. Immediate allergic, hypersensitivity reactions may occur. Reactions similar to other immunoglobulin infusions may occur, including dizziness, flushing, changes in blood pressure, palpitations, chest tightness, dyspnea, abdominal cramps, pruritus, myalgia, and arthralgia. These may be controlled with the rate of infusion. Generally, RSV-IGIV has been well tolerated. In the PREVENT clinical trial of RSV prophylaxis in children with BPD or prematurity, there was no difference in adverse events between placebo and RSV-IGIV treatment.[37]

The efficacy and safety of RSV-IGIV have not been established in children with congenital heart disease (CHD). Data representing the efficacy of RSV-IGIV showed a positive trend but were not statistically significant. In clinical trials, children with CHD with right to left shunts appeared to have an increased frequency of cardiac surgery and a greater frequency of severe and life-threatening adverse events associated with cardiac surgery.[37]

RSV-IGIV is treated with a solvent-detergent viral inactivation procedure to guard against possible transmission of blood-borne viruses.

CLINICAL EFFICACY

RSV-IGIV offers a prophylactic alternative to the treatment of acute RSV infection with aerosolized ribavirin. In studies of RSV prophylaxis, monthly doses of 750 mg/kg of RSV-IGIV were effective in reducing RSV hospitalization in high-risk children with BPD or prematurity. In the PREVENT clinical trial, RSV-IGIV reduced hospitalization resulting from RSV infection by 41% and total days of hospitalization by 53%.

PALIVIZUMAB (SYNAGIS)

Palivizumab represents the new drug class of therapeutic monoclonal antibodies.[44] The drug was approved by the FDA on June 19, 1998, for the prevention and treatment of RSV in premature infants and those with bronchopulmonary dysplasia (BPD).

INDICATION FOR USE

Palivizumab is indicated for the prevention of serious lower respiratory tract disease caused by RSV in children and infants at high risk. Safety and efficacy were established for infants with BPD and infants who had been premature.

DOSAGE AND ADMINISTRATION

The lyophilized drug is reconstituted with 1 ml of sterile water, giving 100 mg/ml. The recommended dose is 15 mg/kg, given intramuscularly once a month throughout the RSV season. The injection should be given in the anterolateral aspect of the thigh rather than the gluteal muscle, to avoid sciatic nerve damage.

MODE OF ACTION

Palivizumab is a humanized monoclonal antibody produced by recombinant DNA techniques, directed against the F protein of the RSV virus. As an antibody against the RSV virus, palivizumab provides neutralizing and fusion-inhibiting activity, preventing viral replication.

ADVERSE REACTIONS

The proportions of subjects in placebo and treatment groups receiving palivizumab who had adverse reactions were similar in clinical trials. Manufacturer's literature states that palivizumab was discontinued in five patients: two with vomiting and diarrhea, one with erythema and moderate induration at the site of the fourth injection, and two because of preexisting medical conditions. Other reactions that occurred in both treatment and placebo groups included upper respiratory infection, otitis media, rhinitis, rash, pain, and hernia, as well as coughing, wheezing, bronchiolitis, and other respiratory complications.

CLINICAL EFFICACY

In a large multicenter trial of infants at high risk of RSV infection, palivizumab given 15 mg/kg intravenously reduced the rate of hospitalization resulting from RSV infection to 4.8%, compared with 10.6% in placebo recipients.[45] Adverse events were again similar in placebo and treatment groups.

AEROSOLIZED TOBRAMYCIN

HISTORICAL BACKGROUND ON USE OF AEROSOL ANTIBIOTICS

The rationale for aerosol administration of antibiotics in respiratory infections is the same in general as for other drug classes: to deliver the drug directly to the target organ (lung), with less systemic toxicity and possibly with less drug, for a given lung level. This was the motivation for aerosolizing penicillin in 1944 for pneumonia reported by Bryson and associates,[46] when wartime demands kept antibiotic supplies in short supply. Krasno and Rhoads[47] reported the inhalation of penicillin dust for a variety of respiratory infections in 1949, using a mask for inhalation through mouth and nose and a plastic mouthpiece device with a surprisingly contemporary appearance.

A variety of antibiotics have been tried as inhaled aerosols, including neomycin and methicillin for *Staphylococcus aureus* in the 1950s and 1960s.[48] The aminoglycosides gentamicin, tobramycin, and amikacin, along with agents from other antibiotic groups, such as colistin, ceftazidime, and amphotericin, also have been nebulized. Aerosol delivery of antibiotics and direct endotracheal instillation were reviewed in the 1974 and 1979 conferences on the scientific basis of respiratory care.[49,50] A listing of selected reports of aerosolized antibiotics, both for cystic fibrosis and other respiratory diseases, is given in Table 13-3.[51-61] Although antibiotics have been administered as inhaled aerosols for years, there was no approved antibiotic for aerosol use until late 1997, when an inhaled formulation of tobramycin became available for general clinical use in cystic fibrosis. O'Riordan and Faris[62] have provided a general review of inhaled antiinfective drug therapy in pulmonary disease, which includes the use of pentamidine and ribavirin, as well as inhaled tobramycin. In their review, they note the reasons why antiinfective therapy has not been previously accepted for general clinical use:

- Acute bacterial infections in the respiratory tract usually have a systemic component, which necessitates systemic drug therapy.
- Respiratory infections, especially with consolidation or cavitation, are thought to have poor regional ventilation, which would prevent aerosol delivery to the affected lung areas.
- A lack of scientific dose-response data exists for aerosol delivery of antibiotics to the lung.

Table 13-3

Reports in the literature of aerosolized antibiotics for cystic fibrosis and other disease states*

STUDY	DRUG AND DOSE	USE
Hodson, 1981[51]	Gentamicin 80 mg, bid	Cystic fibrosis
	Carbenicillin 1 g, bid	
Wall, 1983[52]	Tobramycin 80 mg, bid	Cystic fibrosis
	Ticarcillin 1 g, bid	
Kun, 1984[53]	Gentamicin 20 mg, bid	Cystic fibrosis
Littlewood, 1985[54]	Colomycin 500,000 units, bid	Cystic fibrosis
Stead, 1987[55]	Ceftazidime 1 g, bid	Cystic fibrosis
	Gentamicin 80 mg, bid	
	Carbenicillin 1 g, bid	
Steinkamp, 1989[56]	Tobramycin 80 mg, bid	Cystic fibrosis
Ramsey, 1993[57]	Tobramycin 600 mg, tid	Cystic fibrosis
Eisenberg, 1970[58]	Amphotericin B 10 mg, qid	Coccidioidomycosis
Wright, 1979[59]	Nystatin 100,000 units, tid	Pulmonary aspergillosis
Stockley, 1985[60]	Amoxicillin 500 mg, bid	Bronchiectasis
Ramsey, 1999[61]	Tobramycin 300 mg, bid, 28 days on, 28 days off	Cystic fibrosis

*The first author, dose, and use are given, with full citations provided in the references.

- Because acute respiratory infections are treated with systemic antimicrobial therapy, inhaled antibiotics have been used prophylactically as suppressive treatment in chronic lung diseases. Lack of accurate dose-response data to guide dosing by inhalation with indiscriminate or prolonged use can result in disappointing outcomes or drug resistance.

Before tobramycin was released as an inhaled formulation, there was a need for antibiotic formulations specific to the aerosol route, whether by nebulization or dry powder inhalation. Studies such as those by Hodson and colleagues[51] exemplified a controlled clinical trial, which supported the safety and efficacy of inhaled antibiotics in patients with cystic fibrosis and chronic *P. aeruginosa* infection. Mukhopadhyay[63] noted that, unlike oral drug preparations, inhaled aerosol dosing with antibiotics lacked a scientific basis. Specifically there was no pharmacokinetic data to determine the lung bioavailability from inhaled absorption and distribution, biotransformation, and excretion for most of the doses reported in published studies. As an example, tobramycin had often been given by nebulization using the injectable formulation with a dose of 80 mg per treatment. When inhaled tobramycin was in development for aerosol administration, studies of dose-response for adequate lung levels with a given nebulizer system (PARI LC Plus with DeVilbiss Pulmo-Aide compressor) indicated that a dose of 300 mg per treatment was needed. This is an exception to the usual rule that a lower dose of drug can be given with direct pulmonary targeting compared with systemic drug therapy for pulmonary disease.

CLINICAL USE OF INHALED TOBRAMYCIN

One disease state in which aerosolized antibiotics have been used more consistently for pulmonary infections is cystic fibrosis. Patients with cystic fibrosis are chronically infected with gram-negative organisms, such as *P. aeruginosa,* and the gram-positive bacterium *S. aureus,* as well as other microorganisms. In particular, chronic *Pseudomonas* infection leads to recurring acute respiratory infections. With the exception of the quinolone derivatives such as ciprofloxacin, antibiotics that are effective against *Pseudomonas* do not give sufficient lung levels to inhibit bacteria when taken orally. Antibiotics with poor oral bioavailability for lung tissue include the aminoglycosides, penicillin derivatives, and cephalosporins. Consequently, either the intravenous or inhaled aerosol route must be used.

Baran and colleagues[64] administered 40 mg of gentamicin by aerosol to eight children with cystic fibrosis and found high levels of drug (>20 μg/ml) in the bronchial secretions of seven of the children.[64] Blood levels with the inhaled drug were low, supporting the case for minimal systemic toxicity by aerosol. Similar results with nebulized tobramycin (300 mg) were demonstrated by Le Conte and associates.[65] By contrast, intramuscular injection of 1.5 mg/kg gave low levels of less than 2 μg/ml in bronchial secretions and, in some cases, undetectable levels.[64]

Aerosol administration is attractive because of reduced cost potential and ease of use at home compared with intravenous therapy. Furthermore, fluoroquinolones such as ciprofloxacin or norfloxacin, which are active taken orally, are not as suitable for prolonged maintenance or preventive therapy as the agents given by inhalation, because of the risk of drug-resistant strains of bacteria.[66] A report of the clinical trial establishing the safety and efficacy of inhaled tobramycin (TOBI) in managing *P. aeruginosa* in patients with cystic fibrosis was published in 1999 by Ramsey and colleagues.[61] The use of TOBI is intended to manage chronic infection with *P. aeruginosa* in cystic fibrosis, as follows:

- Treat or prevent early colonization with *P. aeruginosa*
- Maintain present lung function or reduce the rate of deterioration

Efficacy with *Burkholderia cepacia* has not been demonstrated using the inhaled route of administration.

DOSAGE AND ADMINISTRATION

TOBI is recommended for those 6 years old or older. The usual dosage is 300 mg twice daily, approximately 12 hours apart and not less than 6 hours apart, for 28 days consecutively, with the following 28 days off of the drug. This cycle is repeated on a maintenance basis. The drug is formulated as a nebulizer solution with 300 mg in a 5-ml ampule. In clinical trials it was administered using the PARI LC Plus, with a DeVilbiss Pulmo-Aide compressor. Other nebulizer delivery systems must be tested to ensure adequate drug output and particle size.

Patients should be instructed not to mix dornase alfa with tobramycin in the nebulizer. Tobramycin should be inhaled after other therapies usual in cystic fibrosis, such as chest physiotherapy measures, and other inhaled medications including bronchodilators or dornase alfa.

The drug should be stored at refrigerated temperatures of 2° to 8° C (36° to 46° F). After removing

Box 13-2	Side Effects With Aminoglycosides and Tobramycin

Parenteral Administration
Ototoxicity (auditory and vestibular)
Nephrotoxicity
Neuromuscular blockade
Hypomagnesemia
Cross-allergenicity
Fetal harm (deafness)

Inhaled Nebulized Tobramcyin
Voice alteration
Tinnitus
Nonsignificant increase in bacterial resistance

from refrigeration or if refrigeration is not available, the pouches in which the drug is provided can be stored at room temperature less than 25° C for up to 28 days. Drug ampules should not be exposed to intense light. The solution may darken with aging if not refrigerated, although this does not change the drug activity if the manufacturer's guidelines are followed.

MODE OF ACTION

Tobramycin is a member of the aminoglycoside family of antibiotics, so named because of their structure, which consists of amino sugars with glycosidic linkages. This group of antibiotics is effective in treating gram-negative infections and has a bactericidal effect. Tobramycin binds irreversibly to the 30S subunit of bacterial ribosomes. This binding blocks protein synthesis in the bacteria and causes cellular death.

Serum tobramycin levels are approximately 1 μg/ml 1 hour after inhalation in patients with normal renal function.

SIDE EFFECTS

Side effects for both parenteral and inhaled administration of tobramycin are listed in Box 13-2. The adverse effects with *nebulized* delivery are based on the clinical trial of Ramsey and colleagues,[61] and 2 years of experience after the approval of inhaled tobramycin.

PARENTERAL ADMINISTRATION

Adverse effects that can occur with *parenteral* administration of aminoglycosides are reviewed briefly because presence of impaired renal function or other conditions may increase risk of these effects with inhaled administration.

Ototoxicity is associated with parenteral use of aminoglycosides. Ototoxicity is manifested as auditory (cochlear) damage with small loss of hearing at the higher frequencies, or vestibular dysfunction with vertigo, nausea, or nystagmus (involuntary movement of eyeball).

Nephrotoxicity is also possible with aminoglycosides, which are excreted as unchanged drug by glomerular filtration. Although toxicity risk increases with dose, it may occur even with conventional doses in prerenal azotemia or impaired renal function. Because excretion is by the renal system, impaired renal function can also increase risk of the other side effects noted.

Neuromuscular blockade is another side effect resulting from the potential curare-like effect of aminoglycosides on the neuromuscular junction. This can aggravate muscle weakness, can cause further worsening of neuromuscular disorders, or prolong and intensify neuromuscular blockade by curare-like paralyzing agents (see Chapter 18).

Hypomagnesemia can occur in patients who have poor diet or whose diet is restricted.

Cross-allergenicity does exist among the aminoglycosides, and hypersensitivity to one agent in this group constitutes a contraindication to the use of other agents. The side effects cited are more likely with overdosage, poor renal function, and dehydration (resulting from higher renal concentrations with possible nephrotoxicity).

Fetal harm can occur with aminoglycosides, and these drugs can cross the placenta. Irreversible bilateral congenital deafness has been reported in children of mothers who received streptomycin.[37]

SIDE EFFECTS WITH NEBULIZED TOBRAMYCIN

The only adverse experiences reported after the 6-month clinical trial of Ramsey and associates[61] were *tinnitus* and *voice alteration*. There was no hearing loss associated with nebulized use of tobramycin, nor changes in serum creatinine indicative of renal toxicity. There was modest decrease in susceptibility of *P. aeruginosa* to tobramycin in the treatment group but not the placebo group, in Ramsey and colleagues' study. However, this was not associated with a lack of clinical response to inhaled therapy with tobramycin. Use of an alternating schedule of administration may reduce the risk of drug resistance. Ramsey and associates[61,67] noted that their rationale for intermittent administration of tobramycin was the observation that "drug holidays" allow susceptible pathogens to repopulate the airway in patients with cystic fibrosis. Because tobramycin is delivered by inhalation, the airway concentration can be 100 times as high as systemic levels. Thresholds of pathogen susceptibility with parenteral administration do not apply well to direct inhalation doses.

PRECAUTIONS IN USE OF NEBULIZED TOBRAMYCIN

- Inhaled tobramycin should be used with caution in patients with preexisting renal, auditory, vestibular, or neuromuscular dysfunction.
- Admixture incompatibility exists between β-lactam antibiotics (penicillins, cephalosporins) and aminoglycosides when mixed directly together; tobramycin solution should not be mixed with antibiotics in this group, and in general mixing with other drugs is discouraged.
- Factors that could increase risk of hearing damage with prolonged tobramycin use are renal impairment, concomitant dosage of parenteral aminoglycosides, dehydration, and concomitant use of ethacrynic acid, furosemide, or other ototoxic drugs.
- Nebulization of antibiotics during hospitalization should be performed under conditions of containment, as previously described for pentamidine and ribavirin, to prevent environmental saturation and development of resistant organisms in the hospital.
- Aminoglycosides can cause fetal harm if administered to pregnant women; exposure to ambient aerosol drug should be avoided by women who are pregnant or trying to become pregnant.
- *Local airway irritation* resulting in cough and bronchospasm with decreased ventilatory flow rates is a possibility with inhaled antibiotics and seems to be related to the osmolality of the solution.[48,68-70] Peak flow rates and chest auscultation should be used before and after treatments to evaluate airway changes. Pretreatment with a β agonist may be needed.
- *Allergies* in the patient, staff, or family should be considered, if exposure to the aerosolized drug is not controlled. The use of a nebulizing system with scavenging filter, one-way valves, and thumb control could reduce ambient contamination with the drug, as previously described.

CLINICAL EFFICACY

The clinical efficacy of inhaled tobramycin by nebulization was demonstrated in Ramsey and colleagues' randomized controlled study[61] published in 1999. In that study comparing inhaled tobramycin with placebo in 521 patients with cystic fibrosis, 6 months of alternating inhaled tobramycin together with standard therapy for cystic fibrosis resulted in the following:

- Improved pulmonary function (Figure 13-9)
- Decreased density of *P. aeruginosa* in expectorated sputum
- Reduced need for intravenous antipseudomonal antibiotics and hospitalizations
- No development of significant bacterial resistance

GENERAL CONSIDERATIONS IN AEROSOLIZING ANTIBIOTICS

Several points should be noted when nebulizing antibiotic drugs, especially if an injectable formulation is used, although this is *not* recommended for routine clinical use.

- Antibiotic solutions such as gentamicin are more viscous than bronchodilator solutions, and this may affect nebulizer performance. Compressors must be suitably powerful, and high-flow compressors are

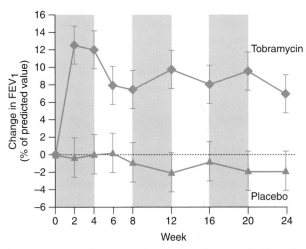

Figure 13-9 The mean change from baseline in FEV_1 for patients receiving inhaled tobramycin versus placebo. Bars represent 95% confidence intervals. (Modified from Ramsey BW and others, Intermittent administration of inhaled tobramycin in patients with cystic fibrosis, *N Engl J Med* 340:23-30, 1999.)

suggested. Flow rates of 10 to 12 L/min have also been suggested for suitably small particle sizes with antibiotic solutions by Newman and assoicates.[71,72]

- Environmental contamination in healthcare agencies and practitioner exposure to aerosolized drug can be reduced by using expiratory filters with one-way valves and a thumb control, as with aerosolized pentamidine.
- Physical incompatibility between some antibiotics has been noted by Hata and Fick.[73] Aminoglycosides such as gentamicin are chemically inactivated by carbenicillin and piperacillin when mixed together. These drugs should be given in separate nebulizer treatments, which has the disadvantage of requiring twice the patient treatment time. Any antibiotic combination, or other drug combinations, should at least be inspected for visible changes such as discoloration or precipitation and not used if this is observed. Ideally drug mixtures for nebulization should be tested for chemical compatibility in addition to a visual macro inspection.

INHALED ZANAMIVIR

CLINICAL USE OF INHALED ZANAMIVIR (RELENZA)

Zanamivir (Relenza) is an antiviral agent approved for use in the treatment of uncomplicated influenza illness in adults, during the early onset (within the first 2 days) of infection. The inhaled formulation of zanamivir was approved for general clinical use by the FDA on July 27, 1999. An oral antiinfluenza agent, oseltamivir phosphate (Tamiflu) is also available as a 75 mg capsule, approved October 27, 1999 by the FDA. This agent is taken as an oral dose of 75 mg twice daily for 5 days, with treatment beginning within 2 days of influenza symptoms. In addition, two older drugs, amantadine and rimantadine, have been used both for prophylaxis and treatment of acute symptoms of influenza. Table 13-4 summarizes information on these four agents, only one of which (zanamivir) is available by inhalation. Prophylactic vaccination against influenza, especially in high-risk patients with cardiovascular or respiratory disease, remains as an unqualified recommendation, despite the availability of drugs to treat acute infection.

DOSAGE AND ADMINISTRATION

Zanamivir is available in a DPI, the Diskhaler device, for oral inhalation. Each blister contains 5 mg of drug, giving a 5 mg per inhalation dose. There are

Table 13-4

Comparative summary of features for antiviral agents used to treat or prevent influenza

DRUG	BRAND NAME	FDA APPROVAL	ACTIVITY	CLINICAL USE	ROUTE OF ADMINISTRATION	ADULT DOSAGE
Amantadine	Symmetrel	1966	Influenza A	Prophylaxis, acute treatment	Oral: tablet, syrup	200 mg/day
Rimantadine	Flumadine	1993	Influenza A	Prophylaxis, acute treatment	Oral: tablet, syrup	100 mg bid
Oseltamivir	Tamiflu	1999	Influenza A and B	Prophylaxis, acute treatment	Oral: capsule, liquid suspension	75 mg bid, for 5 days
Zanamivir	Relenza	1999	Influenza A and B	Acute treatment	DPI: Diskhaler	10 mg (2 inhalations) bid, for 5 days

DPI, Dry powder inhaler; *FDA,* Food and Drug Administration.

four blisters in a Rotadisk, and the drug package contains five Rotadisks with one Diskhaler device. The dose in adults and children 12 years or older is 2 inhalations (two blisters, for a total of 10 mg) taken twice a day, approximately 12 hours apart, for 5 days. The complete drug package has the equivalent of 5 days of treatment, because each Rotadisk contains 1 day's dosage. Patients should finish the entire 5-day course of drug.

MODE OF ACTION

The general mechanism of viral infection was described previously with ribavirin (see discussion of the nature of viral infection). Zanamivir represents a new class of antiviral agent, termed neuraminidase inhibitors, which act by binding to the enzyme neuraminidase and thus blocking the enzyme's action. The influenza virus has an envelope and a protein coat surrounding the viral RNA and targets the respiratory tract. Briefly, as illustrated in Figure 13-10, the virus envelope for both influenza *A* and *B* have two surface glycoproteins, hemagglutinin *(HA)* and neuraminidase *(NA)*. Hemagglutinin binds to a sugary molecule, sialic acid *(SA)*, on the surface of a cell to be infected. This binding leads to fusion of virus and cell membranes and allows adsorption and penetration of the virus into the cell. However, when the newly minted viral particles bud from the cell and are ready to be released, the virus envelope acquires sialic acid from the cell, along with its own hemagglutinin and neuraminidase receptors. Without neu-

raminidase, the virus hemagglutinin would combine with the sialic acid again, "sticking" the viral particles to each other and to the cell surface, preventing further infection. Neuraminidase cleaves part of the sialic acid to prevent HA and SA combination, and prevents viral aggregation (clumping). Neuraminidase is essential for virus release from infected cells, prevents virus aggregation, and may decrease virus inactivation by respiratory mucus. Zanamivir is able to bind to neuraminidase and thereby block the enzyme action. By inhibiting neuraminidase, zanamivir inhibits virus particle separation and cellular release needed for systemic infection to proceed.[74]

Zanamivir is given by inhalation because the drug's binding ability also prevents good absorption when given orally. Inhalation also delivers the drug to the affected organ directly. Approximately 4% to 17% of an inhaled dose is systemically absorbed. Zanamivir has limited plasma protein binding (less than 10%) and is excreted unchanged in the renal system. It is apparently not metabolized to other products in vivo. Serum half-life is 2.5 to 5.1 hours. Any unabsorbed drug is excreted in feces.

ADVERSE EFFECTS

The side effects discussed below have been noted during clinical trials and after release of zanamivir.

BRONCHOSPASM AND DETERIORATION IN LUNG FUNCTION

Patients with underlying respiratory disease such as asthma or chronic obstructive lung disease (COPD)

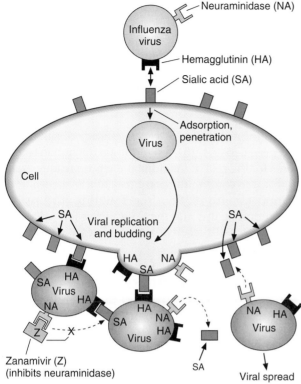

Neuraminidase (NA)

Influenza virus

Hemagglutinin (HA)

Sialic acid (SA)

Adsorption, penetration

Virus

Cell

SA

SA

Viral replication and budding

HA   NA

SA

SA   HA   Virus   HA

NA

HA

SA   NA   HA   Virus

NA   HA   Virus

Z

Zanamivir (Z)
(inhibits neuraminidase)

SA

Viral spread

Figure 13-10   Simplified illustration of the mode of action by which inhaled zanamivir *(Z)* provides its antiviral effect in influenza viral infection. As a sialic acid *(SA)* analogue, zanamivir binds to the enzyme neuraminidase *(NA)* and inhibits its usual inactivation of sialic acid. As a result, the viral hemagglutinin *(HA)* receptor continues to combine with both cell and viral sialic acid, causing viral aggregation and preventing viral release and spread.

may experience bronchospasm after inhaling zanamivir. Respiratory difficulty and wheezing have been reported in a patient with COPD[75] and an asthma patient inhaling zanamivir.[76] Neither patient appeared to have influenza at the time of treatment. A clinical trial of zanamivir by Cass and colleagues[77] in 11 patients with mild to moderate asthma with no influenza showed no symptoms of bronchospasm or airway responsiveness. Such data, however, do not establish the safety of zanamivir in asthmatics *with* influenza infection, which can cause mucosal damage and airway reactivity from the viral inflammation.[78] In ongoing treatment studies in patients with COPD or asthma who had influenza-like illness, more patients on zanamivir than on placebo had a greater than 20% decline in FEV_1 or peak expiratory flow rates.[74] Zanamivir should be discon-

tinued if bronchospasm or a decline in lung function occurs in any patient, and the managing physician should be consulted.

UNDERTREATMENT OF BACTERIAL INFECTION

Bacterial respiratory infections can appear with influenza-like symptoms, and viral respiratory infections can progress to serious bacterial secondary infections.[79] Treatment with an antiviral agent such as zanamivir is not effective against bacterial infection and could possibly allow progression of such infection to serious illness such as pneumonia. Two deaths from bacterial infection in subjects taking zanamivir have been reported,[80] although the reasons have not been determined.[79] In a patient with COPD exacerbation who is treated inappropriately, risk of serious complications and the need for hospitalization can result.[79]

ALLERGIC REACTIONS

As with any drug, patients should be monitored for allergic or allergic-like reactions with zanamivir.

OTHER ADVERSE EFFECTS

Adverse reactions occurring in a small percentage of patients included gastrointestinal (diarrhea, nausea, vomiting) and respiratory (bronchitis; cough; sinusitis; ear, nose, and throat infections) effects, as well as dizziness and headaches. These reactions did not differ substantially from those with placebo and may have been caused by the same lactose vehicle used in active drug and the placebo.

OVERDOSAGE

There have been no reports of overdosage from use of zanamivir.

CLINICAL EFFICACY AND SAFETY

Clinical efficacy of zanamivir has been established in trials that demonstrated that inhaled zanamivir can significantly shorten the duration of influenza symptoms.[78,81,82] With uncomplicated influenza-like illness, treatment with 10 mg of zanamivir twice daily resulted in approximately 1 day of shortening of the median time to improvement in symptoms compared with placebo.[78] The time to improvement in major symptoms was defined as no fever and no or mild headache, myalgia, cough, and sore throat. Among patients who were febrile and began treatment 30 hours or less after onset of symptoms, treatment with zanamivir resulted in a shortening of 3 days in the median time to alleviation of symptoms.[78] There are no data on efficacy when zanamivir is started after more than 2 days of symptoms of influenza (manufacturer's literature).

There was not a consistent difference in treatment effect between patients with influenza A versus influenza B. However, the clinical trials of zanamivir enrolled predominantly patients with influenza A (89% to 11% in one clinical trial). Patients with lower temperature and less severe symptoms in general derived less benefit from treatment with zanamivir.

Clinical trials of zanamivir were performed mainly with previously healthy subjects.[78,81,82] The manufacturer's literature states that safety and efficacy of zanamivir for treating influenza have not been demonstrated in patients with chronic pulmonary disease. In fact, zanamivir may carry risk with patients with COPD or asthma, as indicated in the discussion of side effects. Revised labeling for zanamivir adds a warning that zanamivir is *not generally recommended for patients with underlying airways disease* because of the risk of serious adverse effects.[79]

Zanamivir is not approved for prophylaxis to prevent influenza, nor does it reduce the risk of transmission of the virus to others. However, some data suggest a prophylactic benefit with zanamivir in influenza A and B in university and nursing home communities.[83] Results of a controlled study of inhaled zanamivir for both treatment and prevention of influenza in families in which one member developed influenza-like illness showed that zanamivir did reduce the rate of developing influenza in other family members. The proportion of families in which an initially healthy member developed influenza was 4% with zanamivir compared with 19% with placebo.[84] In the trial, treatment of the index cases with zanamivir in families reduced the median duration of symptoms from 7.5 to 5.0 days, a significant reduction. Oseltamivir (Tamiflu) was approved in early 2001 for prevention of influenza A and B in those 13 years or older who are in close contact with influenza.

A final issue with use of zanamivir or other antiinfluenza agents used in acute treatment is the lack of a clinically easy and inexpensive diagnostic tool to confirm the presence of influenza infection. Zanamivir is of no benefit in persons with infections other than influenza. In the clinical trial of Hayden and colleagues,[78] 262 of 417 total patients (63%) with influenza-like illness had confirmed influenza virus infection.[78] As a result, symptoms alone can result in inappropriate use of antiinfluenza drugs, with attendant risks as outlined in the discussion of adverse effects. Inappropriate use contributes to increased cost.

In summary, the cost versus efficacy of zanamivir has been debated. There is modest reduction in symptoms for the cost of the drug; there is no readily available test to confirm the presence of influenza viral infection for use of the drug resulting in possibly inappropriate use, and the drug carries increased risk in patients with reactive airways disease who might benefit most.

RESPIRATORY CARE ASSESSMENT OF AEROSOLIZED ANTIINFECTIVE AGENTS

The following assessment applies to all of the aerosolized antiinfective agents discussed.

- Assess for the presence of the indication for the agent.
  Pentamidine: Risk of PCP
  Ribavirin: Presence of severe RSV infection in infants or children at risk
  Tobramycin: Chronic *P. aeruginosa* infection compromising lung function in cystic fibrosis
  Zanamivir: Symptoms of acute influenza infection within first 2 days of onset
- Assess the correct configuration and function of aerosol equipment for ribavirin; instruct and verify correct use of aerosol delivery device for other agents.
- On initial aerosol treatment, assess respiratory rate and pattern, pulse and breath sounds; evaluate for the presence of airway irritation resulting in wheezing and bronchospasm.

For pentamidine:

- Monitor for coughing and bronchospasm, and provide a short-acting β agonist or an anticholinergic bronchodilator such as ipratropium if present with inhaled pentamidine.
- Monitor for occurrence rate of PCP, and rate of hospitalizations long term.
- Monitor for presence of side effects (shortness of breath, possible pneumothorax, conjunctivitis,

rash, neutropenia, dysglycemia) or appearance of extrapulmonary *P. carinii* infection.

For ribavirin:

- Monitor signs of RSV infection severity for improvement, including vital signs, respiratory pattern and work of breathing (clinically), level of FIO_2 needed, level of ventilatory support, ABGs, body temperature, and other indicators of pulmonary gas exchange.
- Monitor patient for evidence of side effects such as deterioration in lung function, bronchospasm, occlusion of endotracheal tube if present, cardiovascular instability, skin irritation from the aerosol drug, and equipment malfunction caused by drug residue.

For tobramycin:

- Verify that patient understands that nebulized tobramycin should be given after other cystic fibrosis inhaled medications.
- Check whether patient has renal, auditory, vestibular, or neuromuscular problems or is taking other aminoglycosides or ototoxic drugs. Consider whether tobramycin should be used in the patient based on severity of preexisting or concomitant risk factors.
- Monitor lung function to note improvement in FEV_1.
- Assess rate of hospitalization before and after institution of inhaled tobramycin.
- Assess need for intravenous antipseudomonal therapy.
- Assess improvement in weight.
- Monitor for occurrence of side effects such as tinnitus or voice alteration; have patient rinse and expectorate after aerosol treatments.
- Evaluate for changes in hearing function or renal function during use of inhaled tobramycin.

For zanamivir:

- Assess improvement in influenza symptoms: fever reduction, less myalgia and headache, reduced coughing and sore throat, and less systemic fatigue.
- Monitor for airway irritation and symptoms of bronchospasm, especially during initial use of the dry powder aerosol. Provide a short-acting β agonist if needed or if patient is at risk for airway reactivity (COPD, asthma).

SUMMARY KEY TERMS AND CONCEPTS

- Aerosolized *pentamidine isethionate* is approved for use as second-line prophylactic therapy in patients with AIDS to prevent *P. carinii pneumonia* (PCP). Clinical experience with the aerosolized drug has resulted in significant side effects and less efficacy than with the oral agent *trimethoprim-sulfamethoxazole* (TMP-SMX). TMP-SMX is indicated for prophylaxis of PCP unless side effects are not tolerated, in which case the aerosol drug should be considered.
- The *mode of action* of pentamidine is not fully understood, but seems to involve multiple actions on the organism.
- *Side effects* with aerosolized pentamidine include *local airway effects* such as cough, bronchospasm, dyspnea, and bad taste, as well as *systemic effects.*
- Administration of pentamidine by aerosol should use nebulizers capable of producing *small particle sizes* (1 to 2 μm MMAD), with a *scavenging system* to protect the environment. Precautions against spread of *TB with HIV* patients should be taken, such as containment booths or isolation rooms.
- *Ribavirin* is an aerosolized antiviral drug used with *respiratory syncytial viral* (RSV) infections in children and infants at risk for severe or complicated disease.
- Ribavirin acts as a *nucleoside analogue* to terminate viral DNA replication. The aerosol is administered using a *small particle aerosol generator* (SPAG) unit.
- *Side effects* with ribavirin include pulmonary deterioration and equipment malfunction (ventilator occlusion, endotracheal tube occlusion). *Environmental containment systems* are available to protect caregivers.
- *Respiratory syncytial virus immune globulin* (RSV-IGIV) is available as a monthly infusion of prepared antibody during RSV season, to confer *passive immunity* protection to children at risk, and also as humanized monoclonal antibody, *palivizumab.*
- *Nebulized tobramycin* is used to manage chronic *P. aeruginosa* infection in cystic fibrosis as an alternative to intravenous therapy. The nebulized form is attractive because of poor oral bioavailability for respiratory tract infections.
- *Side effects* with tobramycin include tinnitus and voice changes. Inhaled tobramycin should be used with *caution* in the presence of renal impairment, auditory or vestibular problems, or neuromuscular dysfunction.
- *Zanamivir* is available in a DPI to treat acute symptoms of influenza.
- The *mode of action* of zanamivir is to inhibit viral neuraminidase, causing viral aggregation to the cell and each other.
- *Side effects* include possible bronchospasm or lung deterioration, especially in preexisting airways disease and undertreatment or inappropriate treatment of nonviral bacterial respiratory infections.

SELF-ASSESSMENT QUESTIONS

1. Identify the disease states for which each of these drugs are used when inhaled as an aerosol: pentamidine, ribavirin, tobramycin, zanamivir.
2. Briefly, what is the rationale for aerosolizing an antibiotic such as tobramycin in cystic fibrosis?
3. What is the brand name of aerosol pentamidine?
4. What is the dose and frequency for aerosol pentamidine?
5. What device is approved for aerosolization of pentamidine?
6. Identify the common airway effects with aerosol pentamidine, and suggest a method for preventing or lessening these.
7. What is a major risk to the caregiver when aerosolizing pentamidine to a patient with AIDS?
8. What is the current Centers for Disease Control (CDC) recommended prophylactic treatment for PCP in AIDS patients?
9. What is the brand name and dose for aerosol ribavirin?
10. What is the mode of action of ribavirin?
11. Identify two serious hazards when ribavirin is given to a patient on mechanical ventilation.
12. How, in general, can you prevent environmental contamination when delivering ribavirin to an oxyhood?
13. What is the recommended dosage for inhaled tobramycin?
14. What common side effects have been observed with aerosolized tobramycin?
15. Identify two potential hazards to family members with aerosolized tobramycin at home.
16. Give the brand name and dosage for zanamivir.
17. In one sentence describe the mode of action of zanamivir.
18. What are common hazards in the use of inhaled zanamivir?
19. What factors cause debate over use of zanamivir in treating influenza?

Answers to Self-Assessment Questions are found in Appendix A.

CLINICAL SCENARIO

Mr. P. is a 29-year-old adult male with cystic fibrosis. The history of his disease and its previous treatment is well known to his pulmonary physician. He has been admitted to the hospital with complaints of increasing cough, shortness of breath, and sputum production. He reports that his sputum is greenish. His recent history reveals that his last admission for exacerbation of cystic fibrosis was approximately 6 months ago. He has used albuterol by MDI, with 2 puffs qid, and recently began to use sal-

meterol, 2 puffs bid. He maintains himself on a regular regimen of cystic fibrosis medications, including iron and vitamin supplements and Pancrease. Approximately 3 weeks ago, he complained of increasing pulmonary secretions and noted a mild elevation of his temperature (99.1° F). At that time, his physician prescribed ciprofloxacin, 500 mg orally bid, and he completed a course of 14 days, ending 5 days ago.

He is alert, oriented, and in no acute distress at this time. His skin is warm and dry. His vital signs are BP, 106/66 mm Hg; P, 88 beats/min and regular; RR, 20 breaths/min; and T, 98.9° F. His respiratory pattern is normal, and there is no use of accessory muscles. Auscultation reveals scattered rales and wheezes bilaterally both anteriorly and posteriorly. His cough is nonproductive during the examination.

Chest radiograph shows hyperexpanded lung fields, with linear fibrotic changes bilaterally over the lung fields. Cardiac silhouette shows mild right atrial hypertrophy. No consolidation or pleural effusion is seen. CBC results are hemoglobin, 13.2 g/dl; hematocrit, 38.6%; and WBC count, $13.5 \times 10^3/mm^3$. Remaining blood values are within normal limits. Pulse oximetry measures an 89% saturation on room air. His pulmonary function, measured approximately 2 months ago and available in his chart, shows:

	Observed	Predicted (% predicted)
TLC	7.66 L	6.67 L (115)
FVC	3.52 L	5.23 L (67)
FEV_1	1.41 L	3.51 L (40)
FEF_{25-75}	0.49 L/s	2.93 L/s (17)
ERV	0.94 L	1.69 L (56)
RV	4.0 L	1.54 L (260)

A sputum culture is taken and sent to the laboratory. Mr. P. is admitted for acute exacerbation of his pulmonary symptoms.

Identify key elements of his respiratory care plan that you would suggest. What is the risk of using the ciprofloxacin as an antibiotic to treat his symptoms of infection?

His physician decides to institute a course of tobramycin rather than repeating the ciprofloxacin. Can this antibiotic be given orally as an effective antibacterial agent for Mr. P.'s respiratory infection?

Identify two alternative routes of administration for tobramycin, in this case. Mr. P.'s physician orders intravenous tobramycin as well as by aerosol, 300 mg bid, and he asks you to make a detailed suggestion on administration by nebulizer. What would you suggest?

How would you evaluate (1) the aerosolized antibiotic therapy, and (2) the treatment plan for Mr. P.?

Answers to Clinical Scenario Questions are found in Appendix A.

REFERENCES

1. Waskin H: Toxicology of antimicrobial aerosols: a review of aerosolized ribavirin and pentamidine, *Respir Care* 36:1026, 1991.

2. Montgomery AB and others: Aerosolized pentamidine as sole therapy for *Pneumocystis carinii* pneumonia in patients with acquired immunodeficiency syndrome, *Lancet* 2:480, 1987.

3. Montgomery AB and others: Selective delivery of pentamidine to the lung by aerosol, *Am Rev Respir Dis* 137:477, 1988.

4. Leoung GS and others: Aerosolized pentamidine for prophylaxis against *Pneumocystis carinii* pneumonia, *N Engl J Med* 323:769, 1990.

5. Levine SJ, White DA: *Pneumocystis carinii*, *Clin Chest Med* 9:395, 1988.

6. Corkery KJ, Luce JM, Montgomery AB: Aerosolized pentamidine for treatment and prophylaxis of *Pneumocystis carinii* pneumonia: an update, *Respir Care* 33:676, 1988.

7. Smaldone GC, Perry RJ, Deutsch DG: Characteristics of nebulizers used in the treatment of AIDS-related *Pneumocystis carinii* pneumonia, *J Aerosol Med* 1:113, 1988.

8. Corkery K, Luce JM, Montgomery AB: Characteristics of nebulizers used in aerosolized pentamidine studies, *Respir Care* 33:916, 1988 (abstract).

9. Dolovich M, Chambers C, Newhouse M: Characterization of 3 systems used to deliver pentamidine (P) aerosol, *Am Rev Respir Dis* 141:A153, 1990 (abstract).

10. Vinciguerra C, Smaldone G: Treatment time and patient tolerance for pentamidine delivery by Respirgard II and AeroTech II, *Respir Care* 35:1037, 1990.

11. Mathewson HS: *Pneumocystis carinii* pneumonia: chemotherapy and prophylaxis, *Respir Care* 34:360, 1989.

12. Martinez CM and others: Spontaneous pneumothoraces in AIDS patients receiving aerosolized pentamidine, *Chest* 94:1317, 1988 (letter).

13. Hart CC: Aerosolized pentamidine and pancreatitis, *Ann Intern Med* 111:691, 1989 (letter).

14. Davey RT Jr and others: Digital necrosis and disseminated *Pneumocystis carinii* infection after aerosolized pentamidine prophylaxis, *Ann Intern Med* 111:681, 1989.

15. Quieffin J and others: Aerosol pentamidine-induced bronchoconstriction: predictive factors and preventive therapy, *Chest* 100:624, 1991.

16. Fine JM, Gordon T, Sheppard D: The roles of pH and ionic species in sulfur dioxide and sulfite-induced bronchoconstriction, *Am Rev Respir Dis* 136:1122, 1987.

17. Corkery KJ and others: Airway effects of aerosolized pentamidine isethionate, *Am Rev Respir Dis* 141:A152, 1990 (abstract).

18. Smaldone GC and others: Detection of inhaled pentamidine in health care workers, *N Engl J Med* 325:891, 1991.

19. O'Riordan TG, Smaldone GC: Exposure of health care workers to aerosolized pentamidine, *Chest* 101:494, 1992.

20. Fallat RJ, Kandal K: Aerosol exhaust: escape of aerosolized medication into the patient and caregiver's environment, *Respir Care* 36:1008, 1991.

21. Chaisson RE, McAvinue S: Control of tuberculosis during aerosol therapy administration, *Respir Care* 36:1017, 1991.

22. Centers for Disease Control: Guidelines for preventing the transmission of tuberculosis in health-care settings, with special focus on HIV-related issues, *MMWR* 39:1, 1990.

23. American Respiratory Care Foundation: *Pentamidine aerosols and care giver safety*, Dallas, 1992, AARC.

24. Riley RL, Nardell EA: Clearing the air: the theory and application of ultraviolet air disinfection, *Am Rev Respir Dis* 139:1286, 1989.

25. Centers for Disease Control: Guidelines for prophylaxis against *Pneumocystis carinii* pneumonia for children infected with human immunodeficiency virus, *MMWR* 40:1, 1991.

26. Centers for Disease Control: Recommendations for prophylaxis against *Pneumocystic carinii* pneumonia for adults and adolescents infected with human immunodeficiency virus, *MMWR* 41:1, 1992.

27. Conte JE Jr and others: Intravenous or inhaled pentamidine for treating *Pneumocystis carinii* pneumonia in AIDS: a randomized trial, *Ann Intern Med* 113:203, 1990.

28. Reines ED, Gross PA: Antiviral agents, *Med Clin North Am* 72:691, 1988.

29. Hall CB and others: Aerosolized ribavirin treatment of infants with respiratory syncytial viral infection, a randomized double-blind study, *N Engl J Med* 308:1443, 1983.

30. Hall CB and others: Ribavirin treatment of respiratory syncytial viral infection in infants with underlying cardiopulmonary disease, *J Am Med Assoc* 254:3047, 1985.

31. American Academy of Pediatrics, Committee on Infectious Disease: Ribavirin therapy of respiratory syncytial virus, *Pediatrics* 79:475, 1987.

32. American Academy of Pediatrics Committee on Infectious Diseases: Use of ribavirin in the treatment of respiratory syncytial virus infection, *Pediatrics* 92:501, 1993.

33. Wald ER, Dashefsky B: Ribavirin. Red book committee recommendations questioned, *Pediatrics* 93:672, 1994.

34. Smith DW and others: A controlled trial of aerosolized ribavirin in infants receiving mechanical ventilation for severe respiratory syncytial virus infection, *N Engl J Med* 325:24, 1991.

35. Meert KL and others: Aerosolized ribavirin in mechanically ventilated children with respiratory syncytial virus lower respiratory tract disease: a prospective, double-blind, randomized trial, *Crit Care Med* 22:566, 1994.

36. Demers RR and others: Administration of ribavirin to neonatal and pediatric patients during mechanical ventilation, *Respir Care* 31:1188, 1986.

37. *Drug facts and comparisons,* St Louis, 2000, Facts and Comparisons.

38. Harrison R and others: Assessing exposures of health-care personnel to aerosols of ribavirin: California, *MMWR* 37:560, 1988.

39. Corkery K, Eckman D, Charney W: Environmental exposure of aerosolized ribavirin, *Respir Care* 34:1027, 1989 (abstract).

40. Kacmarek RM: Ribavirin and pentamidine aerosols: Caregiver beware! *Respir Care* 35:1034, 1990 (editorial).

41. Cefaratt JL, Steinberg EA: An alternative method for delivery of ribavirin to nonventilated pediatric patients, *Respir Care* 37:877, 1992.

42. Kacmarek RM, Kratohvil J: Evaluation of a double-enclosure double-vacuum unit scavenging system for ribavirin administration, *Respir Care* 37:37, 1992.

43. Charney W and others: Engineering and administrative controls to contain aerosolized ribavirin: results of simulation and application to one patient, *Respir Care* 35:1042, 1990.

44. Breedveld FC: Therapeutic monoclonal antibodies, *Lancet* 355:735, 2000.

45. Impact-RSV Study Group: Palivizumab, a humanized respiratory syncytial virus monoclonal antibody, reduces hospitalization from respiratory syncytial virus infection in high-risk infants, *Pediatrics* 102:531, 1998.

46. Bryson V, Sansome E, Laskin S: Aerosolization of penicillin solutions, *Science* 100:33, 1944.

47. Krasno LR, Rhoads PS: The inhalation of penicillin dust; its proper role in the management of respiratory infections, *Am Pract* 3:649, 1949.

48. Littlewood JM, Smye SW, Cunliffe H: Aerosol antibiotic treatment in cystic fibrosis, *Arch Dis Child* 68:788, 1993.

49. Williams MH Jr: Steroid and antibiotic aerosols, *Am Rev Respir Dis* 110:122, 1974.

50. Wanner A, Rao A: Clinical indications for and effects of bland, mucolytic, and antimicrobial aerosols, *Am Rev Respir Dis* 122:79, 1980.

51. Hodson ME, Penketh ARL, Batten JC: Aerosol carbenicillin and gentamicin treatment of *Pseudomonas aeruginosa* infection in patients with cystic fibrosis, *Lancet* 2:1137, 1981.

52. Wall MA and others: Inhaled antibiotics in cystic fibrosis, *Lancet* 1:1325, 1983.

53. Kun P, Landau LI, Phelan PD: Nebulized gentamicin in children and adolescents with cystic fibrosis, *Aust Paediatr J* 20:43, 1984.

54. Littlewood JM and others: Nebulised colomycin for early *Pseudomonas* colonisation in cystic fibrosis, *Lancet* 1:865, 1985.

55. Stead RJ, Hodson ME, Batten JC: Inhaled ceftazidime compared with gentamicin and carbenicillin in older patients with cystic fibrosis infected with *Pseudomonas aeruginosa,* *Br J Dis Chest* 81:272, 1987.

56. Steinkamp G and others: Long-term tobramycin aerosol therapy in cystic fibrosis, *Pediatr Pulmonol* 6:91, 1989.

57. Ramsey BW and others: Efficacy of aerosolized tobramycin in patients with cystic fibrosis, *N Engl J Med* 328:1740, 1993.

58. Eisenberg RS, Oatway WH: Nebulization of amphotericin B, *Am Rev Respir Dis* 103:289, 1971.

59. Wright BD, Lee TS, Tseuda K: Pulmonary aspergillosis treated with nystatin aerosol, *Respir Care* 24:150, 1979.

60. Stockley RA, Hill SL, Burnett D: Nebulized amoxicillin in chronic purulent bronchiectasis, *Clin Ther* 7:593, 1985.

61. Ramsey BW and others: Intermittent administration of inhaled tobramycin in patients with cystic fibrosis, *N Engl J Med* 340:23, 1999.

62. O'Riordan T, Faris M: Inhaled antimicrobial therapy, *Respir Care Clin North Am* 5:617, 1999.

63. Mukhopadhyay S: When will nebulized chemotherapy come of age? *Respir Med* 88:245, 1994.

64. Baran D, Dachy A, Klastersky J: Concentration of gentamicin in bronchial secretions of children with cystic fibrosis or tracheostomy, *Int J Clin Pharmacol Biopharm* 12:336, 1975.

65. Le Conte P and others: Lung distribution and pharmacokinetics of aerosolized tobramycin, *Am Rev Respir Dis* 147:1279, 1993.

66. Neu HC: Quinolones: a new class of antimicrobial agents with wide potential uses, *Med Clin North Am* 72:623, 1988.

67. Smith AL, Ramsey B: Aerosol administration of antibiotics, *Respiration* 62(suppl 1):19, 1995.

68. Dickie KJ, de Groot WJ: Ventilatory effects of aerosolized kanamycin and polymyxin, *Chest* 63:694, 1973.

69. Dally MB, Kurrle S, Breslin ABX: Ventilatory effects of aerosol gentamicin, *Thorax* 33:54, 1978.

70. Wilson FE: Acute respiratory failure secondary to polymyxin-B inhalation, *Chest* 79:237, 1981.

71. Newman SP and others: Evaluation of jet nebulisers for use with gentamicin solution, *Thorax* 40:671, 1985.

72. Newman SP, Pellow PGD, Clarke SW: Choice of nebulisers and compressors for delivery of carbenicillin aerosol, *Eur J Respir Dis* 69:160, 1986.

73. Hata JS, Fick RB Jr: *Pseudomonas aeruginosa* and the airways disease of cystic fibrosis, *Clin Chest Med* 9:679, 1988.

74. Gubareva LV, Kaiser L, Hayden FG: Influenza virus neuraminidase inhibitors, *Lancet* 355:827, 2000.

75. Williamson JC, Pegram PS: Respiratory distress associated with zanamivir, *N Engl J Med* 342:661, 2000.

76. Neuraminidase inhibitors for treatment of influenza A and B infections, *MMWR*(RR-14):1, 1999.

77. Cass LM and others: Pulmonary function and airway responsiveness in mild to moderate asthmatics given repeated inhaled doses of zanamivir, *Respir Med* 94:166, 2000.

78. Hayden FG and others: Efficacy and safety of the neuraminidase inhibitor zanamivir in the treatment of influenzavirus infections, *N Engl J Med* 337:874, 1997.

79. FDA: Revised labeling for zanamivir, *J Am Med Assoc* 284:1234, 2000.

80. Yamey G: Drug company issues warning about flu drug, *Brit Med J* 320:334, 2000.

81. O'Riordan TG: Inhaled antimicrobial therapy: from cystic fibrosis to the flu, *Respir Care* 45:836, 2000.

82. The MIST (Management of Influenza in the Southern Hemisphere Trialists) Study Group: Randomised trial of efficacy and safety of inhaled zanamivir in treatment of influenza A and B virus infections, *Lancet* 352:1877, 1998.

83. Dunn CJ, Goa KL: Zanamivir: a review of its use in influenza, *Drugs* 58:761, 1999.

84. Hayden FG and others: Inhaled zanamivir for the prevention of influenza in families, *N Engl J Med* 343:1282, 2000.

CHAPTER 14

Antimicrobial Agents

Manjunath P. Pai • Christopher A. Schriever • Susan L. Pendland

CHAPTER OUTLINE

The antimicrobial properties of fermented beverages, moldy soybean curd, and spices were first described by the Chinese over 2500 years ago.[1] However, dissemination and acceptance of such knowledge did not take root until the early 1900s. The discovery of microscopic "little animals" by Antony von Leeuwenhoek paved the way for Robert Koch to validate that these "little animals," or germs, caused disease. Before Koch's work, almost no one believed that germs caused human disease. Despite the discovery of this important relationship, it would take numerous paradigm shifts and incredible luck before the discovery and usage of antimicrobials transpired.[2]

The sulfanilamides, azo compounds used in the German dye industry, were the first class of agents serendipitously discovered to have antibacterial activity. These compounds were initially unsuccessful and required multiple modifications to reduce their unpleasant side effects. In 1928, Alexander Fleming discovered the first antibiotic, which he named *penicillin*. However, Fleming, like other scientists of the time, did not realize the utility of penicillin for systemic infections. It took a historic 1940 publication entitled "Penicillin as a chemotherapeutic agent" by Chain and colleagues,[3] to set into motion what we now refer to as the "golden age" of antimicrobial chemotherapy.

The realization that living organisms may produce compounds that kill microbes is a relatively new concept. Since this realization, over 30 classes of compounds have been identified from natural sources or created synthetically to treat infections resulting from bacteria, fungi, protozoa, or viruses. Techniques to identify organisms and determine their susceptibility have also evolved over the years and are vital to the choice of the proper antimicrobial agent. In addition, other factors such as the host, antimicrobial pharmacodynamics, antimicrobial combinations, and methods of monitoring therapy are important parameters that need consideration before selecting an antimicrobial agent. This chapter will focus on these basic principles of antimicrobial therapy, provide a synopsis of the mechanism of action and adverse effects, and emphasize the clinical use of the various antimicrobial classes for the treatment of respiratory illnesses.[1]

PRINCIPLES OF ANTIMICROBIAL THERAPY

Several factors require careful consideration before choosing a particular antimicrobial agent. The identification of the organism or organisms responsible for the infection is the first step toward treatment. Once the organism is isolated, antimicrobial susceptibility is performed using standardized methods that can be replicated between laboratories. The susceptibility pattern of the organism narrows the choice of potential agents. Consideration must then be given to host factors such as age, pregnancy, organ function, and site of infection. In addition, drug factors such as available dosage forms, ease of administration, pharmacokinetics, potential adverse events, and economic considerations influence the choice of a specific agent.[4]

IDENTIFICATION OF THE PATHOGEN

The first step to identification of the organism is the collection of potentially infected material for culture. Specimens commonly collected for culture include blood, urine, sputum, cerebrospinal fluid, pleural fluid, synovial fluid, and peritoneal fluid. Several methods are then employed to rapidly identify the pathogens using different chemical stains, immunological assays, and microscopic examination. The simplest and most common preparation is the Gram stain. This stain designates bacteria into two major classes, gram-positive (stain purple) or gram-negative (stain pink). Bacteria stain differently depending on the structural components of their cell wall. These structural components also affect their susceptibility to antimicrobials. Other bacteria such as *Mycobacterium tuberculosis* require the use of an acid-fast stain to penetrate their waxlike cell walls. Mycobacteria require up to 6 weeks for growth on cultures, which makes the acid-fast stain vital for the rapid diagnosis of tuberculosis. Immunological methods such as

enzyme-linked immunosorbent assay (ELISA) and latex agglutination have also been developed to identify pathogens such as viruses, molds, certain bacteria, and protozoa. In many clinical cases the exact identity of the infecting organism is not known. As a result, patients are empirically treated with an antimicrobial agent active against the organism or organisms that are most likely causing the infection. For example, 30% to 40% of patients with community-acquired pneumonia fail to expectorate sputum, which prevents identification of a specific pathogen. However, research has shown that the most common pathogens responsible for community-acquired pneumonia include *Streptococcus pneumoniae*, *Haemophilus influenzae*, and atypical (intracellular) organisms such as *Mycoplasma pneumoniae*, *Chlamydia pneumoniae*, and *Legionella pneumophila*. As a result, empiric therapy for community-acquired pneumonia involves antimicrobials active against this spectrum of organisms. Conversely, identification of an organism from culture material does not necessarily indicate an infection. For example, hospitalized patients often have growth of gram-negative bacilli (rods) in sputum samples. However, these organisms may only represent colonization and not hospital-acquired (nosocomial) pneumonia. Common pathogens and treatment of specific respiratory infections are listed in Table 14-1.[5]

SUSCEPTIBILITY TESTING AND RESISTANCE

Once an organism is isolated, susceptibility test results can usually be obtained within 24 hours. Several methods are commonly used to determine the susceptibility of isolated pathogens. The Kirby-Bauer disk diffusion test involves the use of antibiotic-impregnated disks that are placed on an agar plate heavily inoculated (10^5 colony-forming units [cfu]/ml) with the isolated bacteria. If the organism is susceptible to the antibiotic, then a clear zone of inhibition (no growth of the organism) develops around the disk. The degree of susceptibility or resistance of the organism depends on the diameter of this circular zone of inhibition; that is, a larger diameter indicates greater sensitivity. Another disk diffusion test is the E-test, or elliptical test. The E-test strip is placed on an agar plate heavily inoculated with the isolated organism. The strip creates an antimicrobial gradient, which results in a clear elliptical zone of inhibition. This method allows the determination of the *minimum inhibitory concentration* (MIC). The MIC is defined as the least concentration of antimicrobial that

Table 14-1

Common pathogens and treatment of respiratory infections in adults

RESPIRATORY INFECTION	COMMON PATHOGENS	POTENTIAL ANTIBIOTIC REGIMENS
Sinusitis		
Acute (community)	*Streptococcus pneumoniae, Haemophilus influenzae, Moraxella catarrhalis*	Amoxicillin/clavulanate or cefuroxime axetil or trimethoprim-sulfamethoxazole (TMP-SMX)
Acute (hospital)	*Pseudomonas aeruginosa, Acinetobacter* sp., *Staphylococcus aureus*	Ceftazidime or a carbapenem and vancomycin
Chronic	*Bacteroides* sp., *Peptostreptococcus* sp., *Fusobacterium* sp.	Antibiotics are usually unsuccessful and may require sinus drainage
Bronchitis		
Acute	*Mycoplasma pneumoniae, Chlamydia pneumoniae, Bordetella pertussis*	Antibiotics are usually not indicated
Exacerbation of chronic bronchitis	*S. pneumoniae, H. influenzae, M. catarrhalis*	Value of antibiotics is controversial; doxycycline may be considered
Pneumonia		
Community-acquired	*S. pneumoniae, H. influenzae, M. catarrhalis, M. pneumoniae, C. pneumoniae, Legionella pneumophila*	Azithromycin or clarithromycin or levofloxacin or gatifloxacin or moxifloxacin or (cefuroxime and erythromycin)
Hospital-acquired (nonneutropenic patient)	*S. pneumoniae, P. aeruginosa*	(Cefepime or a carbapenem or ceftazidime or piperacillin) + an aminoglycoside or ciprofloxacin
Hospital-acquired (neutropenic patient)	As listed above and fungi such as *Aspergillus* sp., *Pneumocystis carinii* (especially if HIV-positive)	[(Cefepime or a carbapenem or ceftazidime or piperacillin) + an aminoglycoside or ciprofloxacin] ± vancomycin ± amphotericin B ± TMP-SMX
Aspiration suspected	*S. pneumoniae, Bacteroides fragilis, Peptostreptococcus* sp., *Fusobacterium* sp.	Clindamycin
Patient with cystic fibrosis	*S. aureus, P. aeruginosa, Burk-holderia cepacia*	Aminoglycoside + piperacillin or ceftazidime, ciprofloxacin TMP-SMX (*B. cepacia*)
Empyema	*S. milleri, B. fragilis*, Enterobacteriaceae, *Mycobacterium tuberculosis*	Third-generation cephalosporin + clindamycin (see Table 14-7 for antimycobacterial regimens)

*The potential treatments listed in the table are not listed in the order of superiority. The choice of antimicrobials depend on the individual susceptibility pattern of the suspected organisms within the specific institution.

prevents visible growth. The Kirby-Bauer and E-test methods are illustrated in Figure 14-1.

Other methods include inoculation of the organism into serial dilutions of an antimicrobial in agar containing or, more commonly, in broth culture media (Figure 14-2). Automated systems such as Vitek and MicroScan take advantage of broth microdilution methods to provide efficient and rapid susceptibility results. When susceptibility testing is performed in broth media, a small sample can be re-moved from the test-tubes or microwells with no growth and used to inoculate agar plates. The lowest concentration of antimicrobial agent that prevents growth of the organism on the agar plate after a 24-hour incubation is termed the *minimum bactericidal concentration* (MBC). Drugs that inhibit the growth of bacteria but do not kill them are termed *bacteriostatic.* A *bactericidal* drug is one that kills the bacteria. Examples of bacteriostatic and bactericidal drugs are listed in Box 14-1.

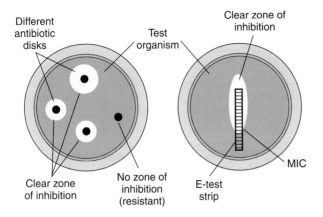

Figure 14-1 Disk diffusion test and E-test methods.

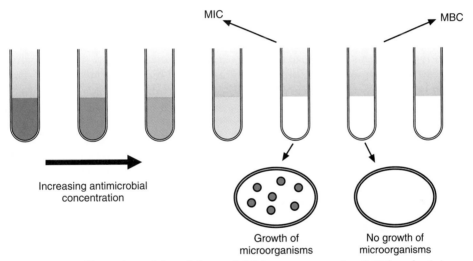

Figure 14-2 Illustration of the minimum inhibitory concentration (MIC) and minimum bactericidal concentration (MBC) by broth macrodilution.

Box 14-1	Examples of Bacteriostatic/Fungistatic and Bactericidal/Fungicidal Antimicrobials
Cidal	**Static**
Penicillins	Tetracyclines
Cephalosporins	Macrolides
Carbapenems	Trimethoprim-sulfamethoxazole
Aminoglycosides	Quinupristin/dalfopristin*
Quinolones	Linezolid*
Metronidazole	Chloramphenicol
Vancomycin*	Clindamycin
Isoniazid	Nitrofurantoin
Rifampin, rifabutin	Azoles
Polyenes	

*Agents that are bactericidal against *Staphylococcus aureus* but bacteriostatic against *Enterococcus* sp.

Susceptibility testing is a critical part of antimicrobial therapy because the empiric regimen may fail when used to treat infections with resistant organisms. Microorganisms, like all living things, have genetic variability that affects their susceptibility to antimicrobials. Selective pressure from extensive clinical and agricultural use of antibiotics is thought to play a primary role in the emergence of resistant bacteria. Mechanisms of bacterial resistance include the production of enzymes that degrade or modify antibiotics, alteration of bacterial cell walls or membranes, upregulation of antimicrobial efflux pumps, and alteration of the site of antimicrobial action. Examples of important emerging resistant bacteria are listed in Table 14-2.[4]

HOST FACTORS

The safety and efficacy of an antimicrobial agent vary based on the population of patients being treated. For example, bone marrow transplant recipients with an active infection may not improve despite use of the ideal antimicrobial agent because of their impaired immune function. Similarly, other immunocompromised hosts such as patients with acquired immuno-

deficiency syndrome (AIDS), recipients of cancer chemotherapy or steroids, and solid organ transplant recipients are also at risk of failing to improve on antimicrobial therapy. Other factors such as the altered pharmacokinetics of an antimicrobial can affect response to therapy. For example, the absorption of certain antimicrobials such as itraconazole (an antifungal agent) are increased in the presence of gastric acid; others, such as penicillin G, are degraded in the presence of acid. The pH of the stomach varies with age; older patients tend to have achlorhydria and young children tend to have a higher gastric pH. As a result, these two populations may have enhanced absorption of penicillin and decreased absorption of itraconazole relative to the rest of the population.

The function of the liver and the kidney also changes with age. These two organs play a major role in the metabolism and elimination of drugs from the body. Premature and newborn children have diminished renal function at birth. Drugs such as the β-lactams and aminoglycosides that are eliminated unchanged in the urine require less frequent dosing because of their reduced clearance. Similarly, renal function declines with age, necessitating dosage reductions in the elderly to prevent potential toxicities from antimicrobial accumulation.

Prevention of toxicity to the fetus or infant while treating a pregnant or nursing mother is also a crucial consideration. In general, most β-lactams and macrolides appear to be safe in pregnancy. The teratogenic potential of most other antimicrobials is simply unknown. However, the tetracyclines have been shown to affect fetal dentition and adversely affect pregnant women. Antimicrobials are often eliminated in breast milk and so have the potential to adversely affect nursing infants. For example, premature babies are often jaundiced at birth because they are unable to efficiently conjugate and eliminate bilirubin. Even a small dose of sulfonamides ingested through breast milk from a treated mother can displace the albumin-bound bilirubin and predispose the child to kernicterus. Kernicterus is marked by a pattern of cerebral palsy with uncoordinated movements, deafness, disturbed vision, and speech difficulties resulting from deposition of bilirubin in the developing brain.

Antimicrobials concentrate in varying degrees within organ systems and can influence the outcome of therapy. Clindamycin achieves excellent bone concentrations and is very useful for treatment of osteomyelitis resulting from susceptible organisms. Sim-

Table 14-2

Emerging resistant bacterial pathogens

CLASS OF BACTERIA	NAME
Gram-positive	Methicillin-resistant *Staphylococcus aureus* (MRSA)
	Vancomycin-intermediate susceptible *Staphylococcus aureus* (VISA)
	Penicillin-resistant *Streptococcus pneumoniae*
	Vancomycin-resistant *Enterococcus* (VRE)
Gram-negative	Multidrug-resistant nonenteric bacilli (*Pseudomonas aeruginosa*, *Stenotrophomonas maltophilia*, *Acinetobacter* sp.)
	Third-generation cephalosporin resistant *Enterobacter* and *Citrobacter* sp.
	Extended-spectrum β-lactamase–producing *Escherichia coli* and *Klebsiella* sp.
	Ampicillin-resistant *Haemophilus* sp.

ilarly, drugs such as the aminoglycosides, most fluoroquinolones, and penicillins achieve very high concentrations in the urine and are useful for the treatment of urinary tract infections. Conversely, certain drugs, although active against the organism in vitro, cannot achieve adequate concentrations at the site of infection. For example, aminoglycosides cannot penetrate the blood-brain barrier to adequately treat meningitis in adults. The blood-brain barrier is the result of tight junctions between the epithelial cells of the capillary wall that prevent drugs from entering the central nervous system.[4]

PHARMACODYNAMICS

Pharmacodynamics refers to the science of understanding the optimal effect of a drug as a function of its concentration and the in vitro activity (MIC) against an organism. The pharmacodynamic properties of an antimicrobial are measured in vitro by using time-kill studies. These studies measure the rate and extent of microorganism killing when exposed to varying concentrations of antimicrobials. If the microbial kill rate increases proportionally with drug concentration, the antimicrobial is said to have a *concentration-dependent* effect. If the microbial kill rate is influenced by the time of drug concentration above the MIC, the antimicrobial is defined as *time-dependent* (or *concentration-independent*). Another pharmacodynamic phenomenon exhibited by antimicrobials is known as the *postantibiotic effect* (PAE). The PAE refers to the sustained suppression of bacterial growth even after the concentration of the antibiotic drops below detectable levels. The length of the PAE varies by the type of organism and the drug. In general, time-dependent drugs, such as the β-lactams, have short PAEs; whereas concentration-dependent drugs, such as the aminoglycosides, metronidazole, and the quinolones, have longer PAEs. Agents with a short PAE should be dosed frequently, and longer dosing intervals should be used for antimicrobials having a long PAE. These pharmacodynamic properties have been demonstrated both in vitro and in numerous animal studies. Clinical trials validating these principles and practical guidelines to incorporate pharmacodynamics in clinical practice are still under study.[4]

ANTIMICROBIAL COMBINATIONS

Empiric regimens must often cover a broad spectrum of organisms, which occasionally requires the use of two or more classes of antimicrobials. Ideally, the regimen should be narrowed once the specific organism has been isolated and susceptibilities are determined. Certain infections are polymicrobial, and in certain settings the use of antimicrobial combinations is justified. When antimicrobials are used in combination, it is important to know whether these agents act synergistically or are antagonistic. Synergy is demonstrated in vitro when the combined effect of two antimicrobials is greater then their added effect (i.e., $1 + 1 > 2$). Antagonism occurs when the effect of the combined drug is lower than the effect expected from either agent alone (i.e., $1 + 1 < 1$). Clearly, antagonism may result in an unfavorable response and such drug combinations should be avoided. A classic example of antagonism was the use of tetracycline and penicillin in children with pneumococcal meningitis. The mortality associated with the use of combination therapy was three times higher than for patients treated with penicillin alone. Conversely, synergistic combinations have played a vital role in the treatment of resistant *Pseudomonas* infections in patients with cystic fibrosis. These patients have recurrent bouts of pseudomonal pneumonia and are often colonized with resistant species. Certain synergistic combinations of β-lactams and aminoglycosides have been shown to curb the development of resistance and improve outcomes.[4]

MONITORING RESPONSE TO THERAPY

Certain laboratory parameters can be monitored to assess the efficacy of an antimicrobial regimen, but ultimately the clinical assessment of the patient is the best measure of response to therapy. Treatment failure may manifest as continued fever spikes, elevated white blood cell count, repeated positive cultures, nonresolution of symptoms, and so on. The reasons for failure can be multifactorial and require consideration of all the aforementioned factors. In addition, noncompliance to the treatment regimen can also play a significant role in treatment failure.

The use of antimicrobials can be associated with significant toxicities. The agent amphotericin B, which is used to treat fungal infections such as pulmonary aspergillosis, can cause significant renal dysfunction. Similarly, other agents can have adverse effects on the liver, gastrointestinal tract, neuromuscular system, hematological system, heart, and lungs. The incidence of these adverse events varies between agents and is often reversible. Monitoring patients receiving antimicrobials carefully can prevent serious and potentially life-threatening adverse events.[4]

ANTIBIOTICS

Numerous antibiotics have been discovered and developed over the last 50 years. A synopsis of the mechanism of action, clinical uses, and adverse reactions of each class will be described.

PENICILLINS

The discovery of penicillin in 1928 by Alexander Fleming ultimately led to the creation of a broad class of antibiotics commonly referred to as the β-*lactams*. The β-lactam antibiotics include the penicillins, cephalosporins, monobactams, and carbapenems. The main constituent of these antibiotics is the β-lactam ring structure. Chemical manipulation of β-lactam side chains led to the development of new agents with enhanced spectrums of antimicrobial activity compared with penicillin. Specific side-chain modifications of penicillin have resulted in a broad class that includes the natural penicillins, aminopenicillins, penicillinase-resistant penicillins, carboxypenicillins, and ureidopenicillins (Table 14-3). Penicillins have also been combined with

Table 14-3

Classification and clinical uses of penicillins

β-LACTAM CLASS (GENERIC NAME)	BRAND NAMES	ROUTE	COMMON USES (MICROORGANISM)
NATURAL PENICILLIN			
Penicillin G (benzylpenicillin)	Pfizerpen	IM, IV	*Streptococcus pyogenes, Neisseria meningitidis,*
Penicillin G (procaine)	Wycillin	IM	*Bacillus anthrasis* (anthrax), *Clostridium*
Penicillin G (benzathine)	Bicillin L-A	IM	*perfringens* (gangrene), *Pasteurella maltocida,*
Penicillin V	PenVee K	PO	*Treponema pallidum* (syphilis)
PENICILLINASE-RESISTANT PENICILLINS			
Oxacillin	Prostaphlin	PO, IM, IV	Methicillin-sensitive *Staphylococcus aureus*
		IM, IV	(MSSA), methicillin-sensitive *Staphylococcus*
			epidermidis (MSSE)
Nafcillin	Unipen	PO	
Cloxacillin	Cloxapen	PO	
Dicloxacillin	Dynapen	PO	
AMINOPENICILLINS			
Ampicillin	Omnipen	PO, IM, IV	*Listeria monocytogenes, Proteus mirabilis, Eikenella*
Amoxicillin	Amoxil, Wymox	PO	*corrodens, Borrelia burgdorferi*
CARBOXYPENICILLINS			
Carbenicillins	Geopen	PO, IM, IV	*Pseudomonas aeruginosa,* Enterobacteriaceae
Ticarcillin	Ticar	IV, IM	
UREIDOPENICILLINS			
Mezlocillin	Mezlin	IM, IV	*P. aeruginosa,* Enterobacteriaceae
Piperacillin	Pipracil	IM, IV	
PENICILLIN PLUS β-LACTAMASE INHIBITORS			
Amoxicillin-clavulanic acid	Augmentin	PO	Increased activity against β-lactamase–
Ampicillin-sulbactam	Unasyn	IM, IV	producing strains *S. aureus, Haemophilus*
			influenzae, Moraxella catarrhalis, Proteus sp.,
			Bacteroides sp.
Ticarcillin-clavulanic acid	Timentin	IV	*P. aeruginosa,* Enterobacteriaceae
Piperacillin-tazobactam	Zosyn	IV	

IM, Intramuscular; *IV,* intravenous; *PO,* oral.

β-lactamase inhibitors to overcome a common mechanism of bacterial resistance. In general, the penicillins are widely distributed throughout the body and are associated with relatively low levels of toxicity. Most penicillin are acid labile (destroyed in the stomach) and therefore are not readily absorbed orally. The majority of drugs in this class are not metabolized and are excreted unchanged in the urine. Therefore most penicillins require reductions in dosage for patients with renal dysfunction.[7]

MECHANISM OF ACTION

The penicillins exert their pharmacological activity by inhibiting cell wall synthesis. Penicillins bind to enzymes (penicillin-binding proteins) located within the cell wall, and prevent cross-linking of the peptidoglycan structure necessary for cell wall development. In addition, penicillins activate an endogenous autolytic system within bacteria, which subsequently leads to cell lysis and death. Penicillins are bactericidal, demonstrate time-dependent killing, and can act synergistically with aminoglycosides against some bacteria (i.e., *Pseudomonas aeruginosa* and enterococci).[8]

CLINICAL USES

Natural Penicillins. Benzylpenicillin (penicillin G) is the parent compound of this class. This agent may be administered by parenteral (IV) or intramuscular (IM) routes. Penicillin G procaine is used for intramuscular dosing only and provides a less painful alternative when sustained serum concentrations are required. Phenoxymethyl penicillin (penicillin V) resists degradation by gastric acid and can be administered orally (PO). The natural penicillins are primarily effective against gram-positive bacteria and anaerobes. Penicillin G is the drug of choice for the treatment of primary and secondary syphilis *(Treponema pallidum)*, along with pharyngitis caused by group A streptococci *(Streptococcus pyogenes)*. Because of increasing frequency of resistance in *Staphylococcus aureus, S. pneumoniae,* and *Neisseria gonorrhoeae,* penicillin G should no longer be considered the agent of choice for infections caused by these organisms.[7]

Penicillinase-Resistant Penicillins. In an attempt to overcome the emergence of penicillinase (β-lactamase)–producing staphylococci, semisynthetic penicillinase-resistant antibiotics were developed. These agents are commonly referred to as *antistaphylococcal* agents because of their excellent activity against *S. aureus.* Methi-

cillin was the first agent in this class of antibiotics, followed by oxacillin, nafcillin, cloxacillin, and dicloxacillin. Chemical modification of penicillin by the addition of an acyl side chain prevents hydrolysis of the agents in the presence of penicillinase. This class has activity against gram-positive cocci (staphylococci and streptococci) and is routinely used in skin and soft-tissue infections. They are not effective in the treatment of infections caused by gram-negative organisms or anaerobes. Until the 1980s, these antibiotics were the mainstay of treatment against staphylococci. However, the emergence of methicillin-resistant staphylococci has greatly reduced the clinical effectiveness of these agents.[7]

Aminopenicillins. Ampicillin and amoxicillin are the primary antibiotics in this class. The aminopenicillins were the first penicillin class developed that were considered clinically active against some gram-negative bacteria *(Escherichia coli, H. influenzae).* Unlike penicillin, ampicillin and amoxicillin are both stable in gastric acid and therefore are suitable for oral administration. Both ampicillin and amoxicillin are frequently used in infections with susceptible organisms of the respiratory *(S. pneumoniae, H. influenzae)* and urinary tracts *(E. coli).*[7]

Carboxypenicillins. With the emergence of more resistant gram-negative bacilli, penicillins with increased gram-negative activity were needed. Carbenicillin was the first penicillin to have activity against *Pseudomonas aeruginosa.* It was also active against most members of the family Enterobacteriaceae, including *E. coli, Enterobacter, Proteus, Morganella,* and *Serratia.* Subsequent modification of carbenicillin resulted in ticarcillin, which has even greater in vitro activity against *P. aeruginosa* and members of the Enterobacteriaceae (including *Klebsiella*). Neither of these agents is considered to have appreciable activity against gram-positive organisms (staphylococci or streptococci). These agents are administered primarily in the intravenous form, because high serum concentrations cannot be achieved with the oral formulations.[7]

Ureidopenicillins. Even though carbenicillin and ticarcillin provided increased gram-negative coverage, antimicrobial agents with enhanced antipseudomonal activity were still needed. The ureidopenicillins were developed to fill this need. Piperacillin is a penicillin antibiotic with enhanced gram-negative activity (especially against *P. aeruginosa*) and with fewer adverse reactions than the carboxypenicillins. In addition, the ureidopenicillins also exhibit activity against strepto-cocci and enterococci, as well as activity against many anaerobes. Piperacillin is the primary agent of this class and has been efficacious in the treatment of pneumonia, bacteremia, infections of the urinary tract, osteomyelitis, and soft tissue infections.[7]

β-Lactam and β-Lactamase Inhibitor Combinations. Certain bacteria have the ability to produce enzymes (β-lactamases) that destroy the activity of penicillins by disrupting the β-lactam structure. β-lactamase inhibitors were developed to overcome this form of resistance. Consequently, combination β-lactam and β-lactamase inhibitors have a large spectrum of activity, making them particularly useful in polymicrobial infections. Currently there are three β-lactamase inhibitors approved for combination with penicillins: clavulanic acid, sulbactam, and tazobactam. The β-lactamase inhibitors enhance the activity of β-lactams against β-lactamase–producing strains of S. aureus, Moraxella catarrhalis, E. coli, H. influenzae, Klebsiella sp., and Bacteroides sp.[7]

ADVERSE REACTIONS AND PRECAUTIONS FOR THE PENICILLINS

The most common adverse reaction to penicillins is hypersensitivity. Approximately 3% to 10% of the population are allergic to penicillin. Reactions may vary in severity from a mild rash to life-threatening anaphylaxis. Patients allergic to a penicillin could be potentially allergic to all classes of β-lactams (cephalosporins, carbapenems). In addition to allergic reactions, hematological reactions such as thrombocytopenia and increased bleeding times have been reported. Hematological disturbances are thought to be higher with carboxypenicillins than the ureidopenicillins. Gastrointestinal disturbances (nausea, vomiting, and diarrhea) are more common with oral dosage forms of the penicillins, especially ampicillin. Interstitial nephritis occurred most commonly with methicillin (not commercially available) but may occur with other penicillins as well. Central nervous system toxicities (i.e., seizures) have been reported with the penicillins. Patients with an underlying seizure disorder and those with renal insufficiency are at greatest risk for developing this complication.[7]

CEPHALOSPORINS

The cephalosporins include a large group of antimicrobials that are structurally related to the penicillins. This class, discovered in the 1940s as a microbial by-product of the fungus Cephalosporium acremonium, is now widely used in clinical practice. Like the penicillins, this class exhibits bactericidal activity, is distributed throughout the body, and produces relatively few adverse effects. Cephalosporins are used for a variety of clinical indications and are available in both oral and intravenous formulations (Table 14-4). Agents from this class have been loosely grouped into "generations" based on their spectrum of activities. Presently there are four generations (classes) of cephalosporins.[9]

MECHANISM OF ACTION

Cephalosporins inhibit bacterial cell wall synthesis in a manner similar to the penicillins. The cephalosporins bind to the penicillin-binding proteins within the cell wall and inhibit the cross-linking of peptidoglycan. This compromises the structural integrity of the bacterial cell wall, resulting in cell lysis (bactericidal).

CLINICAL USES

As a class the cephalosporins are active against a wide variety of organisms. Because of their broad spectrum of activity and low level of toxicity, these agents are commonly used for a wide variety of infections. The spectrum of activity differs for each cephalosporin generation. Notably, all cephalosporins are ineffective against enterococci.[9]

First-Generation Cephalosporins. The first-generation cephalosporin agents are very active against a wide variety of gram-positive organisms, including methicillin-sensitive S. aureus (MSSA) and streptococci. They have moderate activity against community-acquired gram-negative organisms such as E. coli, K. pneumoniae, H. influenzae, M. catarrhalis, and some Proteus spp. They are also considered effective against many oral anaerobes (such as Peptostreptococcus). Commonly used agents within this class are cephalexin, cefazolin, cephalothin, and cefadroxil. These agents are not active against Bacteroides fragilis, P. aeruginosa, and most members of the family Enterobacteriaceae. Generally, first-generation cephalosporins are appropriate for treatment of infections of skin and soft tissue, uncomplicated community-acquired urinary tract infections, streptococcal pharyngitis, and surgical prophylaxis.

Second-Generation Cephalosporins. Second-generation cephalosporins comprise two groups:

Table 14-4

Classification and clinical uses of cephalosporins

CEPHALOSPORINS (GENERIC NAME)	BRAND NAMES	ROUTE	COMMON USES (MICROORGANISM)
FIRST GENERATION			
Cefaclor	Ceclor	PO	MSSA, streptococci
Cefadroxil	Duricef	PO	
Cephalexin	Keflex, Biocef	PO	
Cephradine	Velocef	PO, IM, IV	
Cefazolin	Ancef, Kefzol	IM, IV	
Cephalothin	Keflin	IM, IV	
Cephapirin	Cefadyl	IM, IV	
SECOND GENERATION			
Loracarbef	Lorabid	PO	MSSA, MSSE, *Streptococcus pneumoniae,*
Cefprozil	Cefzil	PO	*Klebsiella* sp., *Escherichia coli, Proteus* sp.,
Cefuroxime axetil	Ceftin	PO	*Haemophilus influenzae*
Cefuroxime	Zinacef, Kefurox	IM, IV	
Cefamandole	Mandol	IM, IV	
Cefonicid	Monocid	IM, IV	
Cefotetan	Cefotan	IM, IV	As above and *Bacteroides fragilis*
Cefoxitin	Mefoxin	IM, IV	
Cefmetazole	Zefazone	IM, IV	
THIRD GENERATION			
Cefixime	Suprax	PO	Better activity than second-generation
Cefpodoxime proxetil	Vantin	PO	cephalosporins against *Klebsiella,*
Ceftibuten	Cedax	PO	*E. coli, Proteus* sp., *H. influenzae*
Cefdinir	Omnicef	PO	*Enterobacter* sp.
Cefotaxime	Claforan	IM, IV	
Ceftriaxone	Rocephin	IM, IV	
Ceftizoxime	Cefizox	IM, IV	
Ceftazidime	Fortaz, Tazidime	IM, IV	As above and *P. aeruginosa*
Cefoperazone	Cefobid	IM, IV	
FOURTH GENERATION			
Cefepime	Maxipime	IM, IV	MSSA, *S. pneumoniae, Klebsiella, E. coli, Proteus* sp., *H. influenzae, P. aeruginosa, Enterobacter* sp.

IM, Intramuscular; *IV,* intravenous; *MSSA,* methicillin-sensitive *Staphylococcus aureus, MSSE,* methicillin-sensitive *Staphylococcus epidermidis; PO,* oral.

the true cephalosporins and the synthetic cephamycins. Cefamandole, cefuroxime, cefaclor, and loracarbef are some of the more widely used true cephalosporins. In contrast to the first-generation cephalosporins, these agents display enhanced gram-negative activity while maintaining comparable gram-positive activity. This group provides improved activity against *H. influenzae, M. catarrhalis, N. meningitidis, N. gonorrhoeae,* and some members of the Enterobacteriaceae. These agents are considered effective in treating the following: community-acquired pneumonia, otitis media, pharyngitis, skin and soft tissue infections, and uncomplicated urinary tract infections. The cephamycins, consisting of cefotetan and cefoxitin, have enhanced activity against gram-negative members of the Enterobacteriaceae, along with anaerobic activity against many *Bacteroides* sp. They are not considered effective against gram-positive organisms such as staphylococci and streptococci. The cephamycins are also useful in the treatment of the following infections: intraabdominal, pelvic and gynecological infections; decubitus ulcers; diabetic foot; and mixed aerobic-anaerobic soft tissue infections.

Third-Generation Cephalosporins. Commonly used agents within the class of third-generation cephalosporins are cefixime, cefpodoxime, ceftibuten, cefoperazone, cefotaxime, ceftazidime, ceftriaxone, and ceftizoxime. These agents are active against most gram-negative organisms. However, only ceftazidime, and to a lesser extent cefoperazone, have activity against *P. aeruginosa*. The third-generation cephalosporins display excellent activity against *S. pneumoniae*, *S. pyogenes*, *H. influenzae*, *N. meningitidis*, *N. gonorrhoeae*, and *M. catarrhalis*. Although activity varies with individual agents, this group is not considered to have significant activity against anaerobes. Ceftriaxone, cefotaxime, and, to a lesser extent, ceftizoxime, achieve clinically significant concentrations within the meninges, making them ideal agents for the treatment of meningitis. Additionally, ceftriaxone has replaced penicillin as the agent of choice in treating all forms of gonococcal *(N. gonorrhoeae)* infection because of the increased prevalence of penicillinase (a β-lactamase)–producing strains. Third-generation cephalosporins are commonly used to treat nosocomial pneumonia, bacteremia, urinary tract infections, osteomyelitis, and soft tissue infections.

Fourth-Generation Cephalosporins. The latest group, fourth-generation cephalosporins, has extended gram-positive and gram-negative coverage. Cefepime is presently the only agent available in the United States. It is parentally administered and active against most gram-negative aerobic organisms, including *P. aeruginosa*. In addition, it has excellent activity against methicillin-sensitive *S. aureus* (MSSA), *Neisseria* sp., *H. influenzae*, *S. pneumoniae*, and *S. pyogenes*. Cefepime has been used primarily in patients for the treatment of uncomplicated and complicated urinary tract infections, skin and soft tissue infections, empiric treatment in patients with neutropenic fever, nosocomial pneumonia, and other serious bacterial infections.

ADVERSE REACTIONS AND PRECAUTIONS FOR THE CEPHALOSPORINS

Similar to the penicillins, the cephalosporins as a group are well tolerated. Hypersensitivity reactions occur in 1% to 3% of patients, with cross-reactivity of cephalosporins in patients with penicillin allergy ranging between 5% and 15%. In general, patients with a penicillin allergy (limited to a rash) may be challenged with a cephalosporin. However, cephalosporin use is contraindicated in patients with a history of anaphylaxis to β-lactams.[10] The process of desensitization should be performed if no therapeutic alternative exists for the use of a cephalosporin. Oral cephalosporins have been associated with minor gastrointestinal complaints such as nausea, vomiting, and diarrhea. Hypoprothrombinemia has been reported, especially with those agents (cefamandole, cefotetan, cefoperazone, and moxalactam) with a methylthiotetrazole (MTT) side chain. The MTT side-chain may also induce a disulfiram-like reaction in patients who concurrently ingest alcohol (disulfiram inhibits the metabolism of alcohol). The symptoms of this uncomfortable reaction include flushing, nausea, thirst, palpitations, chest pain, vertigo, and in some cases even death. Most cephalosporins are eliminated through the kidneys and require dosage adjustment in the presence of renal insufficiency.[11]

CARBAPENEMS

The carbapenems are the newest class of β-lactam antibiotics. Presently two carbapenems, imipenem-cilastatin and meropenem are available for use in the United States. Cilastatin is used to inhibit the metabolism of imipenem within the kidney to prolong the half-life of this agent. Carbapenems are broad-spectrum antibiotics, displaying activity against a wide variety of gram-positive, gram-negative, and anaerobic bacteria.[12]

MECHANISM OF ACTION

The mechanism of action of the carbapenems is similar to that of other β-lactam antibiotics. These agents demonstrate bactericidal activity.

CLINICAL USES

The carbapenems are active against *P. aeruginosa*, multidrug-resistant gram-negative bacilli, and most anaerobes. In addition, carbapenems have activity against gram-positive organisms such as MSSA and *Streptococcus* sp., including pneumococci *(S. pneumoniae)*. They have been used clinically for empiric treatment of bacteremia and sepsis, community-acquired and nosocomial pneumonia, skin and soft tissue infections, complicated urinary tract infections, intraabdominal infections, obstetrical and gynecological infections, osteomyelitis, and infections in patients with cancer and neutropenia. Because of their excellent in vitro activity and broad spectrum of coverage, these agents are often reserved to treat infections that are caused by bacteria resistant to most other agents.

ADVERSE REACTIONS AND PRECAUTIONS

Carbapenems are generally well tolerated, with a low incidence of adverse reactions. Because the carbapenems are structurally related to other β-lactam antibiotics, cross-reactivity may occur when used in patients with allergies to β-lactams. The occurrence of seizures has been reported with the carbapenems, more frequently with imipenem than with meropenem. They are most commonly seen in patients with decreased renal function and those with an underlying seizure disorder. Dosage adjustment is necessary in the presence of renal insufficiency to prevent accumulation of the drug and reduce the potential for seizures.

MONOBACTAMS (AZTREONAM)

Aztreonam is a synthetic monocyclic β-lactam antibiotic. This is the only commercially available agent belonging to the class of antibiotics known as the *monobactams*.[13]

MECHANISM OF ACTION

Aztreonam has a mechanism of action similar to that of other β-lactam antibiotics and demonstrates bactericidal activity.

CLINICAL USES

Aztreonam is only active against gram-negative aerobic bacilli (most Enterobacteriaceae and *P. aeruginosa*). It is not effective against gram-positive and anaerobic bacteria. The strict gram-negative spectrum of aztreonam limits its use as a single agent. It has been used for the treatment of serious urinary tract infections and bacteremia. Aztreonam has more extensive use in combination therapy for treatment of intraabdominal infections, spontaneous bacterial peritonitis, gram-negative osteomyelitis, and hospital-acquired pneumonia and in patients with neutropenic fever.

ADVERSE REACTIONS AND PRECAUTIONS

Aztreonam is well tolerated and is thought to have little to no cross-reactivity to β-lactams. However, rare cases of rashes and even anaphylactic reactions have been reported when aztreonam was used in patients with a β-lactam allergy.

AMINOGLYCOSIDES

Streptomycin was discovered in 1943 and was the first chemotherapeutic agent available to treat tuberculosis. Numerous other aminoglycosides have been developed since and include gentamicin, tobramycin, netilmicin, and amikacin. These agents are used for gram-negative infections, including those caused by *P. aeruginosa*. These antimicrobials have poor gastrointestinal absorption and so require parenteral administration.[14] Table 14-5 lists aminoglycosides and their clinical uses.

MECHANISM OF ACTION

Aminoglycosides bind irreversibly to the 30S bacterial ribosome and inhibit the translation of ribonucleic

Table 14-5

Clinical uses of aminoglycosides

AMINOGLYCOSIDE GENERIC NAME (TRADE NAME)	MOST COMMON CLINICAL USES
Streptomycin	Brucellosis, tuberculosis, endocarditis caused by gentamicin-resistant enterococci
Gentamicin (Garamycin) Tobramycin (Nebcin)	Nosocomial Enterobacteriaceae and *P. aeruginosa* infections, tularemia, brucellosis; endocarditis caused by susceptible enterococci or viridans streptococci, *S. aureus*, *Corynebacterium* sp., penicillin-susceptible *Streptococcus*
Amikacin (Amikin)	Similar to gentamicin and tobramycin but useful against *Acinetobacter* sp., *Nocardia* sp., *Mycobacterium avium-intraceullare*, *M. chelonae*, *M. fortium*
Neomycin (Neosporin)	Prevent wound infections, preoperative gastrointestinal sterilization
Netilmicin (Netromycin)	Similar to gentamicin and tobramycin
Paromomycin (Humatin)	Intestinal amebiasis, tapeworm infestation, *Cryptosporidium* diarrhea

acid (RNA) into proteins. Aminoglycosides also competitively displace cations that link lipopolysaccharides in the outer cell wall of gram-negative bacteria. This destabilization of the cell wall results in increased cell permeability and lysis. Aminoglycosides are bactericidal agents and demonstrate concentration-dependent killing. They are often synergistic when used in combination with β-lactam antibiotics.[15]

CLINICAL USES

Gentamicin and tobramycin have been used for nosocomial gram-negative infections such as ventilator-associated pneumonias. However, aminoglycosides do not achieve high concentrations in bronchial secretions when administered systemically. This is thought to be particularly problematic for patients infected with resistant gram-negative organisms. As a result, aminoglycosides (particularly tobramycin) have been administered by inhalation to control *P. aeruginosa* infections in patients with cystic fibrosis (see the chapter on aerosolized antiinfectives). Amikacin is currently more expensive and is generally reserved for organisms resistant to the other aminoglycosides. Aminoglycosides are used synergistically with β-lactams when treating endocarditis caused by *Streptococcus* sp. and *Enterococcus* sp. Aminoglycosides are also used extensively to treat intraabdominal infections. Streptomycin is used in combination with other antitubercular antimicrobials, especially for multidrug-resistant (MDR) tuberculosis.

ADVERSE REACTIONS AND PRECAUTIONS

The primary toxicities associated with the use of aminoglycosides are nephrotoxicity and ototoxicity. Nephrotoxicity usually develops after at least 5 to 7 days of therapy and occurs more commonly in patients with hypotension, liver disease, advanced age, and coadministration of other nephrotoxic agents. Ototoxicity (both cochleotoxicity and vestibular toxicity) may be irreversible because significant damage must occur before it can be detected. The most common symptoms associated with the development of cochleotoxicity include tinnitus (ringing in the ears); vestibular toxicity manifests as dizziness and nausea. Another serious but rare toxicity is neuromuscular blockade associated with peritoneal irrigation and rapid high-dose aminoglycoside use. Underlying conditions such as myasthenia gravis or concomitant use of neuromuscular blockers may potentiate this side effect, requiring supportive measures such as intubation and possible ventilation support.[16]

TETRACYCLINES

The tetracyclines are broad-spectrum antibiotics with activity against gram-positive and gram-negative microorganisms, as well as many rickettsiae, chlamydiae, mycoplasma, spirochetes, protozoa, and mycobacteria. The most commonly used agent in this class is doxycycline because it can be administered twice daily and is relatively inexpensive. Other available tetracyclines include demeclocycline, minocycline, oxytetracycline, and tetracycline. The agents are available in oral and parenteral formulations.[17]

MECHANISM OF ACTION

Tetracyclines bind reversibly on the 30S ribosome and inhibit the attachment of transfer RNA to an acceptor site on the messenger RNA-ribosome complex. This inhibition blocks protein synthesis and results in a bacteriostatic effect.

CLINICAL USES

Clinical conditions in which tetracyclines are used include respiratory tract infections and other systemic infections. Acute exacerbation of chronic bronchitis and community-acquired pneumonia caused by typical *(S. pneumoniae, H. influenzae)* and atypical *(C. pneumoniae, M. pneumoniae, L. pneumophila)* bacteria can be treated with a tetracycline. Tetracyclines are also useful for the treatment of *C. trachomatis* (sexually transmitted disease), Rocky Mountain spotted fever, Q fever, typhus, brucellosis, Lyme disease, ehrlichiosis, relapsing fever, and cholera. Tetracyclines tend to concentrate in the skin and are useful for the treatment of acne. In addition, tetracyclines have also been used as sclerosing agents for the treatment of malignant and refractory pleural effusions.

ADVERSE REACTIONS AND PRECAUTIONS

Gastrointestinal symptoms such as nausea, vomiting, and diarrhea are the most common side effects associated with the tetracyclines. Tetracyclines bind to growing bone and can temporarily inhibit their growth. The latter side effect makes its use a contraindication during pregnancy, when breast-feeding, and in children less than 8 years of age. Tetracyclines bind to divalent and trivalent cations (calcium, magnesium, aluminum, and iron), which decrease its gastrointestinal absorption when given with antacids, iron supplements, and dairy products. Avoiding the coadministration of tetracyclines with these agents by 1 to 2 hours can prevent this interaction. The prolonged use of minocycline has been associated with vestibular side effects, a blue-black oral pigmentation, and lupuslike symptoms.

MACROLIDES

Erythromycin was introduced in 1952 and was the first agent of this class to be used for infections with atypical organisms and for infections in patients intolerant to penicillin G. Early work with erythromycin involved production of various salt derivatives to improve its gastrointestinal tolerability and absorption. In the last decade, clarithromycin and azithromycin (an azalide) have been introduced. Macrolides exhibit activity against gram-positive (streptococci, MSSA), gram-negative (*H. influenzae, M. catarrhalis)*, and atypical (mycoplasmas, rickettsia, *Legionella* and *Chlamydia*) bacteria. In addition, clarithromycin and azithromycin are active against *Mycobacterium avium*.[18]

MECHANISM OF ACTION

Macrolides inhibit protein synthesis by reversibly binding to the 50S ribosomal subunit and induce the dissociation of transfer RNA from the ribosome during the elongation phase. As a result, bacterial growth is inhibited (bacteriostatic).

CLINICAL USES

Erythromycin is considered the drug of choice for the treatment of pneumonia caused by the atypical pathogens *C. pneumoniae, M. pneumoniae*, and *L. pneumophila*. Erythromycin is considered a safer alternative to the tetracyclines for the treatment of chlamydial *(C. trachomatis)* pelvic infections in pregnant women. Clarithromycin is the preferred agent in combination with ethambutol or rifabutin for the treatment of *M. avium* complex (MAC) in patients with human immunodeficiency virus (HIV) infection. Azithromycin has a superior pharmacokinetic profile to the latter agents by maintaining prolonged intracellular concentrations (long half-life). As a result, azithromycin can be administered once weekly for the prophylaxis of MAC in patients with HIV, compared with clarithromycin, which must be administered twice daily. Similarly a 5-day regimen of azithromycin has been found to be as effective as a 10-day regimen of erythromycin for the treatment of community-acquired pneumonia.

ADVERSE REACTIONS AND PRECAUTIONS

Clarithromycin and azithromycin are generally better tolerated than erythromycin. The most common ad-verse reactions of macrolides include gastrointestinal complaints such as nausea, vomiting, abdominal cramps, and diarrhea (up to 30% of patients on erythromycin). The use of intravenous erythromycin is associated with thrombophlebitis. Ventricular tachycardia and QT prolongation have been reported with the use of the macrolides. Erythromycin and clarithromycin are potent inhibitors of the hepatic drug metabolism system known as the *cytochrome P-450 system* (CYP). As a result, erythromycin and clarithromycin can increase the systemic concentrations of drugs metabolized through CYP. For drugs with narrow therapeutic indices such as theophylline, warfarin, and triazolam, this interaction can lead to potential life threatening complications. Abnormalities in liver function, tinnitus, dizziness, and reversible hearing loss have also been associated with the use of macrolides.[19]

QUINOLONES (FLUOROQUINOLONES)

The fluoroquinolones (Table 14-6) are a semisynthetic group of antimicrobials structurally related to nalidixic acid (quinolone), one of the by-products of chloroquine synthesis. They are widely distributed into most body fluids and tissues (achieve high respiratory tract concentrations). The quinolones are primarily eliminated through the kidneys and achieve high concentrations in the urine. The quinolones currently available in the United States are: norfloxacin, cinoxacin, enoxacin, lomefloxacin, ciprofloxacin, ofloxacin, levofloxacin, trovafloxacin, gatifloxacin, and moxifloxacin. Agents from this class have variable activity against gram-negative, gram-positive, anaerobes, atypical bacteria, and mycobacteria.[20]

MECHANISM OF ACTION

The quinolones exert their antibacterial effect through inhibition of DNA synthesis. They act to inhibit topoisomerase II (DNA gyrase) and topoisomerase IV, which are necessary for bacterial replication. Quinolones are considered bactericidal agents and demonstrate concentration-dependent killing.

CLINICAL USES

Most of the quinolones (excluding norfloxacin, cinoxacin, enoxacin, lomefloxacin) have activity against the common respiratory pathogens, including *S. pneumoniae, H. influenzae, M. catarrhalis, C. pneumoniae, M. pneumoniae*, and *L. pneumophila*. The quinolones have been shown to be effective in the treatment of upper and lower respiratory tract infections,

Table 14-6

Classification and clinical uses of quinolones

QUINOLONES (GENERIC NAME)	BRAND NAME	ROUTE	COMMON USES (MICROORGANISM)
Ciprofloxacin	Cipro	IV, PO	*Pseudomonas aeruginosa*, Enterobacteriaceae, *Neisseria gonorrhoeae*, *Mycoplasma pneumoniae*, *Legionella pneumophila*
Ofloxacin	Oflox	IV, PO	*P. aeruginosa*, Enterobacteriaceae, *N. gonorrhoeae*, *M. pneumoniae*, *Chlamydia pneumoniae*, *L. pneumophila*
Lomefloxacin	Maxaquin	PO	Enterobacteriaceae, *N. gonorrhea*, *C. pneumoniae*
Levofloxacin	Levaquin	IV, PO	*P. aeruginosa*, Enterobacteriaceae, *S. pyogenes*, methicillin-susceptible *S. aureus* (MSSA), *Hemophilus influenzae*, *Moraxella catarrhalis*, penicillin-resistant *Streptococcus pneumoniae*, *M. pneumoniae*, *C. pneumoniae*, *L. pneumophila*
Moxifloxacin	Avelox	PO	Enterobacteriaceae, *S. pyogenes*, MSSA, *H. influenzae*, *M. catarrhalis*, penicillin-resistant *S. pneumoniae*, *M. pneumoniae*, *C. pneumoniae*, *L. pneumophila*
Gatifloxacin	Tequin	IV, PO	Enterobacteriaceae, *S. pyogenes*, MSSA, *H. influenzae*, *M. catarrhalis*, penicillin-resistant *S. pneumoniae*, *M. pneumoniae*, *C. pneumoniae*, *L. pneumophila*
Trovafloxacin	Trovan	IV, PO	Enterobacteriaceae, *S. pyogenes*, MSSA, *H. influenzae*, *M. catarrhalis*, penicillin-resistant *S. pneumoniae*, *M. pneumoniae*, *C. pneumoniae*, *L. pneumophila*, *Bacteroides fragilis*
Norfloxacin	Noroxin	PO	Enterobacteriaceae (only used in treatment of urinary tract infections)
Enoxacin	Penetrex	PO	Enterobacteriaceae, *N. gonorrhoeae* (only used in treatment of urinary tract infections, including uncomplicated urethral or cervical gonorrhoeae)
Cinoxacin	Cinobac	PO	Enterobacteriaceae (only used in treatment of urinary tract infections)

IV, Intravenous; *PO*, oral.

genitourinary tract infections, and skin and skin-structure infections, with results comparable to those found with other antiinfective agents such as cephalosporins, macrolides, and trimethoprim-sulfamethoxazole. The currently available quinolones (except trovafloxacin) do not penetrate the cerebrospinal fluid to any significant extent. Ciprofloxacin has been shown to have the best in vitro activity of the quinolones against *P. aeruginosa* and other gram-negative aerobes. Ciprofloxacin, ofloxacin, and levofloxacin have been used for the treatment of nosocomial pneumonia.

ADVERSE REACTIONS AND PRECAUTIONS

The quinolones are well tolerated and are considered one of the safest antimicrobial classes. Gastrointestinal side effects such as nausea, vomiting, and diarrhea occur in less than 5% of patients treated with quinolones. Prolongation of the QT interval (especially in female patients) has been reported with the use of quinolones. Seizures have been reported with

ciprofloxacin in elderly patients and those with diminished renal function. Trovafloxacin use has been associated with fatal cases of liver toxicity. Currently trovafloxacin use outside the hospital setting for greater than 14 days is not recommended. Studies in immature laboratory animals have demonstrated changes in weight-bearing joints subsequent to quinolone exposure. Although, quinolone-induced arthropathy has not been documented in humans, use of quinolones in children (≤ 18 years of age) should be reserved for cases in which the benefits outweigh the risks. Dosage adjustment of the quinolones (except trovafloxacin) is necessary in the presence of renal insufficiency. Concomitant use of antacids and iron supplements reduces the absorption of quinolones (such as the tetracyclines).

OTHER ANTIBIOTICS

The following agents belong to various classes of antimicrobials with different mechanisms of action and spectrum of activity. The individual agents will be discussed as they represent the clinically used agents of their antimicrobial class.

CHLORAMPHENICOL

Chloramphenicol has been available for use in the United States since 1949. This agent has a broad spectrum of activity against gram-positive, gram-negative, and anaerobic bacteria. Chloramphenicol distributes well into various tissues including the brain. Use of this antibiotic has declined in recent years with the availability of less toxic agents.[21]

MECHANISM OF ACTION

Chloramphenicol inhibits protein synthesis by reversibly binding to the 50S ribosome subunit and essentially has a bacteriostatic effect. With prolonged exposure, chloramphenicol demonstrates bactericidal activity against some organisms by inducing bacterial cell lysis.

CLINICAL USES

Chloramphenicol is highly active against salmonella and has been used for the treatment of gastroenteritis with sepsis, as well as salmonella meningitis. Chloramphenicol has excellent activity against rickettsial diseases such as scrub typhus, murine typhus, and Rocky Mountain spotted fever. However, these diseases are usually treated with tetracyclines, with chloramphenicol reserved for pregnant patients. Anaerobic infections and mixed anaerobic/aerobic infections such as peritonitis and aspiration pneumonia can be treated with chloramphenicol. In addition, chloramphenicol can be used to treat bacteremias caused by *Enterococcus* sp., including some isolates that are resistant to vancomycin.

ADVERSE REACTIONS AND PRECAUTIONS

Because of the possibility of irreversible bone marrow suppression that may lead to serious and fatal blood dyscrasias (aplastic anemia), this agent should not be used when other effective agents are available. Aplastic anemia is a life-threatening complication reported in 1 of every 20,000 patients treated with chloramphenicol. This agent should not be used in premature and newborn infants, who cannot adequately metabolize this drug. The decreased metabolism of chloramphenicol results in high serum concentrations that can lead to gray baby syndrome (vomiting, pallor, cyanosis, circulatory collapse), which has an attributable mortality of 60%. The prolonged use of chloramphenicol in children with cystic fibrosis has been associated with optic neuritis leading to blindness.

TRIMETHOPRIM-SULFAMETHOXAZOLE

Sulfamethoxazole belongs to the class of antibiotics known as the sulfonamides. Trimethoprim is a pyrimidine found to potentiate the activity of sulfamethoxazole. The combination of trimethoprim and sulfamethoxazole (TMP-SMX) was introduced in 1968 and has since gained a place in the treatment of numerous infections. This combination is active against gram-positive (streptococci, MSSA) and gram-negative (*H. influenzae, Burkholderia cepacia, Stenotrophomonas maltophila*) bacteria. In addition, it is active against *Pneumocystis carinii.*[22]

MECHANISM OF ACTION

TMP-SMX exerts antibacterial effects by sequentially blocking bacterial dihydropteroate synthetase and dihydrofolate reductase. These enzymes are responsible for the production of folic acid. Without folic acid, bacteria are unable to synthesize nucleic acid and proteins necessary for growth. TMP-SMX acts synergistically and is considered bacteriostatic.

CLINICAL USES

TMP-SMX is used for the treatment and prophylaxis of *P. carinii* pneumonia (PCP) in patients infected with HIV. TMP-SMX is widely distributed in the body, achieving detectable levels in most tissues. High concentrations are achieved in the urine, making it an ideal agent for the treatment of urinary tract infections (UTIs). In addition, it has been used for treatment of acute exacerbations of bronchitis, traveler's diarrhea caused by enterotoxigenic *E. coli*, otitis media, and shigellosis. In recent years, bacterial resistance to TMP-SMX has increased, creating controversy over the continued use of this combination as a first-line agent for UTIs.

ADVERSE REACTIONS AND PRECAUTIONS

TMP-SMX is relatively well tolerated, with nausea, vomiting, diarrhea, and hypersensitivity being the most common adverse effects. In addition, sulfamethoxazole has side effects that are common to all sulfonamides such as neutropenia, thrombocytopenia, hemolytic anemia, jaundice, hepatic necrosis, and drug-induced lupus. TMP-SMX should be avoided in all patients with "sulfa" allergies or hypersensitivities. Patients who are deficient in the enzyme glucose-6-phosphate dehydrogenase (G6PD) should not receive

TMP-SMX, because this combination can increase the risk of hemolytic anemia. The daily dosage of TMP-SMX should be reduced in the presence of renal insufficiency because both agents are eliminated through the kidneys.

CLINDAMYCIN

Clindamycin, a member of the lincosamide class of antibiotics, has activity against gram-positive and anaerobic bacteria. In addition, this agent is active against *Toxoplasma gondii* and *P. carinii*.[21]

MECHANISM OF ACTION

Like chloramphenicol, clindamycin binds to the bacterial 50S ribosomal subunit to inhibit protein synthesis, resulting in a bacteriostatic effect. This suppression of protein synthesis has been shown to reduce toxin-production in certain strains of *S. aureus* (toxic shock syndrome) and *S. pyogenes* (necrotizing fasciitis).

CLINICAL USES

Clindamycin distributes well in body tissues, but has minimal penetration into cerebrospinal fluid even in the presence of meningitis. Clindamycin is used as an adjunct to agents with gram-negative activity for intraabdominal, pelvic, and diabetic foot infections, all of which tend to be polymicrobial. Anaerobic infections of the respiratory tract such as necrotizing pneumonia, lung abscess, empyema, and aspiration pneumonia are often treated with clindamycin. AIDS-related illnesses such as *Toxoplasma* encephalitis and PCP can also be treated with clindamycin.

ADVERSE REACTIONS AND PRECAUTIONS

Nausea, vomiting, and diarrhea are the most common side effects associated with clindamycin. This diarrhea may be a consequence of *Clostridium difficile*. Discontinuing the offending antibiotic and initiating oral vancomycin or metronidazole therapy treats this mild to life-threatening diarrhea. Prolongation of the neuromuscular blocking effects of pancuronium with the concomitant use of clindamycin has also been reported.

METRONIDAZOLE

Metronidazole is a nitroimidazole that was used initially for its antiprotozoal effects against pathogens such as *Trichomonas vaginalis*, *Giardia lamblia*, and *Entamoeba histolytica*. Its anaerobic properties were discovered after an observation that acute ulcerative gingivitis improved in patients being treated for trichomonal vaginitis.[21]

MECHANISM OF ACTION

The exact mechanism of action is unknown, although it is thought to have different effects in protozoa versus anaerobic bacteria. It is postulated that the microorganisms convert metronidazole into its reduced form. This reduced form causes a loss of the helical structure of DNA and results in DNA strand breaks. Metronidazole is bactericidal against anaerobic pathogens such as *B. fragilis*.

CINICAL USES

Anaerobic infections have been implicated in abscesses within the brain, lung, and intraabdominal cavity. Metronidazole is often added as an adjunct, especially when surgical drainage of the abscess is not possible. Unlike clindamycin, metronidazole penetrates well into the central nervous system and therefore is useful for the treatment of brain abscesses. A key anaerobic pathogen, *B. fragilis* is part of the normal enteric flora and can contribute to sepsis in the event of gastrointestinal disease, surgery, or penetrating trauma. Metronidazole is often added to treat polymicrobial infections, especially where *B. fragilis* is suspected. Bacterial vaginosis caused by *Gardnerella*, *Trichomonas*, and *Bacteroides* sp. is also treated with metronidazole. In addition, diarrhea caused by *C. difficile* can be treated with metronidazole.

ADVERSE REACTIONS AND PRECAUTIONS

An unpleasant metallic taste, nausea, and vomiting are common complaints associated with the use of metronidazole. The prolonged use of this agent, especially with high doses, can lead to peripheral neuropathy. In some rare situations, seizures, encephalopathy, and cerebellar dysfunction has also been noted. Metronidazole can interact with warfarin to potentiate its hypoprothrombinemic effect and lead to significant bleeding. In addition, patients should avoid the use of alcohol while on metronidazole (inhibits alcohol dehydrogenase) because the concomitant use can result in a disulfiram-like reaction.

NITROFURANTOIN

Multiple nitrofuran compounds have been synthesized since their discovery in the early 1940s. The most widely used agent of this class has been nitrofurantoin. This antibacterial does not achieve therapeutic concentrations in body tissues other than the kidney. As a result, it is used only for UTIs.[23]

MECHANISM OF ACTION

Mechanisms such as inhibition of bacterial enzymes, protein synthesis, and damage to bacterial DNA have been implicated. The presence of these multiple inhibitory mechanisms may explain the infrequency of resistance. Nitrofurantoin is bactericidal at the high concentrations achieved in the urine.

CLINICAL USES

Nitrofurantoin is effective for UTIs such as urethritis (urethral infection), cystitis (bladder infection), and pyelonephritis (kidney infection). The most common pathogen associated with these infections is the gram-negative bacterium E. coli.

ADVERSE REACTIONS AND PRECAUTIONS

Nausea and vomiting are common side effects that can require cessation of therapy. Hypersensitivity syndromes such as skin rashes, drug fever, and even asthma have been observed. Nitrofurantoin can accumulate in patients with renal dysfunction and result in serious complications such as peripheral neuritis. In addition, pneumonitis mimicking acute respiratory infection has been reported, but is rapidly reversible with discontinuation of this drug. Chronic pulmonary disease marked by interstitial fibrosis has been reported. This reversible condition may occur in patients who receive nitrofurantoin for longer than 6 months. Hemolytic anemia in patients with glucose-6-phosphate dehydrogenase (G6PD) deficiency can be precipitated with this agent. A disulfiram-like reaction can also occur in patients who consume alcohol while being treated with nitrofurantoin.

VANCOMYCIN

Vancomycin is a glycopeptide antibiotic with activity against gram-positive bacteria. It is not active against gram-negative bacteria. Its use in recent years has escalated as a result of the emergence of methicillin-resistant S. aureus (MRSA).[24]

MECHANISM OF ACTION

Vancomycin inhibits transglycosylation of peptidoglycan by binding to the precursor d-alanine-d-alanine portion. This process prevents the formation of a rigid cell wall structure and results in bacterial cell lysis. Vancomycin is considered bactericidal against gram-positive organisms with the exception of enterococci (bacteriostatic).

CLINICAL USES

Vancomycin is used for infections caused by MRSA, such as bacteremias, endocarditis, pneumonia, peritonitis, and skin and soft tissue infections. Vancomycin also serves as the alternative agent to penicillin for the treatment of viridans streptococcal endocarditis. Vancomycin does not cross the blood-brain barrier efficiently, even in the presence of acute meningeal inflammation. However, pneumococcal meningitis resistant to penicillin can still be treated by these low concentrations of vancomycin. An oral formulation of vancomycin can be used to treat C. difficile diarrhea that is refractory to metronidazole.

ADVERSE REACTIONS AND PRECAUTIONS

A common reaction known as red man or red neck syndrome has been associated with the rapid infusion of vancomycin (related to histamine release). Increasing the time of infusion can prevent this syndrome of skin itch, flushing, angioedema, and hypotension. Ototoxicity and nephrotoxicity have been noted to occur more frequently in patients who receive vancomycin concomitantly with aminoglycosides. Vancomycin is renally excreted and therefore requires dosage adjustment in patients with renal impairment.

QUINUPRISTIN AND DALFOPRISTIN

Quinupristin and dalfopristin (Synercid) are streptogrammins that act synergistically when used together. These agents are active against gram-positive bacteria and are used primarily to treat infections caused by vancomycin-resistant Enterococcus faecium (VREF).[24]

MECHANISM OF ACTION

Dalfopristin blocks peptide bond formation and distorts the ribosome to enhance the binding of quinupristin. The ribosome bound quinupristin inhibits the binding of aminoacyl-transfer RNA to inhibit protein synthesis. The combination is bactericidal against MRSA, but is bacteriostatic against VREF.

CLINICAL USES

Quinupristin-dalfopristin is used primarily for life-threatening VREF infections, but is also indicated for skin and soft tissue infections and pneumonias caused by susceptible gram-positive pathogens. Quinupristin-dalfopristin is not active against most gram-negative bacteria and anaerobes. However, quinupristin-dalfopristin has good in vitro activity against *M. pneumoniae* and *L. pneumophila*.

ADVERSE REACTIONS AND PRECAUTIONS

Quinupristin-dalfopristin is only available as a parenteral formulation and must be administered through a central line (catheter inserted and threaded to the superior or inferior vena cava) because peripheral administration is associated with a high incidence of thrombophlebitis. Arthralgias and myalgias of varying severity have also been reported with the use of these agents in up to 40% of patients. Like erythromycin, quinupristin-dalfopristin is an inhibitor of the CYP system. Therefore drugs (metabolized through the CYP system) with a narrow therapeutic index should be used cautiously in patients on quinupristin-dalfopristin.

LINEZOLID

This antibiotic belongs to a novel class of antibiotics known as the oxazolidinones. Linezolid like quinupristin-dalfoprisitin is active against gram-positive bacteria and is approved for the treatment of severe life-threatening VREF infections. Unlike vancomycin and quinupristin-dalfopristin, linezolid is available as an oral formulation that is completely absorbed from the gastrointestinal tract.[25]

MECHANISM OF ACTION

Linezolid prevents RNA translation by binding to the 23S ribosomal RNA of the 50S subunit to prevent the formation of a functional 70S initiation complex. Use of this novel antimicrobial target for the inhibition of protein synthesis has not been previously exploited.

CLINICAL USES

Linezolid is indicated for the treatment of VREF infections, including cases with concurrent bacteremia. Nosocomial pneumonias and complicated skin and skin structure infections caused by *S. aureus*, including MRSA, may be treated with linezolid. Linezolid lacks significant activity against gram-negative bacteria.

ADVERSE REACTIONS AND PRECAUTIONS

The most common adverse events reported with linezolid include diarrhea, nausea, and headaches. Thrombocytopenia has been reported with the use of linezolid but is associated with prolonged use of the antibiotic ($\geq$2 weeks). Linezolid is a reversible, nonselective inhibitor of monamine oxidase and has the

potential to interact with adrenergic (e.g., dopamine, norepinephrine) and serotonergic (e.g., selective serotonin reuptake inhibitors) agents.

ANTIMYCOBACTERIALS

Tuberculosis has received much attention over the past decade largely because of the increase in cases attributed to the HIV epidemic. Each year millions of individuals are exposed to tuberculosis, many through casual contact. Over 3 million new cases of tuberculosis were reported in the United States for 1996. The Centers for Disease Control (CDC) makes annual recommendations for the prevention and treatment of tuberculosis infection. Nosocomial transmission can be prevented by placing patients with suspected or confirmed tuberculosis in respiratory isolation (negative-pressure room) until they are (1) determined to not have tuberculosis, (2) discharged from the hospital, or (3) confirmed to be noninfectious. Other measures such as use of fitted respiratory masks (by healthcare personnel) can prevent transmission of *Mycobacterium tuberculosis* by aerosolization to caregivers. Treatment consists of multiple antibiotic regimens for 6 to 12 months in duration. Single-agent regimens should never be used for treatment because the likelihood of developing resistance is high. Treatment failures often result from poor patient compliance, as well as resistance to antibiotics. Drugs used in the treatment of tuberculosis can be categorized as either first-line or second-line agents depending on their efficacy and side-effect profiles. Initial therapy generally involves a combination of isoniazid, pyrazinamide, rifampin, and ethambutol. A summary of the clinically used antimycobacterial agents, doses, routes of administration, and side effects are listed in Table 14-7. Addition or subtraction of agents from this regimen is usually based on culture and sensitivity data, along with patient response to treatment. Guidelines for the treatment of active pulmonary tuberculosis are provided in Table 14-8.[26,27]

ISONIAZID

Isoniazid (INH) is well absorbed orally and is distributed throughout the body, especially in the cerebral spinal fluid. Isoniazid is metabolized by the liver, and its metabolite is eliminated by the kidneys.

MECHANISM OF ACTION

Isoniazid inhibits cell wall synthesis by inhibiting synthesis of mycolic acid, a primary component of the mycobacterial cell wall. This agent is bactericidal

Table 14-7

Commonly used antimycobacterials including dose, route, and side-effect profile

ANTIMYCOBACTERIAL	ADULT DOSE	ROUTE	SIDE EFFECTS
Isoniazid	5 mg/kg/day; maximum of 300 mg/day	PO, IM	Hepatotoxicity (symptoms include nausea, loss of appetite, abdominal pain), peripheral neuritis, rash, fever, anemia
Rifampin	10 mg/kg/day; maximum of 600 mg/day	PO IV	Hepatotoxicity, flulike symptoms, discolorations of body secretions to an orange color
Rifabutin	300 mg/day	PO	Hepatotoxicity, flulike symptoms, discolorations of body secretions to an orange color
Pyrazinamide	15-30 mg/kg/day; maximum of 2000 mg/day	PO	Hepatotoxicity, arthralgia, hyperuricemia
Ethambutol	15-25 mg/kg/day; maximum of 2500 mg/day	PO	Optic neuritis (higher in patients receiving >15mg/kg/day)
Streptomycin	15 mg/kg/day; maximum of 1000 mg/day	IM	Ototoxicity (high-frequency hearing loss, vertigo), nephrotoxicity

IM, Intramuscular; *IV*, intravenous; *PO*, oral.

Table 14-8

Guidelines for the treatment of active pulmonary tuberculosis

CLINICAL SCENARIO	TREATMENT REGIMEN
1. INH resistance rate <4%	INH + RIF (or RFB) + PZA + B_6 daily for 2 mo, then INH + RIF (or RFB) + B_6 daily for an additional 4 mo
2. INH resistance rate >4% or unknown	INH + RIF (or RFB) + PZA + ETB or SM + B_6 daily for 2 mo, then INH + RIF (or RFB) + B_6 daily for an additional 4 mo
3. Noncompliant or unreliable patient	Requires directly observed therapy (DOT) INH + RIF (or RFB) + PZA + ETB + B_6 or SM daily for 2 wk, then 2-3 times/wk for 6 wk, then INH + RIF (or RFB) + B_6 2-3 times/wk for 6 mo
4. Known INH resistant or unable to tolerate INH	DOT for RIF (or RFB) + PZA + ETB daily for 18 mo
5. Known RIF resistant or unable to tolerate RIF	INH + PZA + ETB + B_6 daily for 18 mo
6. Pregnancy	INH + RIF + ETB daily for 9 mo
7. HIV infection or AIDS	Treatment as in clinical scenarios 1 and 2 for the first 2 mo, then extend the INH + RIF (or RFB) + B_6 daily for an additional 7 mo

From *MMWR* 9:49(RR-6), 2000.
B_6, Pyridoxine; *DOT*, directly observed therapy; *ETB*, ethambutol; *INH*, isoniazid; *PZA*, pyrazinamide; *RIF*, rifampin; *RFB*, rifabutin.

against replicating tuberculosis bacilli and bacteriostatic against nonreplicating organisms.

ADVERSE REACTIONS AND PRECAUTIONS

An elevation in liver enzymes has been reported in patients receiving isoniazid and is reversible with the discontinuation of the drug. Rare cases of serious hepatitis and death also have been reported. Hepatotoxicity usually occurs between the fourth and eighth weeks of treatment but may occur at anytime. Tests used to measure hepatocellular injury should be performed and include monitoring liver transaminases such as alanine aminotransferase (ALT) and aspartate aminotransferase (AST). In addition, patients should be monitored for the development of symptoms of hepatitis such as nausea, loss of appetite, and abdominal pain. Neurotoxicity has also been reported and occurs more frequently in patients receiving higher dose therapy. Supplementation with pyridoxine (vitamin B_6) has been shown to reduce the frequency of this adverse reaction. Rare miscellaneous reactions such as rash, anemia, and fever also have been reported.

RIFAMPIN AND RIFABUTIN

Rifampin and rifabutin are semisynthetic antibiotics referred to as *rifamycins.* Rifampin and rifabutin have similar structures, as well as spectrums of activity. They are well absorbed orally, with good penetration into most tissues. They do not penetrate the central nervous system well in the absence of inflammation. Rifampin is extensively metabolized through the liver and is an inducer of the CYP system. Rifabutin is also metabolized hepatically; however, it is a weaker enzyme inducer than rifampin. CYP induction is known to decrease plasma concentrations of drugs hepatically metabolized; therefore dosage adjustments of agents metabolized by this system are necessary.

MECHANISM OF ACTION

The rifamycins inhibit bacterial DNA-dependent RNA polymerase. They are bactericidal against actively dividing bacteria

ADVERSE REACTIONS AND PRECAUTIONS

Hepatotoxicity is the major adverse reaction associated with the rifamycins. Elevations in liver transaminases are commonly reported and are usually reversible upon discontinuation of the drug. Patients with preexisting liver damage are more prone to rifamycin-induced hepatotoxicity. Rifamycins are known to change the color of body fluids to a deep orange hue. Patients should be warned that urine, feces, tears, saliva, sputum, and semen might turn an orange color. Uveitis (inflammation of the iris), which manifests as blurry vision has also been reported. Rare reports of flulike symptoms such as fever, chills, nausea, and vomiting have been reported during rifamycin therapy.

PYRAZINAMIDE

Pyrazinamide is a nicotinic acid derivative that is well distributed into most tissues, including the cere-

brospinal fluid. Pyrazinamide is hepatically metabolized and excreted by the kidneys.

MECHANISM OF ACTION

The precise mechanism of action is not known. Mycobacteria convert pyrazinamide to pyrazinoic acid. It is speculated that pyrazinoic acid accumulates in macrophages to lower the intracellular pH and increase the antimycobacterial activity of macrophages in combination with pyrazinamide. Pyrazinamide is bactericidal against mycobacteria when tested in an acidic environment.

ADVERSE REACTIONS AND PRECAUTIONS

Nausea and vomiting are the most common side effect with pyrazinamide treatment. Hepatotoxicity has also been reported in patients receiving pyrazinamide; therefore liver transaminases should be frequently monitored. Patients with preexisting liver abnormalities should be monitored closely. It is not known to induce or inhibit the CYP system to any significant extent.

ETHAMBUTOL

Ethambutol is a synthetic orally administered agent that distributes extensively throughout the body, including the cerebrospinal fluid. It is primarily eliminated unchanged in the urine.

MECHANISM OF ACTION

Ethambutol decreases the synthesis of cell wall polysaccharides such as arabinogalactan to inhibit mycobacterial cell growth. It is a bacteriostatic agent.

ADVERSE REACTIONS AND PRECAUTIONS

Optic neuropathy is the major toxicity associated with the use of ethambutol. Patients usually complain of blurred vision in conjunction with altered color (red-green) perception. Optic neuritis is usually seen with the use of high doses of ethambutol and is slowly reversible upon discontinuation of the drug. Baseline optometric evaluation, followed by periodic examinations is advisable to help monitor for visual changes during treatment. The dose of ethambutol should be adjusted in patients with renal insufficiency.

STREPTOMYCIN

Streptomycin is an aminoglycoside antibiotic that has been in use since the 1940s for the treatment of tuberculosis. It is available in an intravenous formulation only and indicated as an add-on agent in patients with documented or suspected drug-resistant tuberculosis.

MECHANISM OF ACTION

Streptomycin has a similar mechanism of action to that of other aminoglycosides.

ADVERSE REACTIONS AND PRECAUTIONS

Streptomycin, like other aminoglycosides, is associated with nephrotoxicity and ototoxicity. It is eliminated unchanged in the urine and requires dosage adjustment in patients with renal insufficiency.

ANTIFUNGALS

The incidence of fungal infections has increased dramatically over the past two decades. *Candida* sp. are now the fourth most commonly isolated bloodstream pathogens. Candidemia has an attributable mortality of up to 40%. The number of immuno-

compromised patients resulting from AIDS, cancer chemotherapy, and organ transplantation has been increasing. These patient populations have diminished cell-mediated immunity and are predisposed to numerous fungal pathogens that vary in incidence geographically. The treatment of choice for most of these infections has been the polyene amphotericin B. The high incidence of nephrotoxicity associated with this agent served as the impetus for the development of the azoles. Ketoconazole was the first agent of this class, but it has largely been replaced by the triazoles fluconazole and itraconazole. Newer triazoles with improved activity against molds are being developed. In addition a new classes of antifungals known as the echinocandins are now available. A summary of systemically used antifungals including route and clinical uses are provided in Table 14-9.[28]

Table 14-9

Classification of the systemically used antifungals

ANTIFUNGAL CLASS (GENERIC NAME)	BRAND NAME	ROUTE	COMMON USES (MICROORGANISM)
POLYENES			
Amphotericin B	Fungizone	IV, PO*	*Candida* sp., *Aspergillus* sp., *Cryptococcus neoformans, Histoplamsa capsulatum, Blastomyces dermatitidis, Coccidioides immitus*
Amphotericin B colloidal dispersion	Amphotec	IV	*Candida* sp., *Aspergillus* sp., mucormycosis, *C. neoformans*
Amphotericin B lipid complex	Abelcet	IV	*Candida* sp., *Aspergillus* sp., mucormycosis, *C. neoformans*
Liposomal amphotericin B	AmBisome	IV	*Candida* sp., *Aspergillus* sp., mucormycosis, *C. neoforms*, leishmaniasis
AZOLES			
Ketoconazole	Nizoral	PO	*Candida* sp.,† *C. neoformans, H. capsulatum, B. dermatitidis*
Fluconazole	Diflucan	IV, PO	*Candida* sp.,† *C. neoformans*
Itraconazole	Sporanox	IV, PO	*Candida* sp.,† *Aspergillus* sp., *C. neoformans, H. capsulatum, B. dermatitidis, C. immitus, Sporothrix schenckii*
OTHER ANTIFUNGALS			
Caspofungin	Cancidas	IV	*Aspergillus* sp., *Candida* sp.
Flucytosine	Ancobon	PO	*Aspergillus* sp., *Candida* sp., *C. neoformans*
Griseofulvin	Fulvicin	PO	Tinea corporis, tinea cruris, tinea barbae, tinea capitis, and tinea ungium
Terbinafine	Lamisil	PO	Tinea corporis, tinea pedis, tinea manuum, tinea cruris, tinea imbricata, tinea capitis, and tinea ungium

IV, Intravenous; *PO,* oral.
*The oral form of amphotericin B is not absorbed through the gastrointestinal tract.
†*C. krusei* is intrinsically resistant to all azoles.

Polyenes

The polyenes include amphotericin B and nystatin. Amphotericin B has been available for over 50 years and remains the drug of choice for most systemic fungal infections. In recent years, amphotericin B has been formulated into lipid-based products. These lipid-based products alter the distribution of amphotericin B, resulting in a relatively higher uptake of the agent into the reticuloendothelial system (liver, spleen, lymphatics) relative to the kidneys. The net effect of this shift in distribution has been shown to reduce the incidence of nephrotoxicity. Nystatin is only used topically for oral and intertriginous (between skin surfaces) candidiasis. However, a lipid-based formulation of nystatin is currently under investigation.

Mechanism of Action

The polyenes bind to ergosterol (a type of cholesterol) in the fungal cell membrane, creating pores that increase cell membrane permeability. Intracellular potassium and other components escape through the pores, resulting in cell death (fungicidal).

Clinical Uses

The fungicidal activity of amphotericin B has made it the first-line agent for several pathogens causing pulmonary infections, including aspergillosis, blastomycosis, coccidioidomycosis, histoplasmosis, and cryptococcosis. These infections are associated with a high mortality, especially in patients that are neutropenic. Consequently, preventive measures such as amphotericin B prophylaxis and high-dose treatment (through the use of lipid-based formulations) have been sought. However, the optimal dose and treatment duration have been difficult to define because the successful outcome of a systemic fungal infection is largely dependent on recovery of the host immune system.

Adverse Reactions and Precautions

The parenteral administration of amphotericin B is associated with two major types of toxicity. The first is infusion-related and includes flushing, fever, and chills. Pretreating patients (who manifested these symptoms) with antipyretics and antihistamines may minimize these effects. The second major toxicity is renal impairment thought to be a result of diminished renal perfusion. Hydrating the patient with normal saline boluses before and after amphotericin B infusion has been attempted to prevent this toxicity.

The liposomal products such as amphotericin B lipid complex and liposomal amphotericin B have been shown to be less nephrotoxic than the traditional product and allow the administration of higher doses of amphotericin B.

Azoles

The systemically used azoles include ketoconazole, fluconazole, and itraconazole. Ketoconazole was the first oral agent (no intravenous formulation) available to treat systemic fungal infections. This agent is poorly absorbed from the gastrointestinal tract (requires an acidic environment) and has the potential for substantial toxicity. As a result, ketoconazole has largely been replaced by the newer triazoles fluconazole and itraconazole. Fluconazole is available as both an oral and intravenous formulation, is widely distributed, and is relatively nontoxic, but it has a narrow spectrum of activity. Itraconazole has the broadest spectrum of activity of the azoles but is less tolerated than fluconazole.

Mechanism of Action

The azoles inhibit the fungal CYP system responsible for the conversion of lanosterol to ergosterol. The reduction in ergosterol production prevents fungal cell growth (fungistatic).

Clinical Uses

Ketoconazole has been used as a second-line agent to treat candidiasis, blastomycosis, histoplasmosis, and paracoccidioidomycosis. Fluconazole is used primarily for candidiasis and as suppressive therapy for patients with cryptococcal meningitis. In addition, fluconazole has been used to treat coccidioidomycosis. Itraconazole is the drug of choice for the treatment of cutaneous and lymphangitic sporotrichosis. It is also used as prophylaxis and as suppressive therapy for pulmonary aspergillosis. Itraconazole is also used clinically to treat histoplasmosis, blastomycosis, cryptococcosis, coccidioidomycosis, paracoccidioidomycosis, and candidiasis. Of note, candidiasis caused by *C. krusei* (lacks the CYP system) cannot be treated with an azole because this organism is intrinsically resistant to this class of antifungals.

Adverse Reactions and Precautions

Anorexia, nausea, and vomiting are commonly reported with the use of ketoconazole and itraconazole. More serious side effects in men such as impotence, decreased libido, and gynecomastia have been attributed to ketoconazole's inhibition of testosterone synthesis. Both ketoconazole and itraconazole are potent inhibitors of the CYP3A4 system and have a significant potential for drug interactions. Fluconazole is well tolerated and does not have the drug interactions seen with ketoconazole and itraconazole. In addition, fluconazole is not metabolized; it is eliminated unchanged in the urine and so requires dosage adjustment in patients with impaired renal function.

ECHINOCANDINS

Caspofungin is the only agent in this class of antifungals to be approved for clinical use. Several compounds in this class are currently under development. These agents have poor gastrointestinal absorption and require parenteral administration.[29]

MECHANISM OF ACTION

These agents inhibit fungal cell wall synthesis by inhibiting $(1,3)$-β-d-$(+)$-glucan synthase. Echinocandins may be either fungicidal or fungistatic against fungi depending on the isolate.

CLINICAL USES

Caspofungin has demonstrated in vitro and in vivo (animal studies) activity against *Candida* sp. and *Aspergillus* sp., but it is inactive against *Cryptococcus*. Use is currently restricted to the treatment of aspergillosis in patients refractory or intolerant to amphotericin B, lipid-based amphotericin B, and itraconazole.

ADVERSE REACTIONS AND PRECAUTIONS

Data regarding the safety of caspofungin are limited to a small number of patients treated during clinical trials with this agent. In those studies the most common adverse reactions were fever, rashes, and thrombophlebitis. One case of anaphylaxis during the initial administration of caspofungin was reported. Elevations in liver transaminase levels (AST and ALT) were noted with the coadministration of caspofungin and cyclosporine. The concomitant use of these agents is not recommended.

FLUCYTOSINE

Flucytosine acts as an antimetabolite and is used primarily as adjunctive therapy for susceptible fungal pathogens. It is active against *Candida, Cryptococcus,* and *Aspergillus.*[28]

MECHANISM OF ACTION

Flucytosine is converted to flurouracil and competes with uracil during the formation of fungal RNA. Inhibition of RNA formation decreases protein synthesis and prevents cell growth (fungistatic).

CLINICAL USE

Resistance to flucytosine develops rapidly when used as a single agent for systemic fungal infections. As a result, flucytosine has been used in combination with amphotericin B for the treatment of cryptococcal meningitis and aspergillosis.

ADVERSE REACTIONS AND PRECAUTIONS

The most common adverse event associated with this agent is bone marrow suppression leading to anemia, leukopenia, and thrombocytopenia. This toxicity usually results when serum concentrations of this agent exceed 100 μg/ml. Dosage reduction in patients with renal impairment is imperative to prevent this serious complication.

GRISEOFULVIN AND TERBINAFINE

Griseofulvin was one of the first antifungals discovered; however, only dermatophytes (skin fungi) are susceptible to this agent. The absorption of this agent is greatly increased when taken with a high-fat meal. Terbinafine, which was developed recently, has demonstrated more potent activity against dermatophytes. Terbinafine is a highly lipophilic allylamine that concentrates in the stratum corneum, sebum, and hair follicles. This property makes it an excellent agent for cutaneous dermatophytosis ("ring-worm" infection, athlete's foot, etc.) and onychomycosis (fungal infection in nails).[28]

MECHANISM OF ACTION

Griseofulvin is only active against growing dermatophytes. It interferes with microtubule formation of the mitotic spindle, preventing the growth of hyphae. Terbinafine inhibits squalene epoxidase, which reduces ergosterol production and inhibits fungal cell growth.

CLINICAL USES

Griseofulvin and terbinafine are used for fungal infections (tinea) of the skin, hair, and nails. However, the recurrence rates of these infections tend to be higher with griseofulvin relative to terbinafine. Treatment for 12 to 16 weeks with terbinafine has been demonstrated to be superior to griseofulvin for the eradication of finger and toenail fungus.

ADVERSE REACTIONS AND PRECAUTIONS

Heartburn, flatulence, angular stomatitis, glossodynia, and a black-furred tongue are common gastrointestinal side effects of griseofulvin. Headache is also a common side effect of griseofulvin but subsides during the course of therapy. Terbinafine is well tolerated, with the most common side effects reported to be nausea, vomiting, and abdominal cramps. Terbinafine has been associated with transient increases in hepatic transaminases, which revert to normal on discontinuation of the agent. Rash and hypersensitivity reactions have been reported with both of these agents.

ANTIVIRAL AGENTS

Several agents are available for treating viral infections (Table 14-10). All of these agents act by inhibiting steps involved in viral replication, with none inhibiting nonreplicating viruses. Agents used to treat HIV will not be discussed.[30]

ACYCLOVIR AND VALACYCLOVIR

Acyclovir is available in intravenous, oral, and topical formulations. Oral acyclovir is not readily absorbed and so requires frequent daily dosing. Valacyclovir, a prodrug of acyclovir, was developed to improve gastrointestinal absorption of acyclovir. Valacyclovir is only available in oral formulation.[30]

MECHANISM OF ACTION

Acyclovir is a nucleoside analogue, which is phosphorylated and inserted into the replicating viral DNA. Once inserted in the growing chain, viral replication is terminated. Valacyclovir is converted to the active drug acyclovir by enzymatic hydrolysis in the liver and intestine.

CLINICAL USES

Acyclovir and valacyclovir are effective against members of the herpesvirus family. They are most effective against herpes simplex virus (HSV)-1 and HSV-2. In addition, they also have activity against Epstein-Barr virus (EBV), cytomegalovirus (CMV), and varicella-zoster virus (VZV). Acyclovir and valacyclovir are clinically used for the treatment of genital infections caused by HSV and VZV.

ADVERSE REACTIONS AND PRECAUTIONS

Acyclovir is eliminated unchanged in the urine; therefore dosage adjustment is required for acyclovir and valacyclovir in individuals with renal impairment. Cases of nephropathy secondary to acyclovir have been reported in individuals with renal impairment. This adverse event occurs primarily in patients on high doses of acyclovir. Keeping patients well hydrated can prevent nephropathy. The oral formulations are generally well tolerated. The topical formulation of acyclovir may cause transient burning and irritation at the site of application.

Table 14-10

Classification of antivirals

ANTIVIRAL (GENERIC NAME)	BRAND NAME	ROUTE	COMMON USES (MICROORGANISM)
Acyclovir	Zovirax	IV, PO	Herpes simplex (HSV-1 and HSV-2), herpes zoster (HZV), varicella-zoster (VZV)
Valacyclovir	Valtrex	PO	
Penciclovir	Denavir	TOP	HSV-1, HSV-2, HZV, VZV
Famciclovir	Famvir	PO	
Ganciclovir	Cytovene	IV, PO, IO	Cytomegalovirus (CMV)
Valganciclovir	Valcyte	PO	
Cidofovir	Vistide	IV	CMV
Foscarnet	Foscavir	IV	HSV-1, HSV-2, VZV, and CMV that are suspected to be resistant to acyclovir and ganciclovir
Fomivirsen	Vitravene	IVit	CMV
Amantadine	Symadine	PO	Influenza A
Rimantadine	Flumadine	PO	Influenza A
Oseltamivir	Tamiflu	PO	Influenza A and B

IO, Intraocular; *IV*, Intravenous; *IVit*, intravitreal injection; *PO*, oral; *TOP*, topical.

PENCICLOVIR AND FAMCICLOVIR

Penciclovir and famciclovir are similar in structure and activity to acyclovir. Famciclovir is the prodrug of penciclovir that is converted to its active form (penciclovir) in the gastrointestinal tract. Famciclovir is available in oral formulation, and penciclovir is only available in a 1% topical cream. Penciclovir and famciclovir appear to have greater in vitro activity against HSV and VZV than does acyclovir.[30]

MECHANISM OF ACTION

Penciclovir and the prodrug famciclovir are guanine nucleoside analogues, which exert their antiviral effects by incorporating into growing DNA chains, subsequently interfering with viral DNA synthesis and replication.

CLINICAL USES

Penciclovir has activity against viruses from the herpes family. It is effective against HSV-1, HSV-2, and VZV. Like acyclovir, it is less effective against EBV and CMV. In vitro studies have demonstrated some activity against hepatitis B virus (HBV). Penciclovir and famciclovir are clinically used for the treatment of genital infections caused by HSV and VZV.

ADVERSE REACTIONS AND PRECAUTIONS

Both penciclovir and famciclovir are considerably well tolerated. Use of famciclovir has been associated with nausea, vomiting, diarrhea, and headaches. Rare cases of neutropenia have been reported. Penciclovir is eliminated through the kidneys; therefore dosage adjustment of famciclovir is required in patients with moderate to severe renal insufficiency.

GANCICLOVIR AND VALGANCICLOVIR

Ganciclovir is a guanine nucleoside analogue with a similar mechanism of action to acyclovir. Valganciclovir is a newly approved prodrug of ganciclovir that improves ganciclovir absorption. Ganciclovir has a higher affinity for DNA transferase than acyclovir, which increases the intracellular half-life of the drug and allows less frequent dosing. Valganciclovir is available only in oral formulation; ganciclovir is available in oral, intravenous, and intraocular (eye implant) formulations.[30]

MECHANISM OF ACTION

Ganciclovir and the prodrug valganciclovir are both guanine nucleoside analogues. They have a similar mechanism of action as acyclovir. Both agents will incorporate into growing DNA chains, consequently terminating viral DNA synthesis and replication.

CLINICAL USES

Ganciclovir has similar activity to acyclovir against members of the herpesvirus family and VZV. However, ganciclovir has much higher activity against CMV in vitro and in vivo. Ganciclovir is indicated for the treatment and chronic suppression of CMV retinitis and prevention of CMV disease in AIDS and posttransplantation patients.

ADVERSE REACTIONS AND PRECAUTIONS

The most common adverse reaction associated with the use of ganciclovir is bone marrow suppression. In patients with AIDS the incidence of thrombocytopenia and neutropenia may be as high as 20% and 40%, respectively. Dosages should be reduced in the presence of renal insufficiency. In addition to the side effects of myelosuppression, headache, nausea, rash, fever, and liver transaminase elevations have also been reported.

CIDOFOVIR

Cidofovir is an acylic phosphonate nucleoside analogue that has potent antiviral activity against a wide variety of viruses. Unlike the guanine nucleotide analogues, cidofovir has enhanced activity against HSV, EBV, VZV, and CMV. Cidofovir is only available in intravenous formulation.[30]

MECHANISM OF ACTION

Cidofovir exerts its mechanism of action by inhibition of viral replication. Cidofovir is phosphorylated and inserted into the growing DNA chain. Once inserted, viral replication is terminated by inhibition of viral polymerases.

CLINICAL USES

Cidofovir has potent activity against members of the herpesvirus family, EBV, and CMV. It is indicated for use in patients with CMV who failed previous treatments of ganciclovir or foscarnet. It has been used extensively in the treatment of CMV retinitis in patients with AIDS.

ADVERSE REACTIONS AND PRECAUTIONS

Severe dose-dependent nephrotoxicity has been associated with the use of cidofovir. It is contraindicated for use in individuals with renal insufficiency. Saline infusions before and concomitant probenecid administration during cidofovir treatment have been used to help reduce nephrotoxicity. In addition to nephrotoxicity, neutropenia, fever, headache, emesis, rash, and diarrhea have also been reported with cidofovir use.

FOSCARNET

Foscarnet is a pyrophosphonate nucleoside analogue that has potent antiviral activity against HSV, EBV, VZV, and CMV. In addition, foscarnet has demonstrated activity against the hepatitis B and influenza viruses. It is poorly absorbed; therefore it is only available in intravenous formulation.[30]

MECHANISM OF ACTION

Because foscarnet is pyrophosphate analogue, it does not require phosphorylation to become active. Foscarnet works by reversibly blocking viral polymerase phosphorylation, which inhibits viral replication.

CLINICAL USES

Foscarnet has activity against herpesvirus family, along with VZV, EBV, and influenza A and B. Foscarnet is mainly used for the treatment of CMV retinitis in patients with AIDS who are unable to tolerate ganciclovir therapy. However, it is also used for treatment of CMV infections in other immunosuppressed individuals (organ transplantation). In addition, foscarnet has been used to treat HSV and VZV infections that are resistant to acyclovir and ganciclovir. Ganciclovir or acyclovir may act synergistically with foscarnet against some strains of CMV.

ADVERSE REACTIONS AND PRECAUTIONS

Nephrotoxicity is a relatively common side effect occurring in approximately 25% of patients treated. Adequate hydration during foscarnet infusion may reduce the incidence of nephrotoxicity. Dosage reduction is required in those individuals with renal insufficiency. Other adverse reactions include fever, nausea, electrolyte imbalances, vomiting, diarrhea, and headache.

FOMIVIRSEN

Fomivirsen is the first member of a new class of antiretrovirals termed *antisense oligonucleotides.* It is available only as an intravitreal preparation.[31]

MECHANISM OF ACTION

Antisense oligonucleotides are short stretches of DNA or RNA that bind to complementary sequences within the viral nucleic acid. Once bound, viral transcription is terminated. Fomivirsen acts by specifically binding to complementary regions of CMV RNA.

CLINICAL USES

Fomivirsen is indicated only for the treatment of CMV retinitis in patients with AIDS. Fomivirsen has shown to significantly delay the progression of CMV retinitis in AIDS patients. Fomivirsen is administered by intravitreal (into the vitreous humor) injection every week for 3 weeks, then every other week thereafter.

ADVERSE REACTIONS AND PRECAUTIONS

Transient increases in intraocular pressure have been reported along with intraocular inflammation of the anterior and posterior chambers. Topical steroids (eye drops) may be used to alleviate this adverse reaction.

AMANTADINE AND RIMANTADINE

Amantadine and rimantadine are closely related antivirals with activity only against influenza A. In addition, amantadine has also been used in the treatment of Parkinson's disease. Both agents are well absorbed from the gastrointestinal tract and suitable for oral administration.[30]

MECHANISM OF ACTION

Amantadine and rimantadine act by inhibiting viral replication and viral assembly. It is also thought that these agents inhibit the influenza virus from uncoating and entering the mucosal cells of the respiratory tract.

CLINICAL USES

Amantadine and rimantadine have a narrow spectrum of activity because they are only active against influenza A virus. Both agents may be used prophylactically in high-risk patients (i.e., immunocompromised) that are unable to tolerate or benefit from influenza vaccination. In addition, they may also be used in conjunction with vaccination in the same high-risk patient populations. These agents should be initiated within the first 48 hours of onset of symptoms to be effective.

ADVERSE REACTIONS

Amantadine and rimantadine are well tolerated. Central nervous system side effects such as tremor, insomnia, lightheadedness, seizure, cardiac arrhythmias, and agitation have been reported with both drugs (amantadine greater than rimantadine) and appear to be related to higher serum concentrations of these agents. A dosage adjustment of amantadine, but not rimantadine, is required in the presence of renal insufficiency.

OSELTAMIVIR

Oseltamivir belongs to a new class of antivirals known as the *neuraminidase inhibitors.* Oseltamivir is a prodrug, which is converted to its active form (oseltamivir carboxylate) once it is absorbed. It is available only as an oral formulation.[30]

MECHANISM OF ACTION

Oseltamivir specifically inhibits influenza A and B neuraminidase, which prevents influenza viruses from leaving the host cell to infect other cells.

CLINICAL USES

Oseltamivir is only effective for the treatment of influenza A and B infection. It has been shown to clinically reduce the duration of influenza infection. However, therapy must be initiated within 40 hours of the initiation of symptoms to be effective.

ADVERSE REACTIONS AND PRECAUTIONS

Oseltamivir is well tolerated, with nausea and vomiting reported as the most frequent adverse reaction. These symptoms usually occur on the first 2 days of therapy. Dosage adjustment is required in patients with renal insufficiency.

SUMMARY KEY TERMS AND CONCEPTS

- *Antibiotics* are natural compounds produced by microorganisms that either inhibit *(bacteriostatic/fungistatic)* or kill *(bactericidal/fungicidal)* other microorganisms.
- *Antimicrobials* include both natural and synthetic compounds that either inhibit or kill microorganisms.
- The outcome of antimicrobial therapy is dependent on *host factors, susceptibility/resistance* to the antimicrobial, and *pharmacodynamics.*
- The susceptibility of an organism to an antimicrobial is quantified by the *minimum inhibitory concentration (MIC)* and the *minimum bactericidal concentration (MBC).* The science of understanding the optimal effect of an antimicrobial as a function of its concentration to the MIC against the microorganism is known as pharmacodynamics.
- *Antimicrobial resistance* occurs through several mechanisms and continues to be a clinical problem, which can be curtailed through the judicious use of antimicrobials.

- Several antimicrobials exist and have varying activity against *gram-positive, gram-negative, anaerobic,* and *atypical bacteria, mycobacteria, yeast, molds, protozoa,* and *viruses.*
- The β-*lactams* are a large class of antibiotics that include the *penicillins, cephalosporins, carbepenems,* and the *monobactam (aztreonam).*
- Other groups of antibiotics include the *aminoglycosides, tetracyclines, macrolides, quinolones, sulfonamides, glycopeptides, streptogrammins,* and *oxazolidinones.*
- Individual antibiotics that represent sole agents within a class include *chloramphenicol, clindamycin, metronidazole,* and *nitrofurantoin.*
- The most commonly used *antimycobacterials* (treat tuberculosis) include *isoniazid, rifampin, rifabutin, pyrazinamide, ethambutol,* and *streptomycin.*
- The use of *antifungals,* such as the *polyenes, azoles,* and echinocandins, is increasing with the number of immunocompromised patients.
- *Antivirals* (excluding antiretrovirals) mimic nucleosides and inhibit DNA synthesis.

SELF-ASSESSMENT QUESTIONS

1. What is the difference between bacteriostatic and bactericidal antimicrobial agents?
2. Describe the difference between antimicrobial agents that act in a concentration-dependent manner and agents which act in a time-dependent manner.
3. Describe at least three parameters that may indicate antibiotic failure in a patient.
4. Why is it useful to use combination antibiotic therapy? (Be specific.)
5. Describe the mechanism of action of penicillin antibiotics. Name at least two additional antibiotic classes with similar mechanisms of action.
6. Which β-lactam antibiotic is least likely to cause an allergic reaction in a patient with a penicillin allergy?
7. Name three antimicrobial agents that would be useful in the treatment of community-acquired pneumonia.
8. What is the antimicrobial agent of choice for the treatment of *Pneumocystis carinii* pneumonia (PCP)?
9. What agents are considered first-line therapy for the treatment of pulmonary tuberculosis?
10. Which antimicrobial agents are useful for the treatment of nosocomial pneumonia caused by *Pseudomonas aeruginosa?*

Answers to Self-Assessment Questions are found in Appendix A.

CLINICAL SCENARIO

CS is a 61-year-old white male with a history of chronic obstructive pulmonary disease (COPD) and recurrent pneumonia admitted to University Hospital from the community, with complaints of cough with productive yellow-green sputum, fever, chills, and worsening shortness of breath (SOB). The patient states that he has felt relatively well the past 3 to 4 weeks, except for occasional night sweats.

COPD was diagnosed 1995. He also has hypertension (HTN), mild benign prostatic hypertrophy (BPH), and a left below-the-knee amputation (BKA). CS is also allergic to penicillin (anaphylactic reaction).

CS' medications (before admission) are as follows:

Ipratropium 2 puffs q6h (COPD)
Albuterol 2 puffs q4-6h (COPD)
Lisinopril 10 mg qd (HTN)
Terazosin 2 mg hs (BPH)

His vital signs are T, 101.2° F; BP, 158/92 mm Hg; HR, 104 beats/min; RR, 28 breaths/min; weight, 130 lb; height, 65 in; SpO_2, 92% on 4 L O_2, 68% on room air.

CS' physical examination revealed the following (remarkable findings): elderly cachectic male in acute distress; tachycardic, with a regular rhythm; bilateral respiratory crackles; and clubbing and cyanotic nailbeds.

His WBC count is 15.6×10^3 cells/mm^3. Sputum demonstrated many WBCs, few epithelial cells, many gram-positive cocci in chains/pairs; a culture is pending. His chest x-ray film revealed left lower lobe (LLL) infiltrate.

What signs and symptoms of infection in this patient are consistent with the diagnosis of community-acquired pneumonia (CAP)?
What is the most likely pathogen responsible for CAP in this patient?
Name two antibiotics that can be used to treat this patient's CAP.
If the sputum stains are acid-fast positive, what precautions should be taken and what drug therapy should be initiated?

Answers to Clinical Scenario Questions are found in Appendix A.

REFERENCES

1. Chambers HF, Sande MA: General considerations. In Goodman LS, Gilman A, eds: *The pharmacologic basis of therapeutics*, ed 9, New York, 1995, McGraw Hill.
2. Meyer F, Friedland GW: *Medicine's 10 greatest discoveries*, New Haven, 1998, Yale University Press.
3. Chain E and others: Penicillin as a chemotherapeutic agent, *Lancet* 2:226, 1940
4. Thompson RL, Wright AJ: General principles of antimicrobial therapy, *Mayo Clin Proc* 73:995, 1998.
5. Mandell LA, Campbell GD: Nosocomial pneumonia guidelines: an international perspective, *Chest* 113(suppl 3):188S, 1998.
6. Tomasz A: From penicillin-binding proteins to the lysis and death of bacteria: a 1979 view, *Rev Infect Dis* 1:434, 1979.
7. Wright AJ: The penicillins, *Mayo Clin Proc* 74:290, 1999.
8. Selwyn S: The evolution of the broad-spectrum penicillins, *J Antimicrobial Chemother* 9(suppl B):1, 1982.
9. Sanders CC: Cefepime: the next generation? *Clin Infect Dis* 17:369, 1993.
10. Anne S, Relsman RE: Risk of administering cephalosporin antibiotics to patients with histories of penicillin allergy, *Ann Allergy Asthma Immunol* 74:167, 1995
11. Norrby SR: Side effects of cephalosporins, *Drugs* 34(suppl 2):105, 1987.
12. Hellinger WC, Brewer NS: Carbapenems and monobactams: imipenem, meropenem, and aztreonam, *Mayo Clin Proc* 74:420, 1999.
13. Asbel LE, Levison ME: Cephalosporins, carbapenems, and monobactams, *Infect Dis Clin North Am* 14:435, 2000.
14. Gilbert DN: Aminoglycosides. In Mandell GL, Bennet JE, Dolin R, eds: *Mandell, Douglas and Bennett's principles and practices of infectious disease*, vol 1, ed 5, New York, 2000, Churchill Livingstone.
15. Davis BD: Mechanism of bactericidal action of aminoglycosides, *Microbiol Rev* 51:341, 1987.
16. Kahlmeter G, Dahlager JL: Aminoglycoside toxicity: a review of clinical studies published between 1975 and 1982, *J Antimicrob Chemother* 13(suppl A):9, 1984.
17. Smilack JD: The tetracyclines, *Mayo Clin Proc* 74:727, 1999.
18. Piscitelli SC, Danziger LH, Rodvold KA: Clarithromycin and azithromycin: new macrolide antibiotics, *Clin Pharm* 11:137, 1992.
19. Pai MP, Graci DM, Amsden GW: Macrolide drug interaction: an update, *Ann Pharmacother* 34:495, 2000.
20. O'Donnell JA, Gelone SP: Fluoroquinolones, *Infect Dis Clin North Am* 14:498, 2000.
21. Kasten MJ: Clindamycin, metronidazole, and chloramphenicol, *Mayo Clin Proc* 74:825, 1999.
22. Smilack JD: Trimethoprim-sulfamethoxazole, *Mayo Clin Proc* 74:730, 1999.
23. Cunha BA: Nitrofurantoin: an update, *Obstet Gynecol Surv* 44:399, 1989.
24. Fekety R: Vancomycin, teicoplanin, and the streptogramins: quinupristin and dalfopristin. In Mandell GL, Bennet JE, Dolin R, eds: *Mandell, Douglas and Bennett's principles and practices of infectious disease*, vol 1, ed 5, New York, 2000, Churchill Livingstone.
25. Clemett D, Markham A: Linezolid, *Drugs* 59:815, 2000.

26. American Thoracic Society: Targeted tuberculin testing and treatment of latent tuberculosis infection, *MMWR* 9:49(RR-6): 1, 2000.

27. Van Scoy RE , Wilkowske CJ: Antimycobacterial therapy, *Mayo Clin Proc* 74:1038, 1999.

28. Kauffman CA, Carver PL: Antifungal agents in the 1990s: current status and future developments, *Drugs* 53:539, 1997.

29. Walsh TJ and others: New targets and delivery systems for antifungal therapy, *Med Mycol* 38(suppl 1):335, 2000.

30. Keating MR: Antiviral agents for non-human immunodeficiency virus infections, *Mayo Clin Proc* 74:1266, 1999.

31. Perry CM, Barman-Balfour JA: Fomivirsen, *Drugs* 57:375, 1999.

CHAPTER 15

Cold and Cough Agents

Joseph L. Rau

*B*ewildering and in some cases irrational numbers of compounds, both prescription and over-the-counter (OTC), are available for treating symptoms of the common cold.

Common cold: The term "common cold" is used to describe nonbacterial upper respiratory tract infections (URIs), usually characterized by a mild general malaise, and a runny, stuffy nose.

More specific symptoms include sneezing, possible sore throat, cough, and possibly some chest discomfort. Allergic rhinitis is *not* included in this discussion, nor are serious illnesses such as influenza, acute bronchitis, or infections of the lower respiratory tract. Influenza, or the "flu," also caused by viral infection, is associated with symptoms of fever, headache, general muscle ache, and extreme fatigue or weakness. Onset of symptoms is usually rapid. The fever and systemic symptoms with influenza are contrasted with symptoms of the common cold in Table 15-1.

Four classes of agents can be distinguished in cold remedies, used either singly or in combination, as follows:

Sympathomimetics: Decongestion
Antihistamines: Reduce (dry) secretions
Expectorants: Increase mucus clearance
Antitussive: Suppress the cough reflex

These four classes of cold medications target the primary symptoms caused by the cold virus in the respiratory tract. This is illustrated conceptually in Figure 15-1.

Each class is discussed briefly, with representative agents listed. In addition to these four types of ingredients, an analgesic such as acetaminophen may be included, as in Sinutab, which consists of 30 mg of pseudoephedrine (decongestant) and 325 mg of acetaminophen (analgesic).

SYMPATHOMIMETIC (ADRENERGIC) DECONGESTANTS

Sympathomimetic (adrenergic) agents were discussed in their use as bronchodilators in Chapter 6, and the general effects of sympathetic stimulation were outlined in Chapter 5. In cold remedies, sympathomimetics are intended for a *decongestant* effect, which is based on their α-stimulating property and resulting vasoconstriction.

Sympathomimetics such as phenylephrine are found under brand names such as Sinex and Neo-

Table 15-1

Differences in symptoms between the common cold and influenza

SIGNS AND SYMPTOMS	COLD	INFLUENZA
Fever	Rare	Typical, high
Chills	None	Typical
Cough	Present, hacking	Nonproductive, may be severe
Headache	Rare	Prominent
Fatigue	Mild	Early and severe
Myalgia	None or slight	Usual, may be severe
Nasal congestion	Common	Occasional
Sneezing	Common	Occasional
Sore throat	Common	Occasional

Table 15-2

Examples of adrenergic agents used as nasal decongestants

DRUG	ROUTE
Phenylephrine (Neo-Synephrine)	Topical, oral
Epinephrine (Adrenalin Cl)	Topical
Pseudoephedrine (Sudafed, various)	Oral
Ephedrine (Pretz-D)	Topical
Xylometazoline (Otrivin)	Topical
Naphazoline (Privine)	Topical
Tetrahydrozoline (Tyzine)	Topical
Oxymetazoline (Afrin)	Topical

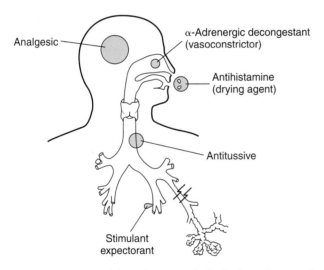

Figure 15-1   Cold medications include four classes of drugs, targeted at the symptoms produced by this upper respiratory viral infection, along with analgesics.

Synephrine and can be used in topical sprays or taken orally. Generally, topical applications require lower dosages than oral use. Problems can occur with either route of administration. Table 15-2 lists sympathomimetic agents used as nasal decongestants in cold remedies.

PHENYLPROPANOLAMINE

In November, 2000, the Food and Drug Administration (FDA) issued an advisory to consumers to avoid OTC products containing phenylpropanolamine (PPA). Manufacturers were advised to stop producing OTC products containing PPA.[1] Results of a 2000 study of men and women found that PPA in appetite suppressants and possibly in cold remedies was an independent risk factor for hemorrhagic stroke in women. The risk of hemorrhagic stroke in women was much greater with use of appetite suppressants containing PPA (odds ratio 16.58) than for use of a cough or cold remedy (odds ratio 3.13). No increased risk of hemorrhagic stroke was found in male subjects with use of cold medications containing PPA, and no men reported use of an appetite suppressant.[2]

TOPICAL APPLICATION

Although onset of action is faster than with oral use, repeated application of these sprays or drops can cause swollen mucosae through rebound nasal congestion, which is the exact problem being treated. Sympathomimetic decongestants should be used for short periods only, of a day or so. Some of the agents such as oxymetazoline (Afrin) can actually create tolerance and physical withdrawal symptoms.

SYSTEMIC APPLICATION

Systemic application has an advantage over topical of giving more extensive decongestant effects involving deeper blood vessels. However, producing nasal vasoconstriction through systemic routes will often lead to other systemic effects of sympathomimetics, such as a rise in blood pressure and increased heart rate.

ANTIHISTAMINE AGENTS

Histamine occurs naturally in the body, and is contained in tissue mast cells and blood basophils. The role of the mast cell in releasing histamine with allergic asthma was discussed in Chapters 11 and 12.

EFFECT OF HISTAMINE

Histamine is an important mediator of local inflammatory responses. Some idea of its effect can be realized from the fact that stinging nettles produce their burning pain because of a high concentration of histamine and acetylcholine. Histamine can cause smooth muscle contraction, increased capillary permeability and dilation, itching, and pain.

Scraping a tongue depressor or blunt pencil across the sensitive skin of the inner arm can illustrate a local inflammatory reaction at least partly mediated by histamine. The result is a *wheal and flare* reaction, also called a *triple response* (local redness, welt formation, and a reddish-white border). The redness and wheal (welt) are caused by dilation and leakage of plasma proteins from skin capillaries. The exudation of plasma causes the swelling. The flare, or reddish-white area surrounding the wheal, is probably due to local axon reflexes from sensory fibers causing dilation of neighboring arterioles.

HISTAMINE RECEPTORS

Histamine (H) produces its inflammatory effects by stimulating specific cell surface receptors. Two types of histamine receptors are distinguished:

H_1 **receptors:** Located on nerve endings and smooth muscle and glandular cells. These receptors are involved in inflammation and allergic reactions, producing wheal and flare reactions in the skin, bronchoconstriction and mucus secretion, nasal congestion and irritation, and hypotension in anaphylaxis.

H_2 **receptors:** Located in the gastric region. These receptors regulate gastric acid secretion, as well as feedback control of histamine release.[3]

A third type of histamine receptor, H_3, has been discovered. This receptor may be an autoreceptor for cholinergic neurotransmission in the airway at the autonomic ganglia, involved in central nervous system functioning and feedback control of histamine synthesis and release.[3,4]

The typical antihistamine found in cold medications is an H_1-receptor antagonist. Examples of these are pyrilamine and chlorpheniramine. H_1-Receptor antagonists block the bronchopulmonary and vascular actions of histamine, to prevent rhinitis and urticaria. H_2-Receptor antagonists are exemplified by cimetidine (Tagamet) or ranitidine (Zantac), which are used to block gastric acid secretion when treating ulcers.

ANTIHISTAMINE AGENTS

All of the antihistamines considered in this chapter are H_1-receptor antagonists. These antihistamine agents are further classified into the major groups given in Table 15-3. The first six groups of antihistamines listed in the table are all first-generation agents

Table 15-3

Major groups of antihistamines, with representative agents by nonproprietary and brand names

GROUP	DRUG
FIRST GENERATION	
Ethanolamine derivatives	Diphenhydramine HCl (Benadryl)
	Clemastine (Tavist)
Ethylenediamine derivatives	Tripelennamine HCl (PBZ)
Piperazine	Hydroxyzine (Atarax)
Piperidine derivatives	Cyproheptadine (Periactin)
	Azatadine (Optimine)
	Phenindamine (Nolahist)
Phenothiazine derivatives	Promethazine HCl (Phenergan)
Alkylamine derivatives	Chlorpheniramine maleate (Chlor-Trimeton)
	Brompheniramine maleate (Dimetapp Allergy)
	Dexchlorpheniramine maleate (Polaramine)
Phthalazinone	Azelastine (Astelin)
SECOND GENERATION	
Nonsedating, long acting	Loratadine (Claritin)
	Fexofenadine (Allegra)
	Cetirizine (Zyrtec)

and can be found in cold preparations. Some of the brand names given may be familiar from OTC preparations readily available in drugstores. Others are found in combination products; these are discussed and listed subsequently. Second-generation antihistamines, which are longer-acting and nonsedating are also listed in Table 15-3.

EFFECTS OF ANTIHISTAMINES

Antihistamines have three major classes of effects: antihistaminic, sedative, and anticholinergic activity. Second-generation agents are selective for H_1 receptors and are less sedating than first-generation agents.

Antihistaminic activity blocks the increased vascular permeability, pruritus, and bronchial smooth muscle constriction caused by histamine. These actions are the reason antihistamines are used to treat allergic disorders such as rhinoconjunctivitis, allergic rhinitis, and urticaria.

The sedative effect of antihistamines is thought to be caused by penetration of the agents into the brain, where inhibition of histamine N-methyltransferase and blockage of central histaminergic receptors occurs. There is also antagonism of other central nervous system receptors, such as serotonin and acetylcholine.[3] The effect of drowsiness with the classic (older) antihistamines can be a major hazard if alertness is required, such as in operating heavy machinery (e.g., a car) or monitoring a patient. This effect can be so pronounced that diphenhydramine HCl is added to acetaminophen in Tylenol PM, and the compound is described as a nonprescription sleep aid.

Finally, the anticholinergic effect produces considerable upper airway drying, just as would occur with an antimuscarinic agent such as atropine sulfate. In addition, effects seen with cholinergic blockade may occur, including central nervous system effects of stimulation, anxiety, and nervousness, as well as peripheral effects of dilated pupils, blurred vision, urinary retention, and constipation.[4] These effects are less likely in occasional use with a cold, but they may be significant with greater use (and dose) for allergic rhinitis or other conditions (e.g., urticaria).

The duration of action of the older antihistamines is generally 4 to 6 hours. However, newer, second-generation agents, often termed "nonsedating," are effective for up to 12 hours or more, depending on dose, and lack the sedating and anticholinergic effects. These newer agents are exemplified by fexofenadine

(Allegra) and cetirizine (Zyrtec). These agents are also listed in Table 15-3. The second-generation agents have little affinity for muscarinic cholinergic receptors and therefore do not cause dry mouth or gastrointestinal side effects. They also lack antiserotonin activity and do not cause appetite stimulation and weight gain, although astemizole and ketotifen may differ in this.[4] These newer drugs may inhibit mediator release from allergic inflammatory cells, in addition to blocking the histamine receptor. Allergic symptoms of sneezing and rhinorrhea are equally well controlled with first-generation and second-generation H_1 antagonists.[4]

STRUCTURE-ACTIVITY RELATIONS

H_1-Receptor antagonists were first discovered in 1937.[5] The chemical structure of histamine, the general structure of the H_1-receptor antagonists, and two examples of H_1 antagonists are given in Figure 15-2. Chlorpheniramine is an antihistamine found in many cold remedies; it represents one of the older, classic H_1-receptor antagonists. Fexofenadine is a newer, nonsedating H_1-receptor antagonist.

The resemblance between histamine and the general formula for the H_1-blocking agents can be seen in the structures shown. In the older agents, exemplified by chlorpheniramine, the R_1 and R_2 attachments are usually a ring structure connected to an ethylamine (C-C-N) group. The presence of the ring structures and other substitutions on the structure make the older antihistamines lipophilic. As a result, the classic first-generation antihistamines readily penetrate into the central nervous system and produce the effect of sedation and drowsiness previously discussed. The newer, nonsedating agents, such as terfenadine, do not readily cross the blood-brain barrier and therefore do not block central H_1 receptors.[5]

USE WITH COLDS

One of the beneficial effects of antihistamine use with a cold is the drying of upper airway secretions, which lessens the rhinitis and accompanying sneezing. There is some question whether the drying of secretions is due to histamine antagonism or to the anticholinergic effect of these agents. How much histamine release occurs with colds is debated. In allergic rhinitis, there is no question that histamine causes much of the inflammatory response, and in fact the newer long-acting agents are particularly helpful with this condition. Blockade of H_1 receptors

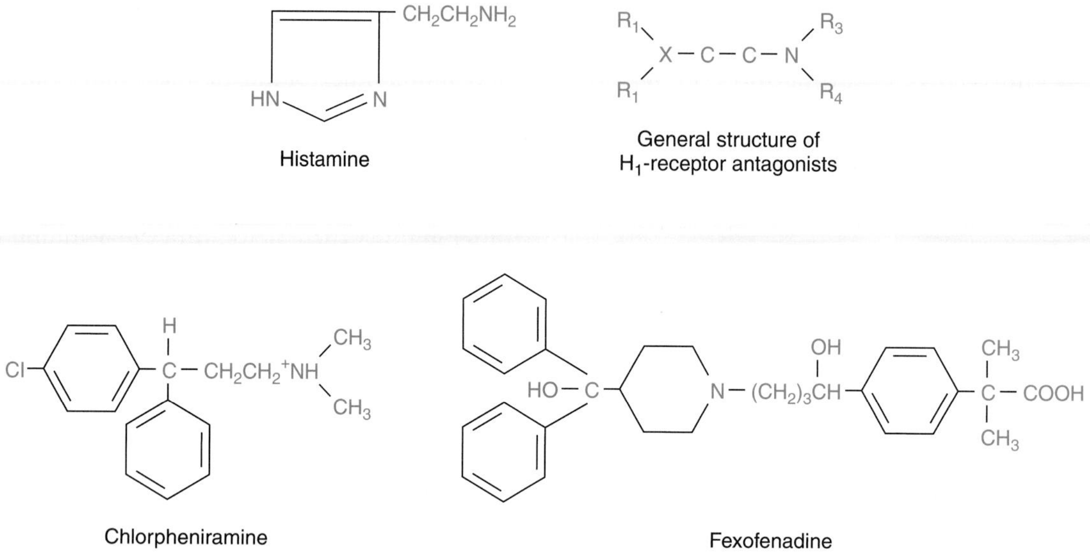

Figure 15-2   The structure of histamine, an inflammatory mediator; the general structure of H_1-receptor antagonists; and the structure of two antihistamines, chlorpheniramine and fexofenadine, are shown. R_1 to R_4 indicate the sites of attachments, with R_1 and R_2 being ring structures in most H_1 antagonists.

prevents the histamine contribution to the symptoms of nasal itching, congestion, sneezing, rhinorrhea, and ocular irritation.

Regardless of the exact effect, the drying of runny nasal secretions is welcomed by cold sufferers, and this coupled with drowsiness can be useful to produce needed rest and sleep at night. Secretions, however, are a defense mechanism with an upper airway viral infection. Antihistamines may cause harm as a result of suppressed secretion clearance and impacted secretions with sinus blockage. Adequate hydration with a cold is always helpful, with or without use of antihistamines.

An alternative to antihistamines for rhinorrhea in a cold is the anticholinergic nasal spray *ipratropium bromide (Atrovent)*, which was discussed in Chapter 7. Ipratropium has been shown to be effective in reducing nasal discharge in viral infectious rhinitis (colds), as well as allergic and nonallergic rhinitis.[6] The drug is well tolerated in a dose of approximately 80 μg divided between nostrils, with no evidence of rebound congestion, mucosal irritation, or significant systemic effects. It can be effective for 4 to 8 hours. An anticholinergic agent applied topically offers an attractive alternative to both vasoconstricting decongestants and antihistamine H_1 antagonists.

TREATMENT OF SEASONAL ALLERGIC RHINITIS

The second-generation H_1-receptor antagonists are more useful in the treatment of seasonal allergic rhinitis, as well as other disorders requiring antihistamine treatment, than in treatment of colds. They are also better tolerated in treating allergic rhinitis than the first-generation agents, because side effects of drowsiness are minimal and duration of action is longer. Agents such as astemizole, loratadine, fexofenadine, and cetirizine are indicated for use in seasonal allergic rhinitis and chronic urticaria. They are intended to relieve symptoms of sneezing; rhinorrhea; itchy nose, palate, and throat; itchy, watery eyes; and pruritus. Categories and examples of agents used in the treatment of seasonal allergic rhinitis are summarized in Table 15-4.[7] Other uses of antihistamines include the treatment of symptoms seen with motion sickness and control of nausea.

EXPECTORANTS

Expectorants are defined as agents that facilitate removal of mucus from the lower respiratory tract. A distinction was made in Chapter 9 (Mucus-Controlling Drug Therapy) between the following types of expectorants:

Table 15-4

Categories of agents used in treating seasonal allergic rhinitis

CATEGORY	EXAMPLE
H_1-Receptor antagonists	Cetirizine
Corticosteroids	Budesonide
Mediator antagonist	Cromolyn sodium
Anticholinergics	Ipratropium bromide
Vasoconstrictors	Pseudoephedrine
Specific immunotherapy	Standardized extracts

Table 15-5

A partial list of expectorants with representative brand names

DRUG	REPRESENTATIVE BRAND
Guaifenesin (glyceryl guaiacolate)	Robitussin, Mytussin, Humibid L.A.
Terpin hydrate*	Various
Iodinated glycerol	Iophen
Potassium iodide	SSKI, various

*No longer approved for use as an expectorant; may still be in distribution.

Mucolytic expectorants: Agents that facilitate removal of mucus by a lysing, or mucolytic, action. Example: Acetylcysteine.

Stimulant expectorants: Agents that increase the production and therefore presumably the clearance of mucus secretions in the respiratory tract. Example: guaifenesin.

Generally the expectorants considered here are stimulants, although the action does not always allow clear distinction. An example is guaifenesin, which is thought to reduce the adhesiveness and surface tension of mucus, and thus increase mucokinesis, that is, movement and clearance of the secretion. Another term used with these agents is *mucoevacuant.*

EFFICACY AND USE

There is controversy over the effectiveness and use of expectorants. The issue is clouded by the following:

- Difficulty in assessing the effectiveness of expectorants and, in particular, lack of objective criteria to demonstrate effectiveness.
- In conjunction with the first point, who would benefit from use of expectorants? In particular, should expectorants be included in treatment of cold symptoms, if a cold involves the upper respiratory tract?

USE IN CHRONIC BRONCHITIS

In 1990, Petty reported the results of a national study evaluating use of the expectorant iodinated glycerol (Organidin).[8] Patients had chronic bronchitis, which is quite different from a common cold. The study concluded that in chronic obstructive bronchitis, iodinated glycerol was safe and effective. Its use improved cough symptoms, chest discomfort, ease in bringing up sputum, and sense of well-being. The duration of acute exacerbations of chronic bronchitis was decreased. It is reasonable that in bronchitis, symptoms and airflow will improve and further infection reduced if mucus clearance can be improved.

MODE OF ACTION

Stimulant expectorants are thought to work by a variety of means, depending on the agent. These mechanisms include the following:

- Vagal gastric reflex stimulation.
- Absorption into respiratory glands to directly increase mucus production.
- Topical stimulation with inhaled volatile agents.

Guaifenesin, also known as glycerol guaiacolate, is classified as a Category I agent, which is safe and effective.[9] Ziment[10] has reviewed the mechanisms of action with iodides, such as iodinated glycerol. Other agents, such as terpin hydrate, sodium citrate, ammonium chloride, or menthols, have no demonstrated efficacy.[9]

Because mucus incorporates water as it is produced, an adequate intake of plain water or other nondiuresing liquids (milk, fruit juices) can help preserve mucus viscosity and clearance, especially with a simple cold.

EXPECTORANT AGENTS

Table 15-5 lists available expectorant agents. Some of these, such as with terpin hydrate, are sold with no brand name. Major agents or groups of agents are briefly characterized.

IODINE PRODUCTS

Potassium iodide is a very old agent that has been used as an expectorant in asthma and chronic bronchitis.[11] It has a direct mucolytic effect in sufficient concentrations. It also has an indirect effect on mucus viscosity by stimulating submucosal glands to produce new, lower-viscosity secretions.

The exact mechanism of action with iodine products is unclear. Iodide appears to distribute to mucous glands, where it is secreted along with increased mucus. Iodide also stimulates the gastropulmonary reflex, has a mucolytic effect, and can stimulate ciliary activity.[10]

Iodides are associated with hypersensitivity reactions in some individuals, and a case of pulmonary edema has been reported with its use.[12]

GUAIFENESIN (GLYCERYL GUAIACOLATE)

Guaifenesin by inhalation is also considered to be an emollient. In experimental animals, doses larger than those used in humans caused an increase in bronchial secretions. Guaifenesin taken orally is thought to reduce the adhesiveness and surface tension of mucus secretions, thereby enhancing mucus clearance. It is considered safe and effective by the FDA.

BROMHEXINE

Bromhexine, a synthetic derivative of the alkaloid vascicine, not available in the United States, has been reported by Thomson and colleagues[13] to increase the rate of mucociliary clearance when taken orally. Other research indicates an increase in sputum volume with an accompanying decrease in viscosity.[14,15]

OTHER EXPECTORANTS

Ziment suggests that chicken broth flavored with garlic and curry may serve as a tasty and effective mucus stimulant via the gastric reflex.[16] The major constituent of garlic is alliin, which has a structure similar to S-carboxymethylcysteine, discussed previously as a mucolytic (Chapter 9). Other ingredients that could have the same potential are pepper sauce (Tabasco), horseradish, and mustard.

TOPICAL AGENTS

This category usually evokes memories of the heated humidifier (vaporizer) with clouds of steam scented with camphor, menthol, or even in the past, chloroform. These agents may still be found in use, but efficacy as an expectorant has not been shown. The burn risk of a hot vaporizer should preclude its use with the young or the old and debilitated.

Some research has shown that so-called bland aerosols of saline do increase sputum volume, possibly through reflex irritation of the bronchi and with increased secretion clearance as a result of coughing.[17] Certainly a particulate suspension may have the potential to function as an irritant to the upper airways.

PARASYMPATHOMIMETICS (CHOLINERGIC AGENTS)

Using parasympathomimetic agents will stimulate mucous gland secretion, but the effect on other muscarinic receptors is too diffuse for practical use as an expectorant. For this reason, a drug such as pilocarpine is not used as an expectorant. Likewise, stimulation of the medulla can increase respiratory tract secretions, but stimulation of the central nervous system is hazardous (see discussion of central nervous system stimulants in Chapter 22).

COUGH SUPPRESSANTS (ANTITUSSIVES)

A fourth category of drugs used with colds and cold symptoms is the cough suppressant. Coughing is a defense mechanism to protect the upper airway from irritants such as dust particles or aerosols, liquids, and other foreign objects. This mechanism is a reflex, coordinated by a postulated cough center in the medulla.

AGENTS AND MODE OF ACTION

Cough suppressants act by depressing the cough center in the medulla. Narcotics (see Chapter 22) possess powerful depressant effects on the medullary centers, including the CO_2 chemoreceptors, and are often used for this purpose. Common agents are codeine or hydrocodone. A commonly used nonnarcotic is dextromethorphan.

Benzonatate (Tessalon), a nonnarcotic, is chemically related to the local anesthetic tetracaine and anesthetizes stretch receptors in the lungs and pleura. This inhibits the cough reflex at its source. There is no inhibitory effect on the central nervous system. The effect begins in 15 to 20 minutes and lasts between 3 and 8 hours.[18] The antihistamine *diphenhydramine* (Benadryl), available in a syrup, may be an effective cough suppressant.

Some cough suppressants, or antitussives, contain *codeine*. In a dose below 15 mg, codeine does not pro-

| Box 15-1 | **Cough Suppressant Drugs** |

Codeine sulfate (various brand names)
Hydrocodone (Hycodan Syrup)
Dextromethorphan (Hold DM, Trocal, Robitussin Cough Calmers, Benylin DM)
Diphenhydramine (Bydramine, Tusstat)
Benzonatate (Tessalon Perles)

duce analgesia in the adult. In the 10- to 20-mg range, there is an antitussive action. Above 30 mg, codeine produces analgesia. *Hydrocodone* produces an antitussive effect with a dose of approximately 5 mg. Box 15-1 lists common antitussive agents, many of which are used in cold compounds. Both dextromethorphan and codeine are available in OTC preparations. These two agents are considered to be preferred cough suppressants based on both safety and efficacy. The need for a prescription antitussive is unusual, especially in a cold, with the availability of OTC preparations.

USE OF COUGH SUPPRESSANTS

Several principles apply to the use of antitussives.

- They are helpful and indicated to suppress dry, hacking, nonproductive irritating coughs, especially if the coughing causes sleep loss. Furthermore, a constant nonproductive cough can cause irritation of the trachea, leading to more coughing.
- Do not suppress the cough reflex in the presence of copious bronchial secretions that need to be cleared. This includes situations of cystic fibrosis and other chronic obstructive lung diseases such as bronchitis. Excess mucus secretions from the lower respiratory tract are not present in an uncomplicated cold (see the definition of a cold) and indicate the need for further evaluation and possible treatment with an antibiotic.
- The combination of an expectorant and an antitussive in a cold medication is questionable. This amounts to suppressing the clearance mechanism while stimulating secretions to be cleared. Use of a single-entity cough preparation, such as Benylin DM (10 mg dextromethorphan per 5 ml) or Robitussin Pediatric (7.5 mg of dextromethorphan per 5 ml), to treat a dry, irritating cough is recommended.

The combination of expectorant and antitussive is based on the rationale that a dry, hacking, frequent cough can be better replaced by a less frequent but productive cough. It can be questioned whether this is needed in an uncomplicated cold. Also, many cold compounds combine an antihistamine to dry secretions with the expectorant that is to stimulate mucus production. The rationale for this is open to question.

COLD COMPOUNDS

A list of selected cold remedies, with the classes of agents included in the compounds, is given in Table 15-6. Table 15-6 includes single-ingredient products, such as Neo-Synephrine, as well as examples of compounds with multiple drug classes, such as Pediacof Syrup. Some of the preparations in elixir form use significant amounts of alcohol as a solvent. For example, Nyquil Nighttime Cold/Flu liquid contains 25% alcohol, and Contac Severe Cold & Flu Nighttime Liquid has 18.5% alcohol. No doubt some subjective sense of improvement reminiscent of the "hot toddy" may be found with such compounds. Another aspect of cold remedies that adds to their confusion is the variation in ingredients, all under the same basic brand name with suffixed initials to indicate substituted or deleted ingredients. For example, Robitussin Cold and Cough, Robitussin A-C Syrup and Robitussin DAC all vary in ingredients, as seen in Table 15-6. Because these compounds change fairly rapidly, no list remains current in terms of what is on the market. However, the basic principle of the typical four classes of ingredients remains, and new compounds can be evaluated for particular uses by considering the effects of these four classes of agents.

Many of these compounds are available as over-the-counter (OTC) preparations, thus requiring no prescription. The possibility of overdosing and abuse by combining prescribed compounds and OTC compounds is very real. Often OTC preparations have the same classes of ingredients but in lower concentrations.

TREATING A COLD

There is no cure for the common cold, and the four classes of drugs used in cold remedies treat only symptoms. Furthermore, their potentially undesirable effects should be considered:

Sympathomimetics: Tremor, tachycardia, and increased blood pressure can be seen, especially when

Table 15-6

Categories of ingredients found in selected cold multicompound medications

TRADE NAME	ADRENERGIC	ANTIHISTAMINE	EXPECTORANT	ANTITUSSIVE
Sudafed Tablets	Pseudoephedrine 30, 60 mg			
Neo-Synephrine	Phenylephrine, 1%			
Chlor-Trimeton Allergy 4 Hours		Chlorpheniramine 4 mg		
Robitussin			Guaifenesin 100 mg/5 ml	
Benylin Adult				Dextromethorphan 15 mg/5 ml
Dimetane Decongestant Caplets	Phenylephrine 10 mg	Brompheniramine 4 mg		
Mytussin DM Liquid			Guaifenesin 100 mg	Dextromethorphan 10 mg
Polaramine Expectorant Liquid	Pseudoephedrine 20 mg	Dexchlorpheniramine 2 mg	Guaifenesin 100 mg	
Hycomine Compound Tablets	Phenylephrine 10 mg	Chlorpheniramine 2 mg		Hydrocodone bitartrate 5 mg
Novahistine DMX	Pseudoephedrine 30 mg		Guaifenesin 100 mg	
Pediacof Syrup	Phenylephrine 2.5 mg	Chlorpheniramine 0.75 mg	Potassium iodide 75 mg	Codeine 5 mg
Robitussin Cold and Cough	Pseudoephedrine 30 mg		Guaifenesin 200 mg	Dextromethorphan 10 mg
Robitussin-DAC	Pseudoephedrine 30 mg		Guaifenesin 100 mg	Codeine 10 mg
Robitussin A-C Syrup		Guaifenesin 100 mg	Codeine 10 mg	

used orally. Rebound congestion can occur if used for longer than a day.

Antihistamines: Can cause drowsiness and impaired responses. Drying of secretions, whether caused by antimuscarinic or antihistamine action may suppress a needed defense reaction of the airways. Nocturnal use is more indicated than around-the-clock use.

Expectorants: Many have questionable efficacy in a cold. The best expectorant, especially with colds, is plain water and juices, avoiding caffeinated beverages such as tea or colas and beer or other alcoholic mixtures.

Antitussives: Useful in the presence of an irritating, persistent, nonproductive cough. However, productive coughs should not be suppressed, and the logic therefore of an expectorant-antitussive combination is questionable.

A combination of all four classes of drugs in one compound does not allow acute or occasional use of the sympathomimetic for decongestion, nocturnal use of antihistamines, and separate use of an expectorant or antitussive, as indicated by symptoms. Single-entity cold medications, such as Sudafed for decongestion or Benylin Adult for cough suppression, are available to treat specific symptoms based on the principles outlined. Fluids and rest remain a basic and rational approach to surviving colds and preventing spread of the rhinovirus, but is probably the least feasible for current lifestyles.

SUMMARY KEY TERMS AND CONCEPTS

- Chapter 15 reviews the four basic ingredients found in cold remedies: *adrenergic decongestants,* such as phenylephrine; *antihistamines,* such as chlorpheniramine; *expectorants,* such as guaifenesin; and *antitussives,* such as dextromethorphan.
- Adrenergic agents act to vasoconstrict and relieve *nasal congestion.*
- Antihistamines *dry secretions* through an anticholinergic effect, as well as by blockade of H_1 receptors.
- Expectorants *stimulate mucus* production, and cough suppressants *depress the cough* reflex. The use of expectorants is questionable in the uncomplicated cold, because the lower respiratory tract is not involved.
- Adrenergic decongestants are useful for nasal clearing, but *rebound congestion* can occur.
- Cough suppressants are useful with a nonproductive, irritating, *dry, hacking cough.*
- Antihistamines dry secretions, but can cause *impaction of secretions* and possible sinus blockage, and should be used sparingly. Use during work should be avoided because of the side effect of *drowsiness.*

SELF-ASSESSMENT QUESTIONS

1. Identify the four classes of ingredients found in cold medications.
2. For each of the following agents, identify the category (e.g., adrenergic, antitussive, etc.): codeine, chlorpheniramine, phenylephrine, dextromethorphan, pseudoephedrine.
3. What is the intended purpose of α-adrenergic agents in cold medications?
4. What is the intended effect of antihistamines (H_1 blockers) in cold medications?
5. Are antihistamines in cold remedies H_1 or H_2 blockers?
6. You drink several beers at a friend's house after taking a dose of Chlor-Trimeton. Should you drive home, and why or why not?
7. Identify the most common expectorant in OTC cold remedies.
8. Briefly explain how guaifenesin stimulates mucus production.
9. List some specific fluids you would recommend to someone with a cold.
10. Differentiate a "cold" from the "flu."

Answers to Self-Assessment Questions are found in Appendix A.

CLINICAL SCENARIO

A 24-year-old respiratory therapy student approaches you after class. He is a previously healthy male, within normal weight limits, and with mild but irregular physical activity. He complains of mild malaise, a runny stuffy nose, sneezing, and a slight sore throat.

What other symptoms would you ask about to differentiate his complaint as a cold versus the flu?

What is your conclusion, at this point?

Based on your information, what would you suggest to him for self-treatment?

Two days later, he complains of a productive cough with yellowish sputum, and his temperature is 99° F. He has chest ache on a deep breath and is feeling very tired. He reports that he had stayed up late the last two nights studying for a pharmacology examination.

What is your assessment now?

Answers to Clinical Scenario Questions are found in Appendix A.

REFERENCES

1. Drug Facts and Comparisons NEWS: PPA to be taken off market, December, 2000.
2. Kernan WN and others: Phenylpropanolamine and the risk of hemorrhagic stroke, *N Engl J Med* 343:1826, 2000.
3. Simons FER, Simons KJ: Second-generation H_1-receptor antagonists, *Ann Allergy* 66:5, 1991.
4. Du Buske LM: Clinical comparison of histamine H_1-receptor antagonist drugs, *J Allergy Clin Immunol* 98:S307, 1996.
5. Woodward JK: Pharmacology of antihistamines, *J Allergy Clin Immunol* 86:606, 1990.
6. Meltzer EO: Intranasal anticholinergic therapy of rhinorrhea, *J Allergy Clin Immunol* 90:1055, 1992.
7. Bousquet J, Chanez P, Michel FB: Pathophysiology and treatment of seasonal allergic rhinitis, *Respir Med* 84(suppl A):11, 1990.
8. Petty TL: The national mucolytic study: results of a randomized, double-blind, placebo-controlled study of iodinated glycerol in chronic obstructive bronchitis, *Chest* 97:75, 1990.
9. Covington TR: OTC cough suppressants/expectorants, *Facts and Comparisons Drug Newsletter* 10:4, 1991.
10. Ziment I: Inorganic and organic iodides. In Braga PC, Allegra L, eds: *Drugs in bronchial mucology,* New York, 1989, Raven Press.
11. Alstead S: Potassium iodide and ipecacuanha as expectorants, *Lancet* 2:932, 1939.

12. Huang T, Peterson GH: Pulmonary edema and iododerma induced by potassium iodide in the treatment of asthma, *Ann Allergy* 46:264, 1981.

13. Thomson ML and others: Bromhexine and mucociliary clearance in chronic bronchitis, *Brit J Dis Chest* 68:21, 1974.

14. Hamilton WFD, Palmer KNV, Gent M: Expectorant action of bromhexine in chronic obstructive bronchitis, *Brit Med J* 3:260, 1970.

15. Brogan TD and others: The effects of bromhexine on sputum from patients with chronic bronchitis and asthma, *Brit J Dis Chest* 68:28, 1974.

16. Ziment I: Expectorants in chronic bronchitis, *Respir Care* 27:1398, 1982.

17. Pavia D, Thomason ML, Clarke SW: Enhanced clearance of secretions from the human lung after the administration of hypertonic saline aerosol, *Am Rev Respir Dis* 117:199, 1978.

18. *Drug facts and comparisons*, St Louis, 2001, Facts and Comparisons.

CHAPTER 16

Selected Agents Used in Respiratory Disease

Joseph L. Rau

CHAPTER OUTLINE

α_1-Proteinase Inhibitor (Human)
   α_1-Antitrypsin deficiency
   Indication for drug therapy
   Dosage and administration
   Hazards and side effects
   Respiratory care assessment of therapy
Smoking Cessation Drug Therapy
   Indication for use
   Drug formulations
   Precautions
   Respiratory care assessment of therapy

Nitric Oxide
   Indication for use
   Dosage and administration
   Pharmacology of nitric oxide
   Effect on pulmonary circulation
   Toxicity
   Contraindications
   Respiratory care assessment of therapy

Chapter 16 presents three groups of drugs that are used for the direct treatment or prevention of respiratory disease. These include α_1-proteinase inhibitor (Prolastin), used in the treatment of congenital α_1-antitrypsin deficiency; nicotine replacement and other agents used in smoking cessation; and nitric oxide, used for pulmonary hypertension states in newborns and in acute respiratory distress syndrome (ARDS) in adults.

α_1-PROTEINASE INHIBITOR (HUMAN)

α_1-Proteinase inhibitor (abbreviated as α_1-PI or simply API) is also known as α_1-antitrypsin (α_1-AT) and is intended for therapy of congenital α_1-antitrypsin deficiency, which leads to emphysema. The proprietary product is known as Prolastin; it is prepared from pooled human plasma from normal donors, with purification and treatment to remove potentially infectious agents. The disease state is usually termed α_1-antitrypsin deficiency, and the deficient protein is termed α_1-proteinase inhibitor. However, the terms α_1-antitrypsin and α_1-proteinase inhibitor are used interchangeably and refer to the same protein.

α_1-ANTITRYPSIN DEFICIENCY

α_1-Antitrypsin deficiency is a genetic defect that can lead to the development of severe panacinar emphysema. This autosomal-recessive disorder is characterized by serum API levels below 35% of normal and presents as panacinar emphysema at age 30 to 50 years. It is estimated that API deficiency accounts for approximately 2% of all emphysema in the United States. It is estimated that there are 60,000 to 100,000 Americans with severe α_1-AT deficiency.[1,2] Among Caucasians, α_1-AT deficiency is as common a genetic disorder as cystic fibrosis.[3] In about 50% of emphysema that results from API deficiency, there is accompanying chronic bronchitis with mucus hypersecretion, perhaps as a result of secretory cell metaplasia caused by unchecked proteases in the epithelial lining fluid.[4] Emphysema caused by API deficiency is worse in the lower lung zones and can be markedly accelerated by cigarette smoking.[1]

The basic pathology of emphysema resulting from an API deficiency is an imbalance between proteases, especially neutrophil elastase (NE), and antiproteases, especially α_1-proteinase inhibitor. The main substrate for API is neutrophil elastase. The pathogenesis of emphysema is described as a process of alveolar wall destruction caused by insufficient protection from the protease neutrophil elastase, an enzyme that can cleave all forms of connective tissue and degrade elastic fiber in the lungs by solubilizing elastin. With inadequate API levels in the lung to balance the protease activity, emphysema results at a significantly earlier age than normally seen. A presentation of severe emphysema at an unexpectedly young age, such as the third or fourth decade, leads to a high suspicion of a genetic defect causing inadequate API blood and subsequently lung levels. The main role of another protease inhibitor, secretory leukocyte protease inhibitor (SLPI), which is secreted by bronchial glands and goblet cells, is to protect the airway epithelium against proteolytic injury. However, Wewers and associates[5] have provided evidence that α_1-proteinase inhibitor (α_1-antitrypsin) is the predominant antiprotease protecting against neutrophil elastase.

GENETICS

α_1-Proteinase inhibitor is a 54-kD glycoprotein, coded by a single gene on chromosome 14. The alleles of the API gene can be categorized as follows[4]:

Normal: Individual has normal serum levels of API.
Deficient: API has altered electrophoretic properties and lower than normal serum concentrations.
Null: Undetectable API levels in the serum.
Dysfunctional: API is present in normal amounts, but does not function normally.

Persons with normal genetic alleles for API (designated by the letter M for the alleles) are termed Pi MM, for protease inhibitor with a pair of the normal alleles. They are homozygous for the normal allele. Normal values for serum API are 150 to 350 mg/dl, based on a commercial standard preparation, or 20 to 48 μM (micromoles), based on a purified laboratory standard. The commercially available standards are about 40% higher in comparison with the purified laboratory standards. Results referenced to the commercial standard are expressed in milligrams per deciliter, whereas the highly purified standard is in micromoles. Commercial standard values can be converted to true standard values by multiplying the commercial value by 0.71.[4,5]

About 95% of persons in the severely deficient category are homozygous for the Z allele, and are designated as Pi ZZ. Serum levels of API range from 2.5 to 7 μM, or a mean of about 16% of normal.[4] The Z allele is rare in Asians and African Americans. Alleles

that do not express API at all are quite rare and are designated as Pi null-null. Individuals with Pi null-null have an absence of measurable API in the serum. Wewers and colleagues[5] describe treatment of a patient with the null-null phenotype and no measurable API serum levels. They were able to show that intravenously administered augmentation therapy with α_1-AT (API) led to normal API levels in the blood, as well as in the lung epithelial lining fluid.

The major risk factor for developing emphysema among Pi ZZ subjects appears to be cigarette smoking, in which emphysema appears much earlier than in nonsusceptible individuals, as previously noted. Other features seen with airflow obstruction in Pi ZZ individuals include a history of pneumonia, episodes of increased cough and sputum production, and a parental history of emphysema.[2]

INDICATION FOR DRUG THERAPY

α_1-Proteinase inhibitor (Prolastin) therapy is indicated for chronic replacement therapy in individuals with congenital deficiency of API, with clinically demonstrable panacinar emphysema. The drug is not indicated for use in patients other than those with Pi ZZ, Pi Z-null, or Pi null-null phenotypes. Subjects with the Pi MZ or Pi MS phenotypes appear to be at small risk for panacinar emphysema.[6] Controlled long-term trials have not been available to show that chronic therapy halts the progression of emphysema because of inherent difficulties in such a trial, including the need for large numbers of patients.[1] Prolastin has only been used in adult subjects. Given the nature of the disease and the action of the drug, the drug cannot reverse damage or improve lung function. The drug is extremely expensive, costing in the range of $25,000 to $40,000 per year for therapy. A cost-analysis of drug therapy concluded that α_1-AT replacement therapy is cost effective in individuals who have severe α_1-AT deficiency and severe chronic obstructive pulmonary disease (COPD).[7]

The American Thoracic Society states that API augmentation therapy should be used for patients with a serum concentration of API less than 11 μmol/L, or 80 mg/dl.[2,8] It is not indicated for patients with cigarette smoking–related emphysema who have normal or heterozygous phenotypes.[4] It is not indicated for individuals with liver disease associated with API deficiency, unless they also have lung disease. The ATS guidelines suggest using augmentation therapy if lung function studies become abnormal and if serial studies show deterioration.

Box 16-1	Summary of Information for α₁-Proteinase Inhibitor (Prolastin)

Use: Panacinar emphysema resulting from congenital α₁-antitrypsin deficiency
Status: Orphan drug
Brand name: Prolastin (Bayer)
Generic name: α₁-Proteinase inhibitor (human)
Manner supplied: 500 mg activity/vial with 20 ml sterile water
1000 mg activity/vial with 40 ml sterile water
Dosage: 60 mg/kg IV weekly, infused at 0.08 ml/kg/hr or greater

DOSAGE AND ADMINISTRATION

The brand of API, Prolastin, is available as single-dose vials, with the total α₁-proteinase inhibitor activity stated on the label of each vial. A summary of drug information is given in Box 16-1. The two approximate strengths are 500 mg and 1000 mg, supplied as a lyophilized concentrate, with 20 ml or 40 ml of sterile water diluent for reconstitution. The drug is designated as an orphan drug.

The recommended dosage of Prolastin is 60 mg/kg of body weight, given once weekly. The dose is given intravenously at a rate of 0.08 ml/kg/min or greater and usually takes about 30 minutes for total infusion. The weekly schedule is determined by the half-life of API, which was measured at 5.2 days for the API infusion reported by Wewers and associates,[5] in treating the individual with the null-null phenotype. The threshold level of API needed to provide adequate antielastase activity in the lungs is given as 80 mg/dl. This figure is based on the commercial standards. Note that the labeled proteinase activity of Prolastin is expressed as actual functional activity, that is, capacity to neutralize porcine pancreatic elastase, and is not equivalent to the commercial standard measurement. Blood levels of α₁-antitrypsin obtained with the commercial standard should not be used to determine dose because the commercial standard measures are greater than the functional (actual) capacity to neutralize elastase.

HAZARDS AND SIDE EFFECTS

Administration of Prolastin is reported to be well tolerated. In a study by Wewers and colleagues[1] with 21 patients receiving the recommended dose of Prolastin in 507 infusions, no severe or acute adverse reactions were reported. An acute fever occurred in three pa-

tients 2 hours after infusion, and one patient had a low-grade fever lasting 48 hours. Tests for hepatitis B virus or human immunodeficiency virus (HIV) were negative.

Potential adverse reactions to infusion with human α₁-proteinase inhibitor include fever, light-headedness, and dizziness. Transient leukocytosis and dilutional anemia several hours after infusion have been reported. Occasional reports of flulike symptoms, chills, dyspnea, rash, tachycardia, or, rarely, hypotension have been noted.

Wewers and colleagues[1] observed no evidence of acute or chronic immunologically mediated reactions associated with infusion therapy. They note that a naturally occurring antibody to α₁-antiproteinase inhibitor has never been described.

The Prolastin preparation is heat-treated in solution at 60° C for no less than 10 hours to reduce the risk of potential transmission of infectious agents. This treatment can destroy hepatitis B virus and HIV and probably inactivates hepatitis non-A, non-B (hepatitis C) virus.[1] Individuals receiving API infusions in Wewers and colleagues'[1] study received both active and passive immunization against hepatitis B.

RESPIRATORY CARE ASSESSMENT OF THERAPY

Respiratory care assessment of α₁-AT replacement therapy is primarily directed at lung function and the rate of change of airflow obstruction in patients.

- Pulmonary function testing of flow rates is used to monitor the degree of airflow obstruction over long-term use of the drug.
- Smoking status should be monitored, and α₁-AT–deficient individuals who smoke should receive both education on the effect of smoking with this disease and direction to resources to aid in smoking cessation (drug therapy, behavior modification assistance).
- Overall pulmonary health should be assessed based on frequency and severity of respiratory infections, cough, sputum production if present, and hospitalization rate.

SMOKING CESSATION DRUG THERAPY

Nicotine, along with lobeline, are naturally occurring alkaloids that are capable of stimulating acetylcholine receptors at the autonomic ganglia of both the sympathetic and parasympathetic systems, as well as the cholinergic nicotinic receptors at skeletal muscle sites (see Chapter 5) and in the brain. The structures of these two agents are shown in Figure 16-1. It is the affinity of nicotine for ganglionic and neuromuscular receptor sites that led to the use of the term *nicotinic* to distinguish them from *muscarinic* receptors, because all of these receptors utilize acetylcholine as a neurotransmitter.

Lobeline is a plant derivative that has less potency than nicotine but a similar spectrum of action. Nicotine itself has greater affinity for ganglionic receptors than for skeletal muscle nicotinic receptors. The response to nicotine stimulation involves simultaneous discharge of both sympathetic and parasympathetic systems. The sympathetic effect predominates in the cardiovascular system, with hypertension, tachycardia, and peripheral vasoconstriction. Part of the sympathomimetic effect is mediated by nicotinic stimulation of receptors on the adrenal medulla, leading to release of epinephrine and norepinephrine. Nicotine produces a parasympathetic effect in the gastrointestinal and urinary tracts, with nausea, vomiting, diarrhea, and urination. Response to nicotine is dose-dependent, and increasing or toxic doses can produce a depolarizing blockade of receptors. Stimulation of neuromuscular receptors causes tremor and loss of hand steadiness.

In addition to stimulating nicotinic receptors at the autonomic ganglia, neuromuscular junction, and adrenal medulla, nicotine binds to receptors in the central nervous system. This causes respiratory stimulation, tremors, convulsions, nausea, and emesis. The last two effects are often seen when nicotine is first inhaled as tobacco smoke, although tolerance rapidly occurs. Nicotine is the chief alkaloid in tobacco products, and addiction to nicotine is the basis for tobacco dependence. In the seasoned smoker, within seconds of inhaling from a cigarette, the internal carotid arteries carry a large bolus of nicotine to the brain, where it binds to nicotine receptors.[9] This binding causes secretion of dopamine, which causes a feeling of pleasure and cognitive arousal. Nicotine also increases levels of norepinephrine, β-endorphin, acetylcholine, serotonin, and other substances in the central nervous system, all of which increase the sensation of euphoria and well-being; enhance concentration, alertness, and memory; and decrease tension and anxiety. Sensitivity and responsiveness to nicotine in the central nervous system is genetically determined and is the basis for forming the physiological addiction to nicotine. Without the proper genetic substrate, a smoker cannot become nicotine dependent. About 10% of smokers lack this substrate and are not physiologically dependent; whereas 90% have the substrate and are nicotine-addicted to various degrees.[9]

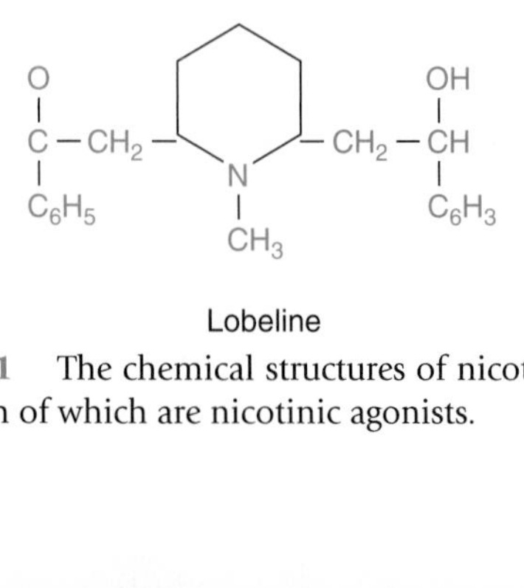

Cigarette smoking is a preventable cause of cardiovascular and lung disease and accelerates the rate of decline of lung function that occurs with aging, as shown in the Lung Health Study.[10] The Lung Health Study concluded that aggressive smoking intervention and cessation reduces the age-related decline in forced expiratory volume in 1 second (FEV_1) in middle-age smokers. Withdrawal from the nicotine in tobacco products is difficult because the stimulatory and reward effects are lost and physical symptoms occur. The latter include craving for nicotine, nervousness, irritability, anxiety, drowsiness, sleep disturbance, impaired concentration, and increased appetite with attendant weight gain. Nicotine replacement therapy, in various dosing formulations, is intended to aid with smoking cessation by allowing initial replacement and then gradual withdrawal of the nicotine found in tobacco. Because nicotine is well absorbed from the skin and mucosa, a transdermal patch, a chewable gum formulation, a nasal spray, and an inhaler have been developed.

INDICATION FOR USE

Nicotine replacement agents are indicated as an aid to smoking cessation to relieve nicotine withdrawal symptoms. Replacement therapy should be used as part of a comprehensive smoking cessation program to increase compliance and reduce relapse. Smokers

Nicotine

Lobeline

Figure 16-1   The chemical structures of nicotine and lobeline, both of which are nicotinic agonists.

with signs of a high physical dependence on nicotine may benefit the most from nicotine replacement therapy. Signs of strong physical dependence are listed in Box 16-2.[9]

DRUG FORMULATIONS

Smoking cessation drug therapy includes various formulations of nicotine and bupropion, an antidepressant found to be useful as an aid to smoking cessation. Table 16-1 lists pharmaceutical details on the

various agents in use at the time of this edition. Ferrill[12] offers a survey and review of smoking cessation agents. Details on the nicotine substitute agents can be found in manufacturers' literature.[11]

NICOTINE POLACRILEX (NICOTINE RESIN COMPLEX)

Nicotine polacrilex, a resin complex, is available as a chewing gum, as a nasal spray, and as an inhaler.

Nicotine polacrilex gum contains nicotine bound to an ion-exchange resin in a chewing gum base. The gum can be difficult to chew, causing jaw ache, and has a bad taste. Absorption of the active nicotine can be inconsistent although it is faster than with the transdermal patch. The absorption of nicotine is reduced if acidic beverages such as coffee, soda, or orange juice are taken simultaneously. Users are instructed to chew the gum until malleable, then "park" it between the cheek and gum, repeating this every few minutes each time the taste is gone. Chewing slowly titrates the dose of nicotine received. Intermittent rather than continuous chewing slows the buccal absorption of the nicotine released. This will also slow the amount of nicotine swallowed, which is not well absorbed from the stomach and can cause gastrointestinal irritation. Each piece of gum (2 mg, 4 mg) delivers about 50% of its nicotine.

Box 16-2	Signs of a High Physical Addiction/Dependence on Nicotine

- Smokes more than 15 cigarettes per day
- Prefers brands with nicotine levels above 0.9 mg
- Has habit of inhaling smoke frequently and deeply
- Smokes within 30 minutes of rising
- Finds it difficult to give up the first morning cigarette and smokes more frequently in the morning
- Finds it difficult to refrain from smoking in smoke-free environments
- Smokes even when ill enough to be bed-ridden

Table 16-1

Smoking cessation drug formulations

CATEGORY	BRAND NAME	DOSAGE
Nicotine transdermal system	Habitrol	21 mg/day for 6 wk, 14 mg/day for next 2 wk, 7 mg/day for last 2 wk
	Nicoderm	21 mg/day for first 6 wk, 14 mg/day for next 2 wk, 7 mg/day for last 2 wk
	Nicotrol	15 mg/day for first 12 wk, 10 mg/day for next 2 wk, 5 mg/day for last 2 wk
	ProStep	22 mg/day for 4 to 8 wk, 11 mg/day for 2 to 4 wk
Nicotine polacrilex	Nicorette (gum)	2 mg if fewer than 25 cigarettes/day; 9-12 pieces/day; maximum of 30 pieces/day
	Nicorette DS (gum)	4 mg if 25 or more cigarettes/day; 9-12 pieces/day; maximum of 20 pieces/day
	Nicotrol NS (nasal spray)	0.5 mg/spray, one each nostril (1.0 mg); 1-2 doses/hr (2 sprays with 1 each nostril is 1 dose), up to 5 doses/hr, or 40 doses/day for 6-8 wk; gradually reduce over next 4-6 wk
	Nicotrol Inhaler	4 mg/use; recommended dosage is 24 to 64 mg (6 to 16 cartridges) per day, up to 12 wk, with gradual reduction over a period up to 12 wk
Bupropion	Zyban	150 mg sustained-release tablets; begin at 150 mg/day for 3 days; increase to 150 mg/day bid, with maximum of 300 mg/day, interval of 8 hr between doses; continue treatment for 7-12 wk

The *nicotine nasal spray* offers the advantage of producing rapid peak plasma levels of nicotine, by delivering the spray directly to the nasal membranes. This may help to reduce or control cravings to smoke. Irritant effects with the nasal spray may include runny nose and nasal irritation, sneezing, cough, and watery eyes. Although rapid relief may be obtained, administration is more obtrusive than with the patch or the gum formulations.

The *nicotine inhaler* offers smokers a "simulated cigarette"; the kit contains a 10-mg/cartridge unit dose, which delivers 4 mg/use, a mouthpiece, blister trays of nicotine cartridges, and a plastic case. The use of a mouthpiece resembling a cigarette holder allows delivery of the nicotine in a manner similar to smoking a cigarette, with oral gratification. This system delivers less nicotine than the other systems. All of the nicotine is absorbed across the oropharyngeal membranes.[9] The inhaler may be most useful in the low-dependency smoker, as an adjunct to the patch to treat sudden cravings, or in combination with bupropion.

Nicotine Transdermal System

The nicotine transdermal system is a multilayered unit that delivers nicotine for 24 hours after application to the skin. Approximately 68% of the nicotine released from the system enters the circulation. Products differ in their kinetics. With Nicoderm, plasma levels rise rapidly and then plateau for 2 to 4 hours, followed by a slow decline. With Habitrol, blood levels peak broadly between 6 and 12 hours, and then decline. The transdermal product provides a more consistent level of nicotine than the gum. This is an easy, convenient, and inconspicuous method of nicotine replacement delivery. A common side effect is skin irritation at the site, but this is minimized by alternating sites. Any skin site that is clean, dry, and hairless can be used. The largest patch (21 mg) is equal to approximately half a pack of cigarettes per day.

Bupropion (Zyban)

Bupropion is an antidepressant found in Wellbutrin; it is also a nonnicotine aid to smoking cessation. The drug is a relatively weak inhibitor of neuronal uptake of norepinephrine, serotonin, and dopamine, which is the basis for its antidepressant effect. The exact mechanism by which bupropion aids in smoking cessation is not known. Bupropion may relieve nicotine withdrawal by slowing the normal reuptake of dopamine or preventing its breakdown in the central nervous system. It has been shown that mood and emotional state are related to the need for smoking and nicotine, although bupropion is effective in smoking cessation even if the smoker is not depressed.[9] Symptoms of nicotine dependence among smokers are correlated with the magnitude of symptoms of depression. Subjects who are negative or depressed are less likely to be able to quit smoking. This would indicate that the antidepressant effect of bupropion assists in smoking cessation. Jorenby and associates[13] found little difference between a placebo group and a nicotine patch group in smoking cessation at 12 months (15.6% versus 16.4%). However, a group receiving bupropion alone achieved a 30.3% cessation rate, and the combination of bupropion and nicotine patch gave the highest cessation rate of 35.5%. This suggests that bupropion added to nicotine substitutes in a program of smoking cessation is helpful. Only about 6% of smokers succeed in quitting with no replacement therapy.[13]

If a patient has not made significant progress toward abstinence from smoking by week 7, it is unlikely that the effort will be successful and bupropion should be discontinued for that attempt. Dose tapering for discontinuation is not required.

Use of bupropion is associated with a dose-dependent risk of seizure. Doses below 300 mg/day are generally safer and have a risk of about 0.1% for seizure.

Coadministration of bupropion with a monoamine oxidase inhibitor (MAOI) or other medications containing bupropion is contraindicated. The drug should not be used in individuals with seizure disorders or with bulimia or anorexia nervosa, which have a higher incidence of seizures.

Precautions

Individuals using nicotine replacement therapy should be instructed that the replacement formulations do contain active nicotine. If used while still using tobacco products, potentially toxic concentrations of nicotine can occur in the blood. Individuals should stop smoking when initiating therapy.

Transference of nicotine dependency from the tobacco product to the replacement product can occur. Use within a program of smoking cessation is encouraged to achieve complete withdrawal. Replacement formulations should be gradually withdrawn and stopped by 3 months.

Use of nicotine replacement therapy should be carefully weighed in patients with cardiovascular disease, including coronary artery disease, cardiac arrhythmias, or vasospastic disease, and in hypertension.

Healthcare workers should avoid handling active nicotine products, such as patches, because nicotine is easily absorbed through the skin. Washing with soap will increase absorption; so only water should be used. Used products must be disposed of properly, so that children or pets are not exposed.

RESPIRATORY CARE ASSESSMENT OF THERAPY

The primary outcome of interest with smoking cessation drug therapy is success in quitting over the long term.

- Monitor abstinence rates at intervals such as 3, 6, or 12 months.
- Monitor for symptoms of nicotine overdosage (possible if subjects continue smoking while using nicotine substitutes), such as nausea, salivation, abdominal pain, vomiting, diarrhea, cold sweat, headache, dizziness, disturbed vision and hearing, mental confusion, or marked weakness.
- Assess bupropion use for improvement in emotional attitude, including reduction in irritability, anxiety, difficulty in concentrating, or depression.
- Assess patients for weight gain, and encourage a program of exercise to prevent relapse caused by desire for appetite control.
- Continue to provide counseling and support throughout treatment for smoking cessation.

NITRIC OXIDE

Nitric oxide (NO) is a product of endothelial cells that acts as a nitrovasodilator. It was investigated for its ability to lower pulmonary vascular resistance in various disease states, such as persistent pulmonary hypertension of the newborn (PPHN) and ARDS. In 1980, Furchgott and Zawadzki showed that endothelial cells in blood vessels elaborate a short-lived vasodilator, which was termed endothelium-derived relaxing factor (EDRF).[14] The neurotransmitter acetylcholine, which can normally dilate blood vessels, has no effect or even vasoconstricts if applied to blood vessels without endothelium. Subsequently, the substance EDRF was identified by Palmer and colleagues[15] and Ignarro and colleagues[16] as nitric oxide. This endogenously produced vasodilator can be inhaled as a gas to cause pulmonary vasodilation. Results of a journal conference on inhaled nitric oxide were published in the February and March, 1999 editions of *Respiratory Care*.

INDICATION FOR USE

Nitric oxide was approved by the Food and Drug Administration (FDA) on December 23, 1999 for use in neonates with hypoxic respiratory failure, to reduce pulmonary artery pressure and increase oxygenation in newborns with pulmonary hypertension and hypoxia.

- *Nitric oxide* is used in conjunction with ventilatory support and other critical care in the treatment of term and near-term (>34 weeks) neonates with hypoxic respiratory failure associated with clinical or echocardiographic evidence of pulmonary hypertension.

Off-label uses of nitric oxide include reduction of pulmonary vascular resistance and pulmonary artery pressure during neonatal cardiac surgery, treatment of hypoxemia or pulmonary hypertension after lung transplantation, and treatment of ARDS. Nitric oxide was approved with an orphan drug designation.

DOSAGE AND ADMINISTRATION

Nitric oxide is supplied in two sizes of gas cylinder: 353 L (delivers 344 L) and 1963 L (delivers 1918 L). The recommended dose is 20 ppm. The treatment should be maintained up to 14 days or until the underlying oxygenation problem has resolved and the neonate can be successfully weaned from nitric oxide. In the Neonatal Inhaled Nitric Oxide Study (NINOS) trial, the majority of patients who failed to improve on 20 ppm and whose dose was increased to 80 ppm, had no response at the higher concentration.[17] The risk of methemoglobinemia and elevated nitrogen dioxide (NO_2) levels increases significantly above 20 ppm, as discussed below.

The safety and effectiveness of nitric oxide were established in patients receiving other critical care support for hypoxic respiratory failure, including vasodilators, intravenous fluids, bicarbonate therapy, and mechanical ventilation. Additional therapies might be needed to maximize oxygen delivery, such as surfactant administration and high frequency oscillatory ventilation. Information about the effectiveness of nitric oxide therapy in infants older than 14 days or adults is not available.

In the clinical trials of nitric oxide, the delivery system used was the INOvent system, which gives a constant concentration of nitric oxide during the respiratory cycle, with minimal nitrogen dioxide generation.

The following summarizes guidelines for the safe administration of nitric oxide based on several sources listed in the references, including a statement by the American Academy of Pediatrics[18,19]:

- Blending and delivery systems should be designed and tested for accurate nitric oxide delivery, minimum nitrogen dioxide production, and capability of administering nitric oxide in constant concentration ranges in parts per million or less throughout the respiratory cycle.
- The delivery system should be calibrated using a precisely defined mixture of nitric oxide and nitrogen dioxide.
- Sample gas for analysis should be drawn before the Y-piece, proximal to the patient.
- Inhaled nitric oxide and nitrogen dioxide should be monitored continuously using chemiluminescence or electrochemical analyzers.
- Oxygen levels in the inspired gas should be measured.
- Blood methemoglobin levels should be measured frequently.
- The minimum effective concentration of nitric oxide should be used.
- Weaning from nitric oxide should be gradual to prevent arterial desaturation and pulmonary hypertension.
- Because inhaled nitric oxide is used in respiratory failure, institutions that offer nitric oxide therapy generally should have extracorporeal membrane oxygenation (ECMO) capability in the event nitric oxide therapy fails. Alternatively, a plan for timely transfer of infants to a collaborating ECMO center should be established prospectively, and transfer should be accomplished without interruption of nitric oxide therapy.

The second-to-last point is particularly significant in the clinical use of nitric oxide to manage pulmonary hypertension. When withdrawing nitric oxide, rebound hypertension occurs, which can be severe and cause oxygen desaturation. This may be due to a downregulating effect on endogenous nitric oxide production in the pulmonary endothelium. The vasodilating effect of inhaled nitric oxide ends with the removal of the gas, because of its short half-life, as subsequently described, as a result of its binding to hemoglobin. An increase in fractional concentration of oxygen in inspired gas (FIO_2) up to 1.0 may be needed as the inhaled nitric oxide is terminated. The

FIO_2 can then be reduced over the next few hours as pulmonary hemodynamics restabilize. Close monitoring of arterial oxygenation is critical when weaning from nitric oxide.

PHARMACOLOGY OF NITRIC OXIDE

The formation, mode of action, and fate of endogenous nitric oxide are diagrammed in Figure 16-2. Nitric oxide is formed endogenously in vascular endothelial cells of the respiratory tract from the precursor amino acid L-arginine by several isoforms of the enzyme, nitric oxide synthase (NOS). Nitric oxide synthase requires the cosubstrates of nicotinamide adenine dinucleotide phosphate (NADPH) and oxygen (O_2). In the reaction, nitrogen is contributed by the arginine, oxygen by the oxygen molecule, and a free electron by NADPH. Nitric oxide synthase is categorized into constitutive NOS (cNOS), including that found in endothelial cells (ecNOS) and in neurons (nNOS), and into inducible NOS (iNOS).[20] The vascular relaxation caused by acetylcholine is due to stimulation of cNOS, which results in an increase in nitric oxide. Histamine, leukotrienes, and bradykinin are other mediators that increase cNOS-mediated nitric oxide and promote vasodilation and lowering of blood pressure. Proinflammatory cytokines, such as interferon-γ (IFN-γ), tumor necrosis factor-α (TNF-α), and interleukin-1 (IL-1) can all induce iNOS to increase endogenous levels of nitric oxide. Glucocorticoids block the induction of

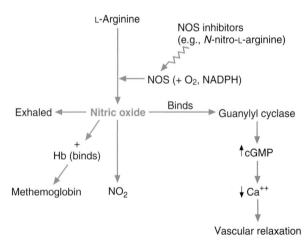

Figure 16-2   Production, physiological effect, and metabolism of endogenous nitric oxide. *cGMP,* Cyclic guanosine monophosphate; *NADPH,* nicotinamide adenine dinucleotide phosphate; *NO₂,* nitrogen dioxide; *NOS,* nitric oxide synthase.

iNOS and inhibit the formation of NO.[20] Nitric oxide is the active form of nitrovasodilators such as nitroglycerin and sodium nitroprusside.[14] Nitric oxide has also been identified as at least one of the neurotransmitters in the nonadrenergic, noncholinergic (NANC) inhibitory nervous system (see Chapter 5).[21] The endogenous production of nitric oxide can be inhibited by L-arginine analogues, which inhibit NOS, for example, N-nitro-L-arginine. The nitric oxide molecule is small and lipophilic, and it has a very short duration of action of 0.1 to 5 seconds in physiological systems.[14,21]

Nitric oxide is generated in vascular endothelial cells and diffuses rapidly into myocytes in the endothelium, binding to guanylyl cyclase. Guanylyl cyclase (also termed guanylate cyclase) stimulates the production of cyclic guanosine-3',5'-monophosphate (cGMP), which causes a decrease in intracellular calcium, and consequent vascular or nonvascular smooth muscle relaxation. The nitric oxide–induced increase in cGMP within the cells also inhibits platelet adherence and aggregation, as well as polymorphonuclear leukocyte chemotaxis.[21] Nitric oxide readily diffuses into the blood vessel itself, as well as into endothelial cells, and enters the red blood cell to bind rapidly with hemoglobin, forming methemoglobin and becoming inactivated in the process. Nitric oxide is also converted in the red blood cell to nitrate, and some endogenous nitric oxide is exhaled from the lung.[21] Because nitric oxide diffuses so readily into the bloodstream and is inactivated by being bound to hemoglobin, its action is limited to the pulmonary vascular endothelium, whether generated endogenously within the lung or inhaled as an exogenous gas. It is thus a selective pulmonary vasodilator. The end products of nitric oxide that enter the systemic circulation are predominantly methemoglobin and nitrate. Nitrite is the predominant nitric oxide metabolite excreted in the urine, accounting for more than 70% of the inhaled dose. A more detailed review of the biology of nitric oxide is given by Aranda and Pearl.[22]

EFFECT ON PULMONARY CIRCULATION

With normal pulmonary hemodynamics (normal vascular resistance), inhalation of NO produces no effect on pulmonary artery pressure or gas exchange.[14] However Frostell and associates[23] reported that hypoxic pulmonary vasoconstriction caused by breathing 12% oxygen in healthy adults increased mean pulmonary artery pressure (PAP) from 14.7 ± 0.8 to 19.8 ± 0.9 mm Hg.[23] This was reversed by adding 40 ppm of ni-

tric oxide to the gas mixture. No change occurred in systemic vascular resistance because nitric oxide was inactivated locally by hemoglobin.

In persistent pulmonary hypertension of the newborn (PPHN), pulmonary vascular resistance is high, which causes right-to-left shunting through the patent ductus arteriosus and foramen ovale. Inhaled nitric oxide dilates pulmonary blood vessels in regions of the lung where ventilation is delivered. This redistributes pulmonary blood flow from areas of low ventilation to those with better ventilation. The improved ventilation-perfusion matching leads to improved partial pressure of oxygen in arterial blood (PaO_2). Because nitric oxide is rapidly and locally inactivated by hemoglobin, no systemic vasodilation or hypotension occurs.[24]

TOXICITY

Toxicity with exposure to nitric oxide can be caused by the nitric oxide itself, by the formation of the nitrite nitrogen dioxide, and the formation of methemoglobin. Nitric oxide can be a mediator of lung injury, for example, with paraquat poisoning, in which inhibition of nitric oxide synthetase actually reduces the amount of lung injury.[25] Nitrogen dioxide is a strong oxidizer that causes lipid peroxidation in cells. The amount of nitrogen dioxide produced depends on the amount of nitric oxide and the amount of surrounding oxygen. The higher the FiO_2, the greater the amount of oxidation of nitric oxide to nitrogen dioxide. Similarly, the higher the concentration of nitric oxide, the shorter time to achieve oxidation to nitrogen dioxide. The lethal effect of nitrogen dioxide is due to pulmonary edema, and short-term exposure to more than 150 ppm of nitrogen dioxide is usually fatal.[21] In the usual doses of nitric oxide, such as 0.5% to 4%, methemoglobinemia is not usually a problem, although this should be monitored.

It is not known whether nitric oxide can cause fetal harm when given to pregnant women, and the manufacturer notes that it is not intended for adults. It is not known if nitric oxide is excreted in human milk. Occupational exposure to nitric oxide is set by the Occupational Safety and Health Administration (OSHA) at 25 ppm and for nitrogen dioxide at 5 ppm (manufacturer's literature).

CONTRAINDICATIONS

Nitric oxide should not be used in neonates who are known to be dependent on right-to-left shunt.

RESPIRATORY CARE ASSESSMENT OF THERAPY

- Because nitric oxide is administered in conjunction with ventilatory support, the usual measures of critical care assessment and in particular ventilator monitoring should be followed.
- Evaluate therapy for a reduction in the oxygenation index (OI = Mean airway pressure in cm H_2O $\times$ FIO_2/PaO_2).
- Evaluate the effect of nitric oxide and monitor the PaO_2 and the overall level of ventilatory support (FIO_2, inspiratory pressure and time, end-expiratory pressure, rate).
- Monitor preductal and postductal pulse oximetry (SpO_2) to evaluate shunting.
- If available, review the echocardiogram to evaluate right-to-left shunting.
- Monitor inspired nitric oxide and nitrogen dioxide, along with methemoglobin.
- Monitor cardiovascular status and stability, including the level of intravenous fluids and vasoactive medications needed.

SUMMARY KEY TERMS AND CONCEPTS

- Three important drugs or groups of drugs used in the treatment and prevention of respiratory disease are *α₁-proteinase inhibitor* (API), *smoking cessation drugs,* and *nitric oxide.*
- α₁-Proteinase inhibitor is given intravenously to individuals with *congenital α₁-antitrypsin deficiency* who exhibit panacinar emphysema at a prematurely early age.
- Individuals who are homozygous (have both recessive alleles) for the defective gene that expresses API lack this enzyme to balance the action of *neutrophil elastase* (NE), another enzyme in the lung that solubilizes connective tissue, causing alveolar wall destruction.
- Smoking cessation agents include nicotine as a transdermal patch, chewing gum, nasal spray, or inhaler as substitute therapy for *smoking cessation* in those with a strong physical addiction and withdrawal symptoms from nicotine absorbed during smoking. A tapered dose regimen allows withdrawal with minimal symptoms and assists in reducing the craving for cigarettes. *Bupropion,* an antidepressant, has been found helpful in smoking cessation.
- Nitric oxide is approved for *pulmonary vascular relaxation* and is used in the treatment of *persistent pulmonary hypertension of the newborn* and investigationally in *acute respiratory distress syndrome* (ARDS) of the adult.

- Nitric oxide is administered as an inhaled gas; it readily diffuses into the vascular endothelium, where it stimulates *guanylyl cyclase* in the cell, *increases cGMP,* and produces smooth muscle relaxation. Nitric oxide also quickly diffuses into the bloodstream, where it is *inactivated by binding to hemoglobin,* producing methemoglobin. Nitric oxide has a *short half-life* of less than 5 seconds because it is quickly bound by hemoglobin. In the presence of oxygen, nitric oxide is converted to *nitrogen dioxide,* a nitrite toxic to the lung.

SELF-ASSESSMENT QUESTIONS

1. What is the disease state in which an α₁-proteinase inhibitor (API) is indicated?
2. What is the route of administration for α₁-proteinase inhibitor?
3. What is the mode of action of α₁-proteinase inhibitor in treating emphysema associated with inadequate API levels?
4. Is treatment with API indicated for age-related emphysema or in general for those who smoke and have emphysema later in life?
5. Identify three pharmaceutical formulations of nicotine that are used as smoking cessation aids.
6. What is the usual effect of nicotine, whether in a smoking cessation aid or in cigarettes, on blood pressure?
7. What is the effect of inhaled nitric oxide?
8. Identify two potentially toxic by-products of inhaled nitric oxide.
9. What is the usual dose of inhaled nitric oxide?
10. Identify two disease states in which nitric oxide has been used to reverse pulmonary hypertension.

Answers to Self-Assessment Questions are found in Appendix A.

CLINICAL SCENARIO

A 42-year-old white female was referred by her family physician to Dr. G, a pulmonologist, with complaints of shortness of breath on exertion and increasing fatigue during her usual activities. On questioning, she reported that she had an uncle who had died "many years previously" in middle age with lung disease, but he had also smoked cigarettes. She admitted that she had been a heavy smoker (around a pack per day) for 5 or 6 years but had quit over 8 years ago. She denied use of alcohol. She described having several attacks of "bronchitis" in the past year, for which her family physician had prescribed antibiotics, with subsequent resolution each time. She also described a small, but increasing production of sputum during the past year, usually clear unless she had an episode of bronchitis. She currently has a cough, with production of a slight amount of greenish sputum on occasion. Her medications include albuterol by metered dose inhaler (MDI), prescribed by her family physician last year.

On physical examination, she is a well-developed, well-nourished appearing individual who exhibits mild respiratory distress. Auscultation of her chest reveals expiratory wheezing, diminished breath sounds bilaterally, and a somewhat prolonged expiratory phase. There is no digital clubbing, cyanosis, pedal edema or jugular distention. Her vital signs are T, 37.1° C; BP, 110/76 mm Hg; P, 76 beats/min; and RR, 24 breaths/min and regular. On room air, her reading on pulse oximetry is 91%.

Given this presenting scenario, what laboratory tests would you recommend Dr. G. obtain to further evaluate her respiratory status?
Based on her clinical picture and the laboratory results, what further test would Dr. G. want now?
With these results, would the use of α_1-proteinase inhibitor therapy be indicated?

Answers to Clinical Scenario Questions are found in Appendix A.

REFERENCES

1. Wewers MD and others: Replacement therapy for alpha$_1$-antitrypsin deficiency associated with emphysema, *N Engl J Med* 316:1055, 1987.
2. Stoller JK: Clinical features and natural history of severe α_1-antitrypsin deficiency, *Chest* 111:123S, 1997.
3. Memorandum: α_1-Antitrypsin deficiency: memorandum from a WHO meeting, *Bull WHO*, 75:397, 1997.
4. Snider GL: α_1-Protease inhibitor deficiency and the preventive therapy of emphysema. In Leff AR, editor: *Pulmonary and critical care pharmacology and therapeutics,* New York, 1996, McGraw-Hill.
5. Wewers MD, Casolaro MA, Crystal RG: Comparison of alpha-1-antitrypsin levels and antineutrophil elastase capacity of blood and lung in a patient with the alpha-1-antitrypsin phenotype null-null before and during alpha-1-antitrypsin augmentation therapy, *Am Rev Respir Dis* 135:539, 1987.
6. Cohen AB: Unraveling the mysteries of alpha$_1$-antitrypsin deficiency, *N Engl J Med* 314:778, 1986.
7. Alkins SA, O'Malley P: Should health-care systems pay for replacement therapy in patients with α_1-antitrypsin deficiency? *Chest* 117:875, 2000.
8. Buist AS and others: Guidelines for the approach to the patient with severe hereditary alpha-1-antitrypsin deficiency, *Am Rev Respir Dis* 140:1494, 1989.
9. Lillington GA, Leonard CT, Sachs DPL: Smoking cessation: techniques and benefits, *Clin Chest Med* 21:199, 2000.
10. Anthonisen NR and others: Effects of smoking intervention and the use of an inhaled anticholinergic bronchodilator on the rate of decline of FEV$_1$: The Lung Health Study, *J Am Med Assoc* 272:1497, 1994.
11. *Drug Facts and comparisons,* St Louis, 2001, Facts and Comparisons.
12. Ferrill MJ: Snuffed out: smoking deterrents, *Drug Newsletter* 15(Nov):83, 1996.
13. Jorenby DE and others: A controlled trial of sustained-release bupropion, a nicotine patch, or both for smoking cessation, *N Engl J Med* 340:685, 1999.
14. Wylam ME: Pulmonary vascular pharmacology. In Leff AR, editor: *Pulmonary and critical care pharmacology and therapeutics,* New York, 1996, McGraw-Hill.
15. Palmer RMJ, Ferrige AG, Moncada S: Nitric oxide release accounts for the biological activity of endothelium-derived relaxing factor, *Nature* 327:524, 1987.
16. Ignarro LJ and others: Endothelium derived relaxing factor produced and released from artery and vein is nitric oxide, *Proc Natl Acad Sci USA* 84:9265, 1987.
17. The Neonatal Inhaled Nitric Oxide Study Group: Inhaled nitric oxide in full-term and nearly full-term infants with hypoxic respiratory failure, *N Engl J Med* 336; 597, 1997.
18. Zapol WM and others: Nitric oxide and the lung, *Am J Respir Crit Care Med* 149:1375, 1994.
19. American Academy of Pediatrics. Committee on Fetus and Newborn: use of inhaled nitric oxide, *Pediatrics* 106:344, 2000.
20. Barnes PJ, Kharitonov SA: Exhaled nitric oxide: a new lung function test, *Thorax* 51:233, 1996.
21. Mizutani T, Layon AJ: Clinical applications of nitric oxide, *Chest* 110:506, 1996.
22. Aranda M, Pearl RG: The biology of nitric oxide, *Respir Care* 44:156, 1999.
23. Frostell CG and others: Inhaled nitric oxide selectively reverses human hypoxic pulmonary vasoconstriction without causing systemic vasodilation, *Anesthesiology* 78:427, 1993.
24. Palevsky HI: Treatment of pulmonary hypertension. In Leff AR, editor: *Pulmonary and critical care pharmacology and therapeutics,* New York, 1996, McGraw-Hill.
25. Martin WJ, Rehm S: Toxic injury of the lung parenchyma. In Leff AR, editor: *Pulmonary and critical care pharmacology and therapeutics,* New York, 1996, McGraw-Hill.

CHAPTER 17

Neonatal and Pediatric Aerosolized Drug Therapy

Ruben D. Restrepo • *Joseph L. Rau*

CHAPTER OUTLINE

Neonatal/Pediatric Drug Labeling
   Legality of off-label prescribing
Aerosol Versus Systemic Drug Delivery in Neonates and Pediatric
  Patients
   Advantages of aerosol delivery

Factors Affecting Neonatal and Pediatric Aerosol Drug Delivery
   Effect of age on the aerosol lung dose
   Effect of small tidal volumes and low flow rates
Studies on Lung Deposition of Inhaled Aerosols
Clinical Response to Aerosolized Drugs in Neonates and Pediatric Patients
Choice of Delivery Device in Neonatal and Pediatric Aerosol Treatment

Substantial differences exist between the adult and neonatal/pediatric airway environment that affect aerosolized drug therapy. The lack of neonatal and pediatric dose labeling for many drugs given by inhaled aerosol complicates aerosol drug dosing for clinicians and can lead to varied dosing among centers. The differences between aerosol drug delivery as a form of topical administration and systemic administration of drugs is not clearly appreciated in many instances, causing aerosol doses to be modified in neonates and children as if they were given systemically. Data on lung deposition and clinical response, especially to bronchodilators, in this population support the use of aerosol drug therapy in young subjects. Differences among aerosol delivery devices should be considered in relation to the age of the subject. All of the considerations in this chapter relate to use of inhaled aerosols for therapeutic use in the lung and not for systemic treatment. The data cited also are based largely on traditional aerosol delivery devices. New and highly efficient delivery systems may lead to different results in the future. Terms used for different age ranges are given in Box 17-1.

NEONATAL/PEDIATRIC DRUG LABELING

Infants, children, and pregnant women are the most common groups in which the labeled use of prescription drugs is lacking. Such use is termed *off-label*, which refers to the fact that a drug lacks Food and Drug Administration (FDA)-approved dosing information for a specific age-group or condition.[1] Even though the drug labeling often states that safety and efficacy in children have not been determined, many of the inhaled aerosol drugs reviewed in this text have clinical indications and uses in the neonatal and pediatric population.

Table 17-1 lists inhaled aerosol drugs and the leukotriene modifiers that currently have an approved age labeling for pediatric use at the time of this edition. Drugs that are not listed in Table 17-1 do not have labeling for pediatric use. For example, this includes terbutaline, bitolterol, pirbuterol, isoetharine, salmeterol (by MDI) and levalbuterol in the inhaled adrenergic group. The anticholinergic bronchodilator ipratropium also lacks pediatric labeling. The nebulizer solution of budesonide is approved for children 12 months to 8 years of age. Ribavirin is the only inhaled agent approved for infants and young children, and there is no inhaled drug approved for neonatal use. Most inhaled drugs are not approved for subjects below 4 to 6 years of age.

In 1994, the FDA's Center for Drug Evaluation and Research issued guidelines *encouraging* pediatric testing of drugs.[2] A subsequent FDA ruling *mandated* that drugs submitted for FDA approval after December 2000 be evaluated in children. Waivers can be given if the drug has no meaningful application in children or is likely to be unsafe or ineffective in pediatric patients.[3]

Box 17-1	Terms and Age Ranges Defining Periods From Birth to Adult

Premature neonate: <37 weeks of gestational age Neonate: First month of postnatal life Infant: 1 to 12 months	Child: 1 to 12 years Adolescent: 12 to 18 years Adult: >18 years

Table 17-1

Pediatric drug labeling for inhaled aerosols and leukotriene modifiers*

DRUG NAME	FORMULATION	AGE LABELING (FDA-APPROVED)
β-ADRENERGIC AGENTS		
Albuterol	MDI	≥4 yr: 2 inhalations q4-6h
	SVN	2-12 yr: 0.1-0.15 mg/kg/dose, titrated to effect; maximum 2.5 mg tid-qid†
	DPI	≥4 yr: 1 capsule inhaled, q4-6h
Epinephrine	SVN	≥4 yr: 0.5 ml of 2.25% solution in 3.0 ml diluent; q3-4h
Metaproterenol	SVN	≥6 yr: 0.1 to 0.2 ml of 5% solution tid-qid
Salmeterol	DPI	≥4 yr: 1 inhalation (50 µg) bid
CORTICOSTEROIDS		
Beclomethasone	MDI (42 µg)	6-12 yr: 1-2 inhalations qid
Budesonide	DPI	≥6 yr: 200 µg (1 inhalation) bid; maximum 400 µg bid
	SVN	12 mo–8 yr: 0.5 mg total daily dose given once, or twice daily, in divided doses; maximum 1 mg total daily as once or 0.5 mg twice daily
Flunisolide	MDI	6-15 yr: 2 inhalations twice daily
Fluticasone	DPI	≥4 yr: 50 µg twice daily up to 100 µg twice daily
Triamcinolone	MDI	6-12 yr: 1-2 inhalations tid-qid or 2-4 inhalations bid
MUCOLYTIC		
Dornase alfa	SVN	Safety and efficacy in children <5 yr have not been studied; usual dose: one 2.5 mg dose daily
NONSTEROIDAL ANTIASTHMA		
Cromolyn sodium	MDI	≥5 yr: 2 puffs qid
	SVN	≥2 yr: 20 mg qid
INHALED ANTIINFECTIVES		
Ribavirin	SPAG	Infants and young children: a 20 mg/ml solution nebulized for 12-18 hr/day for 3-7 days
Tobramycin	SVN	≥6 yr: 300 mg bid, alternate 28 days on, 28 days off
LEUKOTRIENE MODIFIERS		
Montelukast	Tablet (5 mg)	6-14 yr: one 5 mg tab (chewable) daily in evening
	Tablet (4 mg)	2-5 yr: one 4 mg tab (chewable) daily in evening

DPI, Dry powder inhaler; *MDI*, metered dose inhaler; *SPAG*, small particle aerosol generator; *SVN*, small volume nebulizer.
*Additional detail on dosing for adults can be found in previous chapters. Manufacturers' information and other sources on drug administration and dosing should be consulted before use. Drug labeling is current at the time of this edition.
†NAEPP EPR II guidelines give the SVN child dose of albuterol as: 0.05 mg/kg, with a minimum of 1.25 mg and maximum of 2.5 mg q4-6h.

LEGALITY OF OFF-LABEL PRESCRIBING

It is not illegal for a physician to prescribe a drug that has no prescription label for neonatal or pediatric use. The FDA cannot, by law, regulate how a drug is used medically or "interfere with the practice of medicine."[1] If a drug is FDA-approved, it may be prescribed by a duly licensed physician for any indication deemed appropriate. The following points generally apply to such prescribing[1]:

- The drug is prescribed in a manner that conforms to the community's standard of care.
- The therapy is considered reasonable (i.e., the drug use is based on sound physiological principles and pathological need).
- The therapy is safe—the clinician is aware of known side effects, there are means for assessing toxicity, and generally any risk is acceptable and appropriate given the patient situation.
- Parameters to be used in monitoring for side effects and safety, as well as frequency of monitoring, must be decided before drug dosing begins.

Although it is legal for physicians to prescribe off-label use of drugs, drug dosing becomes much more problematic when standardized dose guidelines have not been previously developed during drug clinical trials. Usually drug therapy is based on one of two strategies in dosing, as follows[1]:

Target concentration: Drugs are dosed until a certain blood level is reached; therefore therapeutic effects and side effects are related to the drug concentration in the blood.

Target effect: Drugs are dosed until the desired effect is achieved or unacceptable side effects or toxicity occur.

In general, drug dosing with inhaled aerosols will need to be based on the *target effect strategy:* aerosol doses should be based on the desired effect, with avoidance of toxicity. Data that are now available suggest that in fact aerosol doses to neonates or children are "self-limiting" because of differences between pediatric and adult airways. Aerosol drug dose is not based on body size and blood level, but rather amount reaching the lung.

AEROSOL VERSUS SYSTEMIC DRUG DELIVERY IN NEONATES AND PEDIATRIC PATIENTS

ADVANTAGES OF AEROSOL DELIVERY

The advantages of inhaled aerosol drug delivery with neonates and children are largely the same as in adults, with several additional factors favoring this population:

- Potential for reduced systemic exposure to the drug
- Potential for use of smaller doses by inhaled aerosol compared with other routes of administration (oral, injection)
- Administration painless and generally safe with appropriate monitoring
- Administration feasible in the very young compared with the oral route of administration with pills or tablets
- Provides direct delivery to the target organ
- Avoidance of complicating pharmacokinetic and pharmacodynamic factors in the very young
- A rapid response such as with bronchodilators

The use of inhaled aerosols for therapeutic purposes in treating lung disease is a *topical* form of drug administration. As such, a drug blood level is not required and in fact is undesirable. This factor is basic to discussing the dose or amounts of inhaled drug needed with neonates or children. An aerosol drug is delivered to the airway surface where the effect is desired. For example, an inhaled β_2 agonist has its effect based on topical delivery to β_2 receptors in the airway. The therapeutic effect from an inhaled aerosol drug is a function of the amount of the drug reaching the airway surface or lung topically.[4-6] As a topical form of drug administration, titrating formulas used with oral or parenteral drug administration do not apply well with inhaled aerosol dosing.

A major advantage to using inhaled aerosols to treat the lung is avoidance of systemic factors that can affect oral or injectable drug therapy in neonatal and pediatric use. The effects of many drugs in neonates, infants, and children vary considerably from adults when given by systemic routes of administration. Some of the pharmacokinetic and pharmacodynamic factors causing these differences between adults and younger subjects are reviewed by Christensen and colleagues.[7]

FACTORS AFFECTING NEONATAL AND PEDIATRIC AEROSOL DRUG DELIVERY

The same mechanisms of aerosol penetration and deposition in the lung that were outlined in Chapter 3 apply to aerosol therapy in neonatal and pediatric patients. These are inertial impaction, a function of particle size and velocity, as well as gravitational settling (sedimentation), as a function of mass and residence time. However, the airway environment differs in neonatal and pediatric subjects from that of adults. Table 17-2 outlines functional and structural features of the infant lung that may affect aerosol delivery and deposition.

As suggested by in vitro studies, the increasing upper airway geometry in adults may explain the higher amount of aerosol deposition reaching the lower airway compared with that of the pediatric patient.[9] Therefore the impact of higher upper airway aerosol deposition in infants who are obligate nasal breathers and children wearing face masks on lung deposition should always be in the mind of the clinician. In a study conducted by Olsson,[10] a smaller fraction of the nominal dose of an aerosol reached the lower airways with the child-size oropharynx compared with an adult-size oropharynx. The smaller diameter of neonatal and pediatric lower airways, added to the effects of bronchoconstriction, inflammation,

secretions, and the possible presence of an endotracheal tube, dramatically decreases aerosolized drug deposition in the lungs.[11]

It is also important to clarify the terms and accompanying concepts used in describing aerosol drug administration, to interpret study results correctly. Box 17-2 distinguishes terms with significantly different meanings for an "aerosol dose." As an example of the distinctions in Box 17-2, Agertoft and associates[12] investigated delivery of inhaled budesonide in preschool children ages 3 to 6 years using a PARI LC Jet Plus nebulizer. Their study contained the following "doses":

Nominal dose: The 1.0 mg of budesonide solution placed in the PARI nebulizer

Inhaled or delivered dose: A mean of 25% of the nominal dose, which was measured as the amount of drug deposited on a filter placed between the mouthpiece and the nebulizer; "dose to subject"

Lung dose: Approximately 6% of the nominal dose (or 26% of the "dose to subject"), estimated indirectly from systemic drug levels

The significance of the study by Agertoft and associates is that the "inhaled dose" of 25% is not the "lung dose," which was much less (mean of 6%). In addition, the dose reaching the lungs of children was smaller than the usual 10% to 15% lung dose in adult patients.[4,13] The factors causing this reduction in lung dose are discussed below. Misinterpretation of the "inhaled dose" or "dose to subject" as the "lung dose" would lead to the incorrect conclusion that the nominal dose should be reduced for pediatric subjects.

EFFECT OF AGE ON THE AEROSOL LUNG DOSE

Inhaled aerosol drugs are absorbed into the body from the lung and also from the mouth and stomach if there is oropharyngeal impaction and loss. This is described by the lung/total systemic availability ratio (L/T ratio) presented in Chapter 2. If a fixed fraction

Table 17-2

Comparison of neonatal and adult respiratory parameters

PARAMETER	NEONATE	ADULT
Tracheal diameter	~4 mm	~20 mm
Tracheal length	5-6 cm	10-12 cm
Tidal volume	6 ml/kg	6 ml/kg
Respiratory rate	30-40/min	12-14/min
Minute ventilation	200-300 ml/ kg/min	6 L/min
Dead space	0.75 ml/lb	1.0 ml/lb
Inspiratory flow rate	≤100 ml/sec	~500 ml/sec

From Malinowski C, Wilson B: Neonatal and pediatric respiratory care. In Scanlan CL, Wilkins RL, Stoller JK, eds: *Egan's fundamentals of respiratory care*, ed 7, St Louis, 1999, Mosby.

Box 17-2   Terms to Describe Aerosol Delivery and Administration

Nominal dose: The dose of aerosol drug in the delivery device; usually the total dose charge of a nebulizer or the dose per actuation from an MDI or a DPI.

Inhaled dose: The dose of aerosol reaching the mouth, nose, or artificial airway; usually the same as the "delivered dose," "inhaled drug mass," or "dose to subject"; it is not the same as the lung dose.

Emitted dose: The dose of aerosol produced by an aerosol device when powered or actuated; for an SVN, usually more than the inhaled dose; for an MDI, may be approximately the same as the inhaled (delivered) dose.

Lung dose: The actual amount of drug mass reaching the trachea and beyond.

of an aerosol dose, such as 10% to 15% of the nominal dose, reaches the lungs regardless of age, there would be a risk of higher drug concentrations in the circulation of neonates, infants, and children compared with adults. Systemic side effects rather than local overtreatment in the lung have been the basis for aerosol dose adjustment for age, which is usually based on body weight. An example is the dosage schedule for inhaled albuterol in the 1997 National Asthma Education and Prevention Program (NAEPP) guidelines: 0.05 mg/kg, with a minimum of 1.25 mg and a maximum of 2.5 mg.[14] With this schedule, the full 2.5 mg would be given to a 50-kg child:

$$0.05 \text{ mg/kg} \times 50 \text{ kg} = 2.5 \text{ mg}$$

The need for age adjustment of aerosol doses based on body weight has been clinically debated. The available data at this time suggest that the actual dose of an inhaled aerosol drug in neonates, infants, and young children is *self-limiting* and proportionately less than the traditional 10% to 15% cited for adults.

Anhøj and associates[15] found that an MDI of budesonide with a 250-ml steel NebuChamber having less than 2 ml of dead space delivered the *same* approximate dose to a range of ages from 2 to 41 years. In this study, a face mask was used for 2- to 3-year-olds and a mouthpiece for older subjects. The study confirmed that the inhaled dose and the dose reaching the lung were not the same. The results of this study are graphed in Figure 17-1. The resulting plasma concentration of drug was the same in children and adults. Because the holding chamber removed oropharyngeal/stomach loss and there is high first-pass metabolism of budesonide, plasma drug levels reflect dose in the lung. If the same dose went to the lungs in adults as in 2-year-olds, higher plasma levels would be observed in younger subjects who have smaller circulating blood volumes. Data of Anhøj and associates[15] indicate that inhaled dose need not be adjusted for age to reduce systemic levels and possible toxicity.

The results for lung dose found by Anhøj and associates[15] are confirmed by a clinical study of Oberklaid and colleagues,[16] which compared dose based on body weight with a fixed dose of albuterol in acute asthma in children. In that study, a fixed dose of 2.5 mg by nebulizer was compared with a 0.1 mg/kg bodyweight dose in children 4 to 12 years of age, in acute asthma. The study found no difference between the two dosing protocols in either clinical improvement measured by flows, oxygen saturations, and clin-

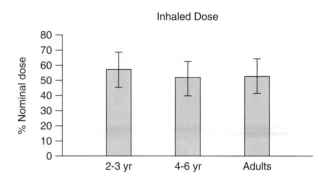

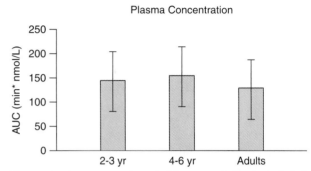

Figure 17-1   Mean values (with 95% CI) for the inhaled dose of budesonide from a metered dose inhaler and steel chamber (NebuChamber), and the area under the curve *(AUC)* of corresponding plasma drug levels for three age ranges. The inhaled dose (dose reaching the patient) is equivalent for various age-groups. Blood levels from lung absorption remain the same in younger subjects, indicating that the dose reaching the lung is proportionately less for younger, smaller subjects. (Data from of Anhøj J and others: Lung deposition of inhaled drugs increases with age, *Am J Respir Crit Care Med* 162:1819, 2000.)

ical score, or cardiovascular and tremor side effects. The fixed dose of 2.5 mg by nebulizer was efficacious and safe.

EFFECT OF SMALL TIDAL VOLUMES AND LOW FLOW RATES

Very low tidal volumes and low inspiratory flow rates would reduce the amount of aerosol drug inhaled from either an SVN or MDI with a reservoir device (holding chamber or spacer). These two factors can significantly alter the inhaled dose in subjects below the age of 6 months.

EFFECT ON SMALL VOLUME NEBULIZER

If we assume a 6 L/min power gas, an adult with inspiratory flow of 500 ml/sec (30 L/min) and a tidal volume of 500 to 1000 ml (500 ml/sec × 1 or 2 sec-

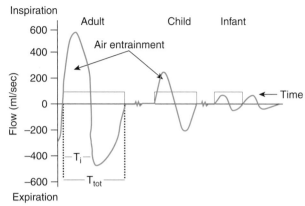

Figure 17-2   Illustration of the amount of nebulizer output inspired with varying inspiratory patterns (volumes, flow rates, times), indicating a smaller fraction of output inspired with low tidal volumes and flow rates in infants compared with adults. T_i, Inspiration time; T_{tot}, total cycle time. (From Collis GG and others: Dilution of nebulised aerosols by air entrainment in children, *Lancet* 336:341, 1990.)

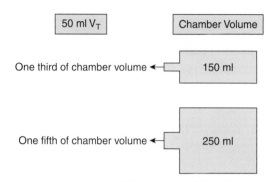

Figure 17-3   Conceptual illustration of the effect of small tidal volumes (V_T) on chamber evacuation with different sized reservoir chambers.

onds) would completely inhale all of a nebulizer output. However, an infant with inspiratory flow of less than 100 ml/sec (<6 L/min) and a tidal volume below 100 ml will not completely inhale all of the nebulizer output during the inspiratory phase (Figure 17-2).

Collis and associates[17] studied the fraction of nebulizer output inspired by infants ages 1 to 12 months, children 3 to 16 years, and adults 20 to 23 years. Infants were sedated with chloral hydrate and tidal breathing recorded by face mask and pneumotachograph. The fraction of nebulizer output inspired was lower in infants below the age of 6 months, then reached a plateau and remained constant above 6 months. Wildhaber and colleagues[18] also found that inhaled aerosol dose from a nebulizer/mask increased with weight in 4- to 12-month-olds and was lower in smaller infants.[18]

EFFECT ON RESERVOIR DOSE

The same effect of low tidal volumes would theoretically reduce the amount of volume and therefore drug mass inhaled from a reservoir chamber (Figure 17-3). The amount of reduction is proportional to the chamber volume for a given infant tidal volume. For a 50-ml tidal volume, approximately one third of a 150-ml chamber and one fifth (20%) of a 250-ml chamber would be inhaled. Even assuming no redistribution of aerosol in the chamber volume, gravitational settling will further reduce available dose within seconds

of MDI actuation into the chamber. The ideal volume for a spacer device is small enough to allow drug inhalation with few breaths for infants with low tidal volumes (<50 ml).

This theoretical prediction is supported by data from Everard and colleagues.[19] Delivery (not lung deposition) of MDI cromolyn sodium by reservoir and face mask with tidal volumes of 25, 50, and 150 ml was measured in vitro using various sizes of chambers.[19] Smaller tidal volumes decreased inhaled drug mass. Higher aerosol concentrations in a smaller chamber enhanced drug delivery with tidal volumes below 150 ml. The same study found that introducing a dead space between the chamber outlet and the filter collecting inspired drug reduced the dose deposited by as much as 50% or more. The results are summarized in Table 17-3. In contrast, an in vivo study by Wildhaber and associates[18] that showed decreasing inhaled dose from a nebulizer with infants as small as 6 to 7 kg also found that there was no effect of size (weight) on inhaled dose for two chamber devices used with an MDI. The two reservoir devices were the Babyhaler (350-ml chamber, 40 ml dead volume) and the NebuChamber (250-ml chamber, no dead volume). The plastic reservoir device (Babyhaler, 350 ml) had the electrostatic charge removed before testing. Turpeinen and colleagues[20] compared the same reservoir devices and found that inhaled mass of budesonide from the Babyhaler did increase with increasing height, weight, and tidal volume, but not with the NebuChamber. Such variation in study results indicates that testing conditions, type of drug, and choice of reservoir device can affect inhaled dose,

Table 17-3

Effect of inspired tidal volumes on mean (range) inhaled aerosol dose in two reservoir devices

DEVICE	TIDAL VOLUME (ML)		
	25	50	150
AeroChamber (150 ml)	0.33 mg (0.29-0.35)	1.15 mg (1.08-1.24)	1.41 mg (1.33-1.46)
Nebuhaler (750 ml)	0.29 mg (0.26-0.32)	0.93 mg (0.91-0.97)	1.55 mg (1.48-1.61)

Data from Everard ML, Clark AR, Milner AD: Drug delivery from holding chambers with attached facemask, *Arch Dis Child* 67:580, 1992.

Box 17-3	**Factors That May Affect the Dose Inhaled From a Reservoir Chamber in Neonatal and Pediatric Subjects**

Mechanical and Design Factors

Chamber volume
Electrostatic charge on plastic devices
Shape of aerosol plume relative to chamber size
Design of inspiratory and expiratory valves, if present
Presence of inspiratory valve
Amount of dead volume in mouthpiece

Patient Factors

Breathing pattern
Inspiratory flow rate
Tidal volume

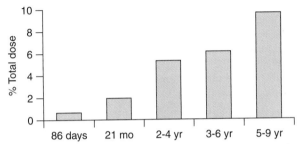

Figure 17-4   Data from four separate studies giving the percent of a total aerosol dose that reaches the lungs of infants and children of varying ages. In each study, aerosol dose was delivered using a metered dose inhaler with reservoir device and a face mask in subjects under 4 years of age. Studies are listed in the references: for 86 days: Fok and colleagues[21]; for 21 months: Tal and colleagues[22]; for 2 to 4 years and 5 to 9 years: Wildhaber and colleagues[23]; for 3 to 6 years: Agertoft and colleagues.[12]

although not necessarily the lung dose. Box 17-3 lists factors in reservoir devices that may affect the inhaled dose to neonates, infants, and small children.

STUDIES ON LUNG DEPOSITION OF INHALED AEROSOLS

The most definitive data for answering the question of how much aerosol drug reaches the lungs of neonates, infants, and children are actual measures of lung deposition for various age-groups. Such data are increasingly available and indicate that the lung dose of an aerosol drug does in fact decrease with age. This is consistent with the data of Anhøj and associates[15] discussed earlier, which found that blood levels of drug, reflecting the dose reaching the lungs, was constant in younger and older subjects, despite the smaller circulating volume of younger patients.

Figure 17-4 summarizes data on lung deposition with inhaled aerosols, compiled from four studies. All of the studies used an MDI with a reservoir device and

a face mask for delivery in subjects below 4 years of age. Values represent the percentage of total dose from the device. Fok and colleagues[21] found that 0.67% (SEM = 0.17) of the total dose of albuterol reached the lungs of infants with a mean age of 86 days (25 to 187 days). Tal and associates[22] found 1.97% (SD = 1.4) as a lung dose of albuterol in patients with a mean age of 21 months (3 months to 5 years). Wildhaber and colleagues[23] found 5.4% (SD = 2.1) and 9.6% (SD = 3.9) of albuterol reached the lungs of 2- to 4-year-olds and 5- to 9-year-olds, respectively. Agertoft and co-workers,[12] using indirect measures of plasma levels, found 6.1% of a budesonide dose reached the lungs of 3- to 6-year-olds. Similar data has been found for aerosol delivery with nebulizers and was listed in Chapter 3 (Table 3-6).

If the amount of aerosolized albuterol reaching the lungs of infants and children in the study by Tal and colleagues[22] is used, it can be shown that the self-

Table 17-4

Calculation of dose per kilogram of aerosolized albuterol for children and adults based on lung deposition data (1.97%) showing equivalence of dose per body size

	ADULT*	CHILD
Weight	80 kg	10 kg
Lung deposition	20%*	2%
Nominal dose	200 μg	200 μg
Dose to lung	40 μg	4 μg
Per-kilogram dose:	0.5 μg/kg	0.4 μg/kg

Data from Tal A and others: Deposition pattern of radiolabeled salbutamol inhaled from a metered-dose inhaler by means of a spacer with mask in young children with airway obstruction, *J Pediatr* 128:479, 1996.
*Percentage lung deposition measured by Tal and colleagues in two adult volunteers in the same study.

limiting effect of younger ages on lung dose results in the same dose per amount of body weight in children as in adults (Table 17-4). The equivalence of dose per body weight illustrated in Table 17-4 and based on lung deposition data argues strongly against the need to adjust the nominal dose of an aerosol drug for age or body size with current aerosol delivery devices. Age and size have a self-limiting effect on lung dose, producing a natural titration of dose. This conclusion may need to be revised pending more efficient aerosol delivery devices.

CLINICAL RESPONSE TO AEROSOLIZED DRUGS IN NEONATES AND PEDIATRIC PATIENTS

The lung deposition data reviewed in the previous section argues that aerosolized drugs do reach the lungs of infants and do so in a self-regulating amount. However, the question of clinical response to aerosol drugs in infants and children is not determined by lung deposition data. The most commonly studied drug class, and one of great interest in neonates and infants, is the adrenergic bronchodilator group. Compared with corticosteroids, the clinical response to bronchodilator occurs within minutes and is more feasible to study in young subjects.

Commonly cited studies from the late 1970s concluded that there was an absence of response to inhaled bronchodilators in infants and children below 18 months of age.[24,25] These studies found no change in respiratory resistance with phenylephrine, epi-

nephrine, or salbutamol (albuterol) in infants and children from 7 to 17 or 18 months of age, using a forced oscillation technique. The authors of the studies speculated that there was either poor development of smooth muscle below 18 months of age or the bronchial obstruction was due to secretions and airway edema rather than bronchoconstriction.

A 1993 study by Turner and associates[26] also found that the level of response to a bronchodilator increases significantly with increasing age in young asthmatics between the ages of 3 and 9 years. However, studies of both ventilated and non ventilated preterm infants have shown dose-related changes in respiratory mechanics, including airway resistance, with aerosolized bronchodilators.[27-31] Table 17-5 lists several studies, and the outcomes measured, that have documented clinical efficacy of aerosolized bronchodilators in infants.

CHOICE OF DELIVERY DEVICE IN NEONATAL AND PEDIATRIC AEROSOL TREATMENT

Box 17-4 gives the age guidelines for use of current aerosol delivery devices in infants and children, based on the 1997 NAEPP guidelines.[14] Either a jet nebulizer or an MDI can be used with suitable auxiliary devices attached. For both the MDI and nebulizer, a face mask is needed in the very young and a reservoir is needed additionally for the MDI. A dry powder inhaler (DPI) is not suitable for young children below the age of 4 or 5 because of their limited inspiratory flow ability and more limited vital capacities.

Studies cited in Chapter 3 (Table 3-5) have shown equivalent clinical response between the MDI-reservoir systems, with or without a mask as needed by age, and jet nebulizers. The MDI delivery system has the advantage of smallness and portability, plus shorter treatment time, even with an increased number of actuations, compared with gas-powered nebulizers, which require a pressurized gas source, bulky equipment, and a 10- to 15-minute treatment time, with additional preparation and cleaning time needed.

It is important to consider changes associated with the use of SVN in-line on pediatric and particularly neonatal ventilated patients, because unexpected changes on both volume and pressure may have deleterious effects. An externally powered nebulizer increases volume and pressure during volume-targeted ventilation, creates a bias flow in the ventilator circuit that may interfere with patient-triggered modes of

Table 17-5

Results of studies examining clinical response to aerosolized albuterol in infants*

AGE	DELIVERY	OUTCOME MEASURED	FIRST AUTHOR
6.6 ± 4.6 wk	MDI via ETT	Improved: dynamic compliance, airway resistance	Holt, 1995[27]
13.3 ± 4.9 days	MDI/spacer via ETT	Improved: respiratory system resistance and compliance	Denjean, 1992[28]
46.7 ± 21.5 days	MDI/reservoir/mask SVN/mask	Improved: respiratory system resistance with both delivery methods	Fok, 1998[29]
37 ± 2.3 wk	MDI/reservoir/mask SVN/mask	Improved: dynamic lung resistance but no change in dynamic compliance for either method of delivery	Gappa, 1997[30]
7.9 ± 5.1 mo	MDI/reservoir/mask SVN/mask	Faster response in clinical score	Rubilar, 2000[31]

ETT, Endotracheal tube; MDI, metered dose inhaler; SVN, small volume nubulizer.
*First author of the studies cited is listed, with complete citation in the references.

Box 17-4	Age Guidelines for Use of Current Aerosol Delivery Devices

Aerosol System	Age-Group
SVN*	≥Neonate
MDI	>5 yr
MDI with reservoir	>4 yr
MDI with reservoir/mask	≤4 yr
MDI with ETT	≥Neonate
Breath-actuated MDI	>5 yr
DPI	≥5 yr

Data from National Asthma Education and Prevention Program, Expert Panel Report II: *Guidelines for the diagnosis and management of asthma*, Bethesda, Md, 1997, National Institutes of Health.
DPI, Dry powder inhaler; ETT, endotracheal tube; MDI, metered dose inhaler; SVN, small volume nebulizer.
*With face mask for those unable to use a mouthpiece.

ventilation,[32] may result in increased airway pressure and unexpected positive end-expiratory pressure (PEEP), and may result in variable FIO_2 levels. The respiratory clinician should also be aware that aerosol delivery may be less effective with manual ventilation versus mechanical ventilation.[33]

The respiratory clinician responsible for management of neonatal and pediatric patients must be aware that the challenge of aerosol administration to this special group rests on the broad spectrum of patients, from premature infants (<1000 g) to adult-size teenagers.

Determination of doses for aerosolized drugs delivered to neonatal and pediatric patients is not completely understood. Despite the differences in all three phases of drug action (drug administration, pharmacokinetic and pharmacodynamic) between adults and children, the selection of the optimal aerosol delivery system plays a role in lung deposition of the drug that should not be underestimated. Identifying the ability of the patient, rather than specific age, is also essential to selecting the most appropriate device in any population.[34]

SUMMARY KEY TERMS AND CONCEPTS

- Many drugs that are given as inhaled aerosols have no labeling for neonatal or pediatric use, and such use is referred to as *off-label* use.
- The advantages with inhaled drugs to treat pulmonary problems in neonates and pediatric patients support the off-label use of these drugs, but there is variation in determining a suitable dose for this population.
- Recent research suggests that *age has a dose-regulating effect* on the amount of aerosol drug reaching the lungs, with less drug reaching the lungs of younger subjects.
- Distinctions are made between the *nominal* dose (dose in the delivery device), the *inhaled* or *delivered dose* (dose reaching the patient's mouth or artificial airway), the *emitted dose* (dose released by the aerosol device), and the *lung dose* (dose actually reaching the trachea and beyond).

- Below the age of 6 months, tidal volumes and inspiratory flow rates can reduce the amount of aerosol drug *inhaled* from nebulizers or MDI/reservoir devices.
- Even when the inhaled dose is the same for pediatric and adult patients, data indicate that the *lung dose* decreases for younger patients. If, as current data suggest, less aerosol drug reaches the lungs of neonatal and pediatric patients compared with adults, the *same nominal dose* can be prescribed for *all* patients.
- Neonatal and pediatric patients should be assessed for *toxic systemic effects* with aerosol drug administration, because of efficient drug absorption from the lung.
- There is *no difference in clinical effect for bronchodilators* between MDI and nebulizer administration. The MDI dose may need to be adjusted upward for normal, pediatric, or adult use because the MDI nominal dose is usually lower than the nebulizer dose.
- There is a *clinical response* to aerosolized *bronchodilator* administration in neonates and very young pediatric patients.

The newborn was supported on pressure-limited, time-cycled, continuous-flow ventilation over the next 10 days and then weaned using continuous positive airway pressure (CPAP) at 5 cm H_2O and an FIO_2 of 0.30. After extubation, and despite use of theophylline, the neonate experienced increasing episodes of bradycardia and desaturation and was then reintubated. After intubation and verification of endotracheal tube placement, auscultation revealed bilateral wheezing, with rales at the lung bases. The neonatologist wishes to institute aerosolized albuterol.

What methods of aerosol delivery are appropriate and available for albuterol?

After the decision was made to use an SVN, a dose of 2.5 mg (0.5 ml of a 0.5% solution) was administered. The neonate's heart rate increased from 168 beats/min to 210 beats/min within 2 to 3 minutes. What would you recommend to the physician?

Answers to Clinical Scenario Questions are found in Appendix A.

SELF-ASSESSMENT QUESTIONS

1. Can an aerosol formulation for oral inhalation be legally administered to neonatal and pediatric patients?
2. Can an adrenergic bronchodilator such as albuterol reduce airway resistance when used in infants and children?
3. Based on the data reviewed in this chapter, does the adult dose of an aerosol drug need to be reduced with pediatric patients, based on weight?
4. What aerosol delivery devices could be used with a 2-year-old child?

Answers to Self-Assessment Questions are found in Appendix A.

CLINICAL SCENARIO

Case courtesy **Robert Harwood, MSA, RRT formerly of Georgia State University**

A 785-g, 24-weeks' gestational age female neonate was born to a 15-year-old, who had presented to the hospital with premature rupture of membranes (PROM). At birth, the neonate was resuscitated with bag/mask ventilation and 100% oxygen. Apgar scores were 4 and 9 at 1 and 5 minutes, respectively. A diagnosis of respiratory distress syndrome (RDS) was made; the neonate was treated with a single dose of beractant (Survanta) and transported to the neonatal intensive care unit (NICU).

REFERENCES

1. Blumer JL: Off-label uses of drugs in children, *Pediatrics* 104(suppl 3):598, 1999.
2. Specific requirements on content and format of labeling for human prescription drugs: revision of "pediatric use" subsecton in the labeling—final rule, *Fed Reg* 59:64240, 1994.
3. Regulations requiring manufacturers to assess the safety and effectiveness of new drugs and biological products in pediatric patients, *Fed Reg* 63:66631, 1998.
4. Zainudin BMZ and others: Comparison of bronchodilator responses and deposition patterns of salbutamol inhaled from a pressurized metered dose inhaler, as a dry powder, and as a nebulised solution, *Thorax* 45:469, 1990.
5. Mestitz H, Copland JM, McDonald CF: Comparison of outpatient nebulized vs. metered dose inhaler terbutaline in chronic airflow obstruction, *Chest* 96:1237, 1989.
6. Newhouse M, Dolovich M: Aerosol therapy: nebulizer vs. metered dose inhaler, *Chest* 91:799, 1987.
7. Christensen ML, Helms RA, Chesney RW: Is pediatric labeling really necessary? *Pediatrics* 104(suppl 3):593, 1999.
8. Malinowski C, Wilson B: Neonatal and pediatric respiratory care. In Scanlan CL, Wilkins RL, Stoller JK, eds: *Egan's fundamentals of respiratory care,* ed 7, St Louis, 1999, Mosby.
9. Berg E: In vitro properties of pressurized metered dose inhalers with and without spacer devices, *J Aerosol Med* 8(suppl):S3, 1995.
10. Olsson B: Aerosol particle generation from dry powder inhalers: can they equal pressurized metered dose inhalers? *J Aerosol Med* 8(suppl):S13, 1995.

11. Dolovich M: Aerosol delivery to children: what to use, how to choose, *Pediatr Pulmonol* 18(suppl):79, 1999.

12. Agertoft L and others: Systemic availability and pharmacokinetics of nebulised budesonide in preschool children, *Arch Dis Child* 80:241, 1999.

13. Newman SP and others: Deposition of pressurized aerosols in the human respiratory tract, *Thorax* 36:52, 1981.

14. National Asthma Education and Prevention Program, Expert Panel Report II: *Guidelines for the diagnosis and management of asthma*, Bethesda, Md, 1997, National Institutes of Health.

15. Anhøj J, Thorsson L, Bisgaard H: Lung deposition of inhaled drugs increases with age, *Am J Respir Crit Care Med* 162:1810, 2000.

16. Oberklaid F and others: A comparison of a bodyweight dose versus a fixed dose of nebulised salbutamol in acute asthma in children, *Med J Australia* 158:751, 1993.

17. Collis GG, Cole CH, Le Souëf PN: Dilution of nebulised aerosols by air entrainment in children, *Lancet* 336:341, 1990.

18. Wildhaber JH and others: Aerosol delivery to wheezy infants: a comparison between a nebulizer and two small volume spacers, *Pediatr Pulmonol* 23:212, 1997.

19. Everard ML, Clark AR, Milner AD: Drug delivery from holding chambers with attached facemask, *Arch Dis Child* 67:580, 1992.

20. Turpeinen M and others: Metered dose inhaler add-on devices: is the inhaled mass of drug dependent on the size of the infant? *J Aerosol Med* 12:171, 1999.

21. Fok TF and others: Efficiency of aerosol medication delivery from a metered dose inhaler versus jet nebulizer in infants with bronchopulmonary dysplasia, *Pediatr Pulmonol* 21:301, 1996.

22. Tal A and others: Deposition pattern of radiolabeled salbutamol inhaled from a metered-dose inhaler by means of a spacer with mask in young children with airway obstruction, *J Pediatr* 128:479, 1996.

23. Wildhaber JH and others: Inhalation therapy in asthma: nebulizer or pressurized metered-dose inhaler with holding chamber? In vivo comparison of lung deposition in children, *J Pediatr* 135:28, 1999.

24. Lenney W, Milner AD: At what age do bronchodilators work? *Arch Dis Child* 53:532, 1978.

25. Lenney W, Milner AD: Alpha and beta adrenergic stimulants in bronchiolitis and wheezy bronchitis in children under 18 months of age, *Arch Dis Child* 53:707, 1978.

26. Turner DJ, Landau LI, LeSouëf PN: The effect of age on bronchodilator responsiveness, *Pediatr Pulmonol* 15:98, 1993.

27. Holt WJ and others: Pulmonary response to an inhaled bronchodilator in chronically ventilated preterm infants with suspected airway reactivity, *Respir Care* 40:145, 1995.

28. Denjean A and others: Dose-related bronchodilator response to aerosolized salbutamol (albuterol) in ventilator-dependent premature infants, *J Pediatr* 120:974, 1992.

29. Fok TF and others: Delivery of salbutamol to nonventilated preterm infants by metered-dose inhaler, jet nebulizer, and ultrasonic nebulizer, *Eur Respir J* 12:159, 1998.

30. Gappa M and others: Effects of salbutamol delivery from a metered dose inhaler versus jet nebulizer on dynamic lung mechanics in very preterm infants with chronic lung disease, *Pediatr Pulmonol* 23:442, 1997.

31. Rubilar L, Castro-Rodriguez JA, Girardi G: Randomized trial of salbutamol via metered-dose inhaler with spacer versus nebulizer for acute wheezing in children less than 2 years of age, *Pediatr Pulmonol* 29:264, 2000.

32. Hanhan U and others: Effects of in-line nebulization on preset ventilatory variables, *Respir Care* 38:474, 1993.

33. Henry WD, Chatburn RL: Effects of manual versus mechanical ventilation on aerosol efficiency, *Respir Care* 33:914, 1988.

34. AARC Clinical Practice Guideline: Selection of an aerosol delivery device for neonatal and pediatric patients, *Respir Care* 40:1325, 1995.

CRITICAL CARE AND CARDIOVASCULAR DRUG CLASSES

CHAPTER 18

Skeletal Muscle Relaxants (Neuromuscular Blocking Agents)

Charles G. Durbin, Jr.

Neuromuscular blocking agents, also termed muscle relaxants, are drugs that cause skeletal muscle paralysis. They do this by interfering with the nerve-to-muscle chemical coupling by acetylcholine at the neuromuscular junction. The two types of neuromuscular blocking agents are as follows:

Nondepolarizing blockers: Exemplified by tubocurarine, in which there is competition for receptors between the agent and endogenous acetylcholine.

Depolarizing blockers: Exemplified by succinylcholine, the only available agent in this class. The drug occupies acetylcholine receptors, depolarizing the postjunctional membrane and rendering it incapable of repolarization.

Neuromuscular blocking agents are used to facilitate elective and emergency tracheal intubation, to provide surgical relaxation, to treat tetanus, and as an adjunct to ventilator management in certain critically ill patients. The history of this class of drugs and the physiology of the neuromuscular junction are briefly reviewed. Modes of action and side effects of nondepolarizing and depolarizing agents are presented. Use of these agents for neuromuscular blockade in critical care and during mechanical ventilation is discussed.

HISTORY AND DEVELOPMENT

Neuromuscular blocking agents have a long and fascinating history. Curare is the generic name for a variety of closely-related agents, most of which were originally used by South American indigenous people as dart and arrow poisons. The paralyzing effect of curare on skeletal muscle ensured food even if the quarry was not killed outright by the arrow itself. Curare become known to Europeans soon after the first European explorers reached the American continents. Late in the sixteenth century, samples of preparations used by the indigenous people were taken to Europe by explorers.[1] Claude Bernard was first to recognize that peripheral muscle paralysis accounted for the lethal effects of the poison, rather than interference with cardiac function and consciousness.[2] The clinical implications of this important observation were not recognized for over 50 years.

Curare can be extracted from several plants, one of which is *Chondodendron tomentosum*, a source of *d*-tubocurarine. The tertiary amine structure of *d*-tubocurarine was identified by King and reported in 1935.[3] A semisynthetic derivative of *d*-tubocurarine is dimethyl tubocurarine (metocurine), which is approximately three times as potent as *d*-tubocurarine in humans.

Griffith and Johnson[4] reported the first trial use of curare as a muscle relaxant in general anesthesia in 1942. Further research on curare-like drugs led to the synthesis of gallamine, reported in 1949, and to the discovery of methonium compounds (hexamethonium, a ganglionic blocker, and decamethonium [Syncurine], a neuromuscular blocker) in 1948 and 1949. Another neuromuscular blocker with a mode of action different from that of curare, and of great clinical use today, is succinylcholine (Anectine, Quelicin). It is interesting that this drug was used experimentally as early as 1906, but because research workers used *curarized* animals for testing succinylcholine, the muscle relaxant actions of succinylcholine were not identified until almost 40 years later.

Uses of Neuromuscular Blocking Agents

The primary clinical uses of neuromuscular blocking agents are as follows:

- To facilitate endotracheal intubation
- For muscle relaxation during surgery, particularly of the thorax and abdomen
- To enhance CO_2 removal in patients who are difficult to ventilate
- To reduce intracranial pressure in intubated patients with uncontrolled intracranial pressure

These agents are usually given intravenously, and their effects on muscle tone are dose related. In the operating room, they are often administered as part of anesthesia induction before endotracheal intubation. They are used in the intensive care unit for elective intubation and management of mechanical ventilation.

A brief review of the physiology of the myoneural junction is given before discussing specific neuromuscular blocking agents.

Physiology of the Neuromuscular Junction

One of the divisions of the peripheral nervous system, the somatic motor system, or skeletal muscle system, controls striated muscle. This is in distinction to the autonomic branch of the peripheral nervous system, which controls the smooth muscle (nonstriated muscle) found in bronchioles, heart, arterioles, and venules. Striated muscles have their contractile elements aligned with the long axis of the muscle fiber and under the microscope can be seen to have striations. Acetylcholine is the neurotransmitter released by all somatic motor nerves; it is also present in autonomic ganglia. This accounts for some of the side effects seen with neuromuscular blockers. Examples of skeletal muscles include the quadriceps, biceps, and diaphragm, which are responsible for motor functions such as movement, lifting, and breathing. The motor functions of the somatic system are under conscious or voluntary control. This is not true for smooth muscles, which are under automatic control of the autonomic nervous system.

Nervous impulses to stimulate skeletal muscle are carried by large myelinated nerve fibers. The cell bodies of these neurons are in the spinal cord or brainstem, and the axons form the peripheral nerves. The termination of the axon on the skeletal muscle fiber is termed the neuromuscular or myoneural junction (Figure 18-1). A single ending of the motor neuron, termed the sole foot, which is one branch of the entire neuron's end plate, is illustrated making a synapse with a special invaginated area on the muscle fiber membrane. Each motor nerve synapses with many motor fibrils. Acetylcholine is the neurotransmitter released at the neuromuscular junction. This process is analogous to that at autonomic ganglia and parasympathetic neuroeffector sites. When the nerve impulse reaches the end of the motor neuron, acetylcholine that has been synthesized and stored in vesicles is

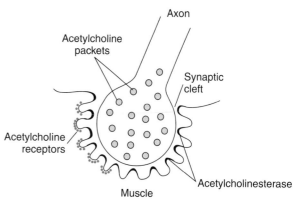

Figure 18-1 Schematic description of the anatomy of the muscle end plate.

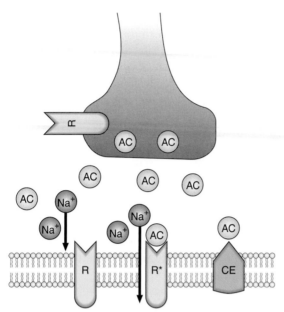

Figure 18-2   Acetylcholine *(AC)* is released into the synaptic cleft, where it is free to bind to postjunctional receptors *(R)*. Binding of two acetylcholine molecules causes a conformational receptor change *(R*)* and opens a pore, reversing the membrane potential and allowing sodium to enter the cell *(Na⁺)*. If enough receptors are activated simultaneously, a muscle action potential is propagated and contraction occurs. Acetylcholine is rapidly broken down by cholinesterase *(CE)*. Prejunctional receptors for AC modify AC release.

released into the synaptic cleft, contacts receptor sites on the muscle fiber membrane, and, within several milliseconds, diffuses out of the synaptic gutter, where it is then inactivated within milliseconds by membrane-bound *acetylcholinesterase* located around the borders of the gutter.

During the short period that acetylcholine is in contact with the muscle fiber membrane, if enough receptors are activated, an end-plate potential is generated. Each acetylcholine receptor has two binding sites to which two acetylcholine molecules must bind to open the pore, illustrated in Figure 18-2. The end-plate potential consists of a depolarization and repolarization phase. In the *depolarization* phase, the muscle membrane becomes permeable to sodium ions and the sodium influx reverses the negative internal and positive external polarity, resulting in a rise in membrane potential. If enough receptors are activated at the same time, a critical threshold is reached and a muscle action potential occurs that propagates in both directions along the muscle fiber

and causes intracellular release of calcium ions that are stored in the sarcoplasmic reticulum. Calcium concentration increases and allows actin and myosin filaments to interact and shorten, and muscle fiber contraction occurs. In the subsequent active *repolarization* phase, the membrane potential returns to its previous level; sodium conductance is blocked once again, potassium is exchanged for sodium, and calcium is sequestered by the sarcoplasmic reticulum. The muscle fiber can now be restimulated by another nerve impulse. Until repolarization is complete, the muscle is refractory to additional depolarization and contraction.

On the basis of the myoneural physiology just described, it is apparent that muscle contraction may be abolished in the following two ways:

1. Competitive inhibition: binding to, blocking, but not depolarizing the acetylcholine receptors; this is the action of *nondepolarizing* agents.
2. Prolonged occupation and persistent activation of the acetylcholine receptors with continued depolarization of the myoneural junction; this is the action of *depolarizing* agents.

Table 18-1 presents an overview of both types of neuromuscular blocking agents, including major chemical families, clinical action, and duration of relaxation from a single bolus. Both depolarizing and nondepolarizing agents resemble the neurotransmitter acetylcholine, each having one or more positively charged quaternary ammonium groups (NH_4^+), which combine with the negatively charged cholinergic nicotinic receptor. The nondepolarizing agents can be grouped into two major families based on structure: the benzylisoquinolines and the steroid derivatives. These differences are important relative to complications and side effects.

NONDEPOLARIZING AGENTS

The earliest group of neuromuscular blocking agents used clinically were those like curare. These agents paralyze skeletal muscle by simple competitive inhibition of acetylcholine at muscle receptor sites. This group is referred to as nondepolarizing because nervous stimulation does not lead to depolarization of the muscle membrane when enough molecules of these blocking agents are present. Chemically, nondepolarizing neuromuscular blockers are either steroidal agents (vecuronium, rocuronium, pipecuronium) or benzylisoquinolin-

Table 18-1

A pharmacological profile of neuromuscular blocking agents

DRUG		DURATION (min)
NONDEPOLARIZING		
Isoquinolone	Tubocurarine	>35
	Metocurine (Metubine)	>35
	Doxacurium (Nuromax)	>35
	Atracurium (Tracrium)	20-35
	Cisatracurium (Nimbex)	20-35
	Mivacurium (Mivacron)	10-20
Steroid	Pancuronium (Pavulon)	>35
	Pipecuronium (Arduan)	>35
	Rocuronium (Zemuron)	20-35
	Rapacuronium (Raplon)*	8-12
	Vecuronium (Norcuron)	20-35
DEPOLARIZING		
	Decamethonium (Syncurine)	20-35
	Succinylcholine (Anectine, Quelicin)	<8

*Rapacuronium bromide (Raplon) was voluntarily withdrawn from the market in 2001 by its manufacturer after several serious adverse bronchospasm events and even some unexplained fatalities.

ium esters (atracurium, mivacurium, doxacurium, rapacuronium).

MODE OF ACTION

Nondepolarizing agents cause muscle paralysis by affecting the postsynaptic cholinergic nicotinic receptors at the neuromuscular synapse. This can be accomplished by blocking the channel externally, occupying the channel pore, or affecting the receptor from the internal side of the muscle membrane, preventing the pore from opening. Different neuromuscular blocking drugs affect the acetylcholine receptor differently, thus accounting for the synergy and prolonged effect often seen when different agents are given together. These agents act competitively, with endogenous acetylcholine, receptor occupancy, and depolarization being a function of the amount of drug and the amount of acetylcholine available at the junction. This is illustrated in Figure 18-3, in which the drug (ND) occupies and then blocks the postsynaptic site at the myoneural junction. Muscle contraction does not occur if enough sites are blocked at any one time. Because nondepolarizing agents act by competitive inhibition, their effect is dose related: larger doses block more receptors. Likewise, this type of blockade can be reversed by making more acetylcholine available to compete for receptor sites.

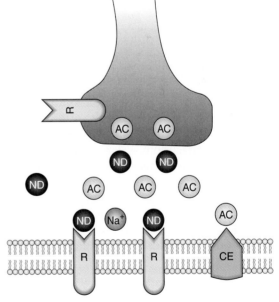

Figure 18-3 Competitive blocking agents, or nondepolarizers (ND), occupy but do not activate acetylcholine receptors (R). Acetylcholine is prevented from receptor occupancy, and muscle contraction fails to occur. Released acetylcholine (AC) is rapidly metabolized by membrane cholinesterase (CE). ND can also bind to prejunctional acetylcholine receptors and modify AC release.

PHARMACOKINETICS OF NONDEPOLARIZING AGENTS

Nondepolarizing neuromuscular blocking agents are ionized as quaternary ammonium drugs, are poorly lipophilic, are poorly absorbed from the gastrointestinal tract, and do not diffuse across the blood-brain barrier. They must be given parenterally, and the intravenous route is preferred for predictable absorption and rapid onset of neuromuscular blockade.

Intravenous injection of curare causes effects within 1 to 2 minutes. These include blurred vision, drooping eyelids, relaxation of the jaw, inability to raise the head, paralysis of the legs and arms, and, finally, loss of respiratory muscles (intercostals, diaphragm). Maximal paralyzing effect is reached between 2 and 10 minutes. Recovery is in reverse order, with recovery of the diaphragm and respiratory muscles occurring first. The sensitivity of individual muscles to paralysis is related to the number of fibers innervated by each motor neuron. Those muscles innervated by nerves with many axons supplying only a few muscle fibrils (e.g., the extraocular muscles) are most sensitive to relaxant effects, whereas those with most diffuse axon arborization are most resistant. The onset of paralysis and the duration of action of the nondepolarizing blockers varies widely among members of this group of drugs. In usual clinical doses, the maximal paralyzing action of *d*-tubocurarine lasts for 35 to 60 minutes and complete recovery may take several hours. Metocurine, pancuronium, pipecuronium, alcuronium, and doxacurium have durations of action similar to that of tubocurarine, and all of these agents are considered to be long-acting neuromuscular blockers. Atracurium, cisatracurium, vecuronium, rocuronium, and mivacurium are redistributed more rapidly and have shorter durations than tubocurarine. These agents are considered intermediate-acting.[4] Rapacuronium, a newer agent, has an onset of action only slightly slower than succinylcholine and about twice the duration of action, 8 to 15 minutes after a bolus dose.[5]

As previously noted, the degree of effect, rate of onset of maximum blockade, and duration of neuromuscular blocking agents is dose-dependent. This is illustrated in Table 18-2 for the drug rocuronium when used in adults. Factors such as advanced age generally increase the time to regression of neuromuscular blockade. Hepatic or renal failure can cause decreased clearance, increased blood levels, and prolonged duration of action for those agents metabolized and eliminated by the liver and kidney.

Table 18-2

Dose-dependent effects of a nondepolarizing blocking agent, rocuronium, used in adults

DOSE (mg/kg)	TIME TO MAXIMUM BLOCK (min)	CLINICAL DURATION (min)
0.45	3	22
0.6	1.8	31
0.9	1.4	58
1.2	1	67

Data from *Drug Facts and Comparisons,* St. Louis, 2001, Facts and Comparisons.

METABOLISM

Neuromuscular transmission is restored by redistribution of the blocking agent from the effector site at the neuromuscular end plate to the rest of the body. When normal conduction returns, as many as 75% of acetylcholine receptors may still be occupied by blocker. This explains why additional boluses of blocker appear more potent and have a markedly prolonged duration of action. After prolonged infusion or repeated boluses, metabolism may be the mechanism for removal of the blocking agent from the neuromuscular junction.

d-Tubocurarine and metocurine are minimally metabolized, and approximately 60% of an injected dose is excreted by the kidneys in urine. The remainder may be excreted in bile. Doxacurium is also eliminated primarily by the kidneys. Steroidal neuromuscular blocking agents (e.g., pancuronium) are metabolized to their 3-hydroxy, 17-hydroxy, and 3,17-dihydroxy products primarily in the liver and are eliminated by the kidneys. Vecuronium is metabolized to *N*-acetyl-vecuronium, a product that is almost entirely dependent on renal excretion and that has neuromuscular blocking effects of about one third of the parent compound. It can accumulate in renal failure and cause prolonged paralysis when given in sufficient dose.

Atracurium and cisatracurium differ from other neuromuscular blocking agents requiring liver metabolism or kidney elimination. These agents are inactivated by a spontaneous self-destruction mechanism that is pH and temperature dependent, but not enzyme dependent, termed *Hoffmann degradation.* Probably more important than Hoffmann degradation, these agents are also rapidly metabolized by ester hydrolysis. Because they do not require liver and kidney elimination, these agents are attractive for use with patients in hepatic or renal failure. One product

Table 18-3

Major metabolic pathways of neuromuscular blockers and effect on duration of action caused by organ failure

AGENT	BRAND NAME	PROLONGATION OF EFFECT WITH RENAL FAILURE	PROLONGATION OF EFFECT WITH HEPATIC FAILURE	ALTERNATIVE METABOLISM
d-Tubocurarine		+	+	
Doxacurium	Nuromax	+++	0	
Pancuronium	Pavulon	+++	+	
Gallamine	Flaxedil	++++	0	
Metocurine	Metubine	++++	0	
Pipecuronium	Arduan	+++	0	
Atracurium	Tracrium	0	0	Hoffman degradation, ester hydrolysis
Cisatracurium	Nimbex	0	0	Hoffman degradation, ester hydrolysis
Vecuronium	Norcuron	++*	+	
Rocuronium	Zemuron	++	0	
Mivacurium	Mivacron	0	0	Plasma cholinesterase†
Rapacuronium	Raplon	++	0	
Succinylcholine	Anectine, Quelicin	0	0	Plasma cholinesterase†

*Metabolic product is one third as potent as parent compound and is entirely removed by renal excretion.
†Atypical pseudocholinesterase may prolong relaxant effect dramatically.

of Hoffmann degradation of atracurium or cisatracurium is laudanosine, a tertiary amine metabolite. Laudanosine is primarily eliminated by the kidneys and only slowly metabolized by the liver, has a long half-life, and can cross the blood-brain barrier. Elevated concentrations have been found in patients with renal failure. Laudanosine is neurostimulatory, and high central nervous system concentrations can cause seizures in animals. Seizures have not been demonstrated with the clinical use of atracurium in humans.[6] Central nervous system excitation and seizures should be considered as a possibility, especially in patients with impaired renal function. Cisatracurium is more potent and results in less laudanosine production than atracurium. The risk of further brain injury from seizures in patients with poor intracranial compliance (e.g., severe head injury) may make these drugs poor choices in these patients. Seizure activity might be masked by pharmacological paralysis, complicating patient assessment.

Mivacurium has a short duration of effect (10 to 20 minutes in usual doses). It is unique among the nondepolarizers in that it is metabolized by plasma cholinesterase, as is succinylcholine, a depolarizing agent. Metabolism of mivacurium is not dependent on the liver or kidneys.[7] However, patients with renal failure or hepatic dysfunction may have decreased plasma cholinesterase, and this may prolong the duration of mivacurium. The effects of organ failure on block duration are illustrated in Table 18-3.

ADVERSE EFFECTS AND HAZARDS

CARDIOVASCULAR EFFECTS

Because the nondepolarizing blocking agents competitively block acetylcholine receptors at autonomic ganglia and the adrenal medulla, they can produce effects on heart rate and blood pressure. They may cause a vagolytic effect, which produces tachycardia, and an increase in mean arterial pressure, by promoting unopposed sympathetic activity.

Pancuronium may cause both these cardiovascular effects; gallamine primarily causes tachycardia. The newer agents, vecuronium, atracurium, cisatracurium, pipecuronium, and doxacurium have minimal effects on heart rate or blood pressure; they do block autonomic ganglia, but this effect is less evident at clinical doses. The cardiovascular stability exhibited by rocuronium and rapacuronium is related to a further separation of the neuromuscular blocking and ganglionic blocking potential of this group of drugs. Mivacurium has been associated with cardiovascular changes, usually a drop in arterial blood pressure.

Table 18-4

Comparison of side effects for a variety of neuromuscular blocking agents

AGENT	HISTAMINE RELEASE	GANGLIONIC BLOCKADE	VAGAL BLOCKADE	VAGAL STIMULATION
d-Tubocurarine	++++	+++	0	0
Doxacurium	+	0	0	0
Pancuronium	+	+	+++	0
Gallamine	++	+	++++	0
Metocurine	++	++	0	0
Pipecuronium	+	0	0	0
Atracurium	++	0	0	0
Cisatracurium	+	0	0	0
Vecuronium	0	0	0	0
Rocuronium	+	0	+	0
Mivacurium	++	0	0	0
Rapacuronium	++	0	0	0
Succinylcholine	+	0	0	+++

HISTAMINE RELEASE

All of the nondepolarizing agents provoke histamine release from mast cells. However, individual agents differ in the degree of this effect. Clinically, histamine release can cause bronchospasm and increased airway resistance to ventilation in the operating room or the intensive care unit. Vasodilation can cause transient hypotension, often seen with these agents. This may give a visible appearance of cutaneous flushing. The degree of histamine release among several agents is indicated in Table 18-4.

d-Tubocurarine is the most potent releaser of histamine and causes the most profound problems with intravenous bolus administration. The histamine-releasing properties of the other agents are less, and, with careful administration, serious consequences from this side effect can usually be avoided.

INADEQUATE VENTILATION

Muscle paralysis of the diaphragm and the intercostals results in total apnea. Adequate airway control and ventilatory support are required until muscle recovery is adequate for spontaneous ventilation. With intensive care unit use in ventilator patients, close patient and machine monitoring are essential to prevent hypoventilation and hypoxemia.

REVERSAL OF NONDEPOLARIZING BLOCKADE

Muscle paralysis caused by nondepolarizing blocking agents can be reversed by use of cholinesterase inhibitors such as neostigmine (Figure 18-3). Neostigmine inhibits the cholinesterase that would normally inactivate the released acetylcholine. This makes more acetylcholine available at the myoneural junction to compete with and displace the blocker and overcome muscle blockade. Clinically useful cholinesterase inhibitors include physostigmine, neostigmine, pyridostigmine, and edrophonium. Physostigmine is very lipophilic and crosses the blood-brain barrier to reverse central anticholinergic symptoms, but it is less efficient in reversing peripheral neuromuscular blockade. Edrophonium is rapid acting but also the shortest duration. Pyridostigmine has a slower onset and is the longest acting; it is often used to treat *myasthenia gravis* and can be given orally. Neostigmine is intermediate in onset and duration of action. Table 18-5 profiles these agents with recommended doses to reverse neuromuscular blockage produced by nondepolarizers.[8]

Because the reversing agents also increase the effects of acetylcholine at parasympathetic ganglia, they all produce cholinergic autonomic side effects. Reversal agents are given with atropine or glycopyrrolate to reduce these unwanted muscarinic effects. Vagolytic agents will prevent the bradycardia, increased salivation, and hyperperistalsis that would result from increased cholinergic activity. The vagolytic agent does not block the reversing effect of the cholinesterase-inhibiting drug at the neuromuscular junction; it only blocks the muscarinic effects at parasympathetic sites.

DEPOLARIZING AGENTS

Depolarizing agents have a mode of action different from that of the curare group, they are shorter acting,

Table 18-5

Agents used for reversal and antimuscarinic effects with nondepolarizing blocking agents

AGENT	DOSE	TIME FOR EFFECT
REVERSAL AGENT		
Edrophonium	0.3-1.0 mg/kg	Rapid onset, short acting
Pyridostigmine	0.1-0.25 mg/kg	Slowest onset, longest acting
Neostigmine	0.01-0.035 mg/kg	Intermediate onset, duration
ANTIMUSCARINIC AGENT		
Atropine	0.008-0.018 mg/kg	
Glycopyrrolate	0.002-0.016 mg/kg	

Data from Buck ML, Reed MD: Use of nondepolarizing neuromuscular blocking agents in mechanically ventilated patients, *Clin Pharm* 10:32, 1991.

and there are no agents that will reliably reverse their blockade. Succinylcholine is the only clinically used agent is this group. After an intravenous dose of 1 to 1.5 mg/kg, total muscle paralysis will occur in 60 to 90 seconds and last from 10 to 15 minutes. Because total paralysis of all muscle fibers results, intubating conditions are better than with any of the nondepolarizing agents. Decamethonium, a depolarizing agent available in Europe, has a slower onset and longer duration of action (30 to 45 minutes). Unlike succinylcholine, decamethonium is not metabolized by pseudocholinesterase but requires hepatic and renal function for terminal elimination.

MODE OF ACTION

The basic action of depolarizing neuromuscular blockers is to first depolarize the postsynaptic muscle membrane in the same manner as acetylcholine and then maintain it in a refractory state. This is illustrated in Figure 18-4, in which a molecule of succinylcholine (S) has occupied the acetylcholine receptor, opened a pore, and allowed the local membrane to become permeable to sodium. If enough receptors are activated, depolarization occurs and is maintained until the succinylcholine leaves the receptor. Further stimulation and contraction of the muscle fiber is not possible until the drug is removed by redistribution and metabolized. Unlike as with curare, there is initial muscle fibril contraction, referred to as *fasciculation*, a classic sign of depolarizing agents such as succinylcholine (Anectine, Quelicin). This is followed by flaccid paralysis. With succinylcholine, there is initially stimulation of autonomic ganglia, causing tachycardia and a rise in blood pressure in adults or, more often, brady-

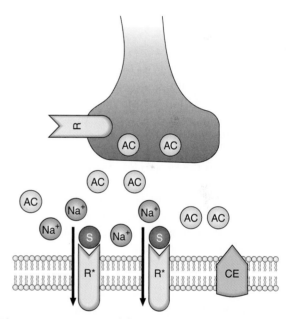

Figure 18-4   Succinylcholine produces a depolarizing block. Molecules of succinylcholine *(S)* occupy and activate the acetylcholine receptor *(R*)*, permitting sodium entry and an initial action potential. Continued occupancy activation prevents repolarization and the next action potential from released acetylcholine *(AC)*. R, Postjunctional receptor. *CE*, Cholinesterase. Activation of prejunctional AC receptors (R) can modify AC release.

cardia and hypotension in babies from vagal stimulation (see Table 18-4). Succinylcholine is metabolized to succinylmonocholine, a weak nondepolarizing blocker that may account for some of the reason why repeated doses produce prolonged blockade. Repeated bolus doses of succinylcholine may produce bradycardia and hypotension in adults. Succinylcholine also provokes histamine release, such as that seen with cu-rare, leading to bronchospasm and hypotension in susceptible individuals.

Normally, plasma cholinesterase will metabolize succinylcholine (a choline ester) within a few min-utes. Generally, depolarizing blockers are shorter act-ing than curare and its analogues.

REVERSAL

Unfortunately, there are no effective antidotes to de-polarizing agents. Use of cholinesterase inhibitors (parasympathomimetics) will result in even more prolonged depolarization because the neuromuscu-lar synapse is already being held in a depolarized state, and further stimulation will simply continue to cause depolarization with no resumption of muscle activity.

USE OF HEXAFLUORENIUM

Hexafluorenium bromide (Mylaxen) is a plasma cholinesterase inhibitor. As just described for such agents, this drug will not reverse blockade from suc-cinylcholine but will in fact prolong the blockade.

Hexafluorenium has been used as an adjunct with succinylcholine to prolong neuromuscular blockade during anesthesia and reduce the muscle fascicula-tions leading to the postoperative muscle pain seen with succinylcholine. Its activity is limited to plasma esterases, and it does not act on junctional cholin-esterase. Hexafluorenium has no effect on conscious-ness or pain awareness. The duration of action is ap-proximately 20 to 30 minutes.

ADVERSE EFFECTS AND HAZARDS

Succinylcholine can cause several side effects, some of which can be life threatening. The significance of these side effects may be of more concern in the in-tensive care unit than for routine operating room use. Use and complications of both depolarizing and non-depolarizing agents in the intensive care unit have been summarized in a review use by Isenstein and associates.[5]

Muscle pain and soreness often follow administra-tion of succinylcholine. The exact mechanism is not known, but it may be caused by the vigorous muscle fasciculations that herald depolarizing block. The use of a small dose of a nondepolarizing blocker (e.g., 3 to 6 mg of *d*-tubocurarine or 0.5 to 1 mg vecuronium) before giving succinylcholine reduces fasciculations and the incidence of pain. This is often referred to as pretreatment with a nondepolarizer, or *defasciculation*.

Higher doses of succinylcholine are needed for com-plete paralysis because pretreatment reduces the effec-tiveness of succinylcholine. Muscle fasciculations can also cause a rise in serum potassium and creatinine phosphokinase, an effect that is also reduced but not totally eliminated by pretreatment.

Succinylcholine causes an efflux of potassium from muscle cells, causing a transient serum potassium el-evation of 0.5 to 1.0 mEq/L in normal individuals.[8] Under some circumstances, an exaggerated rise oc-curs and the resulting hyperkalemia can cause ar-rhythmias or cardiac arrest. Severe hyperkalemia after succinylcholine administration is a risk in burn pa-tients. In addition, patients with spinal cord injury, stroke, or active upper motor neuron lesions are at risk for cardiac arrest from hyperkalemia after suc-cinylcholine use.

Succinylcholine can increase intraocular pressure, probably mediated by contractions of the extraocular muscles. This is partially prevented by defasciculation.

Succinylcholine can dangerously increase intracra-nial pressure in patients with cerebral edema and head trauma, probably as a result of autonomic gan-glionic effects.

Succinylcholine can trigger malignant hyperther-mia, a hypermetabolic state occurring during anes-thesia, resulting in acidosis, cardiovascular collapse, and death. Malignant hyperthermia is caused by a genetic defect of muscle metabolism. Under some types of anesthesia, intracellular calcium remains el-evated, sustained contraction may occur (muscle rigidity results), and runaway metabolism results in metabolic and respiratory acidosis and hyperther-mia.[9] The treatment of malignant hyperthermia is dantrolene sodium (Dantrium), a muscle relaxant (not a neuromuscular blocker) that acts by reducing release of intracellular calcium stored in the sar-coplasmic reticulum.

Succinylcholine may cause *rhabdomyolysis,* or mus-cle necrosis, in patients with Duchenne's and other myopathies or muscular dystrophies. This can lead to renal failure or cardiac arrest from hyperkalemia. Because Duchenne's may not be clinically apparent in early childhood, several cardiac arrests in male children related to succinylcholine administration has led to a warning from the Food and Drug Ad-ministration (FDA) to avoid succinylcholine in male children under the age of 12. The risk of provoking this problem in children must be weighed against the risk of not being able to intubate if succinyl-choline is not used.

SENSITIVITY TO SUCCINYLCHOLINE

At least two types of cholinesterase are found in the body: true cholinesterase, or acetylcholinesterase, which is found at parasympathetic nerve synapses and postsynaptic neuromuscular sites, and pseudo-cholinesterase, or plasma cholinesterase, which is found in plasma.

The pseudocholinesterase in plasma plays no known biological function, but it does rapidly catalyze the hydrolysis of succinylcholine (and mivacurium). It metabolizes most of the administered dose of succinylcholine (95% to 98% of the dose) to an inactive form before arrival at the neuromuscular junction. A small number of individuals have an atypical variant of plasma cholinesterase or no active enzyme at all. The human genetics of these variations have been widely studied.

Individuals with atypical variants of pseudo-cholinesterase do not rapidly hydrolyze succinylcholine within seconds as usual, but may require hours to dispose of the administered drug dose. The effect is that a huge amount of succinylcholine reaches the neuromuscular junction, and a phase II block (see below) occurs. Because reversal is not possible, patients may require hours of supported ventilation because of the prolonged paralysis of the respiratory muscles. Laboratory tests are available to determine atypical cholinesterases. One of these tests is based on a differential inhibition between the atypical and normal cholinesterase by the local anesthetic, dibucaine.[10] At a certain optimum concentration, dibucaine produces a much greater inhibition of the usual plasma cholinesterase than of the atypical enzyme. The percentage inhibition of the cholinesterase enzyme by dibucaine is termed the *dibucaine number*. The normal, or usual, cholinesterase has a number over 70, and the atypical cholinesterase gives a value below 30. Heterozygote individuals give values between 45 and 69, distinguishing them from the normal and atypical homozygotes. Although heterozygotic individuals may have a slight prolongation of relaxation produced by succinylcholine (10 to 20 minutes), this is not clinically significant. Davis and colleagues[11] give a clear discussion of the genetic variations of human cholinesterase, its detection, and clinical implications.

DESENSITIZATION (PHASE II) BLOCK

After repeated use or large doses of succinylcholine, the characteristic of the depolarizing block changes. Instead of showing depolarization characteristics, the block resembles the block produced by nondepolarizers (fade on tetanus and posttetanic facilitation on nerve stimulation; see discussion of monitoring, below). Unlike a nondepolarizing block, this type of block is not reversed by cholinesterase inhibition. This type block, termed *phase II*, or *desensitization block*, has a prolonged and unpredictable duration. Although the mechanism is not fully explained, one theory is that a nondepolarizing block develops after the depolarizing block, as a result of the nondepolarizing blocking effects of succinylmonocholine, the first breakdown product of succinylcholine. Part of the prolonged paralysis produced by succinylcholine in patients with atypical pseudocholinesterase is due to phase II block. The occurrence of a desensitization block must be considered as a possibility in the face of prolonged apnea with succinylcholine. Succinylcholine is rarely repeated or used as a continuous infusion for fear of this outcome.

NEUROMUSCULAR BLOCKING AGENTS AND MECHANICAL VENTILATION

A primary indication for use of neuromuscular blocking agents in ventilator management is to improve asynchronous, spontaneous breathing efforts that interfere with, or "fight," the ventilator-delivered breaths. This dyssynchrony may cause increased intrathoracic pressure, decreased alveolar ventilation, and increased patient work of breathing. The desired goal with these drugs is to improve ventilation and oxygenation and reduce ventilation pressures. Specific disease states in which neuromuscular blockade may be beneficial include the following:

- Status asthmaticus, severe bronchospasm
- Certain modes of ventilatory support (e.g., pressure-controlled inverse ratio ventilation)
- Status epilepticus
- Neuromuscular toxins (e.g., strychnine or methaqualone poisoning)
- Tetanus

The most common clinical uses of muscle relaxation are for facilitating ventilation in *status asthmaticus* and support of severe acute respiratory distress syndrome (ARDS) when pressure-controlled ventilation, with or without inverse ratio ventilation, is used to limit peak airway pressure.

PRECAUTIONS AND RISKS

Neuromuscular blockade is not acceptable without proper *sedation* and *control of pain* to prevent the nightmare of paralysis with full consciousness and sensory perception.

Before subjecting an agitated patient to neuromuscular blockade, *ventilator malfunction* must first be ruled out as the cause of patient agitation, or muscle paralysis could cause death in the face of inadequate machine volume or oxygen delivery.

Eye blinking lubricates and cleans the corneas. Paralysis of eyelid muscles that accompanies use of neuromuscular blockers can result in drying and *abrasion of the cornea* and conjunctiva unless the eyelids are lubricated and taped closed. Corneal abrasions are extremely painful.

With complete paralysis, spontaneous *cough is blocked* as is cough during endotracheal suctioning. The patient can experience pain and discomfort during suctioning if not sedated, and retention of secretions is likely.[5] The incidence of nosocomial pneumonia is probably increased in patients receiving neuromuscular blockade for a prolonged period.

Clinical signs of restlessness, distress, and anxiety are lost with neuromuscular blockade, mandating *close monitoring* of support equipment, intravenous infusions, and vital signs, including continuous cardiac monitoring. Tachycardia or hypertension can indicate anxiety caused by inadequate sedation or lack of pain control, as well as clinical deterioration or machine malfunction.

Alarm systems and continuous observation to detect *accidental disconnection* from the ventilator are mandatory, and alarms to detect hypoventilation and hypoxemia are the standard of care when neuromuscular blockade is employed.

The musculoskeletal system is at risk with continuous neuromuscular blockade. Ankle splinting and side support of the legs or knees can prevent *palsies* or tendon contracture. Frequent turning can help prevent *pressure sores* and decubitus ulcer formation. Physical therapy with range-of-motion exercises may lessen the potential for *muscle atrophy* during prolonged blockade and muscle disuse, which can prolong ventilator weaning.[12] Op de Coul and associates[13] reported prolonged and diffuse muscle atrophy with 1 to 3 weeks of use of pancuronium during mechanical ventilation on 12 adults. Of the surviving patients, seven had full recovery of muscle function and two had only partial recovery within 6 months. Myopathy associated with prolonged use of neuromuscular blocking agents is being more frequently observed. This syndrome, which may take months to resolve, seems to be seen more commonly with the steroid-based neuromuscular blockers (i.e., pancuronium and vecuronium), especially when they are combined with other steroid agents.

CHOICE OF AGENTS

The choice of a neuromuscular blocking agent is situation dependent: the depolarizing agent succinylcholine is well-suited for intubation because of its rapid onset, ideal intubating conditions, and short action. Rapacuronium may be a reasonable substitute for succinylcholine with a better side-effect profile. However, apnea lasts about twice as long, 9 to 15 minutes, and histamine release is greater. The duration of apnea may be shortened significantly with early (within 2 minutes) administration of neostigmine, an option that may be beneficial in patients with difficult airway or failed intubation.[14] The nondepolarizing blocking agents are better suited for long-term use. The kinetics of the nondepolarizing agents lead to a longer duration of action, more gradual onset and off-set of block, and few hemodynamic changes. They can be administered by continuous infusion and, if necessary, the blockade can be antagonized with cholinesterase inhibitors. The characteristics of the perfect neuromuscular blocking agent (not yet developed) are as followed:

- Nondepolarizing block
- Rapid onset of action
- Predictable and controllable duration of action
- Hemodynamic stability at all levels of block and rate of administration
- Predictable kinetics, independent of age or gender
- No active metabolites or toxicity
- Elimination independent of hepatic or renal function
- Inexpensive

The currently available nondepolarizing agents can be compared against these criteria as a guide in drug choice for paralysis in ventilated patients. The choice of agent involves clinical judgment and preference, but the following features of the different nondepolarizing agents can guide a differential choice of agent in a given patient.

There are four important considerations when deciding on a specific nondepolarizing agent for paralysis of a ventilator patient: potential for histamine release, cardiovascular side effects (ganglion and vagal blocking potential), metabolic routes, and cost effectiveness. Tables 18-3 and Table 18-4 compare these factors in several of the neuromuscular blocking agents.

Most nondepolarizing agents release histamine from mast cells. Pancuronium provokes release of the least amount of histamine. Metocurine, vecuronium, rocuronium, and doxacurium are similar to pancuronium and have minimal histamine release relative to the other agents. Atracurium, rapacuronium, cisatracurium, and mivacurium can provoke greater histamine release than pancuronium, but less than tubocurarine, which has significant histamine release. Atracurium can cause cutaneous flushing but usually produces no significant clinical symptoms. Histamine release by these drugs can be minimized by administering a bolus dose slowly over 60 seconds, administering several smaller boluses or giving the agent by slow continuous infusion.

Vecuronium, atracurium, cisatracurium, rapacuronium, and doxacurium have minimal effects on heart rate or blood pressure. Pancuronium and gallamine often produce a transient increase in mean arterial pressure (MAP) and heart rate. Pipecuronium can occasionally cause bradycardia and hypotension or hypotension alone. Rocuronium seems to cause little systemic cardiovascular effect, but an increase in pulmonary vascular resistance has been seen with this drug. Caution is recommended in using this agent with pulmonary hypertension or valvular heart disease. Bolus administration of mivacurium can cause a transient decrease in MAP, usually caused by histamine release.

The method of drug metabolism and excretion is a third factor in selecting an optimal paralyzing agent for a patient on a ventilator. Agents that depend on hepatic and renal paths for elimination are poorly suited for patients with disease or failure of these organs. The potential effects of organ failure on each agent is suggested by the metabolic pathways described in Table 18-3. Atracurium and cisatracurium do not rely on hepatic metabolism or renal excretion, although the metabolite laudanosine may be of concern. Cisatracurium results in less laudanosine than atracurium.[15] Mivacurium is metabolized by plasma cholinesterase, as is succinylcholine.

In general, the nondepolarizing agents with negligible histamine release and few cardiovascular effects include vecuronium and doxacurium. Mivacurium, atracurium, cisatracurium, and rocuronium offer alternative choices for ventilator management, with the first three of these agents having the advantage of alternative metabolic pathways.

Cost is another important consideration. The newer, shorter-acting agents are very expensive, especially if used for a prolonged period in the intensive care unit. Guidelines for relaxant use in the intensive care unit have been published that suggest that cost-effective relaxation can be provided using continuous infusions of pancuronium, if tachycardia is not a concern, or vecuronium in patients with ischemic cardiovascular issues.[16] The clinician is admonished to use peripheral nerve stimulation to titrate administration, reducing the amount of drug used and avoiding prolonged paralysis.

INTERACTIONS WITH NEUROMUSCULAR BLOCKING AGENTS

Several conditions and agents may alter the effect of an administered neuromuscular blocker. Because different blocking drugs may act at different locations on the acetylcholine receptor–pore complex (e.g., external, in the pore, intercellular), combination of agents may be synergistic. Advantage of this potential has been taken to produce mixtures of relaxant drugs to give adequate relaxation with fewer (cardiovascular) side effects. The problem with this approach has been the unpredictability of the duration of relaxation, which tends to be extremely prolonged, especially after repeated mixture administrations. Some classes of drugs and other conditions have neuromuscular blocking effects; these may be additive, antagonistic, or synergistic with neuromuscular blockers. Some of the common interactions are listed in Box 18-1. Important drugs that increase blockade are the aminoglycoside antibiotics. These are often administered to critically ill patients and will potentiate neuromuscular blockade. Occasionally, they will produce weakness or paralysis by themselves. Immunosuppressive drugs may potentiate (e.g., cyclosporine) or antagonize (e.g., azathioprine) relaxation. Theophylline antagonizes neuromuscular blockade and stimulates the respiratory center. Electrolyte imbalances can affect relaxant drug effects.

USE OF SEDATIVES AND ANALGESICS

Although the neuromuscular blocking agents can cause muscle paralysis, they do not affect consciousness or the perception of pain. A classic experiment that established this was performed by the anesthesiologist Smith,[17] who in 1947 allowed himself to be paralyzed with tubocurarine. He reported full awareness during the paralysis, including sensations of choking while he was unable to swallow and shortness of breath even though he was being adequately ventilated.

Box 18-1	Drugs and Conditions That Interact With Nondepolarizing Neuromuscular Blocking Agents

Drugs

Potentiating factors

Potent anesthetic vapors
Antibiotics
   Aminoglycosides
   Clindamycin
   Vancomycin
   Tetracycline
Local anesthetics
Antiarrhythmics
   Procainamide
   Quinidine
   Bretylium
Calcium channel blockers
β-Adrenergic blockers
Cyclosporin
Dantrolene
Cyclophosphamide
Lithium
Mineralocorticoids
Echothiophate
Tacrine
Metoclopramide

Antagonizing factors

Dilantin
Carbamazepine
Theophylline
Anticholinesterase agents
Azathioprine
Ranitidine

Conditions

Potentiating factors

Acidosis
Hyponatremia
Hypocalcemia
Hypokalemia
Hypermagnesemia
Hypothermia
Renal failure
Hepatic failure
Organophosphate poisoning

Antagonizing factors

Alkalosis
Hypercalcemia
Demyelinating injuries
Peripheral neuropathy

Diseases

Potentiating factors

Myasthenia gravis
Muscular dystrophy
Amyotrophic lateral sclerosis
Poliomyelitis
Multiple sclerosis
Eaton-Lambert syndrome

Antagonizing factors

Diabetes mellitus

Feldman S, Karalliedde L: Drug interactions with neuromuscular blockers, *Drug Safety* 15:261, 1996.

In 1942, in Montreal, when Griffith and Johnson[18] used small amounts of curare to enhance abdominal muscle relaxation during laparotomy, anesthesia still relied on spontaneous ventilation. Patients were made weak but not paralyzed while receiving a full inhalation anesthetic. Later, in Liverpool, Gray and others[19] introduced a new technique using curare with much less inhalational anesthetic and much more curare, paralyzing all the skeletal muscles, including the diaphragm. Tracheal intubation and mechanical ventilation were essential with this approach. This dramatic change in practice led to a reduction in mortality from anesthesia. Previously, mortality had been mostly due to the severe cardiac depressant effects of general anesthetics, primarily chloroform. The enormous advantages of this new technique gave it

considerable popularity, which has lasted to the present day. But it also led to the possibility of carrying out surgery on paralyzed, unanesthetised patients, unable to communicate with the outside world.

Before curare was used the depth of anesthesia was reliably judged by close observation of the patient, mostly of movement of skeletal muscle, including the breathing pattern and the reflex responses to surgery. With total paralysis of skeletal muscle there is no reliable method of assessing depth of anesthesia and therefore guaranteeing unconsciousness during surgery. Efforts have recently been made to develop methods of measuring depth of anesthesia in paralyzed patients.[20] So far, these methods are only partially successful,[21] and the goal may well prove to be elusive.[22] The presence of adequate anesthesia is still defined in terms of loss of motor responses to surgical stimuli. Recent reviews of cases of awareness during surgery show that neuromuscular blockers were used in almost all the reported cases; after awareness of sounds, the sensation of paralysis with inability to communicate was the most common recollection (85%) suffered by patients complaining of awareness.[23]

It is absolutely essential to provide sedation and analgesia for ventilator patients undergoing paralysis. Motor responses to pain, such as restlessness, agitation, and movement, are abolished. These clues to patient experience are not available to the caregiver when the patient is undergoing muscle paralysis. The experience of being paralyzed while conscious and aware is extremely anxiety producing and mandates sedation. In their survey, Hansen-Flaschen and others[24] reported that the most commonly used drugs for analgesia and sedation in patients on mechanical ventilation were morphine sulfate, lorazepam, and diazepam. The most common method of administration was intermittent intravenous injection. The drugs most commonly given for sedation by continuous intravenous infusion were midazolam hydrochloride (Versed), fentanyl citrate (Sublimaze), and morphine. It should be noted that diazepam is converted to active metabolites that are very slowly metabolized in the critically ill, producing prolonged and unpredictable effects. Lorazepam would be a better sedative because it has no active metabolites. Sedatives and analgesics should be administered by intravenous injection rather than by oral, intramuscular, or subcutaneous routes. Because the signs of discomfort may be absent under paralysis, a continuous sedative infusion may provide more reliable clinical effects, but because of tolerance the rate may need to be gradually increased to guarantee satisfactory sedation. Other suggestions for sedation and analgesia are presented in Chapter 22, Drugs Affecting the Central Nervous System.

MONITORING OF NEUROMUSCULAR BLOCKADE

The vast experience with neuromuscular blocking agents is in the operating room. The time course of relaxant effect and rate of recovery may not be the same when these drugs are used for extended periods with patients in the intensive care unit to facilitate mechanical ventilation. During brief periods of paralysis, the degree of neuromuscular blockade or the adequacy of return of neuromuscular function can be assessed by simple measures of voluntary muscular abilities. Some of these include subjective assessments, such as hand-grip strength or the ability to hold the head off the bed for 5 seconds; others are more objective and include measurement of vital capacity, negative inspiratory force, and spontaneous respiratory rate. To provide adequate relaxation while avoiding overdose and prolonged paralysis, more precise measures of paralysis are needed.[25] Although clinical signs may be helpful, a more physiological and objective evaluation can be achieved by observing the muscle response to peripheral nerve stimulation.[26]

A common, convenient method of peripheral nerve stimulation uses the ulnar nerve, which innervates the *adductor pollicis* muscle of the thumb. Two small conducting pads are placed on the forearm over the nerve tract, several inches apart. A single discharge from a nerve stimulator to the ulnar nerve will cause a visible thumb twitch. As the amount of paralysis increases, the strength or degree of movement of the twitch decreases. For all relaxants, each individual twitch (separated by at least 10 seconds) will be approximately the same size and the decrement from the twitch with no relaxant will correlate with the degree of receptor occupancy. Neuromuscular transmission occurs with a large margin of safety; that is at least 85% to 90% of receptors must be blocked to see a decrease in twitch strength. Table 18-6 indicates the approximate percentage of occupancy that is predicted by clinical measures of neuromuscular function. Tetanus, a high-frequency stimulation that stresses the neuromuscular junction more than a single twitch, can detect the situation when 50% to 85% of receptors are occupied by a nondepolarizing blocker and twitch has returned to normal. Fade will be seen when a tetanic stimulation is applied. This means the thumb will move rapidly and then relax. A single twitch applied several seconds after a tetanic stimulation demonstrating fade will produce a twitch much greater than the baseline twitch. This is termed *posttetanic facilitation* (PTF). Observation of these phenomena allows a more complete understanding of acetylcholine and neuromuscular blocking kinetics during neuromuscular transmission.

During each nerve depolarization a fixed number of packets (quanta) of acetylcholine are released into the synaptic cleft. Depolarization of only 8% to 10% of acetylcholine receptors are needed to produce muscle depolarization and contraction. If the nerve is repeatedly depolarized (tetanus), the number of acetylcholine packets declines to a readily releasable

Table 18-6

Receptor occupancy associated with various measurements of neuromuscular blockade

RECEPTORS OCCUPIED (%)	TWITCH HEIGHT (%)	TRAIN OF FOUR	CLINICAL OBSERVATIONS
100	0	0	Total paralysis, no voluntary movement of any muscle; no PTF
98-99	0	0	Diaphragm may move; PTF present
95-98	1-5	1-2 twitches	Diaphragm can move minimally; PTF and fade present
90-95	10-25	2-3 twitches	Breathing inadequate
75-90		4 twitches 1st >4th	Tidal volume restored, voluntary movement apparent, can sustain head lift for 5 sec (75%-80% occupancy), NIP >55 cm H$_2$O, vital capacity 60%-70% of normal
50-75	100	4 equal twitches	Normal strength and movement, cough strength decreased; double burst suppression abnormal
<30	100	4 equal twitches	No apparent deficits, double burst suppression normal

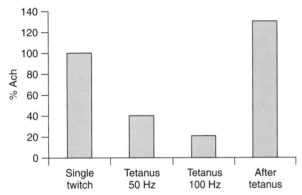

Figure 18-5   The percentage of acetylcholine *(Ach)* released into the neuromuscular junction after each single depolarization during different patterns of stimulation (compared with a single baseline twitch). Actual amount and percentage will vary with specific muscle tested.

baseline pool (Figure 18-5). Without neuromuscular blockers, this still results in normal transmission because so many receptors are available on the postjunctional membrane. However, when 80% to 90% of the receptors are blocked, this smaller amount of acetylcholine will not produce depolarization in some fibrils, accounting for tetanic fade. At the same time, during tetanic stimulation the synthetic processes are markedly increased to resupply the readily releasable pool, resulting in a larger number of packets being produced. When tetanus ceases, this additionally produced pool is then briefly available to be released during the next few depolariza-

tions. This accounts for the posttetanic facilitation observed. Although these methods of stimulation are useful for grossly determining the level of receptor occupancy, they are not as precise as the percentage initial twitch depression. Twitch depression can only be determined by manometric strength determination and comparison with baseline strength. The baseline measurement is often not available, and the techniques for actual strength measurement (rather than movement) are complicated, so this research technique is rarely employed in the clinical environment.

A more practical clinical technique for monitoring blockade is the "train-of-four" (TOF) evaluation. This involves delivery of four supramaximal discharges, one every 0.5 second, equivalent to a short burst of tetanus at a rate of 120 Hz. Comparison of the strength of the fourth and first twitch predicts the degree of receptor occupancy. There are differences in twitch and TOF stimulus responses between depolarizing and nondepolarizing agents, as illustrated in Figure 18-6. The applied electrical stimulus is not painful, and no determination of a baseline twitch without blocker is necessary for TOF monitoring. Clinically, the degree of block can be determined by simply counting the number of twitches seen. Four equal twitches indicate adequate return of neuromuscular function, meaning at most 75% of the receptors are occupied with blocker. Reduced TOF indicates residual paralysis. If only three twitches are seen, approximately 90% of receptors are blocked; if only two, 95% are blocked; and if only one, 98% are blocked.

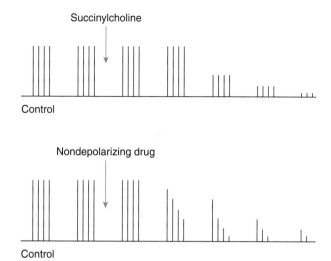

Figure 18-6   The twitch height during train-of-four stimulation shown during paralysis with depolarizing and nondepolarizing blockade. (Modified from Hunter JM: Drug Therapy: new neuromuscular blocking drugs, *N Engl J Med* 332:1691, 1995.)

To avoid overdosing of patients, titration of the neuromuscular blocking drug (bolus or infusion) to maintain at least one twitch is recommended. It is possible that lesser degrees of blockade may be required to achieve the clinical goal of ventilator synchrony. The need for continued paralysis in the patient in the intensive care unit should be assessed at least daily, and, if appropriate, neuromuscular blockade should be discontinued as soon as possible. TOF peripheral nerve stimulation is usually monitored at 15- to 30-minute intervals in the intensive care unit.

SUMMARY KEY TERMS AND CONCEPTS

- *Neuromuscular blocking agents* are used for skeletal muscle paralysis in several clinical situations, including *intubation, surgery,* and *facilitation of ventilation* in certain critically ill patients.
- The most common *examples of ventilated patients* requiring muscle relaxation are severe asthmatics and those requiring "uncomfortable" modes of ventilation such as pressure-control inverse ratio ventilation.
- The two types of neuromuscular blocking agents are *nondepolarizing* and *depolarizing.* Nondepolarizing agents, such as tubocurarine, *competitively block* the cholinergic nicotinic receptor on the postsynaptic muscle fiber, preventing acetylcholine from depolarizing the muscle fiber. Depolarizing agents, such as succinylcholine, act by first depolarizing the muscle fiber and then *prolonging*

the depolarized state to prevent repolarization and further stimulation.
- Nondepolarizing agents have a longer duration of action than the depolarizing agent succinylcholine.
- Nondepolarizing agents can be *reversed* with an indirect-acting cholinergic agent *(cholinesterase inhibitor)* such as neostigmine. There is no reversal agent for succinylcholine.
- *Atypical plasma cholinesterase* metabolizes succinylcholine poorly and prolongs its usually short duration of action.
- Prolonged infusion of succinylcholine can result in a *phase II* (competitive) block.
- Nondepolarizing agents are preferred for *paralysis of ventilator patients* because of the predictability, longer duration of action, and manageable side effects of these agents. Specific agents should be selected based on potential for *histamine release* and *cardiovascular effects,* patient-specific *metabolic pathways,* and *cost.*
- Paralysis of a conscious patient is torture, and *adequate sedation* and *analgesia* are mandatory.
- Titration of drug dose and monitoring of reversal is performed using a *peripheral nerve stimulator* and train-of-four stimulation.

SELF-ASSESSMENT QUESTIONS

1. List four general uses of skeletal muscle relaxants.
2. What are the two types of neuromuscular blocking agents?
3. Identify each of the following agents by type: tubocurarine, vecuronium, succinylcholine, and pancuronium.

4. Which type of neuromuscular blocker can be reversed?
5. What type of drug would you use to reverse vecuronium?
6. Identify another drug that you would want to give before you reverse the vecuronium.
7. Briefly explain why you might need to paralyze a patient receiving mechanical ventilation.
8. Neuromuscular blocking agents do not block consciousness; what two types or classes of drugs would be indicated in a paralyzed patient on a mechanical ventilator?
9. Identify at least two neuromuscular blocking agents that would be preferred for paralysis in a patient receiving mechanical ventilation (assume normal renal and hepatic function).
10. You are called to the recovery room to set up a ventilator for a young woman who has just undergone a hysterectomy and has failed to breathe after a single dose of succinylcholine. What might the problem be?
11. What would you do first to assess a ventilated patient who is restless and "fighting" the ventilator before using a paralyzing agent?

Answers to Self-Assessment Questions are found in Appendix A.

CLINICAL SCENARIO

A 39-year-old white female comes to the emergency department with a complaint of shortness of breath and congestion over the last 3 days. Her problem list includes a history of multiple allergies with asthma and sinusitis and a history of depression. She was admitted 16 months ago with severe asthma. She has had a cough productive of yellow sputum, a postnasal drip, and a "scratchy" throat for the last several days. She is now on amoxicillin and clavulanic acid (Augmentin), albuterol by MDI, fluoxetine, and buspirone.

On physical examination, her vital signs are P, 130 beats/min; BP, 113/80 mm Hg; T, 36.9° C; and RR, 28 breaths/min, with a moderate amount of respiratory distress. On auscultation, wheezing was heard on end-inspiration and during expiration. She exhibits paroxysms of coughing during examination.

An electrocardiogram shows sinus tachycardia, and portable spirometry reveals a forced expiratory volume in 1 second (FEV_1) at 20% of predicted. Pulse oximetry showed 80% saturation on room air. Her chest radiograph is within normal limits. Her WBC count is 18.7 × $10^3/mm^3$, hemoglobin is 15.2 g/dl, and hematocrit is 45.2%. Her electrolytes are within normal limits, except for glucose, which is 154 mg/dl.

What additional drug is immediately indicated, given her laboratory results?
What additional laboratory information would be most helpful in assessing this patient and determining further treatment?
What other drugs would you consider at this point for treating her acute asthma?

After approximately 5 hours of intense treatment, the patient is short of breath and anxious, exhibiting labored breathing with inspiratory and expiratory wheezing. Her HR ranges from 126 to 154 beats/min; RR is 32 to 40 breaths/min; and BP is 118/80 mm Hg, and she is occasionally confused. Arterial blood gas values on a 40% aerosol mask are as follows: pH, 7.32; $PaCO_2$, 45 mm Hg; PaO_2, 90 mm Hg; and SaO_2, 93%.

The decision is made to intubate and support her with mechanical ventilation.

What neuromuscular blocking agent would you consider for a rapid-sequence intubation?

After intubation and placement on the ventilator, the patient's peak airway pressures are excessive (>80 cm H_2O); there is inadequate time for expiration. You attempt to shorten inspiratory times by increasing the inspiratory flow rate, but the maximum pressure limit is continuously reached, terminating inspiratory gas flow. The patient is agitated. You decide to provide neuromuscular blockade.

What agent would you use?
How will you monitor the effectiveness of this therapy?
If the patient were in renal or hepatic failure, what neuromuscular blocking agent would you recommend?

Answers to Clinical Scenario Questions are found in Appendix A.

REFERENCES

1. McIntyre AR: Curare: its history, nature, and clinical use, Chicago, 1947, University of Chicago Press.
2. Bennett AE: The history of the introduction of curare into medicine, *Anesth Analg* 47:484, 1968.
3. King H: Curare alkaloids. I, Tubocurarine, *J Chem Soc,* 1935, p 1381.
4. Griffith HR, Johnson GE: The use of curare in general anesthesia, *Anesthesiology* 3:418, 1942.
5. Isenstein DA, Venner DS, Duggan I: Neuromuscular blockade in the intensive care unit, *Chest* 102:1258, 1992.
6. Zhou TJ and others: Onset/offset characteristics and intubating conditions of rapacuronium: a comparison with rocuronium, *Br J Anaesth* 85:246, 2000.

7. Grigore AM and others. Laudanosine and atracurium concentrations in a patient receiving long-term atracurium infusion, *Crit Care Med* 26:180, 1998.

8. *Drug Facts and comparisons*, St Louis, 2001, Facts and Comparisons.

9. Vakharia N, Hall R: Malignant hyperthermia: a review of current concepts, *Respir Care* 35:977, 1990.

10. Kalow W, Genest K: A method for the detection of atypical forms of human serum cholinesterase: determination of dibucaine numbers, *Can J Biochem Physiol* 35:339, 1957.

11. Davis L, Britten JJ, Morgan M: Cholinesterase: its significance in anaesthetic practice, *Anaesthesia* 52:244, 1997.

12. Kupfer Y and others: Disuse atrophy in a ventilated patient with status asthmaticus receiving neuromuscular blockade, *Crit Care Med* 15:795, 1987.

13. Op de Coul AAW and others: Neuromuscular complications in patients given Pavulon (pancuronium bromide) during artificial ventilation, *Clin Neural Neurosurg* 87:17, 1985.

14. Larijani GE, Zafeiridis A, Goldberg ME: Clinical pharmacology of rapacuronium bromide, a new short-acting neuromuscular blocking agent, *Pharmacotherapy* 19:1118, 1999.

15. Eastwood NB and others: Pharmacokinetics of 1R-cis 1', R-cis atracurium besylate (51W89), and plasma laudanosine concentrations in health and chronic renal failure, *Brit J Anaesth* 75:431, 1995.

16. Shapiro BA and others: Practice parameters for sustained neuromuscular blockade in the adult critically ill patient: an executive summary, Society of Critical Care Medicine, *Crit Care Med* 23:1601, 1995.

17. Smith SM and others: The lack of cerebral effects of *d*-tubocurarine, *Anesthesiology* 8:1, 1947.

18. Griffith HR, Johnson GE: The use of curare in general anesthesia, *Anesthesiology* 3:418, 1942.

19. Gray TC, Halton J: A milestone in anaesthesia? *Proc R Soc Med* 39:400, 1946.

20. Drummond JC: Monitoring depth of anesthesia, with emphasis on the application of the bispectral index and the middle latency auditory evoked response to the prevention of recall, *Anesthesiology* 93:876, 2000.

21. Lubke GH and others: Dependence of explicit and implicit memory on hypnotic state in trauma patients, *Anesthesiology* 90:670, 1999.

22. Jones JG: Perception and memory during general anaesthesia, *Br J Anaesth* 73:31, 1994.

23. Moerman N, Bonke B, Oosting J: Awareness and recall during general anesthesia, *Anesthesiology* 79:454, 1993.

24. Hansen-Flaschen IH and others: Use of sedating drugs and neuromuscular blocking agents in patients requiring mechanical ventilation for respiratory failure: a national survey, *J Am Med Assoc* 266:2870, 1991.

25. Segredo V and others: Persistent paralysis in critically ill patients after long-term administration of vecuronium, *N Engl J Med* 327:524, 1992.

26. Rudis MI and others: A prospective, randomized, controlled evaluation of peripheral nerve stimulation versus standard clinical dosing of neuromuscular blocking agents in critically ill patients, *Crit Care Med* 25:575, 1997.

Cardiac Drugs

Judith Jacobi • Robert D. Warhurst

A wide variety of drugs are used to treat or prevent cardiac problems for patients both inside and outside of the hospital. Many of these drugs have an impact on the respiratory system, either directly or indirectly. In addition, because the cardiovascular and respiratory systems are closely linked, treatment of one organ system may have important implications for the other.

Chapter 19 will review the classes of cardiac drugs used most commonly and highlight some specific agents that have important direct effects on the pulmonary system. The cardiac drugs reviewed are those to increase myocardial contractility, antiarrhythmics, and agents used in cardiac arrest. The pharmacology of other vasoactive agents is discussed in other chapters. Many of these agents can indirectly affect cardiac function, and the reader is encouraged to consult those chapters. Detailed drug and prescribing information will not be provided, and the reader is encouraged to consult the literature provided by the manufacturer for complete prescribing information, as well as the current medical literature. Common terms and abbreviations are listed in Box 19-1.

THE CARDIOVASCULAR SYSTEM

The cardiovascular system functions as independent but related components. This is illustrated in Figure 19-1. Changes in one component of the circuit can influence the function of another (e.g., a change in vascular tone may affect cardiac performance).

FACTORS AFFECTING BLOOD PRESSURE AND CARDIAC OUTPUT

Blood pressure is dependent on vascular tone and cardiac function. Vascular tone is regulated by sympathetic tone and circulating hormones such as epinephrine, angiotensin, and vasopressin. These hormones are secreted in response to a change in tissue perfusion. Several cardiovascular components interact to maintain stable organ and tissue perfusion. These are vascular tone, cardiac contractility, and vascular volume.

Vascular tone is often measured as the systemic vascular resistance (SVR) and is also referred to as afterload. Although SVR may change to maintain perfusion, the blood pressure is usually regulated to stay relatively normal. Mean arterial blood pressure

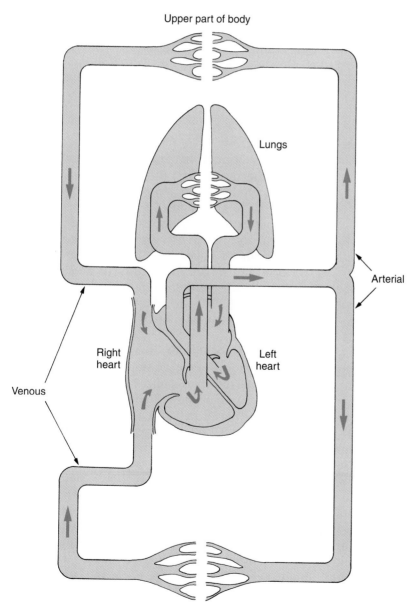

Upper part of body

Lungs

Arterial

Right heart

Left heart

Venous

Lower part of body

Figure 19-1   A simplified view of the integrated cardiopulmonary circuit.

(MAP) is a typical measure of blood pressure as it relates to tissue perfusion. Blood pressure is regulated through changes in cardiac function and vascular tone. Cardiac contractility (as measured by cardiac output [CO]) is also an important determinant of tissue perfusion, as illustrated by the following equation:

$$MAP = CO \times SVR$$

As one component in this equation changes acutely, a proportional change may occur in other components. For example, if cardiac output falls, the SVR must increase to compensate and maintain blood pressure and tissue perfusion.

Cardiac output is dependent on two factors, heart rate and stroke volume (SV), as illustrated in the following equation:

$$CO = HR \times SV$$

Changes in the volume of blood pumped with each beat of the heart are often balanced by changes in heart rate, to maintain a consistent cardiac output. Vascular volume, the third component affecting tissue perfusion, is difficult to measure directly, but influences SV. An indirect measure of vascular volume is the pulmonary capillary wedge pressure (PCWP), also known as *preload.*

Putting these equations together, as follows:

$$MAP = HR \times SV \times SVR$$

illustrates the complex relationship of these components in maintaining cardiovascular stability. Therapies such as fluids, vasopressors, vasodilators, and inotropes can be directed toward each of these components to improve tissue perfusion. This is illustrated in Figure 19-2.

A pulmonary artery catheter is one device that can be used to measure PCWP and cardiac output. The SVR can be calculated from these variables. This monitoring tool can be used to evaluate the cause of severe hypotension (cardiac failure versus vasodilation as in sepsis) and to follow the response to fluids, inotropic agents, and vasoactive therapies. Use of the pulmonary artery catheter is not risk free, because infection, trauma during insertion (pneumothorax), and incorrect interpretation of the data are important complications.

Chronically, the changes in one component of this equation may produce detrimental effects in the other components. Chronic hypertension stimulates remodeling of the ventricular muscle, pro-

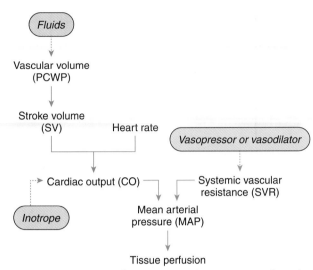

Figure 19-2   Several components interact to produce tissue perfusion. Therapy with fluids, vasoactive agents, or inotropes and where they interact are listed. *PCWP,* Pulmonary capillary wedge pressure.

ducing myocardial hypertrophy. Eventually, a hypertrophic muscle loses efficiency and may become fibrotic, producing a decrease in contractility. Direct injury to the muscle after myocardial ischemia or infarction will acutely decrease cardiac output. Remodeling of muscle tissue after an infarction may decrease its efficiency and produce progressive reductions in cardiac contractility. As an end point, patients will experience symptoms of congestive heart failure (CHF), including hypotension, fatigue, peripheral edema, pulmonary edema, and shortness of breath.

Most patients with heart failure have symptoms related to failure of the left side of the heart and impaired systemic perfusion. Similar hypertrophic changes can occur in the right heart when patients have pulmonary hypertension or chronic obstructive lung disease (COPD). Primary pulmonary hypertension is due to chronic hypoxia, and secondary pulmonary hypertension is often the result of connective tissue diseases, such as systemic lupus erythematosus. In either condition, the right heart eventually fails to adequately perfuse the pulmonary vessels and patients become symptomatic with peripheral edema, hepatic congestion, and jugular distention. Cor pulmonale is the term used to describe right heart failure that develops in patients with chronic lung disease.

Table 19-1

Receptor effects of catecholamines

DRUG	α_2	β_1	β_2	DOPAMINERGIC
Dopamine*	++++	++++	++	++
Dobutamine	+	++++	++	0
Epinephrine	++++	++++	0	0
Isoproterenol	0	++++	++++	0
Norepinephrine	++++	++++	0	0

*Dopamine demonstrates dose-dependent hemodynamic effects.
Number of + indicates relative degree of stimulation.

CARDIOTONIC (INOTROPIC) AGENTS

Stimulation of the myocardium with inotropic agents is an adjunct in the treatment of heart failure. These agents are generally used only for short-term therapy of an acute exacerbation of heart failure. Long-term inotropic therapy may accelerate the myocardial injury as a result of chronic cardiac stimulation. Chronic use of potent inotropic agents has increased mortality, although this detriment must be balanced with the potential for an improvement in the patient's quality of life.

CARDIAC GLYCOSIDES

The cardiac glycoside group of drugs in the digitalis family (digoxin, digitoxin, and ouabain) has been used to treat heart failure for decades. Despite this longevity, data demonstrating a significant impact on heart failure patients are limited. These agents exert a weak inotropic effect and are typically used in combination with vasodilators and other agents shown to improve outcome in heart failure patients, such as aspirin or β blockers.

The cardiac glycosides inhibit the sodium-potassium (Na^+-K^+) ATPase pump, producing an increase in intracellular sodium. This in turn produces an increase in intracellular calcium, thus resulting in increased myocardial contractility. In addition, the digitalis products exert an inhibitory effect on the vagus nerve, potentially slowing heart rate and atrioventricular (AV) conduction. Heart rate reduction is most notable when these agents are used for patients with atrial arrhythmias, although stimulation of the heart through exercise or stress can overcome this effect, limiting the utility.

Accumulation of digoxin occurs in renal insufficiency, because this is the primary route of elimination. Adverse effects of these agents include a variety of nonspecific symptoms such as anorexia, nausea, and diarrhea. More significant are the myriad of cardiac arrhythmias that can result from digitalis toxicity. These include premature ventricular contractions (PVCs), ventricular tachycardia, and a variety of atrial arrhythmias, such as paroxysmal atrial tachycardia (PAT) with block. Bradycardia may be present with digoxin toxicity, but is not a reliable finding in all cases. Serum concentration monitoring is often inadequate to determine the presence of toxicity, because there is significant overlap between symptoms at various serum concentrations. Hypokalemia may exacerbate the risk of digoxin toxicity and potassium replacement should be used to maintain a serum potassium above 4 mEq/L in patients on digoxin.[1] Ironically, severe digitalis overdose can produce hyperkalemia through its effect on the Na^+/K^+ pump. Significant digoxin-induced arrhythmias may be treated with a monoclonal antibody, known as digoxin immune fab that binds digoxin, facilitating its elimination.

β-ADRENERGIC CARDIAC STIMULANTS (CATECHOLAMINES)

The relative effects of the cardiac stimulants on receptors are reviewed in Table 19-1. These agents have very rapid cardiovascular effects but a short duration of effect; usually they are administered as continuous infusions. Stimulation of the α_1 or postsynaptic α_2 receptors by circulating catecholamines produces vasoconstriction. The vasoconstricting agents are discussed in Chapter 20. A positive inotropic effect (improved contractility) and increase in heart rate are achieved with agents that stimulate the β_1 receptor. Stimulation of the β_1 receptor triggers an increase in cyclic adenosine monophosphate (cAMP) that leads to an increase in intracellular calcium and improved myocardial contractility. Bronchodilation and vasodilation are the principal effects achieved with agents that stimulate the β_2 receptor. Stimulation of the dopaminergic receptors increases renal and mesenteric blood flow.

DOBUTAMINE

Dobutamine is a synthetic catecholamine that is the drug of choice for most patients with acute heart failure. Dobutamine directly stimulates the β_1-adrenergic (β_1) receptors at low doses (2.5 to 7.5 $\mu g/kg/min$), causing increase in myocardial contractility. At higher doses (>7.5 $\mu g/kg/min$), there is increasing stimulation of β_2 receptors in addition to the β_1 receptors. The net effect of dobutamine is usually a positive inotropic effect with vasodilating action. The effect of dobutamine on blood pressure depends on the relative improvement in contractility and degree of vasodilation. Hypotension may be the result of greater β_2-stimulated vasodilation. Tachycardia may occur at any dose but is most likely with high-dose therapy. Despite the increase in myocardial contractility, dobutamine is usually well tolerated by patients with ischemic heart disease. Increased coronary perfusion and oxygen delivery is able to compensate for the increased workload. However, if tachycardia develops, cardiac ischemia becomes a greater risk.

One disadvantage of dobutamine is the attenuation of hemodynamic effect after 72 hours of therapy. This tachyphylaxis may be due to downregulation (decreasing availability) of β_1 receptors or decreased production of cAMP.

DOPAMINE

Dopamine is a catecholamine that exerts it effects by directly stimulating adrenergic receptors in a dose-related fashion (i.e., low-, moderate-, and high-dose), in addition to having an indirect effect through release of norepinephrine from adrenergic nerve terminals. At low dosages of 0.5 to 5 $\mu g/kg/min$, dopamine stimulates the dopaminergic$_1$-receptor (DA$_1$), which produces a selective dilation of the renal, mesenteric, cerebral, and coronary vascular beds. At moderate dosages of 5 to 10 $\mu g/kg/min$, dopamine primarily stimulates the β_1 receptors, increasing myocardial contractility and heart rate. There is weaker stimulation of the β_2 receptors (with some dopaminergic$_1$-mediated stimulation), which may slightly reduce systemic vascular resistance. At dopamine dosages above 10 $\mu g/kg/min$, dopamine predominantly stimulates α receptors, producing vasoconstriction.

High-dose dopamine may be detrimental to patients with heart failure by increasing afterload and myocardial workload. Dopamine is more likely to increase heart rate and the risk of tachyarrhythmias than is dobutamine. Dopamine should be administered through a central line whenever possible. Extravasation of dopamine into the tissues will result in a local area of vasoconstriction and necrosis of the tissues.

ISOPROTERENOL

Isoproterenol is a synthetic catecholamine with pure β_1 and β_2 activity. The β_1 receptor stimulation leads to increased myocardial contractility and heart rate. The β_2 activity produces peripheral vasodilation. Isoproterenol is not routinely used in heart failure because of its potent stimulation of heart rate and myocardial oxygen consumption. Isoproterenol is used to treat symptomatic bradycardia.

EPINEPHRINE

Epinephrine is an endogenous catecholamine synthesized from tyrosine in the adrenal medulla. Epinephrine has potent α and β receptor activities. The use of epinephrine in heart failure is limited by its risk of tachycardia and increased myocardial oxygen consumption. Epinephrine also has metabolic effects that may increase serum lactate levels.

PHOSPHODIESTERASE INHIBITORS

Inamrinone (formerly known as amrinone) and milrinone are classed as bipyridines that exert their positive inotropic actions by selectively inhibiting cAMP phosphodiesterase (subclass III), the enzyme that hydrolyzes cAMP. The resultant increase in cAMP concentrations increases intracellular calcium concentrations, producing an increase in myocardial contractility. These agents may augment the effects of the catecholamines, because they both increase cAMP concentrations. In the vascular smooth muscle, the increase in cAMP produces direct vasodilation of arterial smooth muscle as the end point of enhanced muscle activity. The corresponding adverse effect may be hypotension in some patients. These agents are an alternative therapy when dobutamine has caused undesirable tachycardia or tachyarrhythmias.

Inamrinone and milrinone possess longer half-lives for elimination than the catecholamine agents. The time required to achieve steady-state concentrations is up to 24 hours and may be longer in hepatic or renal dysfunction. A loading dose may be used to achieve effective serum concentrations more rapidly.

However, the risk of hypotension is higher with a loading dose. The continuous infusion is also less easily titrated, because changes in rate will not be fully apparent until steady state is achieved. The slow onset and risk of hypotension often make these agents an alternative therapy for treatment of acute heart failure.

Inamrinone is eliminated through hepatic metabolism and milrinone primarily through renal elimination. Dysfunction of these organs will cause accumulation of drug and an increased risk of adverse effects (especially hypotension) if the dosing is not adjusted. Other side effects include an increased risk of tachyarrhythmias, and inamrinone may cause thrombocytopenia and aggravation of underlying arrhythmias.

PULMONARY HYPERTENSION

Pulmonary hypertension is characterized by a progressive elevation of pulmonary artery pressure and vascular resistance. The result is ultimately right heart failure and death. Primary pulmonary hypertension is usually caused by pulmonary arteriopathy or venoocclusive disease. Secondary pulmonary hypertension is the result of lung disease, thromboembolic disease, and connective tissue diseases, such as systemic lupus erythematosus or scleroderma. A variety of treatments may be used to lower pulmonary artery pressure, including high-dose calcium channel blockers (discussed in Chapter 20), anticoagulants, and lung or heart-lung transplantation. High-dose vasodilators may cause systemic hypotension and clinical deterioration. Epoprostenol (also known as prostacyclin) is a potent, short-acting vasodilator and inhibitor of platelet aggregation. A continuous infusion of epoprostenol produces symptomatic and hemodynamic improvement, in addition to improved survival in patients with severe primary pulmonary hypertension. Systemic effects are minimized by rapid elimination of the epoprostenol (half-life 3 to 5 minutes). Adverse effects include jaw pain, diarrhea, flushing, headaches, nausea, and vomiting. The infusion is initiated slowly to minimize side effects, but the dose requirements typically escalate over time. The most serious complication occurs with interruption of the infusion and acute right heart failure. Epoprostenol must be infused without interruption, necessitating a central line and home infusion pump. Alprostadil (prostaglandin E_1) has also been used for the treatment of pulmonary hypertension or right heart failure after cardiac surgery or transplantation. These prostaglandins have also been shown to provide short-term pulmonary vasodilation after aerosol inhalation therapy, but the role of this administration technique remains to be proven.

CARDIAC CONDUCTION

Arrhythmias are disorders of rate, rhythm, impulse generation (automaticity), or conduction of electrical impulses within the heart. Some are asymptomatic and benign, whereas others produce life-threatening changes in hemodynamic stability. Arrhythmias can affect cardiac output by reducing pumping efficiency.

The electrocardiogram (ECG) measures the cardiac impulses and allows interpretation of the arrhythmia. A normal cardiac impulse is generated in the sinoatrial (SA) node, conducted through the atrium, and transmitted through the AV node (with a slight delay) and then through the bundle of His to the apex of the ventricles (Figure 19-3). More detailed mapping of the myocardial electrical activity can also be done in an electrophysiology laboratory by applying electrodes directly to the myocardium. Electrophysiological studies are recommended for difficult to control or frequent, life-threatening arrhythmias.

The electrical activity of individual cardiac cells is dependent on the type of cells and corresponds with the surface electrical activity recorded with an ECG (Figure 19-4, *bottom curve*). Spontaneous pacemakers such as the SA node, the AV node, and the His-Purkinje electrical fibers stimulate contraction of the nearby myocardial cells. The SA node has the fastest rate of spontaneous automaticity, but it is influenced by the autonomic nervous system, through both cholinergic and sympathetic innervation. Electrical activity in cells with spontaneous automaticity is the result of changes in membrane polarization, through Ca^{++} influx (Figure 19-4, *top curve*). Most other cells are stimulated by an impulse conducted through adjoining electrical or myocardial tissue.

From the SA node, electrical activity moves in a wave-front through specialized conducting tissue in the atrium. The impulse passes through the AV node and a large bundle of conducting tissue (bundle of His). The conducting tissues bridging the atria and ventricle are referred to as the *junctional area*. The junctional area is influenced by autonomic tone and possesses a high degree of inherent

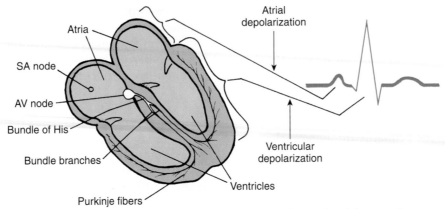

Figure 19-3   Basic cardiac structure and corresponding electrical activity seen in a normal electrocardiographic tracing.

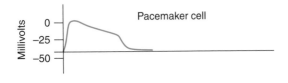

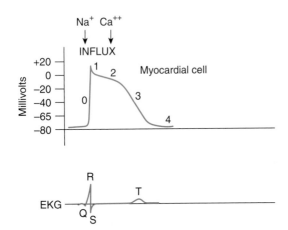

Figure 19-4   The action potentials of pacemaker and myocardial cells, with ion flux and five phases indicated. *AV*, Atrioventricular; *SA*, sinoatrial.

automaticity (but at a slower rate than the SA node). From the bundle of His the cardiac conduction system further bifurcates into several branches: one right bundle branch and two left bundle branches. Beyond the bundles, these nerves branch into an extensive conduction network known as the Purkinje fibers, which reach to the apex of the myocardium.

An understanding of the electrolyte shifts that occur during each impulse allows prediction of the efficacy and potential adverse cardiac effects of an antiarrhythmic. Before cellular excitation of a myocardial cell, an electrical gradient exists between the inside and outside of the cell membrane (cell is polarized) (Figure 19-4, *middle curve*). The electrical gradient just before excitation is referred to as the *resting membrane potential* (RMP). The sodium-potassium pump, specialized ion channels, and ion gates maintain the ionic gradient during the RMP. Each of these ion pathways may be altered by different antiarrhythmic agents. A stimulus that exceeds the threshold for depolarization will result in changes in membrane potential over time, producing a characteristic action potential curve (Figure 19-5). This action potential curve results from the transmembrane shifts of specific ions and is divided into several phases.

Phase 0: During phase 0, a stimulus that exceeds a threshold (approximately 70 mV) triggers a rapid ion shift (depolarization). Rapid influx of Na^+ through specialized "fast response" channels is responsible for the change in polarization.

Phase 1: Near the end of phase 0, an overshoot more than equilibrates the action potential, and chloride influx initiates initial repolarization and phase 1.

Phase 2: During phase 2, calcium begins to move into the intracellular space, causing a slower repolarization. Calcium (Ca^{++}) influx continues throughout phase 2 (plateau phase) and is balanced by K^+ efflux. The calcium entrance provides the critical ionic link to the mechanical properties of the heart. Phase 2 is

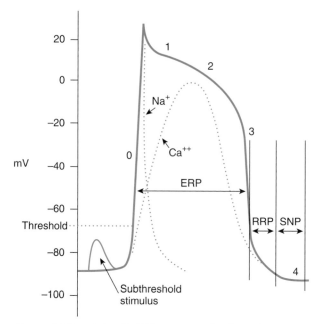

Figure 19-5   A detailed illustration of sodium *(Na⁺)* and calcium *(Ca⁺⁺)* ion exchanges in the five phases of the action potential of a cardiac muscle cell. *ERP,* Effective refractory period; *RRP,* relative refractory period; *SNP,* supranormal period. (From Rau JL Jr: ACLS drugs used during resuscitation, *Resp Care* 40:404, 1995).

the longest portion of the cycle. During phase 2 the cell is effectively refractory (the effective refractory period [ERP]) to further stimulation.

Phase 3: Phase 3 represents the period of repolarization of the membrane through inactivation of the Ca^{++} channels and increased activity of an outward K^+ current. The cell is relatively refractory in this period (the relative refractory period [RRP]) to further stimulation in this phase. During the RRP, the cell can be stimulated by a larger than normal impulse.

Phase 4: In phase 4 the sodium-potassium pump exports sodium from the cell and imports potassium back into the cell, restoring the baseline resting potential of the cell. During a portion of phase 4, a supranormal period (SNP) allows a lower than normal stimulus to trigger another action potential. Late depolarizations that occur in this phase may trigger arrhythmias. During this phase, pacemaker cells have a slow leak of electrolytes that changes the membrane electrical balance until a critical threshold is reached for depolarization and the cycle repeats with phase 0.

Arrhythmias are the result of abnormal impulse generation (automatic tachycardias) or impulse conduc-

tion (reentrant tachycardias). Several factors could contribute to the development of arrhythmias. Myocardial ischemia causes arrhythmias through changes in cellular oxygenation, pH, and the resultant electrolyte abnormalities. Changes in myocardial stretch through volume loading can also precipitate arrhythmias. A surplus of or increased sensitivity to catecholamines, either endogenous or exogenous (vasopressors, decongestants, etc.) can trigger tachyarrhythmias. Also, other chemicals, drugs, toxins, and changes in systemic electrolyte concentrations can increase the risk of arrhythmias. A deficiency of K^+ or magnesium (Mg^{++}) or an excess of Ca^{++} are important arrhythmia triggers. The phases of the electrical activity within an individual cell are important predictors of where and how antiarrhythmic drugs will act.

Arrhythmias may be classified by their rate of firing; bradycardia (<40 beats/min) versus tachycardia (>100 beats/min) and point of origin; supraventricular versus ventricular. Some portions of the conduction tissue serve as latent pacemakers. Normally the latent pacemakers are suppressed by an impulse from the SA node. However, when the SA node is suppressed, these latent pacemakers will discharge, maintaining at least a slow heart rate. Occasionally the latent pacemakers accelerate and the faster rate can override the SA node. Damage to myocardial cells by ischemia or hypoxia or the irritating effect of drugs (digoxin, theophylline, catecholamines) can cause the ectopic pacemakers to fire more rapidly (automatic tachycardia).

Reentry circuits are another common cause of tachycardias. A reentry circuit is created when an impulse is trapped in abnormal myocardial tissue and repeatedly stimulates the surrounding tissue. In the AV node, this results in a rapid SVT, with repeated stimulation of the atrium and then the ventricles. The same model is proposed in other tissues as an explanation for drug-induced tachycardia. Reentry circuits are often triggered by a premature beat that occurs at a critical point in repolarization.

The surface ECG measures the net electrical activity of the myocardium. Basic components of the ECG are the P wave, QRS complex, and T wave (Figure 19-6). Slowing conduction through the AV node will result in prolongation of the PR interval. Prolongation of the refractory period will produce widening of the QRS complex and prolongation of the QT interval. Excessive prolongation of the QT interval may increase the risk of ventricular tachycardia (proarrhythmic effect). Agents that alter conduction between the

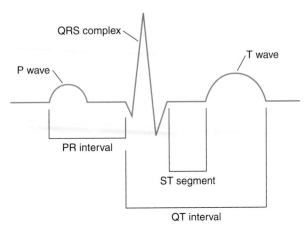

Figure 19-6   The components of the electrocardiogram are identified.

SA node and through the AV node will prolong the PR interval. Antiarrhythmics that slow the rate of phase 0 will produce a prolongation of the QRS complex. The ECG effect of a slowing in phase 3 (repolarization) will cause a prolongation of the QT interval. The ECG effect of an agent can be predicted from its pharmacology. The magnitude of the ECG change may be related to higher concentrations of the antiarrhythmic, but others may be idiosyncratic changes.

ANTIARRHYTHMIC AGENTS

Pharmacological therapy of arrhythmias is the most common approach, although some of these agents may exacerbate arrhythmias and worsen patient outcome. Nonpharmacological approaches such as the use of pacemakers, implantable defibrillators, radiofrequency catheter ablation, and surgical interventions are now common treatments. In addition, correction of underlying causes, such as electrolyte deficiencies (potassium or magnesium), excess (calcium), or reduction of myocardial irritants (e.g., theophylline, dopamine, epinephrine), should be initiated as quickly as possible.

Antiarrhythmics traditionally are divided into classes depending on the predominant electrophysiological action. The Singh–Vaughan Williams classification scheme is commonly used, but several agents possess activity from more than one class. The electrophysiological actions are illustrated in Figure 19-7 and listed in Table 19-2. The ECG effects correlate with the electrophysiological effects and are listed in Table 19-3. Side effects of individual agents are listed in Box 19-2.[1]

DRUG CLASSES

CLASS I ANTIARRHYTHMIC AGENTS

Class I antiarrhythmic agents act by depressing the fast inward sodium currents in myocardial cells to suppress their automaticity and increase resting potential. This class is further subdivided into three levels.

Class IA. Class IA agents have been available for a long time, and the limitations are well described. Proarrhythmic effects are related to QT prolongation, and all may worsen cardiac failure. These agents are metabolized by the liver and can all be monitored with serum concentrations. They have activity against atrial and ventricular arrhythmias.

Disopyramide (Norpace): This agent has limited use because of anticholinergic side effects of dry mouth, constipation, and urinary retention; it also worsens heart failure.

Procainamide (Procan, Pronestyl): The potential for hypotension requires a slow intravenous loading dose. Its active metabolite, *N*-acetylprocainamide (NAPA), will accumulate in renal insufficiency and should be measured, along with the parent compound. Procainamide is a first- or second-line agent in ventricular arrhythmias.

Quinidine: Quinidine is poorly absorbed from the tissue after intramuscular injection. This route is painful, but intravenous therapy must be done cautiously with low doses and close patient monitoring. Use of quinidine is uncommon because of its side-effect potential.

Class IB. Class IB agents are also used commonly and are less likely to have a proarrhythmic effect. Central nervous system toxicity is common. Activity of class IB agents is limited to treatment of ventricular arrhythmias.

Lidocaine: Lidocaine is well tolerated and used frequently for several days after myocardial infarction for treatment of ventricular arrhythmias. It is an alternative to amiodarone in ventricular fibrillation. Side effects are related to a local anesthetic effect and may be transient with a loading dose, but they warrant dose reduction or discontinuation if seen after a prolonged infusion. Serum concentrations may be monitored. Hepatic metabolism is rapid but influenced by perfusion, so elimination is reduced in congestive heart failure or hepatic failure.

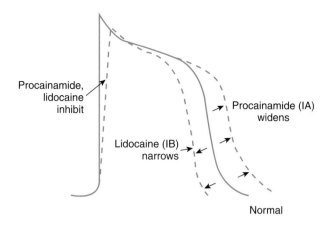

Figure 19-7   The difference in the effect on the action potential duration for the Class IA agent, procainamide, versus the Class IB agent, lidocaine. Both agents inhibit phase 0.

Table 19-2

Antiarrhythmics grouped by Singh–Vaughan Williams class and electrophysiological effects*

CLASS	DRUG	CONDUCTION VELOCITY	REFRACTORY PERIOD	AUTOMATICITY	ION BLOCK
IA	Disopyramide Procainamide Quinidine	↓	↑	↓	Sodium
IB	Lidocaine Mexilitine Tocainide	↔/↓	↓	↓	Sodium
IC	Flecainide Propafenone†	↓	↔	↓	Sodium
II	β Blockers‡	↓	↑	↓	Calcium
III	Amiodarone¶† Dofetilide Ibutilide Sotalol†	↔/↑	↑	↔	Potassium
IV‡	Diltiazem Verapamil	↓	↑	↓	Calcium
Miscellaneous	Digoxin‡	↓	↔/↓	↓	Sodium pump

*The electrophysiological actions are illustrated in Figure 19-7.
†Also has β-blocking effects.
‡Effect in SA and AV nodal tissue only.
¶Also blocks calcium and sodium channels.

Table 19-3

ECG effects of antiarrhythmic agents

ECG EFFECT	MECHANISM	DRUG
Bradycardia	Decreases SA node output	Amiodarone, β blockers, calcium channel blockers, digitalis, propafenone, sotalol
AV Block	Blocks conduction	Adenosine
PR prolongation	Delays AV conduction	Amiodarone, β blockers, calcium channel blockers, digitalis, propafenone, sotalol
QRS prolongation	Delays conduction	Amiodarone, disopyramide, flecainide, procainamide, propafenone, quinidine,
QT prolongation	Delays repolarization	Amiodarone, dofetilide, ibutilide, procainamide, propafenone, quinidine, sotalol

Box 19-2	Antiarrhythmic Agents and Common Adverse Effects*

Adenosine: Transient (30-60 seconds) PAC, PVC, atrial fibrillation, flushing, chest pressure; headache; bronchospasm with preexisting asthma

Amiodarone: Hypotension (IV), gastrointestinal irritation, hepatic injury, pulmonary fibrosis, hypothyroidism, hyperthyroidism; CNS: tremors, ataxia, sleep disturbance, photosensitivity; drug interactions: reduces the metabolism of many other drugs, increasing the risk of toxicity (digoxin, procainamide, warfarin, etc.)

Atenolol: Bradycardia, bronchospasm, heart failure, claudication

Diltiazem: Bradycardia, hypotension, heart failure, constipation

Disopyramide: Anticholinergic (dry mouth, constipation, urinary retention), heart failure, proarrhythmia

Dofetilide: GI upset, headache, proarrhythmic effects

Esmolol: Bradycardia, bronchospasm, heart failure, claudication

Flecainide: CNS: blurred vision, dizziness, headache, anxiety, ataxia; nausea; proarrhythmic potential is high with CHF

Ibutilide: Proarrhythmic effects

Lidocaine: CNS: paresthesias, mental status changes, muscle twitching

Metoprolol: Bradycardia, bronchospasm, heart failure, claudication

Mexiletine: CNS effects common: dizziness, lightheadedness, paresthesias, nervousness, tremor; GI: nausea, dyspepsia

Procainamide: Hypotension with rapid IV administration; lupuslike reaction or positive antinuclear antibody with long-term therapy; GI: nausea, vomiting, diarrhea

Propafenone: Frequent but mild side effects; CNS: dizziness, lethargy, paresthesias, tremor, ataxia; GI: nausea, altered taste, anorexia, constipation; bronchospasm, bradycardia, blurred vision

Propranolol: Bradycardia, bronchospasm, heart failure, claudication

Quinidine: GI: nausea, diarrhea may be severe; CNS: headache, dizziness, cinchonism (tinnitus), hearing loss, blurred vision; thrombocytopenia and hepatic toxicity, proarrhythmia

Sotalol: Bradycardia, proarrhythmic effects; fatigue and dizziness; dyspnea; bronchospasm; nausea/vomiting

Tocainide: CNS effects common: tremor, dizziness, paresthesia, psychosis; GI: nausea; rare but severe agranulocytosis; interstitial pneumonitis; fibrosing alveolitis; pulmonary fibrosis

Verapamil: Bradycardia, hypotension, heart failure, constipation

CHF, Congestive heart failure; *CNS,* central nervous system; *GI,* gastrointestinal; *IV,* intravenous; *PAC,* premature atrial contraction; *PVC,* premature ventricular contraction.
*In addition to ECG effects.

Mexiletine (Mexitil): This agent is a congener of lidocaine for oral therapy only. It is commonly used with another agent to increase its effectiveness. Hepatic metabolism is responsible for clearance, but the rate can vary between patients.

Phenytoin (Dilantin, Cerebyx): This anticonvulsant also has antiarrhythmic effects. It will suppress some automaticity, but its most common use is to shorten the refractory period and speed cardiac conduction in digoxin toxicity. The rate of intravenous loading-dose administration should be controlled to prevent severe hypotension. Oral products are also available. Serum concentrations should be monitored. Hepatic metabolism is responsible for clearance.

Tocainide (Tonocard): Tocainide is a congener of lidocaine for oral therapy only; its use is limited because of side effects. Dose reductions are recommended in renal insufficiency. Pulmonary fibrosis is rare but may be severe.

Class IC. Class IC agents are not commonly used because of their side-effect potential, particularly their proarrhythmic effect. Other agents in this class were discontinued by the manufacturer as a result of their proarrhythmic potential (encainide, moricizine). These agents are used more commonly for supraventricular arrhythmias, but have activity against ventricular arrhythmias.

Flecainide (Tambocor): Use of flecainide is limited to only patients with normal cardiac function because of its proarrhythmic potential. Renal elimination is responsible for flecainide clearance.

Propafenone (Rythmol): This oral agent has class IC activity but also a mild β-blocking effect, which may contribute to its effectiveness. Monitor for potential drug interactions. Hepatic metabolism is responsible for its clearance.

CLASS II ANTIARRHYTHMIC AGENTS

Class II includes the β-blocking agents. These agents are used for the treatment of hypertension, for reduction of infarct size in the periinfarction period, as adjuncts for rate control in atrial fibrillation or flutter, and to convert or prevent SVT. The intravenous agents may be used to treat the arrhythmias acutely. β Blockers inhibit cardiac and pulmonary β receptors, causing bradycardia, decreased contractility, and the potential for bronchoconstriction.

Acebutolol (Sectral): This oral agent is selective for the cardiac β receptors. An active metabolite produced by hepatic metabolism contributes to its effect and is renally eliminated.

Atenolol (Tenormin): Atenolol is available for intravenous or oral therapy. The intravenous form is indicated for periinfarction protection. Renal elimination is the major route of clearance.

Esmolol (Brevibloc): This cardiac-selective ultra–short-acting agent requires a continuous intravenous infusion, so it is usually used only in a monitored setting, such as the intensive care unit. It is used to convert SVT to sinus rhythm. The short duration of effect allows rapid reversal in the event of adverse effects. Esmolol is eliminated via plasma esterases, so is not affected by renal or hepatic dysfunction.

Metoprolol (Lopressor): The liver is the primary route of metabolism for this cardiac-selective β blocker, which is available for intravenous and oral use.

Nadolol (Visken): Nadolol is a long-acting oral agent with extensive renal elimination.

Propranolol (Inderal): Propranolol is available for both intravenous and oral administrations. It has a long elimination rate, primarily through hepatic metabolism.

CLASS III ANTIARRHYTHMIC AGENTS

Class III agents are effective for both supraventricular and ventricular arrhythmias. Another agent in this class, bretylium, is no longer manufactured.

Amiodarone (Cordarone, Pacerone): An intravenous solution is available for acute arrhythmia therapy. It is approved for ventricular arrhythmias

and recommended as a first-line therapy of ventricular fibrillation in cardiac arrest. Amiodarone also has activity against supraventricular arrhythmias and has been used to prevent and treat atrial arrhythmias. The compound is very long acting because of the extensive tissue accumulation and an elimination rate of weeks to months. An active metabolite, desethylamiodarone is also very long acting. Loading doses (either intravenous or oral) are used early in therapy. Many of the long-term side effects are related to drug accumulation in tissues (see discussion of pulmonary toxicity), and the lowest possible dose should be used for long-term therapy. Baseline evaluation of thyroid and liver function is recommended, with periodic monitoring during therapy. Drug interactions are common because of reduction in the metabolism of many other drugs, increasing their risk of toxicity (e.g., digoxin, procainamide, and warfarin). Although classified as a class III agent, amiodarone has very complex electrophysiological effects, with a β-blocking effect similar to the that of the class II agents that can contribute to the development of bradycardia.

Dofetilide (Tikosyn): This oral agent is indicated for the maintenance of sinus rhythm in patients who have had atrial fibrillation/flutter converted to sinus rhythm. It is eliminated via the kidney, and the dose must be adjusted in renal dysfunction. Close monitoring of the ECG effect (QT prolongation) is required during initiation or changes in therapy.

Ibutilide (Corvert): Ibutilide is an intravenously administered agent used as an alternative to electrical cardioversion of atrial arrhythmias to sinus rhythm. The patients are closely monitored for QT prolongation and proarrhythmic effects for up to 4 hours after administration. The principal route of elimination is through hepatic metabolism.

Sotalol (Betapace): This oral antiarrhythmic prolongs the action potential duration, has β-blocking activity, and prolongs the effective refractory period, similar to other agents in this class. As a result, it produces multiple ECG changes. Elimination is influenced by renal function. Sotalol is used for both supraventricular and ventricular arrhythmias.

CLASS IV ANTIARRHYTHMIC AGENTS

Calcium channel blockers are commonly used for the treatment of hypertension, but two of the drugs in this class are also used for the acute treatment of supraventricular arrhythmias and long-term control of ventricular rate in atrial fibrillation or flutter. Both share the potential for hypotension and worsening of congestive heart failure and should be used cautiously in patients with poor cardiac function. A loading dose intravenously precedes a continuous infusion. These agents are also used orally. Both agents are metabolized by the liver, so dose reductions are not needed in renal dysfunction.

Diltiazem (Cardizem): This agent may be less likely to cause a decrease in blood pressure or cardiac contractility.

Verapamil (Isoptin, Calan): Verapamil may have more potent cardiac effects to decrease AV conduction but also may have more side effects than diltiazem.

OTHER AGENTS

Adenosine (Adenocard): Rapid administration of the intravenous agent is used to convert SVT to sinus rhythm through a temporary blockade of AV conduction and reduction in SA node activity. Adenosine may be diagnostic of other atrial arrhythmias during the period of AV block.

Digoxin (Lanoxin): An oral and intravenous agent for control of ventricular rate in atrial fibrillation. It is slower in onset than calcium channel blockers and less effective at rate control during exercise. A loading regimen is used at initiation of therapy because of the long elimination rate and slow accumulation. Dose must be reduced in renal dysfunction. The risk of toxicity (arrhythmias) increases with concurrent hypokalemia or hypomagnesemia.

ARRHYTHMIAS

SUPRAVENTRICULAR ARRHYTHMIAS

Arrhythmias that originate in the atrium or AV node are included in this category and represent the most common arrhythmias. Atrial fibrillation, flutter, and other supraventricular arrhythmias are common. These can be acute, paroxysmal, or persistent. A variety of treatments are available and have been summarized and prioritized.[2]

RATE CONTROL

Treatment of supraventricular arrhythmias includes the use of agents to control the heart rate and agents to convert the arrhythmia to sinus rhythm (suppress ectopy or block reentry). Rate control therapies include digoxin, β blockers, and calcium channel blockers. Rate control is related to slowing of AV

conduction and SA node output, producing ECG changes in the PR segment (see Table 19-3). Digoxin was discussed previously and is limited in benefit because of its slow onset of effect and the inability to control heart rate during exercise, although it may be a useful chronic therapy for patients with concurrent heart failure. The mechanism of digoxin rate control is through an increase in activity of the vagus nerve, increasing cholinergic output and decreasing AV conduction. Potential adverse effects were discussed previously in Box 19-2. Other antiarrhythmics (amiodarone, propafenone, sotalol) possess some β-blocking activity, contributing to rate control and risk of side effects (see Box 19-2).

CONVERSION TO SINUS RHYTHM

The other aspect of supraventricular arrhythmia therapy includes conversion to sinus rhythm. Electrical cardioversion is the most rapid therapy of an atrial arrhythmia causing acute hemodynamic compromise. This mode is also used on an elective basis to convert atrial arrhythmias to sinus rhythm. Elective cardioversion usually requires conscious sedation and appropriate monitoring of ventilation. The use of any modality to convert a patient to sinus rhythm requires bedside ECG monitoring and preparation for the treatment of undesirable cardiac rhythms such as ventricular tachycardia. An agent to control heart rate should be initiated before cardioversion. Patients with chronic atrial fibrillation (>48 hours) should be treated with an antithrombotic agent (heparin, low-molecular-weight heparin, or warfarin) for at least 3 weeks before attempting cardioversion. During atrial fibrillation, clots can form in the atrium and may embolize, causing stroke or other acute arterial occlusion (e.g., mesenteric, renal).

Adenosine is an option for medical cardioversion of some types of SVT. High doses of this endogenous substance cause temporary AV block that interrupts a reentry circuit and restores sinus rhythm. The duration of effect is very short, 15 to 20 seconds. If the patient has an ectopic SVT such as atrial tachycardia or flutter, the arrhythmia will recur when AV conduction is restored. An agent with a longer duration of action to suppress the ectopy (class I or class III agent) is required to eliminate these arrhythmias. Adenosine should not be used for wide-complex tachycardias that may be of ventricular origin. Patients may experience some transient dyspnea or chest pain after adenosine administration (see Box 19-2).

SUPPRESSION OF ECTOPY

Several of the class I and class III agents are used for suppression of ectopy. Class IB agents are effective only against ventricular arrhythmias (discussed below). Class IA, IC, and III agents may be used to suppress both atrial and ventricular arrhythmias.

In nonemergent atrial arrhythmias, ibutilide (class III) is an alternative to electrical cardioversion of atrial fibrillation and flutter. Medical conversion obviates the need for conscious sedation, but patients' ECGs should be monitored closely during and after therapy initiation. Ibutilide is a short-acting intravenous agent; it should be used only after control of the ventricular rate and replacement of potassium and magnesium. Electrolyte deficiencies increase the risk of proarrhythmias related to QT prolongation, polymorphic ventricular tachycardia (torsades de pointes) (see Box 19-2). A chemically similar oral agent, dofetilide, is used for long-term therapy of atrial fibrillation and flutter in selected patients. Initiation of this agent must be done in a hospital setting with close monitoring for QT prolongation or new ventricular arrhythmias (see Box 19-2).

Other agents used for medical cardioversion of ectopic atrial arrhythmias include quinidine, procainamide, amiodarone, sotalol, flecainide, and propafenone. Initiation of medical cardioversion therapy is frequently done in a hospital setting, but may be considered in selected outpatients. Consideration of the risk of adverse events may influence the decision to initiate therapy in a monitored setting (see Box 19-2).

VENTRICULAR ARRHYTHMIAS

Ventricular fibrillation (VF) and unstable ventricular tachycardia (VT) are considered medical emergencies. Rapid electrical defibrillation of VF is the only intervention associated with improved survival after adult cardiac arrest. The outcome of a cardiac arrest worsens for each minute of delay to defibrillation, with only 2% to 5% survival after a 12-minute delay.[3] At least three consecutive shocks with the same or escalating energy should be administered during persistent VF.

Drug therapy of VF is used to prevent recurrence of the arrhythmia after conversion. None of the available agents has been shown to improve outcome of a cardiac arrest. The agents recommended for treatment of VF in the current advanced cardiac life support (ACLS) guidelines include amiodarone, lidocaine, or magnesium for patients likely to be magnesium depleted.[3]

VT may occur at a slow rate and be associated with less severe symptoms. However, cardiac output is inefficient and the rhythm could degenerate into VF. VT may be sustained or nonsustained (three or more consecutive PVCs lasting no more than 30 seconds). Hemodynamically unstable patients should be treated emergently with synchronized electrical cardioversion. As with atrial arrhythmias, correction of underlying causes, electrolyte abnormalities, and concurrent drug therapy should be implemented. Intravenous therapy with agents such as lidocaine, procainamide, or amiodarone may be used to convert sustained VT to sinus rhythm or initiated to prevent recurrence. Patients with sustained VT or high-risk patients with nonsustained VT should be considered for an electrophysiological study. High-risk patients are those with cardiomyopathy or a cardiac ejection fraction less than 35%. Long-term therapeutic options include oral antiarrhythmics such as amiodarone or sotalol or nonpharmacological therapy. Nonpharmacological therapy may include radio frequency catheter ablation of the ectopic source or implantable cardioverter defibrillators (ICD) and is preferred for high-risk patients.[4]

Magnesium is considered the drug of choice for polymorphic VT, such as torsades de pointes, with cardiac pacing or isoproterenol as alternatives. Class I and class III agents should not be used to treat torsades and may precipitate its onset through QT prolongation.

Treatment of PVCs and nonsustained VT remains controversial. Short-term use of lidocaine to suppress ventricular arrhythmias for up to 3 days after a myocardial infarction is common because of its rapid onset and few side effects. However, patients should be monitored for central nervous system side effects such as sedation, excitation, or paresthesias. Long-term use of oral antiarrhythmic agents such as encainide, flecainide, or mexiletine to suppress PVCs may increase the risk of sudden cardiac death in patients with myocardial infarction. Other agents in the same class (disopyramide, procainamide, and quinidine) likely carry the same risk. β Blockers are the only antiarrhythmic agents shown to reduce mortality in post–myocardial infarction patients with symptoms related to PVCs or nonsustained VT, although recent data suggest that amiodarone may also be used safely in these patients.

Amiodarone Pulmonary Effects

Amiodarone is effective for the treatment of a variety of chronic atrial and ventricular arrhythmias. It has extremely complex pharmacology (both class I and class III actions) and potential for side effects. The pulmonary side effects can be very important to recognize and treat because they are associated with up to a 10% mortality risk. Two pulmonary syndromes have been associated with amiodarone and appear to be related to doses above 400 mg per day. Pulmonary side effects are also more common in the elderly and patients with preexisting lung disease. An acute hypersensitivity syndrome has been observed within the first few weeks of therapy. This pneumonitis is associated with fever, shortness of breath, cough, and a lymphocytosis on bronchoalveolar lavage. The treatment requires discontinuation of the amiodarone and initiation of corticosteroids. Rechallenge with amiodarone is not recommended, because the syndrome can recur more quickly and with greater severity. The other syndrome may occur with long-term (7 months to 2 years) amiodarone therapy. It is characterized by an interstitial/alveolar pneumonitis with an insidious onset of nonproductive cough, fatigue, shortness of breath, pleuritic chest pain, and fever. A plain chest radiograph shows diffuse infiltrates or pulmonary fibrosis. After discontinuation of the amiodarone, the symptoms usually begin to resolve after 1 to 2 weeks, but the radiographic changes may be slow to resolve (2 to 4 months). Corticosteroid therapy over the first few weeks may hasten resolution of the symptoms.

Pulmonary function testing and a chest radiograph are recommended at baseline for chronic amiodarone therapy only for patients with preexisting lung disease and should be repeated at the onset of pulmonary symptoms. Routine physical examinations should assess breath sounds, and the patient should be asked about cough or unexplained dyspnea.[5] The lowest effective amiodarone dose should be used to decrease the risk of pulmonary toxicity.

Drugs Used in Advanced Cardiac Life Support

The International Guidelines 2000 Conference on Cardiovascular Resuscitation and Emergency Cardiovascular Care[3] is another step toward its long-term goal: to create valid, widely accepted international resuscitation guidelines based on international science and produced by international resuscitation experts. The recommendations of the Guidelines 2000 Conference attempted to affirm the safety and efficacy of some drug therapies, acknowledge ineffectiveness for other drug therapies, and introduce new treatments based upon an evidence-based evaluation. An overview of the drug therapies for the management of arrhythmias and the use of vasopressors in ACLS will be reviewed. Drugs used in ACLS to control cardiac arrhythmias are summarized in Table 19-4.

It is important to point out that no drug therapy has been shown to improve the outcome of patients who have experienced a cardiac arrest. Defibrillation remains the only therapy demonstrated to improve outcome. Patients who have persistent VF or unstable VT despite defibrillation have received several different therapies in the past, often as a result of anecdotal recommendation. The strength of recommendation of the following therapies is based upon the available science.

Vasopressors

The agents presented in this section will focus primarily on optimizing cardiac output and blood pressure during cardiac arrest. The agents to be reviewed are epinephrine and vasopressin. As a corollary, any agent known to cause vasodilation and hypotension is typically avoided during a cardiac arrest. By maximizing blood pressure pharmacologically, it is hoped that cardiac compressions will achieve an adequate perfusion pressure to sustain vital organs until there is return of spontaneous circulation (ROSC).

Epinephrine

The pharmacology of epinephrine was discussed earlier in this chapter. The purpose for its use in cardiac resuscitation has been for vasoconstriction and cardiac stimulation. The benefit of epinephrine is mediated through both its α and β actions. However, concern has been expressed that excessive myocardial stimulation with epinephrine creates an imbalance between myocardial oxygen supply and demand. The resultant tissue hypoxia and ischemic injury may contribute to a poor outcome. This concern is magnified when discussing the use of high-dose epinephrine, a therapy that has been more strongly recommended in the past. Although high-dose epinephrine may improve ROSC, it has never been shown to improve survival. The recommended epinephrine dose is a 1 mg intravenous push every 3

Table 19-4

Advanced cardiac life support (ACLS) drugs used to control cardiac rate and rhythm

DRUG	DOSE	CLINICAL USE
Amiodarone	300 mg IV push over 1 min	Persistent VF/VT: after defibrillation and vasopressor therapy
Lidocaine	1-1.5 mg/kg IV push; may repeat, up to 3 mg/kg total	Persistent VF/VT: alternative to amiodarone
Magnesium	1-2 g IV push over 1-2 min	Torsades de pointes, alternative in persistent VF/VT
Procainamide	25 mg/min up to 17 mg/kg (rate of infusion is critical)	Recurrent VF/VT: alternative to amiodarone or lidocaine
Atropine	0.5-1 mg IV push; may repeat 1 mg, up to 3 mg total	Bradycardia, asystole
Adenosine	6 mg IV push; may repeat 12 mg IV push	SVT
Diltiazem	0.25 mg/kg IV push; may repeat 0.35 mg/kg IV push, then 5-15 mg/hr infusion	SVT, rate control in atrial fibrillation/flutter
Verapamil	2.5-5 mg IV push; after 10 min may repeat 5-10 mg IV push	SVT, rate control in atrial fibrillation/flutter
Metoprolol	5 mg IV push every 5 min for 3 times	SVT, rate control in atrial fibrillation/flutter, periinfarction protection

Repeat doses administered every 3 to 5 minutes if the underlying problem persists, unless the frequency is otherwise designated.
IV, Intravenous; *SVT,* supraventricular tachycardia; *VF,* ventricular fibrillation; *VT,* ventricular tachycardia.

to 5 minutes. Higher doses of epinephrine (up to 0.2 mg/kg) may be considered when the 1 mg dose has failed.

VASOPRESSIN

Vasopressin is the naturally occurring antidiuretic hormone (ADH). At physiological concentrations, vasopressin's role is to help regulate water elimination by the kidney. However, vasopressin in pharmacologically high doses acts as a nonadrenergic peripheral vasoconstrictor. The peripheral vasoconstriction is mediated by direct stimulation of smooth muscle vasopressin (V_1) receptor. In patients with ventricular fibrillation, vasopressin may have some advantages over epinephrine. First, the half-life of vasopressin is 10 to 20 minutes compared with epinephrine's half-life of 3 to 5 minutes. Because of this difference in half-lives, vasopressin requires less frequent administration than epinephrine. Unlike epinephrine, vasopressin does not increase heart rate and myocardial oxygen consumption. Small clinical trials have indicated the potential benefit of vasopressin in ventricular fibrillation. Vasopressin may be considered as an alternative vasoconstrictor in the management of adult shock-refractory VF. There is insufficient data to recommend its use in other types

of cardiac arrest (pulseless electrical activity or asystole). A dose of 40 U intravenously has been recommended. Adverse effects associated with vasopressin include a reduction of splanchnic blood flow.

ANTIARRHYTHMICS

Antiarrhythmics have been used for patients with persistent VF/VT, after defibrillation and vasopressor use. The pharmacology of these agents was previously discussed. Lidocaine is the traditional first-line agent in this category. However, there are very little clinical data to establish its efficacy. Amiodarone has been shown to be more effective than placebo in out-of-hospital cardiac arrest. The 2000 ACLS Guidelines suggest the use of amiodarone as a 300 mg intravenous push dose in persistent VF/VT, with lidocaine as an alternative. Hypotension and bradycardia are expected adverse effects of amiodarone.

MAGNESIUM

Magnesium is a cation electrolyte with potent myocardial effects. Magnesium deficiency is associated with cardiac arrhythmias and should be considered in patients with persistent ventricular arrhythmias in cardiac arrest. Magnesium is considered to be an effective treatment for torsades de pointes, a type of VT associated with prolonged QT intervals. Most traditional antiarrhythmics are contraindicated in the presence of QT prolongation or torsades.

ATROPINE

Atropine is used for cardiac resuscitation in the case of symptomatic bradycardia or asystole. Atropine is a parasympatholytic agent that increases SA node output and may increase AV conduction. Atropine has a rapid onset and short duration of action, so some patients will require a temporary pacemaker for sustained bradycardia. Atropine may produce excessive tachycardia, which could worsen myocardial ischemia, so therapy should be titrated to a heart rate of approximately 60 beats/min. Atropine is not recommended for patients with bradycardia resulting from severe heart block (type II AV block or complete heart block). Temporary pacing with a transcutaneous or external pacemaker would be the therapy.

SUMMARY KEY TERMS AND CONCEPTS

- Blood pressure is dependent on *cardiac function, vascular tone,* and *vascular volume.*
- *Cardiac drugs* are used to influence cardiac function and include agents to *increase myocardial contractility, regulate arrhythmias,* and *treat cardiac arrest.*
- Vasoactive drugs affecting the vascular component can affect cardiac function (see Chapter 20).
- *Cardiotonic* agents stimulate the myocardium and provide a positive inotropic effect. These agents include the *cardiac glycosides* (digitalis family), *β-adrenergic stimulants, dobutamine, dopamine,* the older agents *isoproterenol* and *epinephrine,* and more recent agents such as the *phosphodiesterase inhibitors* (inamrinone and milrinone).
- *Pulmonary hypertension* (high pulmonary vascular resistance), which may be caused by chronic hypoxemia, can lead to right heart failure, termed *cor pulmonale* in chronic lung disease.
- *Epoprostenol* (prostacyclin) and *alprostadil* (prostaglandin E_1) infusions provide *pulmonary vasodilation.*
- Cardiac arrhythmias impair cardiac function and can be classified by the *cardiac rate* (tachycardia >100 beats/min, bradycardia <40 beats/min) or *point of origin* (supraventricular or ventricular).
- Antiarrhythmic agents are classified into groups based on their electrophysiological action. *Class I agents* depress the fast inward sodium current and are subdivided further in IA, IB, and IC. *Class II agents* are

β-blocking agents. *Class III agents* have complex effects and can prolong the action potential and in some cases exert β-blocking action. *Amiodarone* is included in this group; it has the potential for pulmonary side effects such as pneumonitis and pulmonary fibrosis. *Class IV agents* are calcium channel blockers. Other antiarrhythmic agents include *adenosine,* used to convert supraventricular tachycardia into sinus rhythm.
- Drug groups used in *advanced cardiac life support* (ACLS) include the antiarrhythmics, vasopressors such as epinephrine and vasopressin, the electrolyte magnesium, and atropine for bradycardia or asystole.

SELF-ASSESSMENT QUESTIONS

1. Should pulmonary function testing should be done at baseline for all patients who are started on chronic amiodarone therapy?
2. Should patients with early-onset amiodarone hypersensitivity syndrome continue to receive amiodarone?
3. Is vasopressin an alternative to epinephrine therapy for ventricular fibrillation?
4. What is a positive inotropic effect?
5. What is the general effect on cardiac function of the cardiac glycosides such as digitalis?
6. What effect does milrinone have on cardiac contractility?
7. Which class of cardiac antiarrhythmics includes lidocaine?
8. To which class of antiarrhythmic does esmolol (Brevibloc) belong?
9. What is the mechanism of action for class IV agents such as diltiazem or verapamil?
10. In which type of cardiac arrhythmia would atropine be used?

Answers to Self-Assessment Questions are found in Appendix A.

CLINICAL SCENARIO

Case courtesy **Douglas J. Pearce, M.D.**

A 23-year-old black female is admitted to the hospital with severe dyspnea. The patient states that 5 weeks before presentation, she had a normal spontaneous vaginal delivery of a healthy male infant. Her prenatal course had been fairly unremarkable. She had had some peripheral swelling during her last trimester and elevation of blood pressure, but no eclampsia. Review of her records shows that she is gravida IV, para III, abortus I. She states that she was recovering well from her delivery for the first week and a half or so, but then noticed that her exercise tolerance actually seemed to be diminishing, her weight was increasing, and she noted dyspnea on exertion. Over the last week, she has developed significant lower extremity edema. Over the last 3 to 4 days, she has been unable to sleep without sitting up in a chair. She has not had any chest pain but has had some chest fullness. She also has noted a cough with clear to white secretions. There has been no fever, and she denies nausea, vomiting, or diarrhea. She was initially breast-feeding, but over the last week has felt too ill to breast-feed. She has been pumping her breasts, and there has been no particular erythema or increased tenderness of her breasts.

She admits to 8 pack-years of tobacco use. She tried marijuana as a teenager but denies any recent drugs or alcohol. She reports no allergies and is taking prenatal vitamins.

Examination reveals a mildly obese black female who is tachypneic at rest. Her skin is dry, but her extremities are notably cool. Her vital signs are P, 110 beats/min and regular; RR, 34 breaths/min; and BP, 102/60 mm Hg. Her right jugular vein is clearly distended up to the angle of the jaw. Auscultation of her heart reveals a regular rate with a II/VI tricuspid regurgitation murmur, a II/VI mitral regurgitation murmur, and positive S_3 and S_4. Chest auscultation reveals bilateral rales at least halfway up her lung fields anteriorly and posteriorly. Her abdomen is mildly obese. Bowel sounds are present. She is mildly tender in her right upper quadrant, and her liver span is percussed at 14 cm in the right midclavicular line. There is 2 to 3+ edema in her lower extremities. Pulses are equal bilaterally.

An ECG shows sinus tachycardia, with nonspecific interventricular conduction delay. A chest radiograph (AP) reveals a dilated heart, cephalization of the vessels, and bilateral interstitial infiltrates consistent with pulmonary edema. A two-dimensional ECG with Doppler study shows four-chamber enlargement with severe global hypokinesis of the ventricles. Moderate tricuspid regurgitation and moderate to severe mitral regurgitation are present. Laboratory results are WBC count, 11,500/mm³; hemoglobin, 9.8 g/dl; sodium, 136 mEq/L; potassium, 3.8 mEq/L; magnesium, 1.0 mEq/L; BUN, 19 mg/dl; and creatinine, 0.7 mg/dl. Her SpO_2 on room air is 89%.

This is a 23-year-old female presenting to the hospital with decompensated heart failure. The history, physical examination, and diagnostic studies are consistent with a peripartum cardiomyopathy. The differential diagnosis would include viral cardiomyopathy, idiopathic cardiomyopathy, cardiomyopathy secondary to a toxic agent (e.g., cocaine), or ischemic cardiomyopathy. However, all of these are less likely.

Is oxygen therapy indicated for immediate support of the patient?

The patient received intravenous furosemide 40 mg and 1 hour later an additional intravenous dose of 80 mg. Despite this, urine output has only been 600 ml. Physical examination continues to be consistent with pulmonary edema.

At this point, would initiation of intravenous inotropic therapy to improve cardiac output be a good choice?

Would dopamine be a good choice as an intravenous inotrope in this patient?

What potential side effect of dopamine would be of greatest concern?

Despite receiving dobutamine, she remains symptomatic with pulmonary congestion resulting from heart failure. In addition, she has now developed atrial fibrillation, with a heart rate of 140 beats/min and irregular.

What inotrope may be a better alternative than her current therapy?

What electrolyte therapy would you recommend?

If the tachycardia produces severe hypotension, what therapy would be recommended?

What is the preferred initial drug therapy for control of her ventricular response rate?

Answers to Clinical Scenario Questions are found in Appendix A.

REFERENCES

1. Roden DM: Risks and benefits of antiarrhythmic drug therapy, *N Engl J Med* 331:785, 1994.
2. Agency for Healthcare Research and Quality: Management of new onset atrial fibrillation: executive summary, available at www.ahrq.gov/clinic/atrialsum.htm (accessed Oct, 2000).
3. The American Heart Association in Collaboration with the International Liaison Committee on Resuscitation: Guidelines 2000 for cardiopulmonary resuscitation and emergency cardiac care: an international consensus on science, *Circulation* 102:I1, 2000.
4. Cannom DS, Prystowsky EN: Management of ventricular arrhythmias, detection, drugs, and devices, *J Am Med Assoc* 281:172, 1999.
5. Goldschlager N and others: Practical guidelines for clinicians who treat patients with amiodarone, *Arch Intern Med* 160:1741, 2000.

CHAPTER **20**

Drugs Affecting Circulation

Henry Cohen • Liz Ramos • Maha Sadek

The circulatory system comprises an integral functional part of the cardiopulmonary system. Drug therapy affecting circulation is seen in the acute critical care environment, outpatient care, and home care. Chapter 20 presents four classes of drug therapy, all targeted at the circulatory system. After a brief review of the epidemiology, etiology, and pathophysiology of hypertension, the multiple drug groups used as antihypertensives are described. Drugs used to treat angina pectoris are the second group of drugs described. The third group of drugs affecting the circulation is the vasopressor (vasoconstrictor) group, used in treating shock. The fourth group of agents affecting circulation, the antithrombotic group, is made up of several classes of drugs used to regulate clotting mechanisms.

EPIDEMIOLOGY AND ETIOLOGY OF HYPERTENSION

Over 60 million Americans have high blood pressure ($\geq$140/90 mm Hg). Hypertension adversely affects numerous body organs, including the heart, brain, kidney, and eye. Damage to these organ systems resulting from hypertension is termed *cardiovascular disease* (CVD). Uncontrolled hypertension increases CVD morbidity and mortality by increasing the risk of developing left ventricular hypertrophy, angina, myocardial infarction, heart failure, stroke, peripheral arterial disease, retinopathy, and renal failure. Blood pressure increases with age; thus hypertension is more prevalent in the elderly. Hypertension occurs more frequently in males than females and in more blacks than whites. Hypertension is diagnosed by a minimum of three separate blood pressure determinations on different days. The sixth Joint National Committee on the Prevention, Detection, Evaluation, and Treatment of High Blood Pressure (JNC VI) gives a classification of hypertension (Table 20-1).[1] In almost all cases, hypertension is caused by an unknown etiology and is termed either *primary hypertension* or *essential hypertension*. The prevalence of secondary hypertension is less than 10%, and secondary hypertension may have many disease- and drug-induced etiologies. Disease-induced causes of hypertension include renal disease, hyperthyroidism, hyperparathyroidism, Cushing's syndrome, primary aldosteronism, and pheochromocytoma. Drug-induced causes of hypertension include venlafaxine, cyclosporine, erythropoietin, ephedrine, ma huang, pseudoephedrine,

Table 20-1

Classification of blood pressure for adults ages 18 years and older

CATEGORY	SYSTOLIC (mm Hg)	DIASTOLIC (mm Hg)
Optimal	<120	<80
Normal	<130	<85
High normal	130-139	85-89
Hypertension		
Stage 1	140-159	90-99
Stage 2	160-179	100-109
Stage 3	≥180	≥110

amphetamines, nonsteroidal antiinflammatory drugs (NSAIDs), cyclooxygenase-1 (e.g., ibuprofen, naproxen) and cyclooxygenase-2 (e.g., celecoxib, rofecoxib) inhibitors, estrogens, corticosteroids, high-sodium–containing over-the-counter (OTC) products (e.g., Alka-Seltzer Effervescent Antacids), and chronic alcohol ingestion.[2,3]

PATHOPHYSIOLOGY OF HYPERTENSION

Arterial blood pressure, termed *blood pressure,* is generated by the interplay between blood flow and the resistance to blood flow. Arterial blood pressure reaches a peak during cardiac systole and a nadir at the end of diastole. Arterial blood pressure is defined hemodynamically as the product of cardiac output (heart rate × stroke volume) and total peripheral resistance. Venous capacitance that affects the volume of blood (preload) is a major determinant of cardiac output and systolic blood pressure. Arteriolar capacitance (afterload) is a major determinant of total peripheral resistance and diastolic blood pressure. Antihypertensives elicit actions on some or all of the hemodynamic parameters that define arterial blood pressure.

HYPERTENSIVE CRISIS

A patient with stage 3 hypertension, often referred to as *severe hypertension,* is considered to be in a hypertensive crisis. A hypertensive crisis represents either a *hypertensive urgency* or *hypertensive emergency.* Hypertensive urgencies usually signify diastolic blood pressures greater than 120 mm Hg without signs or symptoms of acute target organ complications. In these situations, reduction in blood pressure may proceed

safely with oral antihypertensives over several hours to several days. Oral captopril, clonidine, and labetalol are routinely used to manage hypertensive urgencies. A hypertensive emergency exists when the elevation of diastolic blood pressure is accompanied by acute or chronic target organ injury. Examples of acute target organ injury include encephalopathy, intracranial hemorrhage, severe retinopathy, renal failure, unstable angina, acute left ventricular failure with pulmonary edema, dissecting aortic aneurysm, and eclampsia. Hypertensive emergencies require invasive arterial blood pressure monitoring and immediate blood pressure reduction with parenteral antihypertensives. Intravenous labetalol and nitroprusside are routinely used to manage hypertensive emergencies.

HYPERTENSION PHARMACOTHERAPY

First-line agents for the treatment of uncomplicated hypertension are thiazide diuretics and β blockers because they are proven to reduce morbidity and mortality.[1] Alternative first-line agents include angiotensin-converting enzyme inhibitors (ACEIs), angiotensin II–receptor blockers (ARBs), α-β blockers and calcium antagonists. Vasodilators, α-blocking agents, α_2 agonists, and antiadrenergic agents are considered second-line antihypertensives.[1] Pharmacotherapy should be initiated with a low dose of a once-daily agent and titrated upward until blood pressure control is achieved or intolerable adverse effects occur. Clinicians should be cognizant that monotherapy achieves effective blood pressure control in only 60% to 70% of patients. Alternatively, a higher response rate may be achieved by initiating low-dose combination antihypertensives. The low-dose combination method may minimize adverse effects and may maximize efficacy and compliance.[4,5] An algorithm for the management of hypertension is depicted in Figure 20-1.[1]

ANGIOTENSIN-CONVERTING ENZYME INHIBITORS

ACEIs act primarily through suppression of the renin angiotensin-aldosterone system. Because of a lack of renal blood flow, renin is released into the circulation, where it acts on angiotensinogen to produce angiotensin I. In the pulmonary vasculature, angiotensin I is then converted by angiotensin-converting enzyme (ACE) to angiotensin II. Angiotensin II is a highly potent endogenous vasoconstrictor that also stimulates aldosterone secretion from the zona glomerulosa cells of the adrenal cortex, contributing to sodium and

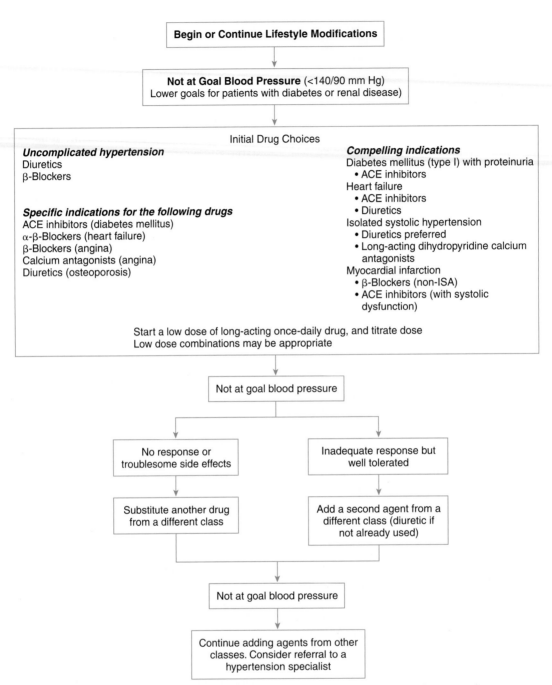

Figure 20-1   Algorithm for the treatment of hypertension. *ACE,* Angiotensin-converting enzyme inhibitor; *ISA,* intrinsic sympathomimetic activity.

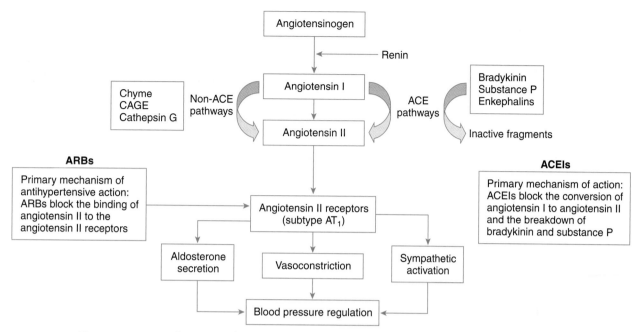

Figure 20-2 Angiotensin II formation and actions. *ACEI,* Angiotensin-converting–enzyme inhibitors; *ARBs,* angiotensin II–receptor blockers; *CAGE,* chymostatin-sensitive angiotensin II–generating enzyme.

water retention.[6] Angiotensin II also stimulates the release of catecholamines from the adrenergic nerve endings and mediates the release of central sympathetic outflow. ACE is abundant in the endothelial cells of blood vessels and to a lesser extent in the kidneys. ACEIs block the conversion of angiotensin I to angiotensin II by competing with the physiological substrate angiotensin I for the active site of ACE (Figure 20-2). The ACEI's affinity for ACE is approximately 30,000 times greater than for angiotensin I. ACEIs also block the degradation of bradykinin and other vasodilating substances, including prostaglandin E_2 and prostacyclin. Because ACEIs are potent antihypertensives in patients with low-renin hypertension, the effects on bradykinin may have an integral role in the mechanism of action of these agents. The hemodynamic effects of ACEIs are a reduction of peripheral arterial resistance, an increase in cardiac output, little or no change in heart rate, an increase in renal blood flow and unchanged glomerular filtration rate (GFR). ACEIs have mild antihyperlipidemic effects.

Nine ACEIs are available on the U.S. market. ACEIs are indicated for hypertension, heart failure, and systolic dysfunction, secondary prevention of myocardial infarction, left ventricular dysfunction, and diabetic nephropathy. ACEIs generally decrease systolic and diastolic blood pressure by 15% to 25%. ACEIs are most effective in normal- or high-renin hypertension; however, they are also effective in low-renin hypertensives. ACEIs are effective alone and in combination with other antihypertensive agents, especially thiazide-type diuretics. With the exception of captopril, all ACEIs are generally administered once or twice daily. Enalaprilat is the only available parenteral ACEI. The pharmacokinetics and dosing guidelines for ACEIs are depicted in Table 20-2.[2,3]

The most common ACEI-induced adverse effect is a persistent nonproductive dry cough (20% to 30%). The cough may be due to ACEI-induced accumulation of kinins, prostaglandins, or substance P in the respiratory tract. The cough may develop within days to 1 year of therapy. Antitussives are ineffective in relieving ACEI-induced cough. Cross reactivity among the ACEIs is absolute; however, ARBs rarely cause cough and may be considered an alternative. ACEI-induced rash is also common; the incidence is 10%, and the reaction is usually transient. The rash often occurs in the upper extremities and is often accompanied by pruritus and erythema. A higher incidence of rash

Table 20-2

Pharmacokinetics and dosing guidelines for angiotensin-converting–enzyme inhibitors

ACEI GENERIC NAME (BRAND NAME)	ELIMINATION TOTAL	ACTIVE METABOLITE	T$_{1/2}$ OF PARENT DRUG (NORMAL RENAL FUNCTION)	DURATION OF ACTION (hr)	DOSE RANGE (mg/day)	DOSE FREQUENCY	EFFECT OF FOOD ON ABSORPTION
Benazepril (Lotensin)	11%-12% bile	Benazeprilat	22	24+	5-80	qd	Slightly reduced
Captopril (Capoten)	95% urine,	N/A	2	6-10	12.5-450	bid-qid	Reduced
Enalapril (Vasotec)	94% urine, and feces	Enalaprilat	11	24	2.5-40	qd	None
Enalaprilat	N/D	N/A	35		1.25-5	q6h	N/A
Fosinopril (Monopril)	50% urine, 50% feces	Fosinoprilat	12-15	24	10-80	qd	Slightly reduced
Lisinopril (Prinivil) (Zestril)	100%	None	13	24	10-40	qd	None
Moexipril (Univasc)	13% urine, 53% feces	Moexiprilat	2-9	24	7.5-30	qd	Markedly reduced
Quinapril (Accupril)	60% urine, 37% feces	Quinaprilat	2-3	24+	20-80	qd	Reduced
Ramipril (Altace)	50% urine, 50% feces	Ramiprilat	11-17	24+	2.5-20	qd	Slightly reduced
Trandolapril (Mavik)	33% urine, 56% feces	Trandolaprilat	24	24+	1-4	qd	Reduced

N/A, Not applicable; *ND,* no data.

with captopril relative to other ACEIs may be due to captopril's sulfhydryl-containing structure. All other ACEIs, with the exception of fosinopril (phosphorus-containing) possess a dicarbocyl group. ACEIs are known to cause dysgeusia (6%) manifesting as a metallic or salty taste or loss of taste perception.

ACEIs may cause a slight increase in potassium that is generally inconsequential. However, the risk of hyperkalemia may be increased with concomitant use of β blockers, heparin, low-molecular-weight heparin (LMWH), trimethoprim, spironolactone, salt substitutes, and patients with diabetes. Orthostatic hypotension is common when initiating ACEI therapy, especially in patients who are in a high-renin state, such as those who are salt or volume depleted (e.g., those with heart failure or receiving diuretics). ACEI-induced blood dyscrasias such as neutropenia and agranulocytopenia occur with an incidence of less than 1% and are more common in patients with connective tissue diseases (e.g., systemic lupus erythematosus). Patients with bilateral renal artery stenosis, unilateral stenosis of a solitary functioning kidney, or

a high-renin state (especially patients with heart failure) are susceptible to developing ACEI-induced acute renal failure. Proteinuria, defined as total urinary protein exceeding 1 g/day and, rarely, accompanied by increases in blood urea nitrogen and serum creatinine, may develop in patients receiving high-dose ACEIs or with average ACEI doses and preexisting renal dysfunction. Angioedema is rare, occurring in about 1 in 1000 patients, but it can be life-threatening when accompanied with dyspnea. Angioedema generally manifests in the upper extremities, primarily the face, lips, tongue, glottis, and larynx. ACEIs should be avoided in females of childbearing age because of the potential for fetal and neonatal morbidity and mortality in the second and third trimesters of pregnancy.

A significant drug interaction occurs when combining ACEIs with NSAIDs. NSAIDs increase renin release by inhibiting renal vasodilating prostaglandins, thereby blunting or negating the antihypertensive effects of ACEIs. The NSAIDs less likely to reduce renal prostaglandins and minimize or circumvent the interaction with ACEIs are sulindac, nabumetone,

Table 20-3

Pharmacokinetics and dosing guidelines for angiotensin II–receptor blockers

ARB GENERIC NAME (BRAND NAME)	ELIMINATION	TERMINAL $T_{1/2}$ (hr)	DOSE RANGE (mg/day)	FREQUENCY	EFFECT OF FOOD ON ABSORPTION
Losartan (Cozaar)	CYP 2C9/3A4	2	25-100	qd	Slightly reduced
Candesartan (Atacand)	Ester hydrolysis/ O-deethylation	9	8-32	qd	No effect
Irbesartan (Avapro)	CYP 2C9/3A4	11-15	150-300	qd	No effect
Telmisartan (Micardis)	Conjugation to acylglucuronide	24	20-80	qd	Slightly reduced
Valsartan (Diovan)	Biliary metabolism	6	80-320	qd	Markedly reduced
Eprosartan (Teveten)	80% unchanged, 20% acyl glucuronide	5-9	400-800	qd	No effect

etodolac, salsalate, and choline magnesium trisalicylate. ACEIs may increase lithium concentrations and have been associated with life-threatening lithium toxicity. ACEI-induced renal sodium depletion may increase lithium renal tubule reabsorption. Patients receiving this combination should be monitored for symptoms of lithium toxicity such as nausea, vomiting, diarrhea, tremor, and mental status changes. Lithium levels should be monitored before and after initiating the ACEI. A quinapril tablet, unlike other ACEIs, contains magnesium carbonate at sufficient concentration to reduce tetracycline absorption up to 40%. The mechanism of this interaction may be chelation and plausibly may occur with fluoroquinolones. To circumvent this interaction, quinapril should be spaced 2 to 6 hours apart from tetracycline and fluoroquinolone antimicrobials.

ANGIOTENSIN II–RECEPTOR BLOCKERS

Several nonrenin and non-ACE pathways are used for the production of angiotensin II (see Figure 20-2). Nonrenin pathways generate angiotensin II from angiotensinogen via tissue plasminogen activator, cathepsin G, and tonin. Non-ACE enzymes that generate angiotensin II from angiotensin I are cathepsin G, chymostatin-sensitive angiotensin II–generating enzyme, and chymase. Hence, ACEIs incompletely block the synthesis of angiotensin II. ARBs are angiotensin II type 1 (AT_1) receptor antagonists. AT_1 receptors are found in many tissues, such as the vascular smooth muscle, myocardial tissue, brain, kidney, liver, uterus, and adrenal glands (cortex and medulla). Many tissues also have an AT_2 receptor; however, it is

not known to have effects on myocardial hemostasis. ARBs have thousands-fold greater affinity for AT_1 receptors than AT_2 receptors. Because ARBs do not inhibit ACE, they do not interfere with the concentrations of bradykinins and substance P. This kinin-sparing effect may explain why the ARBs have a low incidence of inducing cough. However, the beneficial effects of kinins, including blood pressure–lowering potency, may be sacrificed.

Six ARBs are available in the U.S. market. ARBs are indicated for hypertension and can be used for the treatment of heart failure. Limited data are published regarding the ability of ARBs to reduce hypertension-induced morbidity and mortality. In the black population, ARBs as well as ACEIs may be less potent antihypertensives. ARBs, compared with ACEIs, are considered as potent or slightly weaker antihypertensive agents. The inhibition of bradykinin by ACEIs may account for its augmented antihypertensive effect. ARBs are considered second-line agents to ACEIs for both hypertension and heart failure and are indicated when ACEI-induced cough or other adverse effects are intolerable. The ARBs are administered once or twice daily. The pharmacokinetics and dosing guidelines for ARBs are depicted in Table 20-3.[2,3,6]

The side effect profile of ARBs appears to be similar to that of the ACEIs. ARBs may cause orthostatic hypotension, hyperkalemia, neutropenia, nephrotoxicity, and fetotoxicity; however, experience and adverse effect data with these agents are lacking. Similar warnings and precautions exhibited with ACEIs should be undertaken for ARBs. ARBs can cause cough; however, the incidence is significantly less than with ACEIs.

Whether ARBs cause less angioedema than ACEIs is unknown; cross reactivity has been reported. Rash and dysgeusia are rarely reported with ARBs.

Losartan is extensively metabolized by the hepatic cytochrome P450 3A4 (CYP) and 2C9 isoenzymes to an active carboxylic acid metabolite that is predominantly responsible for losartan's AT_1 blockade and antihypertensive effects. Drugs that induce these enzyme systems (e.g., phenytoin, phenobarbital, carbamazepine, and rifampin) may increase losartan's antihypertensive effects by increasing the concentration of the active metabolite. Phenobarbital has been shown to decrease the levels of losartan and its metabolite by 20%. Conversely, drugs that inhibit CYP450 3A4 (e.g., ketoconazole, erythromycin, clarithromycin, fluoxetine, and amiodarone) or 2C9 (e.g., amiodarone, cimetidine, and fluoxetine) may decrease losartan's antihypertensive effects by decreasing the concentration of the active metabolite. However, a study evaluating the effects of cimetidine on losartan did not yield any changes in the disposition of losartan's carboxylic acid metabolite. Telmisartan has been shown to increase digoxin peak plasma concentrations by 50%. Digoxin serum concentrations should be monitored before and after the addition of telmisartan.

CALCIUM CHANNEL BLOCKERS

Vascular smooth muscle and cardiac cell contraction is dependent on the free intracellular calcium concentration. Calcium from the extracellular fluid enters either the high-voltage–gated L-type calcium channels or the low-voltage–gated T-type calcium channels. L-Channel blockade mediates coronary and peripheral vasodilation and may also cause reflex sympathetic activation or a negative inotropic effect. T-channel blockade mediates coronary and peripheral vasodilation and is devoid of a reflex sympathetic activation. The influx of calcium from extracellular fluid into cells triggers a second messenger, *inositol triphosphate,* to release stored intracellular calcium from the sarcoplasmic reticulum. The increase in cytosolic calcium results in enhanced binding to the protein *calmodulin.* A calcium/calmodulin complex activates myosin kinase, which promotes the interaction between actin and myosin, culminating in cellular contraction. Conventional calcium channel blockers inhibit only L-channels. The pharmacodynamic effects of the calcium antagonists on smooth muscle, myocardium, or specialized conduction and pacemaker tissues differ among them because of different receptor distribution and densities and the drug's inherent receptor selectivity and affinity.

Verapamil, the only diphenylalkylamine, and to a lesser extent diltiazem, the only benzothiazepine, lower SA node automaticity and decrease AV node conduction; thus these agents are indicated for the treatment of hypertension, angina, and arrhythmias. Verapamil, and to a lesser extent diltiazem, are potent negative inotropes and may exacerbate heart failure, especially in patients with severe left ventricular dysfunction. The dihydropyridine calcium antagonists are potent vasodilators; these agents include amlodipine, felodipine, isradipine, nicardipine, nifedipine, and nisoldipine. The dihydropyridines, with the exception of nifedipine, have negligible chronotropic effects. Immediate-release nifedipine, especially when administered as a liquid (sublingual), causes a potent reflex tachycardia that increases coronary oxygen demand and has been implicated with an increased risk of myocardial infarction and stroke. Only sustained-release dosage forms of nifedipine are indicated for hypertension. Amlodipine and plausibly felodipine may be used in patients with heart failure because these agents do not decrease cardiac contractility. Calcium antagonists are very effective antihypertensive agents in both elderly and black patients. The pharmacokinetics and dosing guidelines for calcium antagonists are depicted in Table 20-4.[1-3]

The incidence of verapamil-induced constipation is high and often necessitates the use of a stimulant laxative. The dihydropyridines have potent peripheral vasodilating effects, and thus they have a high incidence of palpitations, orthostatic hypotension, flushing, headaches, lightheadedness, and syncope. These adverse effects are minimized with long-acting agents. All the calcium antagonists may cause peripheral edema, gingival hyperplasia, and gastroesophageal reflux.

Diltiazem and verapamil inhibit the CYP 3A4 metabolism and plausibly the *p*-glycoprotein transport of alfentanil, buspirone, carbamazepine, cyclosporine, tacrolimus, methylprednisolone, lovastatin, simvastatin, digoxin, and quinidine, resulting in higher serum levels and potential toxicity. Verapamil and diltiazem inhibit the hepatic metabolism of theophylline. The dihydropyridines have negligible effects on the CYP 450 enzyme system or the *p*-glycoprotein transporter and are not expected to interact with CYP 3A4 substrates. Grapefruit juice inhibits gut CYP 3A4 and may significantly increase the levels of felodipine, nifedipine, and nisoldipine. Because many of the cal-

Table 20-4

Pharmacokinetics and dosing guidelines for calcium antagonists

CALCIUM ANTAGONISTS GENERIC NAME (BRAND NAME)	T½ (hr)	ONSET OF ACTION (ORAL) (min)	DOSE RANGE (mg/day)	DOSE FREQUENCY
Verapamil/SR (Calan, Isoptin, Verelan)	3-7	30	80-480	tid/qd
Diltiazem/SR (Cardizem, Dilacor)	3.5/5	30/60	90-360	bid/qd
DIHYDROPYRIDINES				
Amlodipine (Norvasc)	30-50	N/D	2.5-10	qd
Bepridil (Vascor)	24	60	200-400	qd
Felodipine (Plendil)	11-16	120-300	5-20	qd
Isradipine (DynaCirc)	8	120	2.5-10	bid
Nicardipine/SR (Cardene)	2-4	20	60-120	tid/bid
Nifedipine/SR (Adalat, Procardia)	2-5	20	30-120	tid/qd
Nimodipine* (Nimotop)	1-2	N/D	360	q4h for 21 days
Nisoldipine (Sular)	7-12	N/D	20-60	qd

*Indicated for subarachnoid hemorrhage, not hypertension.
N/D, No data; *SR*, sustained-release.

cium antagonists are significantly metabolized by the CYP 450 system, CYP 450 enzyme inducers such as phenobarbital, carbamazepine, phenytoin, and rifampin may lower their serum concentrations and compromise efficacy.

β BLOCKERS

The antihypertensive effects of β blockers are multimechanistic and are as follows:

- Blockade of the β receptors on the renal juxtaglomerular cells, leading to renin blockade and decreased angiotensin II concentrations
- Blockade of myocardial β receptors, leading to decreased cardiac contractility and heart rate, thus diminishing cardiac output
- Blockade of central nervous system β receptors, leading to decreased sympathetic output from the central nervous system and plausibly blockade of peripheral β receptors, decreasing norepinephrine concentrations

β Blockers with intrinsic sympathomimetic activity (ISA; e.g., pindolol) cause less of a reduction on resting heart rate, cardiac output, and peripheral blood flow. ISA may be beneficial in patients with stable angina and peripheral vascular (arterial) disease. The

α-β blocker carvedilol is indicated for patients with hypertension and for patients with mild to moderate heart failure.

β Blockers are indicated for essential hypertension, angina pectoris, cardiac arrhythmias, secondary prevention of myocardial infarction, congestive heart failure, and pheochromocytoma. β Blockers are also used for migraine prophylaxis, hypertrophic subaortic stenosis, tremors, alcohol withdrawal syndrome, prophylaxis of esophageal varices rebleeding, anxiety, and symptoms of thyrotoxicosis. The pharmacokinetics and dosing guidelines for β blockers are depicted in Table 20-5.[1-3]

β Blockers increase triglycerides and lower high-density lipoproteins (HDL); however, this deleterious effect may diminish after prolonged therapy (1 year). β Blockers may cause hyperglycemia and glucose intolerance. β Blockers can be especially dangerous in diabetics because they mask some of the common symptoms of hypoglycemia such as palpitations, tremors, and hunger. The use of β blockers in patients with hyperlipidemia or diabetes is acceptable if vigilant monitoring of the lipid and glucose profiles takes place. α-β Blockers and agents with ISA are less likely to adversely affect the lipid and glucose profiles.

Table 20-5

Pharmacokinetics and dosing guidelines for β blockers

β BLOCKERS GENERIC NAME (BRAND NAME)	α BLOCKADE	β₁ SELECTIVITY	INTRINSIC SYMPATHOMIMETIC ACTIVITY	LIPID SOLUBILITY	T½ (hr)	DOSE RANGE (mg)	DOSE FREQUENCY
Acebutolol (Sectral)	0	+	+	Low	3-4	200-200	bid
Atenolol (Tenormin)	0	+	0	Low	6-9	25-100	qd
Betaxolol (Kerlone)	0	+	0	Low	14-24	5-20	qd
Bisoprolol (Zebeta)	0	++	+	Low	9-12	25-200	qd
Carteolol (Cartrol)	0	0	+	Low	6	2.5-10	qd
Carvedilol (Coreg)	+	0	0	High	7-10	6.25-50	bid
Labetalol (Trandate, Normodyne)	+	0	0	Moderate	3-5	100-2400	bid
Metoprolol (Lopressor, Toprol XL)	0	+	0	Moderate	3-4	50-200	qd-bid
Nadolol (Corgard)	0	0	0	Low	14-24	20-240	qd
Penbutolol (Levatol)	0	0	+	High	5	20-80	qd
Pindolol (Visken)	0	0	+++	Moderate	3-4	10-60	bid
Propranolol (Inderal)	0	0	0	High	4-6	40-240	bid
Timolol (Blocadren)	0	0	0	Low	3-4	20-40	bid

β-Blocker–induced pulmonary dysfunction may manifest as bronchospasm, bronchial obstruction, rales, wheezing, dyspnea, cough, and exacerbation of previously stable asthma or chronic airway obstruction. Agents with $β_1$-selectivity, such as atenolol and metoprolol, are less likely to cause pulmonary dysfunction; however, they lose their selectivity with increasing doses. β-Blocking agents may exacerbate intermittent claudication and Raynaud's phenomenon, and they may cause central nervous system disturbances such as vertigo, tiredness, fatigue, somnolence, mental depression, and nightmares. A correlation between the individual β blocker's lipid solubility and its ability to penetrate the blood-brain barrier and cause central nervous system adverse effects may exist. Consequently, agents with high lipophilicity, such as propranolol and penbutolol, have a high incidence of central nervous system adverse effects. The β blockers should not be discontinued abruptly, because they will cause a rebound hypertension.

Several β blockers, including bisoprolol, labetalol, metoprolol, pindolol, propranolol, and timolol, are CYP 2D6 substrates. Fluoxetine, paroxetine, and sertraline are potent CYP 2D6 inhibitors and may significantly increase the effect of the substrate β blocker. Because almost all of the β blockers are significantly metabolized by the CYP 450 system, CYP 450 enzyme inducers such as cigarette and marijuana smoking, carbamazepine, phenobarbital, phenytoin, and rifampin may lower their serum concentrations and compromise efficacy. Atenolol is almost entirely renally eliminated and may be used as an alternative to β blockers that interact via hepatic mechanisms.

DIURETICS

The diuretics are divided into five classes: thiazides and thiazide-like agents, loops, potassium-sparing agents, carbonic anhydrase inhibitors (CAIs) (e.g., acetazolamide [Diamox], and osmotics (e.g., mannitol). Thiazides and potassium-sparing agents are the only two classes that are primarily used for the management of hypertension. Thiazides, loop diuretics (except ethacrynic acid), and CAIs are sulfonamide-containing agents and may cross react in patients who have a history of sulfonamide allergy. A significant drug-drug interaction occurs when combining diuretics with NSAIDs and sodium-depleting diuretics with lithium. The mechanisms of these interactions are similar to ACEIs and have been discussed previously in this chapter.

POTASSIUM-SPARING DIURETICS

The potassium-sparing agents are weak hypotensive agents when used alone, but they provide an additive hypotensive effect when used in combination with thiazide diuretics. The two agents used clinically are amiloride (Midamor) and triamterene (Dyrenium). These agents are employed primarily for their antikaluretic effects, to offset the potassium excretion effects of other diuretics. These agents work by blocking sodium channels in the luminal membrane of cells in the distal tubule and collecting duct, thereby attenuating the excretion of potassium, calcium, and magnesium. Both hypokalemia and hypomagnesemia have been implicated as a cause of cardiac arrhythmias; thus there is an advantage to adding these agents to diuretic antihypertensive therapy.

Both agents can cause gastrointestinal side effects such as dyspepsia, abdominal cramps, nausea, and diarrhea; central nervous system side effects such as mental confusion, lethargy, headache, and dizziness; and hematological; dermatological; and musculoskeletal (leg cramps) adverse effects. Triamterene has been associated with interstitial nephritis and nephrolithiases; the incidence may be as high as 1 in 200. Triamterene is photosensitizing, which may be additive when combined with the phototoxic sulfonamide-containing thiazide diuretics. Triamterene may cause hyperuricemia and hyperglycemia.

Spironolactone (Aldactone) is an aldosterone antagonist that exerts its effect on the late distal tubule and collecting duct. Spironolactone is used to spare potassium in combination with diuretics in hypertension, for the management of hepatic cirrhosis (diuretic of choice), primary hyperaldosteronism, and heart failure. Spironolactone's structure resembles that of the corticosteroids and may explain its sexual adverse effects such as impotence, decreased libido, gynecomastia, deepening of the voice, menstrual irregularities, and hirsutism. Other spironolactone-induced adverse effects include diarrhea, gastritis, skin rashes, drowsiness, lethargy, ataxia, headaches, and confusion. Spironolactone, similar to the other potassium-sparing diuretics, may cause hyperkalemia.

THIAZIDE DIURETICS

Thiazide diuretics increase sodium and chloride excretion by interfering with their reabsorption in the distal tubule; a mild diuresis of slightly concentrated urine results. Potassium, bicarbonate, magnesium, phosphate, and iodide excretion are also increased, and calcium excretion is decreased. Although thiazides decrease extracellular fluid volume, antihypertensive activity is primarily caused by direct vasodilation. Thiazides are indicated for hypertension, chronic edema, congestive heart failure, and ascites. Because the thiazides cause hypercalcemia they may be used for the management and prevention of osteoporosis. Chlorthalidone, indapamide, and metolazone do not possess the benzothiadiazide structure; however, they act pharmacologically similar to the thiazide diuretics. Thiazide diuretics lose their antihypertensive potency in patients with a creatinine clearance less than 30 ml/min. Indapamide, however, retains its potency in patients with a creatinine clearance greater than 15 ml/min. Metolazone is the only thiazide-like diuretic that retains potency in patients with a creatinine clearance less than 15 ml/min. The pharmacokinetics and dosing guidelines for the thiazide and thiazide-like diuretics are given in Table 20-6.[1-3]

Common thiazide side effects are hypokalemia, hypomagnesemia, hypercalcemia, hyperuricemia, hyperglycemia, hyperlipidemia, and sexual dysfunction. These abnormalities are dose related and may be minimized by using low-dose agents such as chlorthalidone, 12.5 to 25 mg daily, or hydrochlorothiazide, 12.5 mg twice daily. Less common thiazide-induced adverse effects include dyspepsia, rashes, photosensitivity, thrombocytopenia, and pancreatitis.

LOOP DIURETICS

Loop diuretics, which are often referred to as *high-ceiling diuretics*, act principally at the thick ascending limb of the loop of Henle, where they decrease sodium reabsorption by competing for the chloride site on the Na^+-K^+-$2Cl^-$ symporter (a transport molecule).

Table 20-6

Pharmacokinetics and dosing guidelines for thiazides and thiazide-like diuretics

THIAZIDES AND THIAZIDE-LIKE DIURETICS GENERIC NAME (BRAND NAME)	$T_{1/2}$ (hr)	PEAK EFFECT (hr)	DURATION OF DIURESIS (hr)	DOSE RANGE (mg/day)	DOSE FREQUENCY
Chlorothiazide (Diuril)	1-2	2 (PO)/ 0.5 (IV)	6-12 (PO), 2 (IV)	500-2000	qd-bid
Chlorthalidone (Hygroton)	35-55	2	24-72	15-200	qd
Hydrochlorothiazide (Esidrix, HydroDIURIL, Oretic, Microzide)	2.5-4.5	4-6	6-12	25-100	qd-tid
Indapamide (Lozol)	14-18	2	24-36	1.25-5	qd
Metolazone (Zaroxolyn)	6-20	2	12-24	5-20	qd

Table 20-7

Pharmacokinetics and dosing guidelines for oral loop diuretics

LOOP DIURETICS GENERIC NAME (BRAND NAME)	$T_{1/2}$ (hr)	ONSET (hr)	DURATION (hr)	DOSE RANGE (mg/day)	DOSE FREQUENCY
Bumetanide (Bumex)	0.8 ± 0.2	0.5-1	5-6	0.5-10	qd-bid
Ethacrynic acid (Edecrin)	2-4	0.5	6-8	50-200	qd-bid
Furosemide (Lasix)	0.5-1.1	0.5-1	6-8	40-240	qd-bid
Torsemide (Demadex)	2-4	0.5-1	1	5-200	qd

Excretion of sodium, chloride, potassium, hydrogen ion, calcium, magnesium, ammonium, bicarbonate, and possibly phosphate is enhanced. Diuretics such as the thiazides have a limited diuretic potency with a plateau effect, because they act primarily at sites past the ascending limb, where only a small percentage of the filtered load reaches the more distal sites. Because over 25% of the filtered load is reabsorbed in the ascending limb, loop diuretics are highly efficacious and so termed high-ceiling diuretics.

Loop diuretics are indicated for congestive heart failure, ascites, ascites of hepatic cirrhosis, renal failure, pulmonary edema, hypercalcemia, hypermagnesemia, and syndrome of inappropriate antidiuretic hormone. Loop diuretics are second-line diuretics in the management of hypertension. The pharmacokinetics and dosing guidelines for the oral loop diuretics are depicted in Table 20-7.

Loop diuretics are very potent and as a consequence may cause severe dehydration, hypotension, hypochloremic alkalosis, and hypokalemia. Loop diuretics should not be administered at bedtime because the patient will have to urinate frequently, causing sleep disturbances. Loop diuretics may cause hyperglycemia (not reported with bumetanide), hyperuricemia, dyspepsia, photosensitivity, and ototoxicity. Ethacrynic acid is the most auditory ototoxic loop diuretic and should be considered for cases refractory to other loop diuretics.

ADRENERGIC AGENTS: CENTRALLY ACTING

The α_2 agonists lower blood pressure by affecting both cardiac output and peripheral resistance. The α_2 agonists stimulate brainstem α_2 receptors, resulting in a decrease in sympathetic outflow from the central nervous system. The α_2 agonists are very effective antihypertensives; however, they are not considered first-line therapy because of their side-effect profile. They have a high incidence of anticholinergic side effects, such as blurred vision, dry mouth, and urinary retention, and central nervous system side effects, such as drowsiness, fatigue, headaches, depression, psychosis, and nightmares. Chronic use of these agents results in sodium and fluid retention and almost always necessitates the use of concomitant diuretics. The α_2 agonists are not recommended for

Table 20-8

Pharmacokinetics and dosing guidelines for α_2 agonists

α_2 AGONISTS GENERIC NAME (BRAND NAME)	$T_{1/2}$ (hr)	ONSET OF ACTION	DOSE RANGE (mg/day)	DOSE FREQUENCY
Methyldopa (Aldomet)	1.25	4-6 hr	500-2000	bid-tid
Clonidine (Catapres)	6-20	30-60 min	0.1-2.4	bid-qid
Guanfacine (Tenex)	17	2.6 hr	1-3	qhs
Guanabenz (Wytensin)	7-10	1 hr	4-32	bid

Table 20-9

Pharmacokinetics and dosing guidelines for α_1-adrenergic receptor antagonists

α_1-ADRENERGIC ANTAGONISTS GENERIC NAME (BRAND NAME)	$T_{1/2}$ (hr)	PEAK (hr)	DURATION (hr)	ELIMINATION ROUTES	DOSE RANGE (mg/day)	DOSE FREQUENCY
Doxazosin (Cardura)	11	6	18-36	63% feces, 9% urine	1-16	qd
Prazosin (Minipress)	2	1.5	8-10	90% feces, 10% urine	3-40	bid-tid
Terazosin (Hytrin)	14	2	24	60% feces, 40% urine	120	qd-bid

noncompliant patients and should never be withdrawn abruptly because of the risk of either rebound hypertension or overshoot hypertension (blood pressure higher than pretreatment). The pharmacokinetics and dosing guidelines for the α_2 agonists is depicted in Table 20-8.[1-3]

α_1-ADRENERGIC ANTAGONISTS

The α_1-adrenergic receptor antagonists selectively block the postsynaptic α_1 receptors. Total peripheral resistance is reduced through both arterial and venous dilation; thus these agents decrease both preload and afterload and cause a potent first-dose sympathetic reflex increase in heart rate and renin activity.[8] The α_1-adrenergic antagonists cause a first-dose phenomenon that manifests with orthostatic hypotension, tachycardia, palpitations, dizziness, headaches, and syncope. After several doses, despite persistent vasodilation, tolerance to the first-dose phenomenon develops and heart rate, renin, and cardiac output return to normal. To minimize the first-dose phenomenon, initial doses of α_1-adrenergic antagonists should be low and administered at bedtime. The α_1-adrenergic antagonists have favorable effects on the lipoprotein profile and may decrease triglycerides and low-density lipoproteins and increase HDL by 5% to 10%.

The α_1-adrenergic antagonists are indicated for hypertension, benign prostatic hyperplasia, heart failure,

and Raynaud's vasospasm. However, a recent study of doxazosin compared with other antihypertensives revealed a 25% higher incidence of combined cardiovascular morbidity.[9] A higher incidence of doxazosin-induced stroke, heart failure, angina, and coronary revascularization were reported. Based on the results of this study, α_1-adrenergic antagonists should not be considered for first-line antihypertensive therapy. The pharmacokinetics and dosing guidelines for the α_1-adrenergic antagonists are depicted in Table 20-9.[1-3]

ANTIADRENERGIC AGENTS

The antiadrenergic antihypertensive agents are reserpine, guanethidine (Ismelin), and guanadrel (Hylorel). All three of these agents are second-line antihypertensives. Reserpine works by binding to storage vesicles of peripheral and central postganglionic adrenergic neurons and depleting norepinephrine. Subsequently, reserpine renders the neuronal storage vesicles dysfunctional. Reserpine may cause sedation, depression, suicidal ideation, psychosis, peptic ulcer disease, and nasal stuffiness. Reserpine's side effects can be minimized with low yet effective antihypertensive doses (0.25 mg or less). Guanethidine and guanadrel are postganglionic sympathetic inhibitors that produce a selective block of efferent peripheral sympathetic pathways. Guanethidine and guanadrel act as *substitute neurotransmitters* by replacing norepinephrine in the neuronal storage vesicle. Guanethidine and guanadrel cause similar adverse effects, such as orthostatic hypotension, sexual dysfunction, and diarrhea that can be occasionally explosive. The antihypertensive effects of these agents may be diminished when combined with tricyclic antidepressants, amphetamines, and ephedrine.

VASODILATORS

The two common vasodilators used in the management of hypertension are hydralazine (Apresoline) and minoxidil (Rogaine, Loniten). Hydralazine is also indicated for heart failure and has been used for angina. These agents reduce total peripheral resistance by a direct action on vascular smooth muscle increasing intracellular concentrations of cyclic guanosine monophosphate (cGMP). These vasodilators are so potent that they cause a profound activation of baroreceptors, leading to reflex tachycardia, renin release, and an increase in cardiac output. To minimize tachycardia and fluid retention, these agents are often administered concomitantly with a β blocker and a loop diuretic, respectively. Hydralazine has been associated with peripheral neuropathy and drug-induced systemic lupus erythematosus–like syndrome. When hydralazine is administered with food its bioavailability may double and may cause cardiac toxicity. Hydralazine should be administered consistently with or without food. Minoxidil-induced adverse effects include hirsutism, nausea and vomiting, and pericardial effusions.

ANGINA

Ischemic heart disease can present as many clinical variants such as stable exertional angina; unstable (rest, preinfarction, crescendo) angina; coronary vasomotion; vasospasm associated with atypical, variant, or Prinzmetal's angina; silent myocardial ischemia; or a myocardial infarction. Angina pectoris (chest pain) is a symptom or marker of myocardial ischemia. Ischemia is defined as a lack of oxygen and decreased or no blood flow to the myocardium. Angina pectoris can present with a heavy weight or pressure on the chest, a burning sensation, or shortness of breath. The chest tightness or pressure can occur over the sternum, left shoulder, and lower jaw. Chest pain can be precipitated by exercise, cold environment, physical exercise, or emotional stress (anger). The duration of pain intensity may range from a few minutes to half an hour. During angina an

imbalance of myocardial oxygen supply and myocardial oxygen demand occurs. Factors that increase myocardial oxygen demand include increased heart rate, increased systolic wall force or tension, or increased contractility. Factors that decrease myocardial oxygen supply include a decrease in the concentration of oxygen (e.g., anemia), a decrease in coronary blood flow (e.g., thrombus), or the myocardium's inability to extract oxygen from the blood.

Pharmacotherapy for angina pectoris includes the nitrates, β blockers, and calcium antagonists. All patients with angina should receive daily aspirin for prophylaxis of a myocardial infarction.[10,11] For the management of vasospastic and chronic stable angina, diltiazem, verapamil, amlodipine, and nifedipine are indicated. For the management of angina, β blockers are usually dosed to achieve a resting heart rate of 50 to 60 beats/min and a maximal exercise heart rate of 100 beats/min.

NITRATES

Nitroglycerin reduces myocardial oxygen demand by causing venodilation of coronary arteries and collaterals, resulting in decreased end-diastolic pressures. Venous effects predominate; however, nitroglycerin can affect arteries at high doses. The nitrates' cellular mechanism of action is depicted in Figure 20-3. Nitrates are indicated for acute treatment or prophylaxis of angina, acute myocardial infarction, acute heart failure, low-output syndromes, and hypertension (intravenous). Nitrates may be administered by various routes and are readily available in multiple preparations, including oral, intravenous, ointment, transdermal, translingual, and sublingual tablets. Sublingual nitroglycerin is indicated for acute anginal relief. Sublingual nitroglycerin has an onset of action of minutes and duration of action of 30 minutes. Sublingual nitroglycerin should be administered every 5 minutes until relief is obtained. If pain relief is not achieved after three doses in 15 minutes, emergency care should be sought. Sublingual tablets must always be stored in their original container or they may lose potency. Additionally, unused tablets should be discarded 6 months after the original container is opened, because a loss of potency may have occurred. Other forms of nitroglycerin are isosorbide dinitrate (Isordil) and isosorbide mononitrate (Imdur).

Serious adverse reactions to nitrates are uncommon and mainly involve the cardiovascular system. The most frequent adverse effects include tachycardia, palpitations, postural hypotension, dizziness, flushing,

Nitrates $\longrightarrow$ Nitric oxide $\xrightarrow{\text{Guanylyl cyclase}}$ cGMP $\longrightarrow \downarrow Ca^{++} \longrightarrow$ Smooth muscle relaxation

Figure 20-3 Mechanism of action of nitrates on smooth muscle relaxation. The nitrates are converted intracellularly (denitration) to nitric oxide and 5-nitrosothiol. Nitric oxide interacts and activates guanylyl cyclase to increase intracellular concentrations of cyclic guanosine monophosphate results in phosphorylation of various proteins that reduces calcium release from the sarcoplasmic reticulum, subsequently causing smooth muscle relaxation.

and headache. Case reports of clinically significant methemoglobinemia are rare at conventional doses. Methemoglobinemia formation is dose related and occurs by the nitrite ion reacting with the ferrous hemoglobin. Tolerance to the vascular and antianginal effects may occur with prolonged use. Because most evidence supports the central role of cGMP stimulation in nitrate-induced vasodilation, it has been suggested that the tolerance results from sulfhydryl depletion at the nitrate receptor. Sulfhydryl depletion leads to reduced S-nitrosothiol production and therefore a decreased production of cGMP. Theoretically, administration of a sulfhydryl donor, such as *N*-acetylcysteine or captopril, may restore vascular response to nitrates. Increasing doses of nitroglycerin overcome tolerance, but this is short-lived. To circumvent nitrate tolerance, a nitrate-free interval of 10 to 14 hours is suggested.

VASOPRESSORS AND INOTROPES

Shock occurs when the circulatory system fails to maintain adequate cellular perfusion despite volume resuscitation, leading to tissue and organ hypoperfusion. Vasopressors and inotropes are sympathomimetic agents used in shock to treat hypoperfusion and provide hemodynamic support. Vasopressors and inotropes increase myocardial contractility, constrict capacitance vessels, and dilate resistance vessels. The vasopressors and inotropes routinely used for hemodynamic support are dopamine; dobutamine; norepinephrine and, to a lesser extent, epinephrine; and phenylephrine. (For additional review of the pharmacological properties of these agents see Chapter 19.)

DOPAMINE

Dopamine is an endogenous catecholamine and a precursor of norepinephrine and epinephrine. At low doses, dopamine exerts an effect on vascular D_1-dopaminergic receptors in the renal, mesenteric, and coronary beds. At intermediate doses, dopamine exerts a positive inotropic effect by stimulating myocardial β_1 receptors, resulting in an increase in systolic blood pressure and pulse pressure. At high doses, dopamine stimulates α_1-adrenergic receptors, resulting in vasoconstriction. Dopamine is often the first vasopressor used in septic shock. Dopamine has an onset of action of 5 minutes and a half-life of 2 minutes.

During a dopamine infusion, patients may experience nausea, vomiting, tachycardia, and arrhythmias; however, with downward dosage adjustment these effects are short-lived. As a result of local vasoconstriction, dopamine may cause necrosis and sloughing at the site of injection. The effect of dopamine and other β-mediated vasopressors (e.g., norepinephrine, epinephrine) may be diminished when combined with β-adrenergic blockers (e.g., propranolol and atenolol). The effects of dopamine and other α-mediated vasopressors may be diminished when combined with α-adrenergic blockers such as prazosin, terazosin, haloperidol, phenothiazine, and tricyclic antidepressants.

DOBUTAMINE

Dobutamine is structurally similar to dopamine. Dobutamine predominantly exerts its effect by stimulating myocardial β_1 receptors while producing mild chronotropic and vasodilatory effects. Dobutamine has minor α_1 (vasoconstriction) and β_2 (vasodilation) effects. It is indicated for short-term inotropic support in patients with ventricular dysfunction. Dobutamine increases cardiac output and stroke volume with a minimal chronotropic effect. It has an onset of action of 5 minutes and a half-life of 2 minutes. Tolerance to the effects of dobutamine is common, generally occurring within 72 hours. Peripheral adverse effects include ectopic heartbeats, increase in heart rate and blood pressure, chest pain, and angina. Central adverse effects include throbbing headaches and paresthesias.

EPINEPHRINE

Epinephrine is a potent α- and β-adrenergic agonist. Epinephrine is used as a refractory agent in shock management. Epinephrine causes profound increases in systolic and, to a lesser extent, diastolic blood pressure. Epinephrine may cause anginal pain and must be used with extreme caution in patients with a history of coronary artery disease. A high dose and rapid administration of intravenous epinephrine have been associated with significant increases in blood pressure, cardiac arrhythmias, and cerebral hemorrhage. Adverse effects commonly seen are anxiety, fear, restlessness, headache, tremor, dizziness, lightheadedness, and weakness. Epinephrine, similarly to norepinephrine and phenylephrine, may cause lactic acidosis.

NOREPINEPHRINE

Norepinephrine is a potent α-adrenergic agonist with less pronounced β-adrenergic agonist effects. Norepinephrine increases mean arterial pressure as a result of vasoconstrictive effects, with minor effects on heart rate and cardiac output. The vasoconstrictive effects of norepinephrine lead to increased systemic vascular resistance. The adverse effects of norepinephrine are analogous to epinephrine; however, they are less pronounced, transient, and less common. Norepinephrine is an extravasant that may cause local vasoconstriction and severe tissue necrosis at the site of injection.

PHENYLEPHRINE

Phenylephrine is a potent postsynaptic selective α$_1$-adrenergic receptor agonist with little effect on myocardial β receptors. Phenylephrine is a potent vasoconstrictor with a rapid onset and short duration of action. Phenylephrine is relatively devoid of β-mediated effects, making it an attractive alternative in the management of shock. However, there is a paucity of data documenting phenylephrine efficacy in shock. Phenylephrine-induced adverse effects include tachyarrhythmias, nervousness, weakness, dizziness, tremor, respiratory distress, and pallor.

ANTITHROMBOTIC AGENTS

Currently, three categories of *antithrombotic agents* are available: anticoagulant, antiplatelet, and thrombolytic. The anticoagulant agents work by preventing the formation of the fibrin clot and preventing the further clot formation in already existing thrombi. Antiplatelet agents inhibit the action of the platelets in the clotting process. Thrombolytics lyse thrombi by degrading fibrin. Box 20-1 lists the antithrombotic agents.[12]

FORMATION AND ELIMINATION OF AN ACUTE CORONARY THROMBUS

Under normal conditions the body maintains an equilibrium state between clot formation (thrombosis) and clot breakdown (fibrinolysis).[13] Thrombosis is initiated by an injury to the endothelial wall of a coronary vessel. When injury occurs, the anticoagulated endothelial surface is disrupted and the highly procoagulant subendothelium surface is exposed. Instantaneously, platelets will be attracted and adhere to the subendothelial vessel surface, representing the initial step in clot formation. Platelet adhesion is mediated mainly by von Willebrand factor. Von Willebrand factor is present in the subendothelium and is

Box 20-1	**Antithrombotic Agents**

Anticoagulant Agents
Heparin
Enoxaparin (Lovenox)
Dalteparin (Fragmin)
Danaparoid (Orgaran)
Ardeparin (Normiflo)
Tinzaparin (Innohep)
Lepirudin (Refludan)
Warfarin (Coumadin)
Anisindione (Miradon)

Antiplatelet Agents
Aspirin
Dipyridamole (Persantine)
Aspirin and dipyridamole (Aggrenox)

Ticlopidine (Ticlid)
Clopidogrel (Plavix)
Cilostazol (Pletal)
Abciximab (ReoPro)
Tirofiban (Aggrastat)
Eptifibatide (Integrilin)

Thrombolytic Agents
Alteplase (Activase)
Reteplase (Retavase)
Urokinase (Abbokinase)
Streptokinase (Streptase)
Anistreplase (Eminase)
Tenecteplase (TNKase)

actively recruited when the subendothelium is injured. Adhered platelets are exposed to many subendothelial proteins, such as collagen and thrombin. Collagen and thrombin promote platelet activation. Activated platelets release platelet agonists such as adenosine diphosphate, norepinephrine, serotonin, and arachidonic metabolites, mitigating and amplifying platelet aggregation and forming an unstable thrombus or platelet plug. The most important consequence of platelet activation is the expression of platelet receptor glycoprotein (GP) IIb/IIIa on the platelet's surface allowing binding to fibrinogen. Fibrinogen then binds to the two GP IIb/IIIa molecules, causing a cross-linking of receptors on adjacent platelets and initiating platelet aggregation. Triggers affecting platelet aggregation and their antagonists are depicted in Figure 20-4. Fibrinogen is then converted into fibrin monomers by the action of thrombin; this is the final step in clot formation. Homeostasis is complete when the fibrin clot becomes insoluble within the vessel. This stable fibrin clot is the end result of the coagulation cascade. Under normal conditions, multiple inhibitors and control mechanisms keep these reactions localized to the site of the injury.

The fibrin clot ultimately must be removed for hemostasis to remain. Activation of the fibrinolytic system by plasminogen activators, which are present in most body fluids and tissues (t-PA), results in the conversion of plasminogen to plasmin, initiating the dissolution of fibrin and fibrinogen. The breakdown of fibrinogen and fibrin results in polypeptides termed *fibrin split* or *fibrinogen degradation products* (FDPs). FDPs are anticoagulant substances that can cause bleeding if fibrinolysis becomes uncontrolled and excessive. *d*-(+)-Dimers are fragments of plasmin digested, cross-linked fibrin that rise in concentration after the onset of fibrinolysis. The extrinsic and intrinsic pathways of the coagulation system are depicted in Figure 20-5.[2,3,11]

ANTICOAGULANT AGENTS

HEPARIN

Heparin is indicated for the prevention and treatment of venous thromboembolism, prevention and treatment of pulmonary embolism, treatment of atrial fibrillation with embolization, diagnosis and treatment of disseminated intravascular coagulation, and prophylaxis and treatment of peripheral arterial embolism. Heparin is a complex mucopolysaccharide that is extracted from porcine intestinal mucosa or bovine lungs. Heparin binds to antithrombin III, accelerating its ability to inactivate thrombin (factor IIa) and factors IX, X, Xa, XI, and XII and inhibit the conversion of fibrinogen to fibrin. Heparin also prevents the formation of a stable fibrin clot by inhibiting the activation of factor XIII.

Unfractionated heparin has a high molecular weight of approximately 15,000 daltons. Fractionated heparin has a low molecular weight of approximately 5000 daltons. High-molecular-weight heparins are cleared faster and require more frequent dosing or

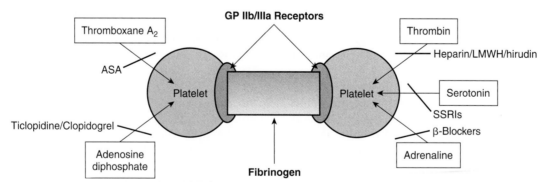

Figure 20-4 Triggers affecting platelet aggregation and their antagonists. Numerous agonists can mitigate platelet activation, which can be inhibited by drugs with corresponding mechanisms of action. However, the expression of the platelet receptor GB IIb/IIIa on the platelet surface causes fibrinogen to bind to the platelet and subsequent linking of the two platelets (aggregation). This is the final common pathway to platelet aggregation. *ASA,* Aspirin; *GP,* glycoprotein; *LMWH,* low-molecular-weight heparin; *SSRIs,* selective serotonin reuptake inhibitors.

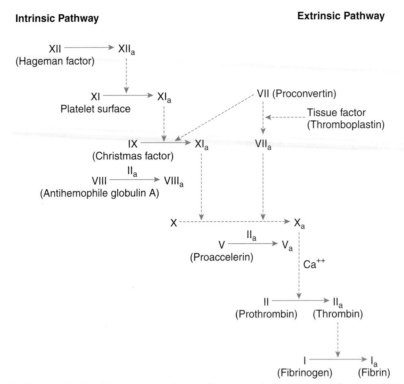

Figure 20-5   Extrinsic and intrinsic pathway of the coagulation system. The coagulation system is divided into the intrinsic pathway and extrinsic pathway. The intrinsic, or contact, activation pathway is activated by trauma or infection, which causes inflammatory proteins to be released in the circulation. The extrinsic pathway's main role is initiating coagulation during hemostasis. The activated forms of factors X and V catalyze in the presence of calcium the conversion of prothrombin to thrombin.

continuous infusions. Low-molecular-weight heparins, relative to unfractionated heparin, exert a greater inhibitory effect on factor Xa but have less antithrombin III activity. Unfractionated heparin binds extensively to plasma proteins such as glycoproteins, vitronectin, lipoproteins, fibrinogen, platelet proteins such as platelet factor 4, acute-phase reactant proteins, and endothelial cells. Extensive protein binding yields poor heparin bioavailability and an unpredictable effect. Heparin-induced thrombocytopenia is dependent on platelet factor 4 binding. Ostensibly, the risk of thrombocytopenia is greatest with unfractionated heparin and lowest with low-molecular-weight heparins.

Low-molecular-weight adverse effects and unfractionated heparin-induced adverse effects include bleeding, hematoma, early thrombocytopenia, delayed thrombocytopenia with or without white clot syndrome, hyperkalemia, osteoporosis, and an increase in liver enzyme tests (LETs). An increase in LETs may occur in up to 30% of patients receiving low- or high-molecular-weight heparins. However, the increase in LETs appears to be benign and has not been associated with any cases of hepatic sequelae. Early-onset heparin-induced thrombocytopenia manifests with a decrease in platelets of approximately 50,000/mm³. The decrease in platelets is transient and inconsequential. Delayed-onset heparin-induced thrombocytopenia is due to the formation of antiplatelet antibodies between days 6 and 12. These platelet antibodies aggregate and form a paradoxical heparin-induced white clot syndrome. White clot syndrome may manifest as pulmonary embolism, myocardial infarction, stroke, renal or hepatic thrombosis, or skin necrosis and gangrene. Low-molecular-weight heparin cannot be administered as an alternative to heparin because of greater than 95% cross reactivity.

The antidote for heparin is protamine sulfate. Protamine sulfate is derived from the sperm of mature testes of salmon and related species. Protamine is electropositive and will rapidly bind to the electronegative heparin to form salts that have no anticoagulant effect. Additionally, protamine will also cause a dissociation of heparin-antithrombin III complexes in favor of a heparin-protamine complex. The recommended neutralizing dose of protamine is 1 mg for every 100 units of heparin. Protamine should be administered by slow intravenous infusion to prevent hypotension, bradycardia, or dyspnea. Excessive protamine may act as an anticoagulant, resulting in bleeding complications; therefore a careful underdosing strategy is suggested. The activated partial thromboplastin time (APTT) is used to monitor heparin's effects because it is sensitive to the inhibitory effects of thrombin, factor Xa, and factor IXa and correlates with heparin levels. The goal of heparin therapy is to balance the prevention of unwanted clotting without an increased risk of hemorrhage. This may be accomplished by maintaining the APTT between 2 and 2.5 times the control value. APTT should not be used to monitor low-molecular-weight heparins. The effect of low-molecular-weight heparins may be monitored with anti–factor Xa levels.

COUMARIN (WARFARIN)

Coumarin (Warfarin) is indicated for the prophylaxis and treatment of venous thrombosis, pulmonary embolism, and thromboembolic complications associated with atrial fibrillation and cardiac valve replacement and as an adjunct in the treatment of coronary occlusion. Coumarin is also used to reduce the risk of death, reinfarction, and thromboembolic events such as stroke or systemic embolization after myocardial infarction. Coumarin administration is indicated after the initial course of heparin therapy, to prevent further thromboembolic complications. Coumarin interferes with the hepatic synthesis of vitamin-K dependent factors II, VII, IX, and X and proteins C and S. Inhibition of coagulation factors begins 12 to 24 hours after administration; however, the antithrombotic effects of coumarin may not occur until 2 to 7 days after initiation of therapy.

The International Normalized Ratio (INR) is the standard for monitoring coumarin therapy. Utilizing prothrombin time (PT) as a tool for monitoring coumarin therapy is problematic because thromboplastin reagents vary in their responsiveness to coumarin-induced reduction in clotting factors, a variability that is dependent on their method of preparation. The INR is a *mathematical correction* of the results of the one-stage PT time that standardizes the reporting of PT determinations worldwide. The INR takes into account the sensitivity of the thromboplastin used in each specific laboratory to determine the PT. The target INR range for coumarin in most clinical scenarios is 2 to 3. Coumarin is a racemic mix; the S-isomer has a half-life of 2 days, and the less potent R-isomer has a half-life of 1.3 days and thus is dosed once daily.

Hemorrhage is the most common adverse effect associated with coumarin. Hemorrhage may manifest as ecchymosis, petechiae, melena, hematochezia, hematuria, hemoptysis, hematemesis, epistaxis, or gingival bleeding. Because coumarin inhibits protein C (half-life 8 hours) and protein S (half-life 30 hours), which have shorter half-lives than factors II (half-life 60 hours), IX (half-life 24 hours), and X (half-life 72 hours), there is a risk of a paradoxical thrombus and skin necrosis with gangrene. Purple toe syndrome, caused by the release of atheromatous plaque emboli and cholesterol-rich microembolization, occurs approximately 3 to 10 weeks after initiation of coumarin therapy. This reversible syndrome is typically characterized by a purplish or mottled discoloration of the plantar surfaces and sides of the toes that blanches on moderate pressure and fades with elevation of the legs. Oral or parenteral Vitamin K_1 (phytonadione) may be administered to reverse the anticoagulation effects of coumarin. Table 20-10 lists selected significant coumarin drug interactions.

ANTIPLATELET AGENTS

ASPIRIN

In platelets, the prostaglandin derivative thromboxane A_2 is a major inducer of platelet aggregation and vasoconstriction. Aspirin is hydrolyzed to salicylic acid and inhibits prostaglandin production by acetylating cyclooxygenase, the initial enzyme in the prostaglandin biosynthesis pathway. This inhibition of platelet aggregation lasts for the life of the platelet, which is approximately 7 to 10 days. By inhibiting platelet aggregation, aspirin will increase bleeding times. Low doses of aspirin inhibit platelet aggregation, whereas larger doses inhibit cyclooxygenase in arterial walls, which interferes with prostacyclin production. Prostacyclin is a potent vasodilator and inhibitor of platelet aggregation. Lower doses therefore plausibly may be more effective than higher doses in preventing coronary heart disease; however, this has not been proven clinically. Aspirin is indicated for reducing the risk of recurrent transient ischemic attacks

Table 20-10

Selected significant drug interactions with coumarin

PRECIPITANT DRUG	MECHANISM
Amiodarone Cimetidine Lovastatin Metronidazole Omeprazole Quinidine Trimethoprim-sulfamethoxazole	These agents may increase the anticoagulant effect of coumarin by the inhibition of coumarin's hepatic cytochrome P450 (CYP 2C9, CYP 3A4, or CYP 1A2) metabolism. The risk of bleeding may be increased.
Chloral hydrate Loop diuretics Nalidixic acid NSAIDs	These agents may increase the anticoagulant effect of coumarin by displacement from protein binding sites (albumin). The risk of bleeding may be increased.
Antimicrobials NSAIDs Salicylates	These agents may increase the anticoagulant effect of coumarin either by inhibition of gastrointestinal vitamin K or by inhibiting platelet aggregation. The risk of bleeding may be increased.
Barbiturates Carbamazepine Etretinate	These agents may decrease the anticoagulant effect of coumarin by the induction of coumarin's hepatic cytochrome P450 (CYP 2C9, CYP 3A4, or CYP 1A2) metabolism. A lack of coumarin efficacy and thrombosis may occur.
Glutethimide Rifampin Cholestyramine Estrogens	These agents may decrease the anticoagulant effect of coumarin by various mechanisms. A lack of coumarin efficacy and thrombosis may occur.
Oral contraceptives Spironolactone Sucralfate Thiazide diuretics Vitamin K	

NSAIDs, Nonsteroidal antiinflammatory drugs.

or stroke and reducing the risk of death or nonfatal myocardial infarction in patients with previous infarction or unstable angina. Aspirin-induced adverse effects include peptic ulcer disease, renal dysfunction, increased blood pressure, tinnitus, pulmonary dysfunction, and bleeding.

DIPYRIDAMOLE

Dipyridamole is a vasodilator and platelet adhesion inhibitor. It has been postulated that patients with prosthetic heart valves have abnormally shortened platelet survival time. Dipyridamole lengthens the abnormally shortened platelet survival time in a dose-dependent manner. Dipyridamole inhibits platelet function by inhibiting phosphodiesterase, which leads to increased cellular concentrations of cyclic 3',5'-adenosine monophosphate (cAMP) within platelets. This effect is mediated by inhibiting red blood cell uptake of the platelet activity inhibitor adenosine or inhibiting the formation of thromboxane A_2. Dipyridamole is only indicated as an adjunct to coumarin anticoagulants in the prevention of postoperative thromboembolic complications of cardiac valve replacement. Adverse reactions to dipyridamole are transient and include dizziness, hypotension, and abdominal distress.

Aggrenox is a combination extended-release gelatin capsule of 200 mg dipyridamole and 25 mg aspirin. Aggrenox is indicated to reduce the risk of stroke for patients who have had transient ischemic attacks or completed ischemic strokes. The second European Stroke Prevention Study (ESPS-2) has shown that dipyridamole modified-release formulation, 200 mg given twice daily, is effective in the secondary prevention of stroke and transient ischemic attack compared with placebo and that the coadministration with aspirin, 25 mg twice daily, provides an additive benefit.[14] ESPS-2 showed that the relative risk reduction for stroke with aspirin administration was 18.1% ($P = 0.013$); for dipyridamole, modified-release was 16.3% ($P = 0.039$); and with the combination, it was 37% ($P < 0.001$), when compared with placebo.

CILOSTAZOL AND PENTOXIFYLLINE

Cilostazol is a quinolone derivative that selectively and reversibly inhibits cellular phosphodiesterase III by increasing the levels of cAMP, resulting in vasodilation and inhibition of platelet aggregation. Cilostazol is indicated for intermittent claudication in patients with peripheral arterial disease. Cilostazol allows for increased walking distances and improves symptoms and quality of life in patients with intermittent claudication. The only alternative to cilostazol for intermittent claudication is pentoxifylline (Trental); however, its efficacy has not been proven. Pentoxifylline is a xanthine agent with rheological properties that decrease blood viscosity and improve erythrocyte flexibility. Cilostazol is associated with a high incidence of transient adverse effects such as headache, diarrhea, dizziness, and palpitations. In patients with heart failure, oral phosphodiesterase inhibitors such as milrinone have been associated with increased mortality resulting from arrhythmias; thus cilostazol is contraindicated in patients with heart failure and should be used prudently in patients with coronary artery disease. Indeed, cilostazol has been associated with increases in heart rate and reductions in PR, QRS, and QT intervals on electrocardiography. Cilostazol is a CYP 3A4 and 2C19 substrate and has been associated with significantly elevated levels when combined with the CYP 3A4 inhibitors diltiazem and erythromycin.

TICLOPIDINE

Ticlopidine (Ticlid), a phenoperidine, is a platelet aggregation inhibitor that interferes with platelet membrane function by inhibiting adenosine diphosphate (ADP)-induced platelet-fibrinogen binding and subsequent platelet-platelet interactions. Ticlopidine's effect on platelet function is irreversible and lasts for the life of the platelet. Ticlopidine is indicated for stroke. The Ticlopidine Aspirin Stroke Study (TASS) showed that the ticlopidine group had a 21% greater relative risk reduction for stroke compared with aspirin and a 9% greater reduction in stroke, myocardial infarction,

or vascular death at 3 years.[15] The Canadian American Ticlopidine Study (CATS) showed that ticlopidine reduced the relative risk of stroke, myocardial infarction, or vascular death by 30% compared with placebo, 10.8% ($P = 0.006$).[16]

Because of the risk of life-threatening blood dyscrasias such as thrombotic thrombocytopenic purpura (TTP) and neutropenic/agranulocytosis, ticlopidine is a refractory agent reserved for patients who are intolerant or allergic to aspirin or clopidogrel or failed therapy with these agents. The onset of TTP occurs after 3 to 4 weeks of therapy, and the onset of neutropenia occurs after 4 to 6 weeks of therapy. The incidence of TTP may be as high as 1 case in every 1600 to 4000 patients. Signs and symptoms of TTP include renal dysfunction, hemolytic anemia, purpura, petechiae, fever, weakness, difficulty speaking, seizures, jaundice, dark or bloody urine, and pallor. Ticlopidine may cause gastrointestinal disturbances such as diarrhea, nausea, and vomiting in up to one third of patients. Rare cases of rash that may progress to Stevens Johnson's syndrome and cholestatic jaundice have occurred with ticlopidine use.

CLOPIDOGREL

Clopidogrel (Plavix) is a prodrug thienopyridine derivative that inhibits platelet aggregation by the same mechanism as ticlopidine. Clopidogrel is indicated for the reduction of atherosclerotic events in patients with a history of myocardial infarction, stroke, or PAD. Clopidogrel is slightly more effective than aspirin in reducing the combined risk of ischemic stroke, myocardial infarction, or vascular death in patients with atherosclerotic vascular disease.[17] Clopidogrel has a lower incidence of rash, gastrointestinal disturbances, neutropenia, and plausibly TTP. Cholestatic jaundice has not been reported with clopidogrel.

GLYCOPROTEIN IIB/IIIA INHIBITORS

The GP IIb/IIIa inhibitors are indicated for the treatment of patients with acute coronary syndromes—unstable angina or non–ST-elevation acute myocardial infarction, including patients who are medically managed and those undergoing percutaneous coronary intervention. The management of unstable angina or non–ST-elevation acute myocardial infarction includes the use of aspirin, heparin, and the GP IIb/IIIa inhibitor. This combination has led to a decrease in the composite end points of a new myocardial

Table 20-11

Characteristics of glycoprotein IIb/IIIa inhibitors

DRUG	PHARMACOLOGY	ORIGIN	BINDING TO PLATELETS	ELIMINATION HALF-LIFE	PLATELET FUNCTION RECOVERY	ELIMINATION
Abciximab (ReoPro)	Chimeric human-murine mono-clonal antibody Fab fragment GP IIb/IIIa inhibitor	Antibodies from immunized mice	Irreversible	30 min	~48 hr	Renal, lymphatic system
Tirofiban (Aggrastat)	Non–peptide GP IIb/IIIa inhibitor	Chemically derived	Reversible	2 hr	~4 hr	65% Renal, 25% biliary
Eptifibatide (Integrilin)	Cyclic heptapeptide	Active component of snake venom peptides	Reversible	2.5 hr	~4 hr	50% Renal, 30% metabolized in plasma into amino acids

GP, Glycoprotein.

infarction or death.[18] The most common adverse effect reported during therapy was bleeding. The incidence of major bleeding manifesting as gastrointestinal, genitourinary, or intracranial hemorrhage with the three-drug combination was only slightly greater than with aspirin and heparin alone, thus illustrating the safety of the GP IIb/IIIa inhibitors. Although minor bleeding with the GP IIb/IIIa is common (10%) it is generally inconsequential. Because these agents may cause thrombocytopenia, daily platelet, hemoglobin, and hematocrit monitoring is required. The pharmacological characteristics of the GP IIb/IIIa inhibitors are depicted in Table 20-11.

THROMBOLYTIC AGENTS

Thrombolytics are indicated for the management of ST-segment-elevation acute myocardial infarction. Thrombolytics reduce the incidence of heart failure and death associated with an acute myocardial infarction. Thrombolytics restore coronary blood flow by dissolving the thrombus, thus limiting the extent of ischemia and necrosis. Thrombolytics convert plasminogen to plasmin. Subsequently, the proteolytic enzyme plasmin initiates clot lysis and produces FDPs.

Eligible patients should receive thrombolytic therapy within 12 hours of symptom onset. Streptokinase may be the agent of choice in patients who present after 6 hours of symptom onset. Controversy exists regarding which agent is the drug of choice. The most common adverse effect associated with these agents is major and minor bleeding. Sites of major bleeding include gastrointestinal, genitourinary, respiratory tract, retroperitoneal, and intracranial hemorrhage. Minor bleeding often manifests as superficial or surface bleeding as a result of arterial punctures and surgical intervention. Thrombolytic-induced hemorrhagic stroke in those greater than 75 years of age occurs more often with alteplase than streptokinase. Patients greater than 75 years of age should receive streptokinase rather than alteplase. Alteplase is the only thrombolytic indicated for the management of acute ischemic stroke for those who present within 3 hours of symptom onset.[19] Alteplase and tenecteplase are known to be fibrin-specific because they promote the conversion of plasminogen into plasmin in the presence of clot-bound fibrin only, with limited systemic proteolysis. The increased fibrin specificity is believed to induce less extensive systemic depletion of clotting factors such as fibrinogen and plasminogen. The clinical relevance of thrombolytic fibrin specificity has not been elucidated. The pharmacological properties of the thrombolytic agents are depicted in Table 20-12.[20]

Table 20-12

Pharmacological properties of thrombolytic agents

DRUG	SOURCE	MOLECULAR WEIGHT (daltons)	TYPE OF AGENT	PLASMA HALF-LIFE (min)	FIBRINOLYTIC ACTIVATION	ANTIGENIC
Streptokinase	Streptococcal culture	47,000	Bacterial proactivator	12-18	Systemic	Yes
Urokinase	Heterologous mammalian tissue culture	32,000-54,000	Tissue plasminogen activator	15-20	Systemic	No
Alteplase	Recombinant DNA technology using heterologous mammalian tissue culture	70,000	Tissue plasminogen activator	2-6	Systemic	No
Anistreplase	Streptococcal culture	131,000	Bacterial activator	46-60	Systemic	Yes
Reteplase	Recombinant DNA technology using *Escherichia coli*	N/A	Tissue plasminogen activator	13-16	Systemic	Yes

DNA, Deoxyribonucleic acid; *N/A,* not available.

SUMMARY KEY TERMS AND CONCEPTS

- Hypertension is defined as a blood pressure of 140/90 mm Hg or greater.
- When the cause is unknown, hypertension is termed *primary* or *essential* hypertension.
- Arterial blood pressure is a product of cardiac output (heart rate times stroke volume) and total peripheral vascular resistance.
- Stage 3 hypertension, with a systolic pressure of 180 mm Hg or greater and a diastolic pressure of 110 mm Hg or greater is a hypertensive crisis.
- First-line drug groups used to treat hypertension include the thiazide diuretics, β blockers, angiotensin-converting–enzyme inhibitors (ACEIs), angiotensin II–receptor blockers (ARBs), α-β blockers, and calcium antagonists.
- Second-line antihypertensives include α_2 agonists, vasodilators, and antiadrenergic agents.
- Angina pectoris is a marker for myocardial ischemia.
- Pharmacotherapy for angina includes the nitrates (e.g., nitroglycerin), β blockers, and calcium antagonists.
- Antithrombotic agents include anticoagulants (heparin, coumarins), antiplatelet agents (aspirin, dipyridamole, cilostazol, pentoxifylline, ticlopidine, clopidogrel, and glycoprotein IIb/IIIa inhibitors) and thrombolytic agents (agents to lyse clots, e.g., streptokinase, alteplase).

SELF-ASSESSMENT QUESTIONS

1. List the adverse effects associated with angiotensin-converting–enzyme inhibitors (ACEIs).
2. Which of the β blockers possess intrinsic sympathomimetic activity (ISA)?
3. Which of the β blockers possess selective β_1-blocker activity?
4. List the adverse effects associated with α_1-adrenergic antagonists.
5. What are the most common side effects of nitrates?
6. List the metabolic effects associated with thiazide diuretics.
7. List five medications that may cause drug-induced increases in blood pressure.
8. Which calcium channel blocker is most likely to cause constipation?
9. What is the best parameter available to monitor the effects of coumarin?
10. What is the antidote for heparin?
11. What is the mechanism of action of coumarin?
12. Name the pharmacological class responsible for inhibiting the final pathway in platelet aggregation.
13. Which thrombolytic is recommended for patients greater than 75 years of age who present with ST-segment-elevation myocardial infarction?

14. Name the only ACEI that is available in a parenteral dosage form.
15. What is the best parameter available to monitor the effects of heparin?

Answers to Self-Assessment Questions are found in Appendix A.

CLINICAL SCENARIO

A 75-year-old male presents to the emergency department complaining of chest pain of 1 hour in duration. He has had intermittent chest pain for the past week. He describes experiencing substernal pain that radiates down his left arm. The pain is associated with diaphoresis and is not relieved by change in body position. He has a history of hypertension for the past 10 years. He has no history or family history for coronary artery disease. He is currently taking labetalol, 200 mg twice daily, and an enteric-coated aspirin, 81 mg daily. He has no known allergies.

On physical examination, he appears anxious and is complaining of chest pain. His vital signs are BP, 140/70 mm Hg; P, 74 beats/min; and RR, 20 breaths/min. His heart sounds are normal, with no murmurs or gallops present. His lungs are clear on auscultation, and his abdomen, extremities, and funduscopic examination are unremarkable. His skin is cool and clammy.

Electrocardiography displays evidence of sinus bradycardia with a heart rate of 49 beats/min. His cardiac enzymes all were elevated (CK, 200 U/L; CK-MB, 20 U/L; and troponin$_T$, 2).

In summary, this 75-year-old male, based on his history, physical examination, and ECG, is diagnosed with a non-ST-segment elevated myocardial infarction.

Is this patient a candidate for immediate administration of a glycoprotein IIb/IIIa inhibitor?
Is this patient a candidate for immediate administration of thrombolytic therapy?

Answers to Clinical Scenario Questions are found in Appendix A.

REFERENCES

1. The Sixth Report of the Joint Committee on detection, evaluation and treatment of high blood pressure (JNC-VI), *Arch Intern Med* 157:413, 1997.
2. *Drugs facts and comparisons*, St Louis, 2000, Drugs Facts and Comparisons.
3. Oates J: Antihypertensive agents and the drugs therapy of hypertension. In Hardman J, Limbrid L, eds: *Goodman & Gilman's the pharmacological basis of therapeutics*, ed 9, New York, 1995, McGraw-Hill.
4. Weir M: When antihypertensive monotherapy fails: fixed-dose combination therapy, *South Med J* 93:548, 2000.
5. Psalty B and others: Health outcomes associated with antihypertensive therapies used as first-line agents, *J Am Med Assoc* 227:739, 1997.
6. Weber M, Messerli F, Bruner H: Angiotensin II receptor inhibition, *Arch Intern Med* 156:1957, 1996.
7. Grossman E and others: Should a moratorium be placed on sublingual nifedipine capsules given for hypertensive emergencies and pseudoemergencies, *J Am Med Assoc* 276:1328, 1996.
8. Veelken R, Schimieder R: Overview of α1-adrenegic antagonism and recent advances in hypertensive therapy, *Am J Hypertens* 9:139S, 1996.
9. Davis B and others: Major cardiovascular events in hypertensive patients randomized to doxazosin vs chlorthalidone: the antihypertensive and lipid lowering treatment to prevent heart attack trial (ALLHAT), *J Am Med Assoc* 283:1967, 2000.
10. Thandani U: Treatment of stable angina, *Curr Opin Cardiol* 14:349, 1999.
11. Williams G: Hypertensive vascular disease. In Fauci A and others, eds: *Harrison's principles of internal medicine*, ed 14, New York, 1998, McGraw-Hill.
12. Mathis AS: Newer antithrombotic strategies in the initial management of non-ST-segment elevation acute coronary syndromes, *Ann Pharmacother* 34:208, 2000.
13. Heesen M and others: What the neurosurgeon needs to know about the coagulation system, *Surg Neurol* 47:32, 1997.
14. Diener HC and others: European Stroke Prevention Study 2: dipyridamole and acetylsalicylic acid in the secondary prevention of stroke, *J Neurosci* 143:1, 1996.
15. Gent M and others: The Canadian-American Ticlopidine Study (CATS) in thromboembolic stroke, *Lancet* 1:1215, 1989.
16. Hass WK and others: A randomized trial comparing ticlopidine hydrochloride with aspirin for the prevention of stroke in high-risk patients (TASS), *N Engl J Med* 321:501, 1989.
17. Gent M and others: A randomized, blinded, trial of clopidogrel versus aspirin in patients at risk of ischaemic events (CAPRIE), *Lancet* 348:1329, 1996.
18. Latour-Perez J: Risk and benefits of glycoprotein IIb/IIIa antagonists in acute coronary syndrome, *Ann Pharmacother* 35:472, 2001.
19. Albers GW and others: Antithrombotic and thrombolytic therapy for ischemic stroke, *Chest* 119:300S, 2001.
20. Ohman EM and others: Intravenous thrombolysis in acute myocardial infarction, *Chest* 119:253S, 2001.

Diuretic Agents

Erkan Hassan

The main purpose of diuretics, or agents that increase urine output, is to eliminate excess fluid from the body.

Diuretic: Any substance that increases urine flow; specifically those agents whose therapeutic purpose is to cause a net loss of water from the body.

The above definition excludes agents that promote urine output without a *direct* action on the kidney. For example, digitalis is not considered a diuretic, although it can increase urine output by restoring cardiac output, which improves circulation and renal perfusion. Renal function is reviewed briefly with an emphasis on acid-base balance. The major groups of diuretics and their modes of action are each summarized. These include osmotic diuretics, carbonic anhydrase inhibitors, thiazides, loop diuretics, and potassium-sparing agents.

RENAL STRUCTURE AND FUNCTION

The kidneys are paired retroperitoneal organs found on either side of the spinal cord at the level of the umbilicus. In the adult, each kidney weighs approximately 160 to 175 g and is 10 to 12 cm long. Perfusion of the kidney is via the renal artery, and approximately 21% of the cardiac output goes to the renal system. This is a perfusion of 1000 to 1250 ml/min in the normal adult. Like the heart and brain, the kidney is an active organ (not a passive filter) with a high oxygen consumption. For this reason, impaired circulation can cause renal damage or failure.

Figure 21-1 illustrates the kidney and its functional unit, the nephron, which is analogous to the alveolus as the functional unit in the lung. Each kidney contains around a million nephrons, 75% of which can be lost before problems arise. The nephron is made up of the glomerulus, proximal tubule, loop of Henle, distal tubule, and collecting tubule.

The renal artery branches into the afferent arteriole, which enters and forms the capillary tuft of the glomerulus. This blood flow then leaves in the efferent arteriole, which then forms the capillary network around the tubules and loop of Henle. This capillary network rejoins to form the renal vein.

The glomerulus is supported and surrounded by an epithelial-lined capsule named Bowman's capsule. The glomerular capsule is actually the beginning of the proximal tubule, and filtration of fluid from the blood to the tubule occurs in the glomerulus. This fluid is the glomerular filtrate, which empties into the proximal convoluted tubule; goes through the descending and ascending loops of Henle, into the distal convoluted tubule and then the collecting duct;

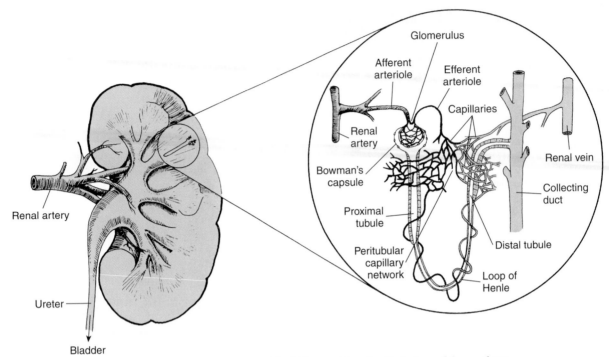

Figure 21-1   Basic structure of the kidney, with a detailed view of the nephron.

and finally empties into the ureter to be stored in the bladder.

Nephron Function

Beginning in the glomerulus, the nephron forms a cell-free ultrafiltrate, with a relatively small amount of protein, which has the same ionic concentration (Na^+, Cl^-, HCO_3^-, etc.) as plasma. Of the blood going to the nephron, around one fifth of the volume, or about 130 ml/min, is filtered through the glomerulus. In the passage through the nephron, over 99% of the glomerular filtrate is reabsorbed in the tubules, and less than 1% of the fluid is excreted as urine. Out of the 130 ml/min filtered, 129 ml/min will be reabsorbed. *Diuretics interfere, in various ways, with the reabsorption of water in the tubules of the nephron.*

Usually, the nephron accomplishes the following:

- Keeps blood protein and cells out of the glomerular filtrate
- Maintains the alkaline reserve of the blood by bicarbonate reabsorption and hydrogen ion excretion, using bicarbonate, phosphate, and ammonia buffers
- Excretes nitrogenous wastes such as urea and uric acid

- Eliminates drugs and their breakdown products from the body

Electrolyte Filtration and Reabsorption

The following important ions are filtered and exchanged in the tubules:

Sodium: Eighty percent of the sodium in the filtrate is reabsorbed in the proximal tubules and 20% in the distal tubules. There is an exchange of Na^+ for H^+ or K^+ in the distal tubules.

Potassium: Most filtered K^+ is reabsorbed in the proximal tubules. The K^+ found in the urine is that secreted by the distal tubule.

Chloride and bicarbonate: These are passively reabsorbed in the proximal and distal tubules.

Water is also passively reabsorbed or excreted, depending on the concentration of electrolyte, primarily sodium, in the filtrate. By inhibiting sodium reabsorption, a diuretic causes more water to remain in the filtrate and be excreted.

Aldosterone is a mineralocorticoid secreted by the adrenal cortex, which increases sodium and water reabsorption in the distal tubule. A diuretic such as spironolactone can increase sodium and water loss by inhibiting aldosterone.

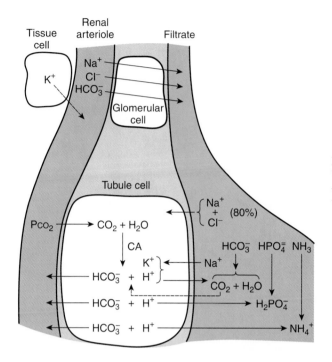

Figure 21-2 The basic mechanisms for kidney retention of bicarbonate with hydrogen ion buffering. Sodium exchange with chloride and for hydrogen is also indicated. *CA,* Carbonic anhydrase.

ACID-BASE BALANCE

Because a fundamental function of the kidney is control of buffering substances, especially bicarbonate, diuretics may cause acid-base imbalances to occur as they increase water loss. Figure 21-2 illustrates the hydrogen and bicarbonate pathways that regulate pH. The filtration and reabsorption of Na^+, Cl^-, and HCO_3^-, described previously, can be seen in Figure 21-2. The important exchange for acid-base balance is that of sodium. Sodium is reabsorbed in the tubules by several means, as follows:

- Reabsorption with *chloride* to preserve electrical neutrality
- Exchange of sodium for hydrogen or *potassium*, again preserving neutrality

Either *low chloride* (hypochloremia) or *low potassium* (hypokalemia) will force sodium to exchange for hydrogen, producing a loss of H^+ and metabolic alkalosis.

$$\left.\begin{array}{l}\text{Hypochloremia}\\\text{Hypokalemia}\end{array}\right\} \rightarrow \text{Metabolic alkalosis}$$

Finally, preventing the bicarbonate in the *filtrate* from forming CO_2 and water will lead to a loss of bicarbonate buffer in the urine and metabolic acidosis.

DIURETIC GROUPS

There are five major groups of diuretics, as well as a sixth group of miscellaneous, older agents that are briefly described in this chapter. Figure 21-3 illustrates the site of action of each of the five major groups of diuretics commonly used. Each group of diuretics acts at a different site in the nephron, as shown in Figure 21-3.

1. *Carbonic anhydrase inhibitors* block the reabsorption of sodium and bicarbonate from the proximal tubule.
2. *Osmotic diuretics* block the reabsorption of water in the proximal tubule and descending loop of Henle.
3. *Loop diuretics* block sodium and chloride reabsorption in the ascending loop of Henle.
4. *Thiazide diuretics* block sodium and chloride reabsorption in the distal tubule.
5. *Potassium-sparing diuretics* block sodium reabsorption in the late distal tubule and in the collecting duct.

Use of more than one type of diuretic agent can lead to a *sequence of nephron blockade,* because of these different sites of action. A more complete description of the mode of action of each class of diuretic will be given as the class is discussed. Diuretic groups of most

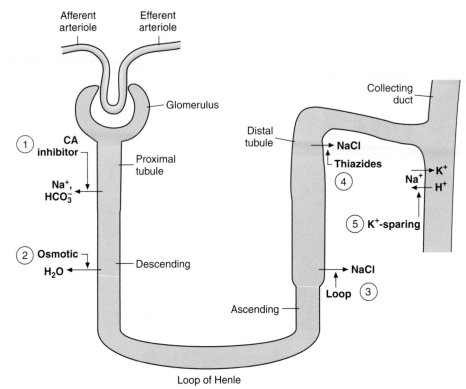

Figure 21-3   An illustration of the nephron, from glomerulus to collecting duct, showing the various sites of action for the diuretic groups. *CA*, Carbonic anhydrase.

immediate relevance to respiratory and critical care clinicians are those used in treatment of heart failure and hypertension.

OSMOTIC DIURETICS

Osmotic diuretics (Table 21-1) are freely filtered at the glomerulus but are not reabsorbed. These agents remain in the tubule lumen and impair the proximal tubule and thick ascending limb from reabsorbing sodium. However, the resultant increased delivery of sodium and chloride to the distal tubule results in increased exchange of sodium for potassium, producing a net kaluresis.

Of the four currently available osmotic diuretics (glycerin, isosorbide, mannitol, and urea), mannitol is the typically selected agent because of its lower toxicity. Mannitol has a relatively short half-life and therefore manifests with a rapid onset and quick offset of action. To maintain a continued diuretic action, the drug is frequently administered via continuous infusion.

CARBONIC ANHYDRASE INHIBITORS

The primary site of action of carbonic anhydrase inhibitors is within the proximal tubule. The enzyme carbonic anhydrase is responsible for the hydration of bicarbonate, which is then reabsorbed. Sodium is reabsorbed along with the bicarbonate. Therefore inhibition of carbonic anhydrase inhibits the reabsorption and increases the diuresis of sodium bicarbonate (Figure 21-4). The resulting loss of bicarbonate produces a metabolic acidosis.

Because the majority of filtered sodium is reabsorbed in the proximal tubule, one would expect the use of carbonic anhydrase inhibitors to result in a dramatic diuretic effect. However, as a group, the carbonic anhydrase inhibitors are poor diuretics because the sodium reabsorption inhibited in the proximal tubule is presented to and reabsorbed at the thick ascending limb of the loop of Henle. Their weak diuretic properties coupled with the development of a metabolic acidosis limits the usefulness of these agents.

Table 21-1

Characteristics of diuretics

DRUG	ROUTE	ONSET (min)	PEAK (hr)	DURATION (hr)	HALF-LIFE (hr)	ORAL BIOAVAIL-ABILITY (%)	TYPICAL DOSE
OSMOTIC							
Glycerin	PO	10-30	1-1.5	4-5	0.5-0.75		1-2 g/kg
Isosorbide	PO	10-30	1-1.5	5-6	5-9.5		1-3 g/kg
Mannitol	IV	30-60	1	6-8	0.25-1.5	N/A	50-100 g
Urea	IV	30-45	1	5-6	N/A	N/A	1-1.5 g/kg
THIAZIDE							
Bendroflumethiazide	PO	120	4	12-16	3-4	100	5 mg
Benzthiazide	PO	120	4-6	16-18	N/D	N/D	50-100 mg/day
Chlorothiazide	PO	120	4	12-16	0.75-2	10-21	0.5-2.0 g/day
	IV	15	0.5	12-16			
Chlorthalidone	PO	120-180	2-6	24-72	40	64	50-100 mg/day
Hydrochlorothiazide	PO	120	4-6	12-16	50.6-14.8	65-75	50-200 mg/day
Hydroflumethiazide	PO	120	4	12-16	17	50	25-200 mg/day
Indapamide	PO	60-120	<2	36	14	93	1.25-5 mg/day
Methylclothiazide	PO	120	6	24	N/D	N/D	5 mg
Metolazone	PO	60	2	12-24	N/D	65	5-20 mg/day
Polythiazide	PO	120	6	24-48	25-37	N/D	2-4 mg/day
Quinethazone	PO	120	6	18-24	N/D	N/D	50-100 mg/day
Trichlormethiazide	PO	120	6	24	2.3-7.3	N/D	2-4 mg/day
LOOP							
Bumetanide	PO	30-60	1-2	4-6	1-1.5	72-96	0.5-2.0 mg
	IV	5	0.25-0.5	0.5-1			
Ethacrynic acid	PO	30	2	6-8	1	100	50-100 mg
	IV	5	0.25-0.5	2			
Furosemide	PO	60	1-2	6-8	2	60-64	20-80 mg
	IV	5	0.5	2			
Torsemide	PO	60	1-2	6-8	3.5	80	5-20 mg
	IV	10	<1	6-8			
POTASSIUM SPARING							
Amiloride	PO	2 hr	6-10	24	6-9	30-90	5-20 mg/day
Spironolactone	PO	24-48 hr	48-72	48-72	20	73	25-400 mg/day
Triamterene	PO	2-4 hr	6-8	12-16	3	30-70	200-300 mg/day

IV, Intravenous; *N/A*, not applicable; *N/D*, no data; *PO*, oral.

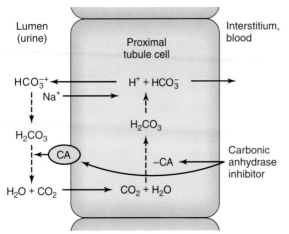

Lumen (urine)

Interstitium, blood

Proximal tubule cell

HCO_3^{-+} ← H⁺ + HCO_3^- →

Na⁺

H_2CO_3

H_2CO_3

CA

−CA ←

Carbonic anhydrase inhibitor

$H_2O + CO_2$ → $CO_2 + H_2O$

Figure 21-4   The effect of carbonic anhydrase inhibitor diuretics such as acetazolamide, which block the availability of hydrogen to exchange for sodium in the proximal tubule, causing a loss of sodium, bicarbonate, and water, along with reduced bicarbonate reabsorption into the cell and the blood. *CA,* Carbonic anhydrase.

Other potential uses of carbonic anhydrase inhibitors include glaucoma, metabolic alkalosis, and altitude sickness. Carbonic anhydrase is an important enzyme in the formation of intraocular fluid. Therefore carbonic anhydrase inhibitors effectively decrease intraocular pressure and treat glaucoma. Short-term carbonic anhydrase inhibitors may also correct a metabolic alkalosis as a result of the acidosis they produce. Finally, carbonic anhydrase inhibitors have been shown useful against altitude sickness, although the exact mechanism of action is not known. The most common adverse effect of carbonic anhydrase inhibitors is hypokalemia resulting from the increased amount of sodium presented to the collecting duct, which is then reabsorbed in exchange for potassium excretion.

LOOP DIURETICS

Loop diuretics (see Table 21-1) inhibit the reabsorption of chloride at the thick ascending limb of the loop of Henle. Sodium and water follow the chloride. Normally, 20% to 30% of filtered sodium is reabsorbed at the site of action. Loop diuretics are capable of preventing almost all of the filtered sodium from being absorbed.[1]

When administered intravenously, loop diuretics produce an acute hemodynamic effect independent of their diuretic properties. Within 5 minutes after the administration of intravenous loop diuretics to cardiac

patients, an acute vasodilatory effect is observed. This effect is manifested by a decrease in pulmonary capillary wedge pressure, blood pressure, and systemic vascular resistance. The effect seems to be derived from the renal release of vasodilating prostaglandins.[2,3] Because the diuretic effect of intravenous loop diuretics is typically not seen for 15 to 20 minutes after administration, patients with acute pulmonary edema may derive a clinical benefit from intravenous loop diuretics before the onset of diuresis. The hemodynamic effect is short lived, with all measurements returning to baseline once diuresis has begun. The acute hemodynamic effect has also been reported to activate the sympathetic nervous system, resulting in an adverse hemodynamic profile characterized by increased afterload and diminished cardiac function before the onset of diuresis.[4] This effect is also short lived and dissipates with the onset of diuresis.

After intravenous administration, loop diuretics have a diuretic onset of approximately 15 to 20 minutes and may last several hours. Therefore several doses per day may be required to maintain a net diuretic effect for 24 hours. Patients requiring frequent bolus doses may benefit from a continuous infusion.

Administration of loop diuretics to patients with renal dysfunction results in less total drug reaching the site of action within the nephron; therefore the administration of larger doses are required to achieve a therapeutic effect.[5-7] In these patients, differences exist among the effects of furosemide, bumetanide, and torsemide. Furosemide may have a more prolonged effect in patients with renal dysfunction. However, patients may be resistant to furosemide compared with bumetanide. Because loop diuretics are the most potent diuretics, they are effective at very low creatinine clearance levels. Loop diuretics as single agents should be considered as first-line therapy in patients with creatinine clearance values below 40 ml/min. If this dose is inadequate to produce a diuresis within 20 minutes, the dose can be doubled every 20 minutes until a response occurs or until a maximum dose is reached. Various studies have reported a ceiling effect to furosemide of approximately 250 mg.[8,9] Therefore increasing the dose above this ceiling dose may not produce an increased response.

Although patients with renal dysfunction require larger doses to deliver diuretics into the urine, the remaining nephrons in these patients continue to function normally. Overall, sodium excretion may be limited as a result of diminished sodium filtration. To overcome this relative resistance, an effective response may occur by administering a large enough effective dose several times a day.

Certain disease states result in a diminished response that does not improve by administering larger doses. Although the mechanism for this effect is unknown, it has been reported in patients with congestive heart failure, cirrhosis, or nephrotic syndrome.[10] In these patients, multiple doses should be given rather than larger single doses. This finding implies a modest ceiling dose of loop diuretics in patients with congestive heart failure and cirrhosis.[10]

THIAZIDE DIURETICS

Thiazide diuretics (see Table 21-1) block sodium chloride reabsorption at the distal tubule and early collecting duct.[11] Thiazide diuretics also inhibit carbonic anhydrase in the proximal tubule. The clinical impact of thiazide diuretics actions in the proximal tubule are negligible, with the diuretic properties predominately being a result of the distal tubule mechanism.[12]

Thiazide diuretics are less potent agents than loop diuretics because only 5% of filtered sodium is reabsorbed in the distal tubule. Therefore these agents are used in patients with mild edematous states. Thiazide diuretics are effective down to a creatinine clearance of approximately 30 ml/min. Compared with loop diuretics, thiazide diuretics have a limited dose response curve. This results in a narrow difference between the maximum and minimum effective doses. Doses above 50 mg may not produce a greater diuresis, but they may predispose the patient to increased toxicity.

Doses above 50 mg may, however, be useful in the treatment of hypertension. The use of thiazide diuretics in the treatment of hypertension produces an effect initially as a result of diuresis-induced decreases in blood volume.[10] Long-term benefits of thiazide diuretics in hypertension are most likely not due to a diuretic response. One proposed mechanism is decreased peripheral vascular resistance.[13] Although the exact mechanism of action is unknown, hypertensive patients may respond to thiazide diuretic doses above 50 mg per day.

POTASSIUM-SPARING DIURETICS

The potassium-sparing diuretics (see Table 21-1) work in the distal tubule. Three agents are in this category: amiloride, spironolactone, and triamterene. Sodium reabsorption in the distal tubule occurs by mechanisms dependent upon and independent from aldosterone. These agents block sodium reabsorption by slightly different mechanisms of action. Spironolac-

tone blocks the receptor for aldosterone, whereas amiloride and triamterene block the entry of sodium into the kidney lumen. Based on the mechanism of action, spironolactone is specifically used for conditions known to have elevated aldosterone concentrations, such as hyperaldosteronism (primary and secondary), cirrhosis and ascites, adrenal hyperplasia, and renal artery stenosis. The most common use is in patients with cirrhosis and ascites. Because the duration of effect of spironolactone is 1 or more days, the dose should be increased every 3 or 4 days until the desired level of diuresis is attained.[14]

In the distal tubule, sodium is exchanged for potassium and hydrogen. Therefore the use of one of these agents blocks this exchange. Based on this effect, these agents are known as *potassium-sparing diuretics*, although they are not very potent diuretics. Potassium-sparing diuretics are frequently used in combination with thiazide diuretics. The rationale for the combination is that thiazide produces a better diuresis, whereas the potassium-sparing agent diminishes the potassium loss from the thiazide. This thought process is flawed.[10] Only about 5% of patients receiving thiazide diuretics become potassium depleted. In addition, the potassium-sparing agents may produce hyperkalemia, which is a more life-threatening situation than potassium depletion. Therefore prophylactic use of these agents should be discouraged.

Several variables may predispose patients receiving potassium-sparing diuretics to develop hyperkalemia. These include coadministration of the following:

- Potassium supplements
- Angiotensin-converting enzyme inhibitors
- Nonsteroidal antiinflammatory agents

In addition, patients with diminished renal function are likely to retain potassium.

Triamterene is a short-acting agent requiring multiple doses per day. Triamterene must be converted to an active metabolite by the liver; therefore this agent may be a poor choice in patients with liver dysfunction.[15] Amiloride has a moderately long half-life and does not require metabolic activation.

DIURETIC COMBINATIONS

Various diuretic combinations may be used in an attempt to obtain additive or synergistic effects in patients who respond poorly to one agent. By using agents with different sites of action within the nephron, the diuretic response may be enhanced. The most common combination is of a loop diuretic and a thiazide.[16] Although not consistently effective, combinations occasionally may result in a pronounced diuresis.

DIURETIC COMPLICATIONS

Diuretics have been used successfully for over 40 years, and, like all therapeutic agents, they have the potential to cause side effects. The majority of complications associated with diuretic use can be anticipated as an extension of their pharmacological activity, with volume depletion and electrolyte abnormalities being the most common. Other adverse effects are rare or idiosyncratic and cannot be anticipated nor prevented.

VOLUME DEPLETION

Because diuretics promote sodium and fluid excretion, elimination may exceed intake, resulting in volume depletion. Certain situations may predispose a patient to volume depletion (Box 21-1). Diuretic-induced volume depletion should be treated by discontinuation of the diuretic. Mild cases of volume depletion may respond to liberalization of sodium intake, whereas more severe cases will require intravenous saline replacement.

HYPOKALEMIA

Potassium is exchanged for sodium in the distal convoluted tubule and collecting duct. Any diuretic that increases sodium delivery to those regions may potentially induce hypokalemia. In addition to a direct potassium loss, diuretic-induced volume depletion produces reabsorption of sodium via release of aldosterone in the distal tubule in an effort to bolster intravascular volume. This additional sodium reabsorption also contributes to potassium excretion. Dietary sodium intake and chloride depletion may also influence potassium excretion.

Box 21-1	Causes of Volume Depletion With Diuretics

- Initiation of treatment or increased dose
- Improved compliance
- Reduced dietary sodium intake
- Development of diarrhea or enteric fluid loss (diarrhea)
- Drugs that impair diuretic administration
- Improved underlying disease state not requiring diuretics

Diuretic-induced hypokalemia appears to be dose related, with loop diuretics having a lower incidence than thiazide diuretics.[17] Although studies have tried to identify the incidence of diuretic-induced hypokalemia, it is impossible to predict whether a particular patient will develop hypokalemia.[18-20] The issue of potassium supplementation is also controversial. Who to treat, when to treat, and how to treat hypokalemia are all unresolved questions. At the center of this unresolved issue is whether hypokalemia poses a risk for arrhythmias or sudden cardiac death. Supplemental potassium should be considered in patients with a history of cardiac disease, patients with symptoms indicating hypokalemia, patients with a serum potassium level less than 3.0 mEq/L, and patients on digitalis therapy.[21]

Potassium-sparing diuretics may induce a hyperkalemic state in up to 8.6% of patients receiving spironolactone and up to 23% of patients receiving a potassium-sparing diuretic and potassium supplementation.[20,22]

ACID-BASE DISORDERS

With diuresis and volume depletion, hypokalemia and hypochloremia may result. This state may then cause a metabolic alkalosis, which is responsive to potassium and chloride replacement therapy. The exceptions are carbonic anhydrase inhibitors, whose use may result in metabolic acidosis.

BLOOD GLUCOSE CHANGES

Loop and thiazide diuretics have been associated with hyperglycemia. The average rise in serum glucose is between 6.5 mg/dl to 9.6 mg/dl, although cases of diabetic ketoacidosis have also been reported.[23,24] The severity of glucose elevation in these reports was related to the dose of diuretic used, as well as the drop in potassium levels. Although the cause of the hyperglycemia is not completely understood, several possible etiologies have been postulated. These include decreased pancreatic insulin release and insulin resistance with impaired uptake of glucose in response to insulin.

OTOTOXICITY

The loop diuretics may cause a dose-related ototoxicity consisting of tinnitus and clinical or subclinical hearing loss. The ototoxicity results from anatomical and chemical abnormalities produced within the inner ear.[21] Ototoxicity is related to the blood level of these agents. Therefore rapid infusion and drug accumulation with large parenteral doses in renal failure both predispose patients to ototoxicity. Reducing the infusion rate or administering the drug orally may alleviate the hearing loss.[25,26]

The majority of ototoxicity is reversible; however, cases of irreversible hearing loss have occurred. Ethacrynic acid has a higher likelihood of causing irreversible hearing loss.[26,27] Limited data on bumetanide indicate that it may have a lower incidence of ototoxicity than furosemide and ethacrynic acid.

To minimize diuretic induced ototoxicity, ethacrynic acid should be avoided. In addition, chronic doses greater than 500 mg in patients with advanced renal disease and repetitive dosing in patients with acute renal failure and rapid infusions should be avoided.

SUMMARY KEY TERMS AND CONCEPTS

- *Diuretics* represent a class of agents with a wide therapeutic index with a high propensity to cause toxicity if not properly used and monitored.
- *Effective use* of diuretics requires knowledge of the pharmacology of each class of agent, as well as an understanding of the patient's disease state.
- Diuretics have a wide array of *possible uses,* some of which are not related to net fluid losses.
- *Volume* and *electrolyte* disorders are the most likely and predictable consequences of diuretic use and can be anticipated based on the specific agent used.
- Other *adverse effects* are related to the entire class. Monitoring the patient may help mitigate these effects in some instances.

SELF-ASSESSMENT QUESTIONS

1. What is a diuretic?
2. Identify the five major groups of diuretics used clinically.
3. If an agent such as one of the loop diuretics causes a loss of potassium, how will this lead to a metabolic alkalosis?
4. Which diuretics would preserve potassium?
5. What is the potential effect of a carbonic anhydrase inhibitor on acid-base balance?
6. Explain how a diuretic such as furosemide can be helpful in acute congestive heart failure with pulmonary and vascular edema?

Answers to Self-Assessment Questions are found in Appendix A.

CLINICAL SCENARIO

Case courtesy **Douglas J. Pearce, MD, cardiologist**

A 73-year-old white male presents to the emergency department with a chief complaint of severe dyspnea that began about 8 hours before presentation. The patient's history is significant for long-standing hypertension and coronary artery disease. In 1985, he had an inferior myocardial infarction and then in 1989 had another myocardial infarction of unknown location. After this, he underwent a coronary artery bypass graft procedure. His left internal mammary artery was used to bypass the left anterior descending artery, a saphenous vein graft was placed to the posterior descending artery, and a sequential saphenous vein graft was placed to the first and second obtuse marginal arteries. Cardiac catheterization before bypass grafting revealed inferior wall akinesis with global hypokinesis of the remaining walls. His left ventricular ejection fraction was estimated to be 40%. Since his bypass surgery, he has not had any further angina or infarctions, but he has had two admissions for acute pulmonary edema. Both episodes were felt to have been precipitated by medical noncompliance, but this could not be confirmed. At this presentation, the patient again denies chest pain. He states that he began feeling dyspneic the night before presentation and then awoke about 5 AM severely dyspneic and coughing up white, foamy phlegm. When queried about his compliance with his medicines, he admits that he sometimes forgets to take his clonidine.

The patient has chronic renal insufficiency and has had right inguinal hernia repair. He denies any allergies.

The patient is on the following medications: clonidine 0.1 mg PO bid; atenolol 50 mg PO qhs; aspirin 325 mg PO qd; transdermal nitroglycerin 0.4 mg qh (he places a patch on in the morning and takes it off at bedtime); and furosemide 40 mg PO q AM.

Physical examination reveals an elderly white male in obvious respiratory distress. His vital signs are P, 120 beats/min and regular; RR, 32 beats/min; and BP, 230/140 mm Hg, and he is afebrile. His neck shows positive jugular venous distention. Heart auscultation reveals a regular rate, with an I/VI systolic ejection murmur, negative S_3, and positive S_4. His lungs demonstrate bibasilar rales half of the way up the thorax. His abdomen is flat and bowel sounds are present; no masses or tenderness are identified. His extremities are slightly cool, and pulses are felt in all extremities, but are somewhat thready.

The patient's laboratory results are Na^+, 138 mEq/L; K^+, 3.6 mEq/L; BUN, 40 mg/dl; and creatinine, 2.8 mg/dl. His ECG shows sinus tachycardia, with inferior Q waves and lateral Q waves of questionable significance. A chest radiograph shows mild cardiomegaly with bilateral infiltrates consistent with pulmonary edema.

This is a 73-year-old white male with ischemic heart disease, hypertension, and chronic renal insufficiency. His history, physical examination, and diagnostic data are consistent with acute pulmonary edema. His blood pressure is markedly elevated. There is a history of possible medical noncompliance, which would make one suspicious that he has not taken his clonidine. Acute hypertension in the face of already impaired left ventricular systolic function is a common cause of acute pulmonary edema. Of note, the patient does have some evidence of renal insufficiency with an elevated creatinine. His potassium is at the lower end of normal, probably secondary to his furosemide.

True or False: In addition to oxygen and morphine sulfate 2 mg intravenously, a thiazide-type diuretic should be administered immediately.
If the patient fails to respond to furosemide 80 mg intravenously, should another loop diuretic be tried?
True or False: When the patient begins to diurese, close observation of the potassium level will be needed.

Answers to Clinical Scenario Questions are found in Appendix A.

REFERENCES

1. Chennavasin P and others: Pharmacodynamic analysis of the furosemide-probenecid interaction in man, *Kidney Int* 16:187, 1979.
2. Dikshit K and others: Renal and extrarenal hemodynamic effects of furosemide in congestive heart failure after myocardial infarction, *N Engl J Med* 288:1087, 1973.
3. Bourland WA, Day DK, Williamson HE: The role of the kidney in the early nondiuretic action of furosemide to reduce elevated left atrial pressure in the hypervolemic dog, *J Pharmacol Exp Ther* 202:221, 1977.
4. Francis GS and others: Acute vasoconstrictior response to intravenous furosemide in patients with chronic heart failure, *Ann Intern Med* 103:1, 1985.
5. Hammarlund-Udenaes M, Benet LZ: Furosemide pharmacokinetics and pharmacodynamics in health and disease: an update, *J Pharmacokinet Biopharm* 17:1, 1988.
6. Beerman B, Leinfelder J, Anderson SA: Clinical pharmacology of torsemide, a new loop diuretic, *Clin Pharmacol Ther* 42:187, 1987.
7. Brater DC: Diuretics. In Williams RL, Brater DC, Mordenti J, eds: *Rational therapeutics: a clinical pharmacologic guide for the health professional*, New York, 1989, Marcel Dekker.
8. Voelker JR and others: Comparison of loop diuretics in patients with chronic renal insufficiency: mechanism of difference in response, *Kidney Int* 32:572, 1987.
9. Rudy DW and others: The pharmacodynamics of intravenous and oral torsemide in patients with chronic renal insufficiency, *Clin Pharmacol Ther* 56:39, 1994.
10. Brater DC: Pharmacology of diuretics, *Am J Med Sci* 319:38, 2000.
11. Seely JF, Dirks JH: Site of action of diuretic drugs, *Kidney Int* 11:1, 1977.
12. Kanau RT, Weller DR, Webb HL: Clarification of the site of action of chlorthalidone in the rat nephron, *J Clin Invest* 56:401, 1975.
13. van Brummelen P, Man in't Veld AJ, Schalekamp MADH: Hemodynamic changes during long-term thiazide treatment of essential hypertension in responders and non-responders, *Clin Pharmacol Ther* 27:328, 1980.
14. Ochs HR and others: Spironolactone, *Am Heart J* 96:389, 1978.
15. Villenuve JP, Rocheleau F, Raymond G: Triamterene kinetics and dynamics in cirrhosis, *Clin Pharmacol Ther* 35:831, 1984.
16. Sica DA, Gehr TWB: Diuretic combinations in refractory oedema states, *Clin Pharmacokinet* 30:229, 1996.
17. Carlsen JE and others: Relation between dose of bendrofluazide, antihypertensive effect, and adverse biochemical effects, *Br Med J* 300:975, 1990.
18. Schnaper HW and others: Potassium restoration in hypertensive patients made hypokalemic by hydrochlorothiazide, *Arch Intern Med* 149:2677, 1989.
19. Toner JM, Ramsay LE: Thiazide-induced hypokalemia: prevalence higher in women, *Br J Clin Pharmacol* 18:449, 1984.
20. Widmer P and others: Diuretic-related hypokalemia: the role of diuretics, potassium supplements, glucocorticoids and beta 2-adrenoceptor agonists: results from the Comprehensive Hospital Drug Monitoring Programme, Berne (CHDM), *Eur J Clin Pharmacol* 49:31, 1995.
21. Greenberg A: Diuretic complications, *Am J Med Sci* 319:10, 2000.
22. Greenblatt DJ, Koch-Weser J: Adverse reactions to spironolactone: a report from the Boston collaborative drug surveillance program, *J Am Med Assoc* 225:40, 1973.
23. Amery A and other: Glucose intolerance during diuretic therapy: results of trial by the European Working Party on Hypertension in the Elderly, *Lancet* 1:681, 1978.
24. Savage PJ and others: Influence of long-term, low-dose, diuretic-based, antihypertensive therapy on glucose, lipid, uric acid, and potassium levels in older men and women with isolated systolic hypertension, *Arch Intern Med* 158:741, 1998.
25. Dormans TP, Gerlag PG: Combination of high-dose furosemide and hydrochlorothiazide in the treatment of refractory congestive heart failure, *Eur Heart J* 17:1867, 1996.
26. Rybak LP: Ototoxicity of loop diuretics, *Otolaryngol Clin North Am* 26:829, 1993.
27. Seligmann H and others: Drug-induced tinnitus and other hearing disorders, *Drug Saf* 14:198, 1996.

CHAPTER 22

Drugs Affecting the Central Nervous System

Charles G. Durbin, Jr.

The most widely used drugs, both therapeutic and recreational, are those affecting the central nervous system. Humans are intrinsically concerned with and perhaps even defined by the processes of thinking and feeling. These processes originate within the brain. Thoughts and feelings, although poorly understood, reside primarily with neurochemical interactions and balance in the brain. Drugs that affect neurotransmitters are used to affect perception and mood. Whereas the gross anatomy of the brain has been elegantly described, the complex interaction of various brain areas and individual neurons is less well understood.

In general, the cortex, or outer covering, of the brain is considered to be the location of thought, memory, self-awareness, and personality. Perception of sensation and control of body movement, including speech, are also represented in specific areas of the cortex. The midbrain functions as a relay station for information traveling to and from the cortex. It also integrates and modulates autonomic functions; this function occurs primarily in the hypothalamus. The brainstem, or medulla, contains the control areas for autonomic functions such as breathing and cardio-vascular control, as well as the areas responsible for alertness, the reticular activating system. The spinal cord enters the brain at the brainstem, and the cerebellum, immediately behind the brainstem, affects fine motor control and coordinates movement. Much of our understanding of brain organization and function comes from removing areas of brain and identifying resulting deficits in animals. Some information has been acquired by studying humans who have had strokes or destructive brain surgery. These observations have led to a general understanding of functional neuroanatomy and recognizing that the brain can recover significant function after damage to important areas.

More complicated than the gross anatomy would suggest, individual neurons have a wide array of connections with many different neurons in diverse areas of the brain. These patterns are different in different individuals and also change with time in the same individual. It is apparent that many functions are represented in multiple ways, making them resistant to damage. Although the number of individual neurons does not increase after adulthood is reached, the brain is able to change and increase the number of connections

411

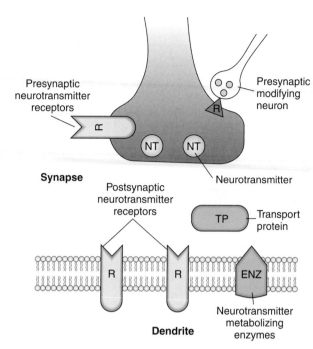

Figure 22-1   Schematic of the components of neuron-to-neuron communication. Neurotransmitter is synthesized in the nerve and transported and stored in the nerve terminal. Other components of neurotransmission include transport proteins *(TP)* in the synapse, receptors *(R)* on the postjunctional membrane, receptors *(R)* on the prejunctional membrane, membrane-bound enzymes *(ENZ)*, and modifying neurons.

and complexity of the neuronal circuitry throughout life. Although each neuron releases only a single neurotransmitter and occasionally a coneurotransmitter, the actual effect of these neurotransmitters on the next neuron is modified by additional presynaptic and postsynaptic neurons, which may inhibit or augment the primary neurotransmitter's effect.

Several diseases appear related to loss of particular neurons with specific neurotransmitters. For example, Parkinson's disease is caused by a loss of dopamine-containing neurons in the *substantia nigra* area of the midbrain. It is characterized by resting tremor; rigidity; bradykinesia, or slowness in effecting movement; gait disturbances; and postural instability. Treatment of the disease involves increasing the amount of dopamine contained in and released from the remaining neurons.[1,2] Some forms of depression are believed to be caused by reduced activity of norepinephrine neurons in the brain, particularly those in the *locus ceruleus*.[3] There appears to be a decrease in both the preganglionic augmentation effects of serotonin and direct stimulatory effects of norepinephrine. Treatment is to restore more normal activity of the norepinephrine neurons by inhibiting the reuptake of serotonin by modulating neurons, enhancing the amount of norepinephrine released, and increasing the duration of its effects in the synapse.

It is clear from the diversity of neuronal connections and the plasticity of the central nervous system that drugs used for central nervous system therapy will have widespread and varying effects. This functional and chemical complexity of the brain and peripheral nervous system explains why side effects and toxicities are common with central nervous system drug therapy.

NEUROTRANSMITTERS

Each neuron releases predominantly one type of neurotransmitter from its axon to synapse with the next neuron. If enough receptors are activated on the postsynaptic membrane, electrical depolarization occurs and a signal is passed to the next neuron. The functional anatomy and components of neurotransmission are illustrated in Figures 22-1 and 22-2. Released neurotransmitters are bound to and transported by proteins in the synapse, taken back up by the releasing nerve terminal, repackaged into vesicles, and recycled. Bound neurotransmitters are not available for receptor interactions, and alterations in the transport proteins in amount or affinity affect the signal propagation potential. Some of the released neurotransmitter is metabolized by membrane-bound enzymes on the postsynaptic cell membrane. The resulting constituent components are taken up presynaptically

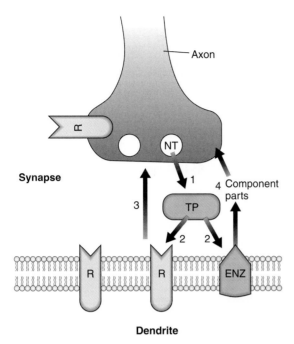

Figure 22-2   Schematic for the pathways that neurotransmitters follow after release into the synapse. After axonal depolarization, the stored neurotransmitter *(NT)* is released in the synapse *(1)*, where it is bound to the transport or carrier protein *(TP)*. NT is transported to and binds with postjunctional receptors *(2)*, is metabolized by membrane-bound enzymes *(2)*, is actively taken up by the releasing neuron *(3)*, or is released and binds to prejunctional receptors. NT substance that is degraded to its component parts is taken up by the releasing neuron to be resynthesized and reused *(4)*.

Table 22-1

Central nervous system chemicals that function as neurotransmitters

CHEMICAL CLASS	NEUROTRANSMITTER
Biogenic amines	Norepinephrine
	Epinephrine
	Dopamine
	Acetylcholine
	Histamine
	Serotonin (5-hydroxytryptamine)
Amino acids	γ-Aminobutyric acid (GABA)
	Glutamate
	Glycine
	Aspartate
Nucleotides and nucleosides	Adenosine triphosphate
	Adenosine
Peptides	Thyrotropin-releasing hormone
	Enkephalins
	Angiotensin II
	Oxytocin
	Vasopressin
	Bradykinin
	Dynorphin
	Substance P
	Substance K
	Neuropeptide Y
	β-Endorphin
	Luteinizing-hormone–releasing factor
	Corticotropin-releasing factor
	Somatostatin
	Secretin
	Melanocyte-stimulating hormone

and used as precursors for neurotransmitter synthesis. Receptors on both the presynaptic membrane and the postsynaptic membrane specific for the released chemicals, as well as for other chemicals from modulating and neighboring neurons, affect the activity of the neuron.

Examples of chemicals that behave as neurotransmitters are listed in Table 22-1. The effect of the neurotransmitter released is determined by many factors, including the amount of neurotransmitter released, type and quantity of transport proteins, previous release of neurotransmitters, presence of modifying substances, efficiency of reuptake processes, and activities of modulating interneurons. Specifics of this transmission modulation system differ for various brain areas, mental functions, and neurotransmitters. Central nervous system–active drugs may have effects on specific parts of a neurotransmitter system or have generalized effects on brain function. Augmentation or inhibition of neurotransmission can result from drug interaction at any of the sites illustrated in Figures 22-1 and 22-2.

DRUGS THAT ALTER MOOD

ANTIDEPRESSANTS

Depression is one of the most common psychiatric disorders and a major cause of worldwide disability. In the United States the 1-month prevalence of a major depressive episode has been estimated to be more than 2% of the population.[4] The Global Burden

Table 22-2

Drugs used to treat depression

CLASS	GENERIC DRUG	U.S. BRAND NAMES
Tricyclic antidepressants (TCAs)	Amitriptyline	Elavil, Endep
	Clomipramine	Anafranil
	Desipramine	Norpramin
	Doxepin	Sinequan, Adepin
	Imipramine	Tofranil
	Nortriptyline	Aventyl HCL, Pamelor
	Protriptyline	Vivactil
	Trimipramine	Surmontil
Tetracyclic antidepressants	Maprotiline	Ludiomil
Monoamine oxidase inhibitors	Brofaromine*	
	Moclobemide*	
	Phenelzine	Nardil
	Tranylcypromine	Parnate
Selective serotonin reuptake inhibitors (SSRI)	Citalopram	Celexa
	Fluoxetine	Prozac, Luvox
	Paroxetine	Paxil, Paxil CR
	Sertraline	Zoloft
Serotonin and norepinephrine reuptake inhibitors	Mirtazapine	Remeron
	Venlafaxine	Effexor, Effexor XR
	Milnacipran*	
Serotonin receptor antagonists	Retanserin*	
	Nefazodone	Serzone
Serotonin receptor agonists	Felsinoxan*	
	Gepirone*	
	Ipsaprone*	
	Tandospirone*	
GABA-mimetics	Fengebine*	
Dopamine reuptake inhibitor	Bupropion	Wellbutrin, Zyban
Herbal remedy	Hypericum	St. John's wort
Miscellaneous drugs	Amoxapine	Asendin
	Trazodone	Desyrel

*Not currently available in the United States.

of Disease Study found unipolar depression to be the fourth leading cause of worldwide disability, even after excluding deaths from suicide.[5] The prevalence of major depressive disorder may be on the increase, and it is predicted that by 2020, unipolar major depression will be the second leading cause of disability worldwide.[6] Although genetic factors are important, most cases of depression are believed to be caused by reduced activity of norepinephrine neurons, particularly those in the limbic system. Therapy has been to increase the activity of these neurons directly or by increasing the preganglionic stimulatory neurotransmitter, serotonin.

The classes of drugs used to treat depression are listed in Table 22-2 and include the tricyclic antidepressants (TCAs), the monoamine oxidase inhibitors (MAOI), the selective serotonin uptake blockers (SSRI), and unrelated other drugs that have a variety of structures and actions. The side effect profile of the different groups varies widely. The side effects for some antidepressant drugs are listed in Table 22-3. TCAs, which have been used for over 50 years, have widespread effects in the central and peripheral nervous system. They are relatively toxic and have serious side effects. A major side effect of the TCAs is

Table 22-3

Incidence of various side effects of commonly used antidepressants

MEDICATION	SEDATION	AGITATION	ANTICHO-LINERGIC EFFECTS*	POSTURAL HYPO-TENSION	GASTRO-INTESTINAL UPSET	SEXUAL DYSFUNCTION	WEIGHT GAIN	WEIGHT LOSS
SEROTONIN AND NOREPINEPHRINE REUPTAKE INHIBITORS								
Tricyclics (Tertiary Amines)								
Amitriptyline	++++	0	++++	+++	+	+	++	0
Doxepin	++++	0	++++	+++	+	+	+	0
Imipramine	++++	0	++++	+++	+	+	+	0
Tricyclics (Secondary Amines)								
Desipramine	+++	0	+++	++	+	+	+	0
Nortriptyline	+++	0	+++	++	+	+	+	0
Bicyclic								
Venlafaxine†	++	+	++	0	+++	++	0	+
SELECTIVE SEROTONIN REUPTAKE INHIBITORS								
Citalopram	0	0	+	0	++	+	+	+
Fluoxetine	+	++	+	0	++	++	+	+
Paroxetine	++	0	+	0	++	++	+	+
Sertraline	+	+	+	0	++	++	+	+
SEROTONIN ANTAGONIST								
Mirtazapine	+++	0	++	+	0	0	++	0
NOREPINEPHRINE REUPTAKE INHIBITOR, DOPAMINE REUPTAKE INHIBITOR								
Bupropion	+	++	++	0	++	0	+	++
SEROTONIN ANTAGONISTS AND REUPTAKE INHIBITORS								
Nefazodone	++	0	++	+	+	0	0	0
Trazodone	++++	0	++	+	+	0	+	+

From Whooley MA, Simon GE: Managing depression in medical outpatients. *New Engl J Med* 343:1947, 2000.
0, None; +, minimal (<5% of patients); ++, low frequency (5% to 20%); +++, moderate frequency (21% to 40%); ++++, high frequency (>40%).
*Side effects may include dry mouth, dry eyes, blurred vision, constipation, urinary retention, tachycardia, or confusion.
†Venlafaxine may cause a dose-related elevation in diastolic blood pressure; monitoring of blood pressure is recommended.

cholinergic blockade. This may result in tachycardia, dry mouth, blurred vision, constipation, urinary retention, and orthostatic hypotension. Acute effects include sedation; toxic overdose is characterized by central nervous system stimulation, including seizures; and cardiac tachyarrhythmias, including *torsade de points*. Both TCAs and MAOIs have been associated with an increase in cardiovascular complications, especially in depressed patients who have preexisting cardiac disease. These complications are less likely to occur when a therapeutic dosage is ad-

ministered. Injuries because of falls are more likely in elderly, depressed patients as a result of orthostatic hypotension from TCAs. Because the intestinal mucosa is rich in MAO enzymes, limiting the uptake of dietary catecholamines, MAOIs can cause problems with hypertension, including hypertensive crisis when patients consume food with a high concentration of tyramine (e.g., cheese and red wine), a precursor of serotonin.

The SSRIs differ structurally and in side-effect profile from TCAs and MAOIs. They appear to be effective for treatment of depression and are much safer than TCAs and MAOIs. Other classes of drugs listed in Table 22-2 have varying effects on the norepinephrine-serotonin system, and have been developed to have fewer and less severe side effects (see Table 22-3).

PSYCHOTHERAPEUTIC AGENTS

Psychotic illnesses are differentiated from neuroses primarily by the degree of dysfunction and the presence of severe derangement of thought and perception. In addition to psychotherapy, they often require pharmacological treatment, usually directed at reducing the effect of the neurotransmitter dopamine in the limbic system of the midbrain. The drugs used are termed *neuroleptics,* literally meaning, "taking hold of the brain." *Neuroleptic* refers to the effects on cognition and behavior of this group of antipsychotic drugs, which produce a state of apathy, lack of initiative, and limited range of emotion in nonpsychotic individuals. These drugs are sometimes referred to as *major tranquilizers.* In psychotic patients, they cause a reduction in confusion and agitation and normalization of psychomotor activity. Some of these drugs are used to control agitation in hospitalized patients not affected by a specific psychosis. A list of some of the common neuroleptics is found in Table 22-4.

Side effects of the neuroleptic drugs are related to blocking of dopamine, and to a lesser extent, other neurotransmitters in other areas of the brain. By blocking cholinergic neurons, they produce tachycardia, dry mouth, blurred vision, constipation, and urinary retention. In the chemotactic trigger zone (vomiting center) they may suppress nausea and vomiting. Some neuroleptic agents are used clinically for this effect. In the basal ganglia, dopamine inhibition causes rigidity and ataxia much like Parkinson's disease. Neuroleptic agents can cause orthostatic hypotension by peripheral α-blockade. Intentional or accidental overdose can result in cardiovascular compromise and respiratory muscle failure. Treatment is supportive and may need to be provided for a prolonged time because of the extremely long half-lives of these agents.

ANXIOLYTICS

The benzodiazepines are a group of agents that have been used to reduce anxiety under a variety of circumstances. They are also used as amnesics, preventing conversion of short-term experience into

Table 22-4

Drugs that are used in the management of psychotic disorders

CLASS	GENERIC DRUG	BRAND NAMES
Phenothiazine	Acetophenazine	Tindal
	Chlorpromazine	Thorazine
	Fluphenazine	Prolixin
	Mesoridazine	Serentil
	Perphenazine	Trilafon
	Prochlorperazine	Compazine
	Promazine	Sparine
	Thioridazine	Mellaril
	Trifluoperazine	Stelazine
	Triflupromazine	Vesprin
Thioxanthenes	Chlorprothixene	Taractan
	Thiothixene	Navane
Butyrophenones	Droperidol	Inapsine
	Haloperidol	Haldol
Miscellaneous agents	Clozapine	Clozaril
	Loxapine	Loxitane
	Molindone	Moban
	Olanzapine	Zyprexa
	Pimozide	Orap
	Quetiapine	Seroquel
	Risperidone	Risperdal
	Lithium	
Cholinesterase inhibitors	Donepezil	Aricept
	Tacrine	Cognex

permanent memory. By themselves, they cause no change in respiration; however, they may augment the depression induced by opioids. They have little effect on cardiac function and are very safe agents from this standpoint. Benzodiazepines are excellent induction agents when providing general anesthesia and are useful in preventing unpleasant recall during uncomfortable interventions. They may be used as somnifics. These agents are used to terminate seizures and will elevate seizure threshold. Benzodiazepines exert their effects by binding to benzodiazepine receptors in the γ-aminobutyric acid (GABA) receptor complex on neurons, increasing the GABA chloride channel permeability, which hyperpolarizes the neuron, making depolarization less likely (Figure 22-3). A specific antagonist, flumazenil (Romazicon) can reverse the sedative effects of the benzodiazepines.

Several other drugs are used to treat anxiety and other neuroses. Some of these are listed with the ben-

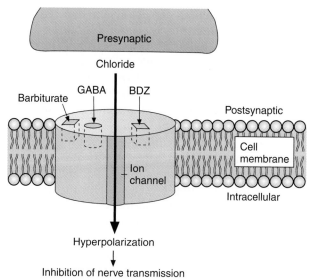

Figure 22-3 The mode of action by which barbiturates and benzodiazepines *(BDZ)* depress central nervous system function; stimulation of receptors on the chloride ion channel facilitates γ-aminobutyric acid (GABA)-induced inhibition of neuronal function.

zodiazepines in Table 22-5. Their mechanisms of action are not related to interactions with the benzodiazepine receptor or the GABA system. Some of the drugs in Table 22-5 are used to promote sleep; these and other nonrelated sleep-inducing agents are listed in Table 22-6. Although they induce sleep, benzodiazepines and other drug classes interfere with the normal sleep-cycles by reducing the amount of time spent in rapid eye movement (REM) sleep.

BARBITURATES

One of the oldest group of sedative drugs, the barbiturates, is a derivative of barbituric acid. Because of their toxic potential and rapid development of tolerance, they have largely been replaced by the benzodiazepines, except for a few specialized uses. Several ultra–short-acting barbiturates are used for anesthetic induction (thiopental, thiamylal, methohexital), as hypnotics (pentobarbital, secobarbital), and for seizure control and prophylaxis (phenobarbital). Use of barbiturates as hypnotics is limited by rapid development of tolerance and reduction in the quality of sleep (decreased amount of REM). They are potent inducers of the CYP 450 drug metabolizing system that can alter the levels of many other drugs. Although many of the barbiturates' therapeutic effects are

Table 22-5
Drugs used to treat anxiety and neuroses

CLASS	GENERIC DRUG	U.S. BRAND NAMES
Benzodiazepines	Alprazolam	Xanax
	Clorazepate dipotassium	Tranxene
	Chlordiazepoxide	Librium
	Diazepam	Valium, Dizac
	Estazolam	Prosom
	Flurazepam	Dalmane
	Halazepam	Paxipam
	Lorazepam	Ativan
	Midazolam	Versed
	Oxazepam	Serax
	Temazepam	Restoril
	Triazolam	Halcion
	Prazepam	Centrax
Benzodiazepine antagonist	Flumazenil	Romazicon
Other anxiolytics	Buspirone HCl	BuSpar
	Chlormezanone	Trancopal
	Doxepin HCl	Sinequan
	Hydroxyzine	Atarax, Vistaril
	Meprobamate	Equanil, Miltown
Barbiturates		

Table 22-6
Medications used to induce sleep

CLASS	GENERIC DRUG	BRAND NAMES
Benzodiazepine	Estazolam	Prosom
	Flurazepam HCl	Dalmane
	Quazepam	Doral
	Temazepam	Restoril
	Triazolam	Halcion
Barbiturate	Secobarbital	Seconal
	Pentobarbital	Nembutal
	Butabarbital	Butisol
Antihistamine	Cyproheptadine	Periactin
	Diphenhydramine	Benadryl
	Hydroxyzine	Atarax, Vistaril
Miscellaneous	Acetylcarbromal	Paxarel
	Chloral hydrate	
	Ethanol	Alcohol
	Ethinamate	Valmid
	Glutethimide	Doriden
	Paraldehyde	Parnal
	Zaleplon	Sonata
	Zolpidem	Ambien

mediated by a specific receptor at the GABA-mediated inhibitory receptor, they have widespread depressive effects on neuron activity. Intentional or accidental overdose results in respiratory arrest and cardiovascular collapse because of brain control center depression. This drug class also carries a high risk of addiction and abuse. Severe withdrawal symptoms, including seizures, occur after abruptly stopping chronic barbiturates.

OTHER HYPNOTICS

Difficulty sleeping is a common clinical complaint that frequently results in the prescription of a hypnotic. In addition to the short-acting benzodiazepines and barbiturates mentioned above, several other sedatives are used for inducing sleep. Unfortunately, all disrupt sleep patterns and may not improve overall well-being. Hypnotics to induce sleep are generally recommended for brief periods (1 or 2 weeks). However, some patients remain on these medications continually for years. In addition to drugs interacting with the GABA complex, many medications generally depress brain function and cause sedation and induce sleep. Commonly referred to as hypnotics (meaning sleep-inducing, not to be confused with "hypnosis") or soporifics, medications used for sleep enhancement are listed in Table 22-6.

ETHYL ALCOHOL

Alcohol is a by-product of sugar fermentation. It is used as a socially acceptable nonprescription, sedative-hypnotic agent. Ingested to excess, it behaves like a general anesthetic, depressing all brain areas, resulting in loss of voluntary muscle control and consciousness. At toxic levels (400 to 600 mg/dl, blood alcohol level) the respiratory center is affected and death as a result of respiratory arrest is likely. The disinhibiting effects of modest alcohol intoxication result from depression of higher cortical behavior control centers, probably by decreasing the GABA receptor effects of endogenous mediators. At higher levels, diffuse membrane disruptive effects occur, causing generalized neurological depression. When combined with other sedative-hypnotic drugs, the degree of intoxication is additive. Chronic alcohol ingestion results in upregulation of GABA receptors and other brain functions, with the development of tolerance to the intoxicating and toxic depression caused by alcohol. Abrupt withdrawal after prolonged use may result in the syndrome of *delirium tremens* (DTs),

characterized by central nervous system hyperactivity, including hyperthermia, increased blood pressure, muscle twitching, hallucinosis, and seizures. The mortality from DTs is high, ranging from 5% to 10% if seizures occur. The withdrawal syndrome can be prevented or treated with any of the sedative-hypnotic drugs, and usually a benzodiazepine is chosen because of its relative safety.

Because alcohol is a carbohydrate, if ingested in large quantities, it replaces many of the dietary calories and decreases appetite. Protein, fat, and vitamin malnutrition are often seen with chronic alcohol abuse. Alcohol is metabolized to CO_2 and H_2O, producing acetaldehyde in the process. Because it is a food, ethyl alcohol saturates the metabolic enzyme system and undergoes first-order elimination kinetics. This means that a constant amount of alcohol is removed per unit time, rather than a fixed percentage of the blood concentration as with most other drugs. In the average person, this results in about 10 to 12 g of alcohol removed per hour.

PAIN TREATMENT

Pain is a common human problem. Because pain is a subjective, unpleasant experience, it is difficult objectively to observe and quantitate. Recognition of the physiological and psychological consequences of inadequate pain treatment has led to increased attention to pain control in patients. In hospitalized patients, estimation of pain has been raised to the level of a vital sign, on par with blood pressure or respiratory rate. Pain is now often referred to as the "fifth vital sign." Besides the difficulty of estimating the amount of pain, it is well known that many factors alter patients' responses to a given degree of discomfort. Physiological, social, and psychological factors profoundly alter patients' perception and tolerance of pain.[7,8] The meaning of pain to the individual can affect the reported pain and the response of the pain to treatment. It is helpful to view the pain experience as composed of at least two components: the sensation of *pain* as mediated by the central nervous system receiving nociceptive input from peripheral pain receptors; and *suffering*, the negative, personal emotional response to the pain experience. The integration and expression of these two components produces the pain behavior, which influences the patient's analgesic requirements. Medications may be directed at the origin, integration, or interpretation of the pain experience. Often combinations of medications are more effective than a single approach to this common problem.

Nonanalgesic drugs also affect perception and tolerance of pain. Sedative drugs such as the barbiturates and benzodiazepines appear to reduce pain tolerance, actually increasing the amount of pain perceived and reported by patients receiving them. This probably occurs by reducing cortical modulation of the pain perception, thereby increasing pain behaviors. These agents, when combined with analgesics, however, seem to decrease the painful experience and enhance analgesia. When interviewed after resolution of the pain episode, patients do not usually report having experienced pain of the extreme magnitude that was perceived by caregivers.

Another factor that must be taken into account when assessing pain is that patients have poor pain memories. With time, ability to recall the severity and characteristic of pain diminishes. This applies to the effects of treatment as well. Patients asked whether past pain treatment was effective almost always report improvement in pain, even if objective evaluation at the time documents no change or even worsening pain.[9] Antidepressants combined with analgesics are used to treat chronic pain states. They may be effective by modifying the depressed mood that accompanies chronic discomfort.

Although there are external clues to the presence and magnitude of a person's pain, personal reports are the only way to judge the presence and magnitude of pain. Visual or numerical analog pain scales (VAS) are the most commonly employed methods for estimating the magnitude of pain. The simplest and most common pain scale employed is an 11-point scale with 10 being the worst imaginable pain and 0 being totally without pain. Patients are asked to rate their pain from the "worst imaginable pain" as a "10" to "no pain at all" at "0." These scales appear to have internal and external validity.[10-12] The numerical rating is convenient and recognizable, and it lends itself to frequent repetition and consistent reporting. In children, a series of smiling and frowning faces, such as the Wong/Baker Rating Scale, may be used to allow the child to report the degree of pain.[13] These scales help in assessing the adequacy of analgesia and also create a shorthand way for patients to communicate their need for additional analgesia to the bedside caregiver.

Caregivers must integrate VAS reports, patient pain behaviors, and vital signs with their own biases[14] as to the degree of pain that "should" be present to decide whether to administer additional analgesic drugs.[15] It appears that caregivers often deliver inadequate amounts of analgesics.[16] Inappropriate expectations of the degree of pain in both the patient and caregiver contribute to this reluctance to administer potent analgesics. Acute pain remains undertreated in many patients.

NONSTEROIDAL ANTIINFLAMMATORY DRUGS

One of the frequently used analgesic classes, nonsteroidal antiinflammatory drugs (NSAIDs), is employed to treat moderate pain (Table 22-7). NSAIDs work by affecting the hypothalamus and by inhibiting the production of inflammatory mediators, primarily prostaglandins, at the peripheral site of the painful stimulus. The salicylates are the oldest member of this class and have been known for over 100 years for their effects as antipyretics. Aspirin is a common component of over-the-counter (OTC) analgesics and cold remedies. Aspirin decreases the synthesis of prostaglandin by irreversibly inhibiting both of the cyclooxygenase enzymes 1 and 2 (COX-1 and COX-2). COX-1 is primarily located on tissues, including blood vessels, kidney, and gastric mucosa, and COX-2 is primarily associated with inflammation. Unlike aspirin, others in this group reversibly inhibit these enzymes and may have fewer or less severe side effects. Selective COX-2 agents appear to have similar efficacy and a better safety profile.

Gastric irritation and ulceration are major problems with administering NSAIDs. Renal injury can result from prolonged use and high dosage of these medications. They also inhibit platelet aggregation and this compounds the problem of gastrointestinal bleeding. The antiplatelet effects are used therapeutically either after or to prevent cardiac thrombosis. Aspirin use in childhood febrile illness has been associated with an increased incidence of Reye's syndrome, an often fatal rise in intracranial pressure associated with massive hepatic dysfunction.[17,18] Allergic reactions to this class of drugs is common. Rashes, urticaria, angioneurotic edema, asthma, and anaphylaxis have been seen.

Acetaminophen (Tylenol), although a weak inhibitor of the cyclooxygenase system, has no significant antiinflammatory effects but is effective in relieving mild to moderate pain. It does not inhibit platelets or cause gastric ulcers. In large doses, it can cause lethal hepatic necrosis. Because it is used in many nonprescription cold preparations, accidental

Table 22-7

Nonsteroidal antiinflammatory drugs

CLASS	GENERIC DRUGS	BRAND NAMES
Nonspecific cyclooxygenase inhibitors		
Salicylates	Aspirin	
	Choline salicylate	
	Diflunisal	Dolobid
	Magnesium salicylate	
	Salsalate	Amigesic, Disalcid
	Sodium salicylate	
	Sodium thiosalicylate	
Aniline derivatives	Acetaminophen	Tylenol, Tempra
	Phenacetin	
Indoles	Etodolac	Lodine
	Indomethacin	Indocin
	Sulindac	Clinoril
Propionic acid derivatives	Ibuprofen	Advil, Motrin
	Fenoprofen	Nalfon
	Flurbiprofen	Ansaid
	Ketoprofen	Orudis
	Naproxen	Naprosyn, Naprelan, Anaprox
	Oxaprozin	Daypro
Piroxicam derivative	Piroxicam	Feldene
Pyrazolone derivative	Phenylbutazone	
Miscellaneous	Diclofenac	Voltaren, Cataflam, Arthrotec
	Ketorolac	Toradol
	Meclofenamate	Meclomen
	Mefenamic acid	Ponstel
	Nabumetone	Relafen
	Tolmetin	Tolectin
COX-2 inhibitors	Celecoxib	Celerex
	Meloxicam	Mobic
	Rofecoxib	Vioxx

overdose from combined dosing during self-medication occasionally occurs.

Recently, selective COX-2 inhibitors have been released into clinical practice. They should have fewer gastrointestinal side effects and fewer effects on platelet and white blood cell function. Their role in treatment of pain is yet to be determined. Patients with sulfa allergies and asthma must be cautious with these as well as all of the NSAIDs.

OPIOID ANALGESICS

Opioids or narcotic analgesic are derivatives of the naturally occurring drug mixture opium, derived from the poppy flower. These agents are used for treatment of moderate to severe pain. They act by binding to opioid receptors in the brain and spinal cord. They modify pain pathways at the spinal level, as well as profoundly influencing the subjective response to pain at the cortical level. Endogenously occurring opioids, the endorphins and enkephalins, are neuromodulators affecting pain perception and mood. Opioids exert their effects and side effects by binding at receptors for these naturally occurring agents. There are at least three distinct opioid receptors, termed: *mu* (μ), *kappa* (κ), and *delta* (δ), and several subtypes. Agonist drugs may bind at one or more of these receptors, accounting for some of the differences seen in their effects. Besides pain relief, high enough doses of opioids can result in loss of consciousness and, because of a profound dose-dependent depression of respiratory drive, respiratory arrest. The opioids produce a euphoric effect on mood, making them popular drugs of abuse. Tolerance develops rapidly and withdrawal is very painful and unpleasant. These factors contribute to the highly addictive potential of the opioids.

The μ-receptor is responsible for the analgesic effects in the central nervous system and spinal cord. It also accounts for respiratory depression, constipation, nausea and vomiting (from the chemotactic trigger zone receptors), and antitussive effects. κ-Receptors located in the spinal cord and, to a lesser extent, in the central nervous system, mediate analgesia. They may be the receptors responsible for the analgesic effects of the mixed agonist-antagonist drugs. The δ-receptor is the receptor for the naturally occurring mediator enkephalin; its role in analgesia is not clear. It may be important in the spinal mediation of pain perception. This is just the outline of the opioid receptor system; there are other types and subtypes of receptors. Their actual function in human health is not understood. The effect of various opioids can be

Table 22-8
Opioid drugs

EFFECT AT THE OPIOID RECEPTOR	GENERIC DRUG	BRAND NAMES
Agonist	Morphine	MSIR, MS Contin
	Opium	Paregoric, Pantopon
	Codeine	
	Alfentanil	Alfenta
	Dihydrocodeine	Synalgos, Compal
	Fentanyl	Sublimaze, Actiq, Duragesic
	Heroin	
	Hydrocodone	Hycodan
	Hydromorphone	Dilaudid
	Levomethadyl	ORLAAM
	Levorphanol	Levo-Dromoran
	Meperidine	Demerol
	Methadone	Dolophine, Methadose
	Oxycodone	Roxicodone, OxyContin
	Oxymorphone	Numorphan
	Propoxyphene	Darvon
	Remifentanil	Ultiva
	Sufentanil	Sufenta
Mixed agonist-antagonist	Buprenorphine	Buprenex
	Butorphanol	Stadol
	Dezocine	Dalgan
	Nalbuphine	Nubain
	Pentazocine	Talwin
Antagonist	Nalmefene	
	Naloxone	Narcan
	Naltrexone	Trexan

explained by their actions at one or more of these receptors.

Opioids are listed in Table 22-8. Some have pure agonist effects, acting as the endogenous mediators at the receptors, and others antagonize the endogenous mediators but have a small agonist effect (mixed drugs or agonist-antagonist drugs). There are several strictly antagonist agents. These drugs are used to reverse the analgesic and respiratory depressive effects of the opioids. The most serious side effect of the opioid antagonists is respiratory depression, which is mediated by decreased sensitivity of the respiratory center to elevations in

Pa_{CO_2}. Miosis (small pupils) is pathognomonic for opioid drug administration and is a consequence of effects on the sympathetic nervous system. Constipation results from opioid depression of motility of the stomach and intestines. Nausea and vomiting are a direct effect on the brainstem effectors. Cough suppression results from a direct central effect of the opioid.

Because of their effects on pain perception, narcotics are often used as part of a "balanced" anesthetic. Doses that cause profound depression of respiration have minimal or no effect on cardiac function. Because of this safety, opioids are the basis for anesthesia for the seriously cardiovascular-compromised patients. By themselves, opioids have no effect on consciousness or memory. Combined with small doses of benzodiazepines or gaseous anesthetics, they can be used to provide surgical anesthesia.

Strong opioid drugs are often referred to as *narcotics*, from the Greek word for "stupor." The word *narcotic* has significant legal overtones. For this reason, its use has been avoided in this section. *Opiates* are compounds derived from opium and are a small number of the drugs discussed above. *Opioids*, as used in this section, implies simply that the agents interact with one or more of the opioid receptors.

ROUTES OF OPIOID ADMINISTRATION

As discussed above, pain is a subjective experience. Inadequate analgesia is a common complaint voiced by patients. This is especially true after surgery. Fear of respiratory depression is often given as the reason caregivers are reluctant to administer more opioids. Novel ways of treating pain have been developed to improve treatment of pain. Patient-controlled analgesia (PCA) is a method by which patients can self-administer a predetermined intravenous bolus of an opioid at a set interval. This avoids the delay in getting a dose requested from and later delivered by a nurse. More total analgesia drug is needed if pain is allowed to intensify between drug doses. It is more effective to keep control of pain than to regain control of it. Continuous administration of a background opioid rate also may help with this problem. Patients using PCAs for postoperative pain use less total opioid and report subjectively less pain than patients receiving scheduled or as-needed opioids delivered by nurses.

OPIOID INHALATION

Opioids are occasionally administered by inhalation. This route has been suggested to be more effective than systemic opioids for decreasing the sensation of dyspnea in patients with advanced respiratory failure. Opioid receptors have been found in lung tissue, but their exact function in modifying the sensation of dyspnea has not been determined. Inhaled (nebulized) opioids may affect dyspnea by a central mechanism because these drugs are rapidly absorbed from the lung. No controlled studies have demonstrated improved effectiveness of opioids when administered by inhalation; however, this route may be an alternative when intravenous access is not available.[19] Terminal cancer patients without lung disease have been given their systemic doses of analgesics through this route with good clinical effect.

LOCAL ANESTHETICS

Pain treatment can be achieved by blocking transmission of the pain impulse from the damaged area. Local anesthetics are used to interrupt these nervous signals. Local anesthetics produce nerve conduction block by blocking sodium channels. These are located all along the cell, including the axon. When depolarization occurs, the impulse is propagated down the axon by an abrupt increase in the membrane's sodium permeability. When the drug binds to and occludes the channel pore, sodium is unable to enter the cell and propagation of the electrical impulse is stopped. All local anesthetics consist of a lipophilic part and a hydrophilic, amide part connected by either an amide or ester linkage. This is illustrated in Figure 22-4. Several of the common agents are listed in Table 22-9. Sodium channel blockade makes some of these drugs useful in terminating cardiac conduction abnormalities, as well as providing analgesia. Some evidence suggests that systemic administration or inhalation may also enhance bronchodilation in asthma, as well as suppress irritant tracheal cough responses. At toxic levels, central nervous system excitation occurs and frank seizures may result. Epinephrine is often added to a local anesthetic for vasoconstriction to delay its absorption, thus prolonging its effect and decreasing blood levels and potential toxicity. Bupivacaine is very cardiotoxic, and a toxic dose may result in profound and prolonged cardiac depression or arrest.

EPIDURAL ANALGESIA

Continuing epidural infusions for analgesia has improved postoperative pain therapy. There is evidence that patient outcome may also be improved with epidural infusions of local anesthetics, opioids, or both.[20,21] This is especially true for the very ill.[22-25] The quality of the analgesia and the ability to eliminate

pain in many body areas is superior with local anesthetic infusion compared with systemic analgesics. Minimal effects on normal sensory and motor function can be achieved with very dilute local anesthetics. Addition of opioids to the mixture permits even less local anesthetic to be infused. If sympathetic blockade produces unacceptable hypotension, local anesthetics can be eliminated completely, with significant analgesia obtained with narcotic infusion alone. Pain modulation from epidural opioids occurs at receptors at the spinal cord segmental level. The major side ef-

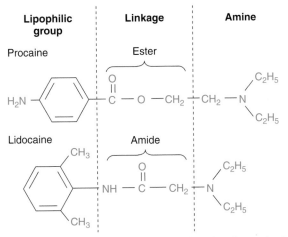

Figure 22-4   Chemical structures of the local anesthetics procaine and lidocaine, showing their respective ester and amide linkages, location of the lipophilic group, and the ionizable amine group.

Table 22-9

Examples of local anesthetics

CLASS	GENERIC DRUG	BRAND NAMES
Ester	Benzocaine	
	2-Chloroprocaine	Nesacaine
	Procaine	Novocain
	Tetracaine	Pontocaine
Amide	Bupivacaine	Marcaine, Sensorcaine
	Levobupivacaine	Chirocaine
	Etidocaine	Duranest
	Lidocaine	Xylocaine
	Mepivacaine	Carbocaine, Polocaine
	Prilocaine	Citanest
	Ropivacaine	Naropin

fects of epidural analgesia using local and/or opioid infusions are listed in Box 22-1.

COMBINATIONS OF ANALGESIC CLASSES

Another strategy to improve analgesia and reduce the likelihood of opioid overdose is to combine several different classes of analgesics. Prescription combina-

tions of NSAIDs and opioids are widely available. Some of these are listed in Table 22-10. The concept of attacking pain at several places is useful, but the fixed combinations of drugs with different effects, toxicities, and half-lives makes titration to an individual patient's need difficult with these agents. Use of the separate agents independently titrated may improve this problem but makes taking of many medications more difficult for patients.

CHRONIC PAIN SYNDROMES

Surgery or trauma causing acute pain can lead to central sensitization and persistence of pain after the peripheral lesion has resolved. It is not known how frequently this problem leads to a chronic pain syndrome, but information is accumulating suggesting that specific treatment in the acute period may reduce the likelihood of a neuropathic problem later.

Neuropathic pain may start with nerve injury, which results in axon degeneration and regeneration. Associated with this process in animal models are abnormal discharges at the spinal cord level, leading to sensitization, abnormal sensation, phantom pain, and rapid changes in the functional architecture of the

Box 22-1 Side Effects of Agents Used for Epidural Analgesia

Local Anesthetics
Motor weakness
Numbness
Hypotension
Difficulty diagnosing epidural hematoma

Opioids
Respiratory depression (equal to or less than systemic opioids)
Reduced gastrointestinal motility (greater than systemic opioids)
Nausea and vomiting (equal to systemic opioids)
Difficult micturition (greater than systemic opioids)
Pruritus (much greater than systemic opioids)

Table 22-10
Some examples of combinations of NSAIDs and opioid analgesics

NSAID	DOSAGE	OPIOID	DOSAGE	BRAND NAME
Acetaminophen	650 mg	Propoxyphene	100 mg	Darvocet N100
Acetaminophen	650 mg	Propoxyphene	50 mg	Darvocet 50
Aspirin	325 mg	Codeine	30 mg	Empirin #3
Aspirin	325 mg	Codeine	60 mg	Empirin #4
Acetaminophen	500 mg	Hydrocodone	5 mg	Hyco-Pap
Acetaminophen	650 mg	Hydrocodone	10 mg	Lorcet 10/650
Acetaminophen	650 mg	Hydrocodone	7.5 mg	Lorcet Plus
Acetaminophen	500 mg	Hydrocodone	2.5 mg	Lortab
Acetaminophen	500 mg	Hydrocodone	5 mg	Lortab ASA
Acetaminophen	650 mg	Oxycodone	10 mg	Percocet 10/650
Aspirin	325 mg	Oxycodone	4.5 mg	Percodan
Aspirin	325 mg	Oxycodone	2.25 mg	Percodan-Demi
Acetaminophen	325 mg	Oxycodone	5 mg	Roxicet
Acetaminophen	650 mg	Pentazocine	25 mg	Talacen
Acetaminophen	300 mg	Codeine	15 mg	Tylenol #2
Acetaminophen	300 mg	Codeine	30 mg	Tylenol #3
Acetaminophen	300 mg	Codeine	60 mg	Tylenol #4
Acetaminophen	500 mg	Oxycodone	5 mg	Tylox
Acetaminophen	500 mg	Hydrocodone	5 mg	Vicodin
Ibuprofen	200 mg	Hydrocodone	7.5 mg	Vicoprofen
Acetaminophen	650 mg	Propoxyphene	65 mg	Wygesic

pain pathways at the level of the spinal cord and lower brain. Hyperesthesia (increased and unpleasant sensitivity to all sensory modalities), hyperpathia (increased unpleasant abnormal feeling from mildly uncomfortable stimuli), and allodynia (painful feeling from gentle stimuli) can be demonstrated to occur soon after acute painful trauma in some patients, especially after surgery on or near major nerve trunks. In some patients, this process may persist and advance to result in a chronic pain syndrome. The characteristics of neuropathic pain include evidence of a primary injury; pain involving (but not confined to) a body area with a sensory deficit; burning, electric, or shooting character to the pain; dysesthesias in the area; pain spreading beyond the cutaneous nerve distribution; sympathetic hyperactivity; and allodynia, hyperpathia, and hyperalgesia. In some complex regional pain syndromes, the autonomic deregulation results in skin changes, edema, and nail and hair loss. This syndrome may lead to severe suffering and incapacitation. Once established, neuropathic pain is poorly responsive to analgesic treatment, but may respond to sympathetic interruption or α-receptor blockade.[26] It is possible that modification of the initial pain input may decrease the incidence or reduce the severity of the syndrome that develops over time.

Preemptive analgesia is the delivery of adequate and appropriate analgesia before initiation of nociceptive input from the surgical incision. By totally abolishing the painful stimulus, the potential for chronic pain syndromes should be reduced. Although general anesthetics and opioids do modify the central sensitization to some extent, regional analgesia, anti-inflammatory agents, central α receptor blockers, and N-methyl-d-(+)-aspartate (NMDA) receptor antagonists, alone or in combination, offer hope of actually preempting pain and eliminating postoperative pain syndromes.

ANESTHESIA

The state of general anesthesia is a drug-induced absence of perception. Stronger stimuli may require deeper anesthesia. Anesthetics are usually administered by inhalation or intravenously because of the more predictable time course of drug actions. Often, combinations of drugs are used to achieve the state of anesthesia. The ideal anesthetic would include the following:

- A pleasant and rapid induction and emergence
- Rapid changes of depth of anesthesia to match surgical demands
- Skeletal muscle relaxation to facilitate surgical exposure
- A wide margin of safety
- No toxic or adverse effects

The first and most common anesthetic agents are the gases and volatile liquids. These are listed in Table 22-11. Dosage and potency are compared by using the concept of minimal alveolar concentration (MAC), which is the amount necessary for achieving the anesthetic state. This is a statistical concept, much like the ED_{50} (effective dose for 50% of subjects to respond), based on the measured agent concentration in exhaled gas (which is in equilibration with the blood) sufficient to prevent movement on surgical incision in half of the subjects. The mechanisms by which anesthetic gases and vapors exert their effects is poorly understood but may be receptor mediated (the GABA receptor being a top candidate) or may be more diffuse, temporary disruption of nerve cell communication. The facts that anesthetic vapor potency is linearly related to fat solubility and that anesthetics can be reversed by high pressures (50 to 100 atmospheres) suggest that cell wall swelling from the agent dissolving in the lipid membrane is an important contributor to the anesthetic state.

Volatile anesthetics by themselves achieve some of the characteristics of the "ideal" anesthetic in that depth of anesthesia can rapidly be changed, induction and emergence is rapid (with some agents), and there are few toxic concerns. These agents do not reliably provide muscle relaxation. Neuromuscular blockers and other adjuvant drugs are often titrated to create

Table 22-11

Gases and volatile liquids used to produce general anesthesia

AGENT	COMMON OR BRAND NAME
Nitrous oxide	Laughing gas
Halothane	Fluothane
Isoflurane	Forane
Enflurane	Ethrane
Sevoflurane	Ultane
Desflurane	Suprane
Diethyl ether*	Ether
Cyclopropane*	
Chloroform	
Methoxyflurane*	Fluoromar

*No longer used for anesthesia in the United States.

the desired anesthetic state and prevent potent agent overdose. Neuromuscular blockers are discussed in Chapter 18. Their use in anesthesia includes facilitation of tracheal intubation (often a short-acting agent) and surgical relaxation, necessary for intrathoracic, intraabdominal and other procedures. Pharmacological reversal of the long-acting neuromuscular blocking agents is also discussed in Chapter 18. Because volatile anesthetics provide little analgesia, narcotic and nonnarcotic analgesics are often a part of the anesthetic mixture. Analgesics may reduce the amount of volatile agent necessary to achieve "anesthesia." The use of a mixture of agents to achieve the anesthetic state is often referred to as *balanced anesthesia*, in which each element is provided in balance and by a different drug. Induction of general anesthesia is usually facilitated by a rapidly effective, sedative-hypnotic agent, although inhalation induction with a newer volatile agent (sevoflurane) is rapid and not unpleasant. Intravenous induction agents commonly used are listed in Table 22-12.

Depth of anesthesia is determined by patient response to painful stimuli and is often judged by the sympathetic response, that is, a change in heart rate or blood pressure. Because other factors may influence these signs, determination of anesthetic depth is much more of an art than a science. Monitors are available that are based on the processed electroencephalogram that are touted to predict depth of anesthesia (BIS monitor), but these devices are subject to other influences as well. During the course of surgery and anesthesia, the degree of surgical stimulus and the depth of anesthesia varies, and one function of the anesthesiologist is to match these two. Analgesia may be needed intraoperatively, as well as part of pain management in the postoperative period. In medically compromised patients, the main activity of the anesthesiologist is to obtain and maintain stability and prevent death; the anesthetic may simply consist of preventing pain and abolishing recall of interoperative events. The entire cardiovascular armamentarium may be used as part of anesthetic management for these critically ill unstable patients.

CONSCIOUS SEDATION

Fear and pain are frequent side effects of many clinical interventions. The pain experience, which includes the physical and emotional components, associated with clinical interventions is unnecessary and may increase morbidity and mortality. For these reasons, minimizing fear and pain is an important part of clinical care.

Besides general anesthesia, many approaches are available to modify the unpleasant experience of diagnostic and therapeutic procedures. Patient preparation, education, relaxation exercises, hypnosis, and drugs may be useful. "Conscious sedation" is the term applied to the pharmacological modification of painful and frightening experiences during medical procedures. As implied in the name, sedated patients should remain "conscious" and able to communicate, protect their own airway, and breathe adequately. Improved patient comfort and outcome is a goal of sedation. However, because of variations in patient responses, consciousness as well as the patients' ability to maintain an unobstructed airway may be lost during sedation.

Institutional standards for safe and effective provision of conscious sedation are required by the Joint Commission for Accreditation of Health Care Organizations and other regulatory agencies. These standards must be adhered to throughout the institution, whether sedation is provided by a nurse, respiratory therapist (RT), anesthesiologist, or other healthcare provider. Many concerned groups have developed guidelines for providing safe conscious sedation. RTs should understand sedative and analgesic pharmacology and may actively participate in provision of conscious sedation.[27,28] Because most of the serious complications of conscious sedation relate to airway compromise, RTs are uniquely qualified to safeguard patients and improve outcomes during conscious sedation.

STANDARDS FOR PROVIDING CONSCIOUS SEDATION

Most conscious sedation guidelines and many clinical reports differentiate several levels of sedation. Often a clear distinction is drawn between "conscious" and "deep" sedation.[29] However, the progression from "conscious sedation" to "deep sedation" to

Table 22-12

Anesthetic induction agents

CLASS	GENERIC DRUG	BRAND NAMES
Barbiturates	Methohexital	Brevital
	Thiamylal	Surital
	Thiopental	Pentothal
Benzodiazepines	Diazepam	Valium
	Lorazepam	Ativan
	Midazolam	Versed
Miscellaneous agents	Etomidate	Amidate
	Ketamine	Ketalar
	Propofol	Diprivan

Table 22-13

Levels of sedation and recommendations for monitoring

LEVEL OF SEDATION	DEFINITION	SUGGESTED MONITORS
Conscious sedation	Minimally depressed level of consciousness retaining the patient's ability to maintain the airway independently and continuously and to respond to physical stimulation and verbal commands	Dedicated monitoring assistant Pulse oximetry IV access Blood pressure measurement every 15 min
Deep sedation	Depressed consciousness accompanied by partial loss of protective reflexes and inability to respond purposefully to verbal command	Skilled airway person Monitoring and recording person IV access Pulse oximetry Continuous ECG monitoring Blood pressure measurement every 5 min
General anesthesia	Unconsciousness accompanied by partial or complete loss of protective reflexes and inability to maintain an airway independently	Anesthesia personnel Anesthesia assistant IV access Pulse oximetry Carbon dioxide measurement device Continuous ECG monitoring Blood pressure measurement every 5 min Other requirements dictated by the patient's physiological condition

ECG, Electroencephalogram; *IV,* intravenous.

"general anesthesia" is difficult to control clinically and each deeper level implies increased risks and mandates more intensive monitoring and increased level of support. The definitions of these states and suggested requirements for monitoring are given in Table 22-13.

All published conscious sedation "standards" insist on the presence of *more than one* person during the period of sedation (at least the operator and a monitoring assistant). Several guidelines suggest that deep sedation and general anesthesia are *indistinguishable* and at least three qualified people must be continually present during the sedation period.[30] The standards also suggest that one person must have, *as sole responsibility,* continual monitoring of the patient and recording of vital signs. When providing conscious sedation, it is necessary to continually assess and ensure oxygenation, ventilation, and temperature maintenance. Although some conscious sedation guidelines suggest how to monitor these vital functions, the decision to use a particular device and frequency of repeated observations is left to the responsible clinician.[31] What is not left to the discretion of the clinician is the number of personnel necessary and

that they must be specially qualified and assigned *only* to monitor one patient's vital functions and the progress of sedation. There must be resuscitation equipment immediately available and individuals trained to use it. To be competent at providing conscious sedation requires a didactic understanding of pharmacology of the drugs discussed in this chapter and a performance-based competency including intravenous therapy, monitor use, and supervised clinical practice.[32]

CENTRAL NERVOUS SYSTEM AND RESPIRATORY STIMULANTS

In contrast to most of the sedative drugs discussed in this chapter, some drugs can *increase* activity of the brain rather than depressing it. Such drugs are termed *analeptic* drugs. If the effects are primarily on the respiratory center, the agent may be a respiratory or ventilatory stimulant. Stimulant drugs are used for treatment of narcolepsy, attention-deficit hyperactivity disorder (ADHD), obesity, and, to a lesser extent, respiratory failure. Some of these drugs are listed in Table 22-14. Most of the stimulant drugs are sympa-

Table 22-14

Central and peripheral nervous system stimulating drugs

CLASS	USE	GENERIC DRUG	BRAND NAMES
Sympathomimetics	Diet	Benzphetamine	Didrex
		Diethylpropion	Tenuate
		Fenfluramine	
		Mazindol	Mazanor, Sanorex
		Mephentermine	
		Phenmetrazine	
		Phendimetrazine	Adipost, Bontril, etc.
		Phentermine	Fastin, Zantryl, etc.
		Phenylpropanolamine	Dexatrim, etc.
		Nabilone	Cesamet
		Sibutramine	Meridia
	Diet and CNS stimulant	Amphetamine	Adderall
	Diet and CNS stimulant	Methamphetamine	Desoxyn
	CNS stimulant	Dextroamphetamine	Dexedrine
Xanthines	CNS stimulant	Aminophylline	
		Caffeine	
Miscellaneous	ADHD	Methylphenidate	Ritalin
		Pemoline	Cylert

ADHD, Attention-deficit hyperactivity disorder; *CNS,* central nervous system.

thomimetics, acting directly on α and β receptors. Their abuse potential is great and their side effects are predictable. They interfere with sleep and are used (and abused) to promote wakefulness and weight loss.

Some drugs can increase ventilation. Doxapram has been used in the past as a treatment for acute and chronic respiratory failure. It was given intravenously and would cause a transient increase in rate and depth of ventilation. It is rarely used as no sustained improvement of respiratory failure has been demonstrated. Methylxanthines, used to promote bronchodilation, also increase catecholamines and increase ventilation. Caffeine, a common component in popular beverages, is used therapeutically in apnea-bradycardia syndromes of premature births. Agents causing metabolic acidosis such as salicylate toxicity or carbonic anhydrase inhibitor diuretics can increase ventilation in response to the systemic acidosis that develops. This increase in minute ventilation is not, however, considered "therapeutic." Progesterone can cause a sustained increase in ventilation and fall in $PaCO_2$ and is occasionally used in treating chronic elevations in CO_2 from advanced obstructive lung disease. Hormonal effects on mood and breast development limit its usefulness.

Respiratory failure resulting from sedative or opioid drug overdose should be treated with specific antagonists, flumazenil and naloxone, rather than the nonspecific effects of the analeptic drugs. Respiratory stimulants have little or no clinical role in treating respiratory failure. Elevated $PaCO_2$ caused by muscle fatigue from increased work of breathing as a result of chronic obstructive pulmonary disease (COPD), acute respiratory distress syndrome (ARDS), or severe bronchospasm, would not be expected to improve with catecholamine stimulating agents. Mechanical ventilation, muscle rest, and bronchodilators are more appropriate approaches.

SUMMARY KEY TERMS AND CONCEPTS

- Drugs that affect the *central nervous system* are *commonly prescribed.* They exert their effects by interacting with *neurotransmission;* affecting neurotransmitter *release, metabolism,* or *uptake;* or acting at primary or modifying receptors or *transport proteins.*
- The clinical effects of central nervous system drugs depend on the localization of specific neurotransmitters in specific brain areas.

- Because the organization of the central nervous system is complex, the main cause of side effects of this class of drugs is their interaction in diffuse brain areas.
- Central nervous system drugs may increase or decrease individual neuronal activity. The balance of activity of different types of neurons seems to affect brain function and mood. Restoration of this balance is the goal of treatment of mood disorders.
- *Depression* is a common *mood disorder*. Several classes of drugs, including the *tricyclic antidepressants* (TCAs), *monoamine oxidase inhibitors* (MAOIs), and *selective serotonin reuptake inhibitors* (SSRIs), are used for this disorder and exhibit a wide range of side effects.
- Other *psychotherapeutic* drugs include the *major tranquilizers* and *sedative-hypnotic* drugs.
- *Depression* of *respiratory drive* is an important *side effect* of several classes of central nervous system drugs, including the general anesthetics and *opioid analgesics.*
- *Hypnotic drugs* primarily *activate the GABA receptor–*mediated chloride channel, hyperpolarizing the cell and decreasing consciousness, anxiety, and recall.
- GABA channel activation may also be important in production of general anesthesia and sleep. Sleep is a complex activity and induction of sleep can be pharmacologically influenced by sedative drugs; however, the quality of the sleep so induced is poor.
- *Antagonism* of the *benzodiazepine effects* on this channel can be accomplished with *flumazenil,* which binds to the receptor site, but does not activate the channel.
- *Opiate effects* can be antagonized with *naloxone* or *naltrexone.*
- *Pain* may be relieved by *local anesthetics* blocking sensory transmission, by *nonsteroidal antiinflammatory drugs* (NSAIDs) modifying peripheral inflammation and central integration, and *opiates* by modifying the spinal cord transmission, brainstem processing, and cortical perception of pain.
- *Local anesthetics* consist of a *hydrophilic end* connected to an active *amino end* connected by an *amide* or *ester* linkage.
- Local anesthetics block *sodium channels* in axons and abolish neural transmission.
- Inadequate pain relief has been identified as a serious problem. Many pain control options are available to hospitalized patients.
- *Patient controlled (opioid) analgesia* (PCA), *epidural analgesia* with local anesthetics and opioids, and combinations of analgesic classes can result in excellent postoperative pain relief.
- *Conscious sedation* is a technique using sedatives and analgesics to prevent patient discomfort during invasive procedures. To prevent catastrophe, a *dedicated individual* must *monitor* the progress of sedation and be prepared to correct airway and cardiovascular problems.
- *Central nervous system–stimulating* drugs include the *methylxanthines* (caffeine and aminophylline) and doxapram. These agents have little clinical usefulness in treating respiratory failure or drug-induced respiratory depression.
- Specific antagonists for benzodiazepine sedative drugs and opioids are more useful for reversing drug-induced hypoventilation.

SELF-ASSESSMENT QUESTIONS

1. What is the difference between sedation and analgesia?
2. Identify the general class of each of the following agents
   (sedative-hypnotic, analgesic, tranquilizer, anesthetic, antipsychotic):
   lorazepam, phenobarbital, doxapram, chloral hydrate, thiopental, midazolam, nitrous oxide, chlorpromazine, halothane, morphine, ibuprofen.
3. You are planning to extubate and remove a patent from the ventilator. However, the nurse administers a large dose of lorazepam (Ativan) for anxiety. What problem may occur if you proceed?
4. What is the most serious side effect of tranquilizers, sedatives, or analgesics (especially opioids)?
5. You have two patients, both of whom have overdosed on central nervous system depressants.
   Patient 1: Comatose, cyanotic, dilated pupils
   Patient 2: Comatose, cyanotic, pinpoint pupils
   Which patient may have taken a barbiturate and which a narcotic analgesic?
6. Identify your initial priorities as a respiratory therapist in caring for a subject with an overdose of tranquilizers.
7. What is the mode of action of the benzodiazepines?
8. Identify an agent that can reverse the effects of benzodiazepines such as midazolam and triazolam.
9. Will barbiturates be helpful in managing pain in a ventilator patient?
10. Would meperidine be helpful to prevent or lessen perception of pain?
11. For a patient with a bleeding disorder, such as hemophilia, or one who is on anticoagulants such as warfarin, suggest an analgesic for minor pain.
12. Are there any serious side effects to use of a ventilatory stimulant such as doxapram?

Answers to Self-Assessment Questions are found in Appendix A.

CLINICAL SCENARIO

Case courtesy **Robert Aranson, MD, Pulmonologist/ Intensivist, formerly of Emory University School of Medicine, Grady Memorial Hospital, Atlanta, Ga.**

A 35-year-old black male was admitted to the hospital with lethargy, after being found in his apartment by a friend. An empty bottle of amitriptyline pills was lying next to the man. In the emergency room, the patient became more lethargic to the point of unresponsiveness and developed hypopnea and bradypnea. He was subsequently intubated and mechanically ventilated with a volume-cycled ventilator. The patient had a history of depression, but had been in good physical health. He was taking amitriptyline, which was prescribed by his psychiatrist for his depression. In an act of despair, he had taken an overdose of his medication. The man has no allergies, and his past medical history and family history are unremarkable.

Physical examination reveals a mesomorphic male appearing his stated age, markedly sedated, intubated, and mechanically ventilated. His vital signs are T, 39° C rectally; P, 140 beats/min; RR, 12 breaths/min on an assist/control (A/C) rate of 12 breaths/min; BP, 110/60 mm Hg, right arm, supine. HEENT is unremarkable except for oral endotracheal tube (ETT) in place. His chest is normoresonant to percussion and his lungs have clear breath sounds bilaterally. Cardiovascular examination revealed that on palpation, the point of maximal impulse was located normally in the fifth intercostal space in the midclavicular line. Auscultation revealed a normal S_1 and S_2 without murmurs, gallops, or rubs. He has normal jugular venous pressure, and his pulses were 2+ throughout. The man's abdomen is mildly distended with absent bowel sounds. No masses or organomegaly are present. His extremities are unremarkable, and his skin is very warm and dry. He is unresponsive to visual, auditory, or tactile stimuli, and his pupils are equally dilated and sluggishly responsive to light. All of his extremities are flaccid, and his reflexes are 1+ throughout. His plantar reflexes are downgoing.

Laboratory results reveal normal hemogram, electrolytes, BUN, creatinine, and liver function tests. The tricyclic antidepressant (TCA) level was in the toxic range. His chest radiograph is normal. The ETT is approximately 2 cm above the carina. The ECG showed sinus tachycardia at 140 beats/min, with prolonged PR and QRS intervals. Arterial blood gas (ABG) on A/C ventilation at 12 breaths/min, V_T, at 800 ml; FIO_2, 1.0 resulted in a pH of 7.44, $PaCO_2$, 38 torr; PaO_2, 550 torr.

The patient was diagnosed with a TCA overdose, and admitted to the medical intensive care unit (MICU), where he was treated with activated charcoal 30 g via nasogastric tube q6h, along with normal saline hydration intravenously. After the first dose of charcoal, his heart rate dropped to approximately 120 beats/min, and his FIO_2 was eventually tapered to 0.35, with a resulting ABG of pH, 7.43; $PaCO_2$, 40 torr; and PaO_2, 175 torr. Several hours after the second charcoal dose, he awoke and was able to write notes to the MICU staff, stating that he was anxious to be extubated. The staff wanted to oblige and placed him on a T-piece with 35% O_2 from a large-reservoir nebulizer. About 2 hours later, the patient fell asleep while on the T-piece, and an ABG at that time revealed pH, 7.36; $PaCO_2$, 48 torr; and PaO_2, 165 torr. An astute respiratory therapist noticed the marked change in the ABG parameters, and placed the patient back on the ventilator. The patient was eventually able to be extubated uneventfully several hours after the fourth dose of charcoal. He was transferred in stable medical condition to the psychiatry service the day after extubation.

What are the toxic side effects of TCAs, and what class of drugs (and what drug in particular) do they mimic in this regard?

How is TCA overdose typically treated?

Why did the patient awaken and then fall back asleep in between doses of activated charcoal?

What implications does this phenomenon have for respiratory therapists in freeing TCA-overdosed patients from the ventilator? When would it have been deemed safe to extubate this patient?

What did the ABG on T-piece imply regarding the patient's ventilatory status? Could the patient have been extubated with this particular ABG? Why or why not?

Was supplemental oxygen ever needed for this patient? Why or why not?

Answers to Clinical Scenario Questions are found in Appendix A.

REFERENCES

1. Olanow CW and others: The effect of deprenyl and levodopa on the progression of Parkinson's disease, *Ann Neurol* 38:771, 1995.

2. Lozano AM and others: New developments in understanding the etiology of Parkinson's disease and in its treatment, *Curr Opin Neurobiol* 8:783, 1998.

3. Ressler KJ, Nemeroff CB: Role of norepinephrine in the pathophysiology and treatment of mood disorders, *Biol Psych* 46:1219, 1999.

4. Regier D and others: One month prevalence of mental disorders in the United States, *Arch Gen Psych* 45:977, 1988.

5. Murray C, Lopez A: Global mortality, disability, and the contribution of risk factors: Global Burden of Disease Study, *Lancet* 349:1436, 1997.

6. Murray C, Lopez A: Alternative projections of mortality and disability by cause 1990-2020, *Lancet* 349:1498, 1997.

7. Chen AC and others: Human pain responsivity in a tonic pain model: psychological determinants, *Pain* 37:143, 1989.

8. Carragee EJ and others: Pain control and cultural norms and expectations after closed femoral shaft fractures, *Am J Orthop* 28:97, 1999.

9. Feine JS and others: Memories of chronic pain and perceptions of relief, *Pain* 77:137, 1998.

10. Chambers CT and others: Development and preliminary validation of a postoperative pain measure for parents, *Pain* 68:307, 1996.

11. McGrath PA and others: A new analogue scale for assessing children's pain: an initial validation study, *Pain* 64:435, 1996.

12. Colwell C, Clark L, Perkins R: Postoperative use of pediatric pain scales: children's self-report versus nurse assessment of pain intensity and affect, *J Ped Nur* 11:375, 1996.

13. Wong DL, Baker CM: Pain in children: comparison of assessment scales, *Pediatr Nurs* 14:9, 1988.

14. Todd KH, Samaroo N, Hoffman JR: Ethnicity as a risk factor for inadequate emergency department analgesia, *J Am Med Assoc* 269:1537, 1993.

15. Sjostrom B and others: Assessment of postoperative pain: impact of clinical experience and professional role, *Acta Anaesth Scand* 41:339, 1997.

16. Beauregard L, Pomp A, Choiniere M: Severity and impact of pain after day-surgery, *Can J Anaesth* 45:304, 1998.

17. Hurwitz ES and others: Public Health Service study of Reye's syndrome and medications: report of the main study, *J Am Med Assoc* 257:1905, 1987.

18. Forsyth BW and others: New epidemiologic evidence confirming that bias does not explain the aspirin/Reye's syndrome association, *J Am Med Assoc* 261:2517, 1989.

19. Manning HL: Dyspnea treatment, *Respir Care* 45:1342, 2000.

20. Ballantyne JC and others: The comparative effects of postoperative analgesic therapies on pulmonary outcome: cumulative meta-analyses of randomized, controlled trials, *Anesth Analg* 86:598, 1998.

21. McNeely JK and others: Epidural analgesia improves outcome following pediatric fundoplication: a retrospective analysis, *Reg Anesth* 22:16, 1997.

22. Yeager MP and others: Epidural anesthesia and analgesia in high-risk surgical patients, *Anesthesiology* 66:729, 1987.

23. Pelton JJ, Fish DJ, Keller SM: Epidural narcotic analgesia after thoracotomy, *South Med J* 86:1106, 1993.

24. Ackerman III WE, Molnar JM, Juneja MM: Beneficial effect of epidural anesthesia on oxygen consumption in a parturient with adult respiratory distress syndrome, *South Med J* 86:361, 1993.

25. Kirsch JR and others: Preoperative lumbar epidural morphine improves postoperative analgesia and ventilatory function after transsternal thymectomy in patients with myasthenia gravis, *Crit Care Med* 19:1474, 1991.

26. Hayes C, Malloy AR: Neuropathic pain in the postoperative period, *Int Anesth Clin* 35:67, 1997.

27. Anonymous: Administration of sedative and analgesic medications by respiratory care practitioners: a position statement from the American Association for Respiratory Care, *Respir Care* 43:655, 1998.

28. Durbin Jr CG: Respiratory therapists and conscious sedation, *Respir Care* 44:909, 1999.

29. Phero JC: Pharmacologic management of pain, anxiety, and behavior: conscious sedation, deep sedation, and general anesthesia, *Pediatr Dent* 15:429, 1993.

30. Rosenberg MB, Campbell RL: Guidelines for intraoperative monitoring of dental patients undergoing conscious sedation, deep sedation, and general anesthesia, *Oral Surg Oral Med Oral Pathol* 71:2, 1991.

31. Matthews RW and others: Pulse oximetry during minor oral surgery with and without intravenous sedation, *Oral Surg Oral Med Oral Pathol* 74:537, 1992.

32. Glassman P, Garrison R: A suggested curriculum for teaching conscious sedation in advanced general practice programs: GPR and AEGD, *Special Care Dent* 13:27, 1993.

Answers to Assessment Questions and Clinical Scenarios

CHAPTER 1

SELF-ASSESSMENT QUESTIONS

1. What is the definition of the term *drug*?
   Answer: A *drug* may be defined as any chemical that alters an organism's function.
2. What is the difference between the generic and the trade name of a drug?
   Answer: The generic name of a drug is non-proprietary, whereas the brand name is the name given by a particular manufacturer of the drug. If a physician prescribes a particular brand of the drug, the pharmacist must sell that brand unless generic substitution is indicated on the prescription.
3. What part of a prescription contains the name and amount of the drug being prescribed?
   Answer: The inscription.
4. A physician's order reads as follows: "gtts iv of racemic epinephrine, c̄ 3 cc of normal saline, q4h, while awake." What has been ordered?
   Answer: Four drops of racemic epinephrine with 3 cc of normal saline, to be given every 4 hours while the patient is awake.
5. The drug salmeterol was released for general clinical use in the United States in 1994. Where would you look to find information on this drug, such as the available dosage forms, doses, properties, side effects, and action?
   Answer: Several sources of information would be available on a new drug, Mosby's Drug Consult, in addition to research reports in the journal literature: the package insert with the drug, the PDR, and the USP-NF. Usually a new drug release is accompanied by marketing literature from the manufacturer that is available from drug representatives or at conferences.

CLINICAL SCENARIO

Where could you find information on the drug, Primatene Mist, that he was taking?
Answer: Primatene Mist is a good example of the need for problem-solving in seeking drug information. A first reference to check would be the PDR; however, you will not find Primatene Mist listed there because this is an old agent in long use. If you cannot find a drug listed in the PDR, other sources would be the package insert on the agent, obtained from a pharmacy, or a current compendium of agents available in the United States, such as Mosby's Drug Consult and *Drug Facts and Comparisons*. All of these sources will provide information on the drug, including its pharmacokinetics (onset, duration) and side effects. Finally, textbooks featuring respiratory care drugs, such as this one, provide the same information in the appropriate chapter.

In general, what is the fundamental error this person displayed?
Answer: Failure to seek medical help while self-treating with an OTC drug product. He probably did not realize (1) that Primatene Mist is epinephrine, which is short-acting (1 to 2 hours' duration), and will not control the full development of an asthma attack termed the *late-phase* reaction; and (2) a progressive asthma episode can cause serious obstruction of the airway and often worsens in the evening or night. Given his continued symptoms, he required more aggressive therapy than Primatene Mist.

CHAPTER 2

SELF-ASSESSMENT QUESTIONS

1. If a drug is in liquid solution, what routes of administration are available for its delivery, considering only its dosage form?

Answer: Oral, injection, inhalation (nebulization), topical (possibly). The type of drug, pharmacokinetics, and intended effect will further narrow the choice of route of administration.

2. Although generic drug equivalents all have the same amount of active drug, will formulations of the same drug from different manufacturers all have the same ingredients?

    Answer: No, not necessarily. Other ingredients than the active drug may differ. For example, in a tablet preparation, the substances used to form the active drug into a molded tablet may vary.

3. If 200 mg of a drug results in a plasma concentration of 10 mg/L, what is the calculated volume of distribution (V_D)?

    Answer: V_D = 200 mg/(10 mg/L) = 20 L.

4. If the V_D of a drug such as phenobarbital is 38 L/70 kg and an effective concentration is 10 mg/L, what loading dose would be needed for an average adult (assuming total bioavailability)?

    Answer: Dose = V_D × Concentration = 38 L × 10 mg/L = 380 mg.

5. If an inhaled aerosol has zero gastrointestinal absorption of active drug, and only lung absorption, what is the L/T ratio?

    Answer: 1.0; L/T = lung availability/(lung + stomach availability); and stomach = 0.

6. True or False: A patient uses a reservoir device with an inhaled aerosol and there is no swallowed portion of the drug; therefore there will be no side effects systemically.

    Answer: False; systemic drug levels are due to *total* drug absorbed, from the gastrointestinal tract and lungs. Sufficient lung absorption of active drug could produce extrapulmonary side effects.

7. Which receptor system signal mechanism is responsible for the effects caused by β receptor activation, such as those seen with adrenergic bronchodilators, terbutaline, or albuterol?

    Answer: G protein linked receptors.

CLINICAL SCENARIO

What may be a likely cause of the patient's respiratory symptoms?

Answer: The pharmacokinetics of the drug are not suitable for a qid schedule. Assuming there is no other complication developing (and that should be ruled out by assessing the patient), the duration of the drug's effect is too short. The improvement in airway resistance has declined, and the patient is working harder to breathe again.

What solutions could you offer?

Answer: You could administer the isoetharine more frequently on a q3h schedule instead of the qid schedule. However, a better choice might be to identify a longer-acting bronchodilator with 4 to 6 hours' duration, such as one of the noncatecholamine agents (see Chapter 6) if the qid schedule is maintained. Less-frequent dosing is more cost effective for an in-hospital patient as well.

CHAPTER 3

SELF-ASSESSMENT QUESTIONS

1. What are the three most common aerosol generating devices used to deliver inhaled drugs?

    Answer: Small volume nebulizer (SVN), metered dose inhaler (MDI) with or without a reservoir device, and dry powder inhalers (DPI).

2. Describe the inspiratory pattern you would instruct a patient to use with an MDI.

    Answer: Exhale to end tidal volume; begin to inhale slowly through the mouth and simultaneously actuate the MDI; continue to inhale to total lung capacity, and hold the breath for 5 to 10 seconds.

3. What are three advantages offered by a reservoir device used with an MDI?

    Answer: Reservoir devices can modify the aerosol plume from an MDI in three ways: (1) allow time/distance between actuation and inhalation for particle evaporation and reduced particle size; (2) allow distance for the high initial particle velocity to slow; and (3) somewhat simplify the hand–breathing coordination required with MDI use. The net effect of the first two influences reduces oropharyngeal impaction and loss.

4. Would a dry powder inhaler be appropriate for a 3-year-old child with asthma?

    Answer: No. These devices require an inspiratory flow rate of 60 L/min or more for optimal use. This probably exceeds the capability of most 3-year-old children. DPIs are not recommended for children younger than 5 years.

5. What is meant by the term *dead volume* in an SVN?

    Answer: The dead volume is the residual amount of solution left in a nebulizer when the nebulizer "sputters" and is no longer able to generate aerosol. This is usually around 0.5 to 1.0 ml in most disposable nebulizers.

6. What is the optimal filling volume and power gas flow rate to use with an SVN?

    Answer: For most disposable nebulizers, the optimal filling volume is 3 to 5 ml and the power gas flow rate is 8 to 10 L/min. A flow rate of 8 L/min probably gives the maximal particle size penetrating the lower respiratory tract and therefore the maximal drug mass able to reach the airway. However, a flow rate of 10 L/min will reduce particle size further and decrease the treatment time.

CLINICAL SCENARIO

What would you do to analyze this situation and ensure that the MDI is functioning properly?

Answer: First check to be sure there are in fact no obstructions in the mouthpiece of the actuator. After shaking well, discharge a dose to room air (away from everyone) to see if there is a visible plume. If possible, you might compare the aerosol plume from his canister to another MDI, to see if they appear to be comparable. If you have a laboratory (e.g., in the hospital) try to have the canister weighed to ensure adequate fullness. Short of analyzing the aerosol, you cannot guarantee a correct dose of albuterol, but you can measure the person's peak expiratory flow with a peak flow meter or his FEV_1 with a portable spirometry screening unit before and after use. If he exhibits his usual amount of reversibility, this is indirect evidence of drug delivery. Also, ask him if he obtains relief when he uses the MDI during wheezing or chest tightness.

Assuming the MDI appears functional based on the preceding check, how would you explain the situation with HFA albuterol to the patient?

Answer: The HFA formulation of albuterol has a higher plume temperature and a lower plume force on actuation. It is a softer and gentler spray. Patients who may have used a CFC formulation of albuterol by MDI often think they are not getting the usual dose because they cannot feel the colder forceful blast they experienced with the CFC formulation.

CHAPTER 4

SELF-ASSESSMENT QUESTIONS
PREPARED-STRENGTH DOSAGE CALCULATIONS

1. A bottle is labeled Demerol (meperidine) 50 mg/cc. How many cc are needed to give a 125 mg dose?

    Answer: 50 mg/1 cc = 125 mg/x cc; x = 2.5 cc.

2. Promazine HCl comes as 500 mg/10 ml. How many milliliters are needed to give 150 mg?

    Answer: 500 mg/10 ml = 150 mg/x ml; x = 3 ml.

3. Hyaluronidase comes as 150 U/cc. How many cc for a 30 U dose?

    Answer: 150 U/cc = 30 U/x cc; x = 0.2 cc.

4. Morphine sulfate 4 mg is ordered. You have a vial with 10 mg/ml. How much do you need?

    Answer: 10 mg/ml = 4 mg/x ml; x = 0.4 ml.

5. A dosage schedule for the surfactant poractant calls for 2.5 ml/kg birth weight. How much drug will you need for a 800-g baby?

    Answer: 800 g × 1 kg/1000 g = 0.8 kg; 2.5 ml/kg × 0.8 kg = 2 ml.

6. Diphenhydramine (Benadryl) elixer contains 12.5 mg of diphenhydramine HCl in each 5 ml of elixir. How many milligrams are there in one-half teaspoonful dose (1 tsp = 5 ml)?

    Answer: ½ teaspoon = 2.5 ml.
    12.5 mg/5 ml = x mg/2.5 ml; x = 6.25 mg.

7. A pediatric dose of oxytetracycline 100 mg is ordered. The dosage form is an oral suspension containing 125 mg/5 cc. How much of the suspension contains a 100 mg dose?

    Answer: 125 mg/5 cc = 100 mg/x cc; x = 4 cc.

8. How much heparin is in 0.2 ml, if you have 1000 U/ml?

    Answer: 1000 U/ml = x units/0.2 ml; x = 200 U.

9. Albuterol syrup is available as 2 mg/5 ml. If a dose schedule of 0.1 mg/kg is used, how much syrup is needed for a 30-kg child? How many teaspoons is this?

    Answer: 30 kg × 0.1 mg/kg = 3 mg
    2 mg/5 ml = 3 mg/x ml; x = 7.5 ml
    7.5 ml × 1 tsp/5 ml = 1.5 tsp

10. Terbutaline is available as 2.5 mg tablets. How many tablets do you need for a 5 mg dose?

    Answer: 2.5 mg/1 tab = 5 mg/x tab; x = 2 tablets.

11. If Tempra is available as 120 mg per 5 ml, how much dose is there in one-half teaspoon?

    Answer: ½ teaspoon = 2.5 ml; 120 mg/5 ml = x mg/2.5 ml; x = 60 mg.

12. Theophylline is available as 250 mg/10 ml, and is given intravenously as 6 mg/kg body weight. How much solution do you give for a 60-kg woman?

    Answer: 60 kg × 6 mg/kg = 360 mg; 250 mg/10 ml = 360 mg/x ml; x = 14.4 ml.

13. Terbutaline sulfate is available as 1 mg/ml in an ampule. How many milliliters are needed for a 0.25 mg dose?

    Answer: 1 mg/ml = 0.25 mg/x ml; x = 0.25 ml.

14. A patient is told to take 4 mg of albuterol four times daily. The medication comes in 2 mg tablets. How many tablets are needed for one 4 mg dose?
    Answer: 2 mg/tab = 4 mg/x tab; x = 2 tablets.
15. Metaproterenol is available as a syrup with 10 mg/5 ml. How many teaspoons should be taken for a 20 mg dose?
    Answer: 1 tsp = 5 ml.
    10 mg/5 ml = 20 mg/x ml; x = 10 ml.
    10 ml × 1 tsp/5 ml = 2 tsp.
16. If you have 3 mg/ml of d-(+)-tubocurarine, how many milliliters are needed for a dose of 9 mg?
    Answer: 3 mg/ml = 9 mg/x ml; x = 3 ml.
17. If a dosage schedule requires 0.25 mg/kg of body weight, what dose is needed for an 88-kg person.
    Answer: 0.25 mg/kg × 88 kg = 22 mg.
18. If theophylline is available as 80 mg/15 ml, how much is needed for a 100 mg dose?
    Answer: 80 mg/15 ml = 100 mg/x ml; x = 18.75 ml.
19. How much drug is needed for a 65-kg adult, using 0.5 mg/kg?
    Answer: 0.5 mg/kg × 65 kg = 32.5 mg.
20. Pediatric dosage of an antibiotic is 0.5 g/20 lb of body weight, not to exceed 75 mg/kg/24 hr.
    a. What is the dose for a 40-lb child?
    Answer: 0.5 g/20 lb × 40 lb = 1.0 g.
    b. If this dose is given twice in 1 day, is the maximum dose exceeded?
    Answer: 2 doses = 2 × 1.0 g = 2.0 g = 2000 mg.
    40 lb × 1 kg/2.2 lb = 18 kg.
    2000 mg/18 kg = 111.1 mg/kg.
    Yes, two doses give 2000 mg per 40 lb, which is 2000 mg per 18 kg, or 111.1 mg per kg a day.

PERCENTAGE-STRENGTH PROBLEMS

1. How many grams of calamine are needed to prepare 120 g of an ointment containing 8% calamine?
   Answer: 0.08 = x g/120 g; x = 9.6 g.
2. One milliliter of active enzyme is found in 147 ml of solution. What is the percentage strength of active enzyme in the solution?
   Answer: x = 1 ml/147 ml; x = 0.0068 = 0.68%.
3. If theophylline is available in a 250 mg/10 ml solution, what percentage strength is this?
   Answer: x = 0.25 g/10 ml; x = 0.025 = 2.5%.

4. You have epinephrine 1:100. How many milliliters of epinephrine would be needed to contain 30 mg of active ingredient?
   Answer: 0.01 = 0.03 g/x ml; x = 3 ml.
5. A dose of 0.4 ml of epinephrine HCl 1:100 is ordered. This dose contains how many milligrams of epinephrine HCl (the active ingredient)?
   Answer: 0.01 = x g/0.4 ml; x = 0.004 g = 4 mg.
6. If you administer 3 ml of a 0.1% strength solution, how many milligrams of active ingredient have you given?
   Answer: 0.001 = x g/3 ml; x = 0.003 g = 3 mg.
7. A drug is available as a 1:200 solution and the maximum dose that may be given by aerosol for a particular patient is 3 mg. What is the maximal amount of solution (in milliliters) that may be used?
   Answer: 1:200 = 0.5% = 0.005; 3 mg = 0.003 g; 0.005 = 0.003 g/x ml; x = 0.6 ml.
8. Epinephrine 1:1000 contains how many milligrams per milliliter?
   Answer: 1:1000 = 0.1% = 0.001; 0.001 = x g/1 ml; x = 0.001 g = 1 mg.
9. How many milligrams per milliliter are there in 0.3 ml of 5% strength metaproterenol?
   Answer: 0.05 = x g/0.3 ml; x = 0.015 g = 15 mg.
10. How many milligrams of sodium chloride are needed for 10 ml of a 0.9% solution?
    Answer: 0.009 = x g/10 ml; x = 0.09 g = 90 mg.
11. If you have 5 mg/ml of Xylocaine, what percentage strength is this?
    Answer: x = 0.005 g/ml; x = 0.005 = 0.5%.
12. A 0.5% strength solution contains how many milligrams in 1 ml?
    Answer: 0.005 = x g/ml; x = 0.005 g = 5 mg.
13. Cromolyn sodium contains 20 mg in 2 ml of water. What is the percentage strength?
    Answer: x = 0.02 g/2 ml; x = 0.01 = 1%.
14. How much active ingredient of acetylcysteine (Mucomyst) have you given with 4 cc of a 20% solution?
    Answer: 0.2 = x g/4 cc; x = 0.8 g = 800 mg.
15. You have 20% acetylcysteine; how many milliliters do you need of this to form 4 ml of 8% solution?
    Answer: 0.08 = 0.2(x) ml/4 ml; 0.2(x) = 0.32; x = 1.6 ml, and saline qs for 4 ml.
16. The recommended dose of metaproterenol 5% is 0.3 cc. How many milligrams of solute are there in this amount?
    Answer: 0.05 = x g/0.3 cc; x = 0.015 g = 15 mg.

17. Mucomyst brand of acetylcysteine was marketed as 10% acetylcysteine with 0.05% isoproterenol. How many milligrams of each ingredient were in a 4 cc dose of solution?
    Answer: Acetylcysteine: $0.10 = x\,g/4\,cc$; $x = 0.4\,g = 400\,mg$.
    Isoproterenol: $0.0005 = x\,g/4\,cc$; $x = 0.002\,g = 2\,mg$.

18. Which contains more drug: $\frac{1}{2}$ cc of 1% drug solution with 2 ml of saline, or $\frac{1}{2}$ cc of 1% drug solution with 5 ml of saline?
    Answer: They each contain the same amount of drug: 5 mg ($0.01 = x\,g/0.5\,cc$; $x = 0.005\,g = 5\,mg$). The different amounts of diluent (2 ml, 5 ml) will change the resulting percentage strength and the total amount of new solution, but not the amount of drug.

19. How many milligrams per milliliter are in a 20% solution?
    Answer: $0.20 = x\,g/ml$; $x = 0.2\,g = 200\,mg$.

20. On an emergency cart, you have sodium bicarbonate solution ($NaHCO_3$), 44.6 mEq/50 ml. A physician orders an aerosol of 5 cc and 3.25% strength. How many milliliters of the bicarbonate solution do you need?

    > 1 mEq = 1/1000 GEW; GEW = gram formula wt/valence.
    > Atomic weights: Na = 23; H = 1; C = 12; O = 16.

    Step 1: Percentage strength of 44.6 mEq/50 cc:

    Answer: $NaHCO_3$ − GEW = 84 g/1 = 84 g.
    1 mEq = 0.084 g. 44.6 mEq × 0.084 g/mEq = 3.75 g.
    Percentage strength = 3.75 g/50 cc = 0.0075 = 7.5%.

    Step 2: Calculate how much of a 7.5% solution is needed to form 5 cc of 3.25% strength using formula for dilute solution:

    $$0.0325 = 0.075\,(x)/5\,cc.$$
    $$x = 5(0.0325)/0.075 = 2.17\,ml.$$

    Take 2.17 ml of the bicarbonate solution and add saline qs for a total of 5 cc. Resulting strength will be 3.25%.

INTRAVENOUS INFUSION RATES

1. You wish to give a solution of 500 mg/L of dobutamine at a rate of 10 µg/kg/min, to a 50-kg woman. What drip rate will you need?
   Answer: Dose = 10 µg/kg/min × 50 kg = 500 µg/min.
   Concentration = 500 mg/L = 0.5 mg/ml = 500 µg/ml.
   Flow rate (drops/min) = 500 µg/min × 1 ml/500 µg × 15 drops/ml = 15 drops/min.

2. If you have 2 mg of isoproterenol in 500 ml of solution, and you wish to deliver 5 µg/min intravenously, what drip rate is needed?
   Answer: Concentration = 2 mg/500 ml = 0.004 mg/ml = 4 µg/ml.
   Flow rate (drops/min) = 5 µg/min × 1 ml/4 µg × 15 drops/ml = 18.75 drops/min.

3. You have 250 mg of dobutamine in 1 L of solution. You want to deliver 5µg/kg/min to a 60-kg man. What infusion rate in milliliters per minute and in drops per minute, is needed?
   Answer: Concentration = 250 mg/1000 ml = 0.25 mg/ml = 250 µg/ml.
   Dose = 5 µg/kg/min × 60 kg = 300 µg/min.
   Flow rate (ml/min) = 300 µg/min × 1 ml/250 µg = 1.2 ml/min.
   Flow rate (drops/min) = 1.2 ml/min × 15 drops/ml = 18 drops/min.

4. You have 250 ml of D_5W and a drip rate of 15 drops/min. How long will the bag of solution last?
   Answer: Flow rate (ml/min) = 15 drops/min × 1 ml/15 drops = 1 ml/min.
   Time (min) = 250 ml × 1 min/ml = 250 min.

5. You have epinephrine solution, 1 mg 250 ml. What drip rate is needed to deliver 4 µg/min?
   Answer: Concentration = 1 mg/250 ml = 0.004 mg/ml = 4 µg/ml.
   Flow rate (drops/min) = 4 µg/min × 1 ml/4 µg × 15 drops/ml = 15 drops/min.

6. If you wish to deliver 500 ml of a solution in 1 hour and 40 minutes, what drip rate should you set?
   Answer: 1 hour, 40 minutes = 100 minutes.
   Flow rate (ml/min) = 500 ml/100 min = 5 ml/min.
   Flow rate (drops/min) = 15 drops/ml × 5 ml/min = 75 drops/min.

7. A recommended dose of intravenous epinephrine is 15 ml/hr, using a solution of 4 µg/ml. What drip rate is needed to achieve the recommended infusion rate?
   Answer: Flow rate (ml/min) = 15 ml/hr × 1 hr/60 min = 15 ml/60 min = 0.25 ml/min.
   Flow rate (drops/min) = 0.25 ml/min × 15 drops/ml = 3.75 drops/min.

CLINICAL SCENARIO

Can you use the 1 N solution as diluent, unchanged?
Answer: A 1 Normal (N) solution contains 1 g equivalent weight (GEW) of solute per liter of solution. If we calculate the percentage strength of a 1 N solution

of NaCl, we can compare this to 0.9% to determine equivalence or lack of equivalence. The molecular weights of sodium (Na) and chlorine (Cl) are 23.0 and 35.5, respectively. A GEW is the molecular weight divided by the valence of the elements. So,

$$1 \text{ GEW, NaCl} = 58.5 \text{ g}/1 = 58.5 \text{ g.}$$
$$1 \text{ N solution} = 1 \text{ GEW/L} = 58.5 \text{ g/L or}$$
$$= 5.85 \text{ g}/100 \text{ ml.}$$
$$= 5.85\%.$$

Therefore a 1 N solution of NaCl is 5.85% strength and is not the same concentration as normal saline, which is 0.9% strength. A 0.9% solution would be 0.9 g/100 ml, not 5.85 g/100 ml. Use of the more concentrated 1 N solution, which is hypertonic relative to body fluid, may cause bronchial irritation in a nebulizer solution for inhalation.

CHAPTER 5

SELF-ASSESSMENT QUESTIONS

1. Which portion of the nervous system is under voluntary control: the autonomic or the skeletal muscle motor nerve portion?
   Answer: The skeletal muscle motor nerve portion.
2. What is the neurotransmitter at each of the following sites: neuromuscular junction, autonomic ganglia, most sympathetic end sites?
   Answer: Neuromuscular junction—acetylcholine.
   Autonomic ganglia—acetylcholine.
   Most sympathetic end sites—norepinephrine.
3. Where are muscarinic receptors found?
   Answer: At parasympathetic nerve terminal sites.
4. What is the effect of cholinergic stimulation of airway smooth muscle?
   Answer: Bronchoconstriction.
5. What is the effect of adrenergic stimulation on the heart?
   Answer: Increased rate and force of contraction.
6. Classify the drugs pilocarpine, physostigmine, propranolol, and epinephrine.
   Answer: Pilocarpine—direct-acting cholinergic.
   Physostigmine—indirect-acting cholinergic.
   Propranolol—adrenergic-blocking agent (β_1 and β_2).
   Epinephrine—adrenergic agonist (stimulates α and β receptors).
7. How do indirect-acting cholinergic agonists (parasympathomimetics) produce their action?

Answer: Indirect-acting parasympathomimetics, such as neostigmine, inhibit the cholinesterase enzyme, which increases the amount of acetylcholine available to stimulate postsynaptic sites at the nerve terminal.

8. What effect would the drug atropine have on the eye and on airway smooth muscle?
   Answer: Atropine is a competitive blocking agent for muscarinic receptors. The drug would block the eye circular iris muscle to dilate the pupil (mydriasis), paralyze the ciliary muscle to flatten the lens (cycloplegia), and antagonize cholinergic induced bronchoconstriction in the airway.
9. What is the general difference between α and β receptors in the sympathetic nervous system?
   Answer: The α receptors generally cause an excitatory effect (e.g., vasoconstriction), and β receptors generally produce inhibition (e.g., airway smooth muscle relaxation).
10. What is the primary mechanism for terminating the neurotransmitters acetylcholine and norepinephrine?
    Answer: Acetylcholine is metabolized by cholinesterase enzymes; norepinephrine is reabsorbed back into the presynaptic neuron.
11. What is the predominant sympathetic receptor type found on airway smooth muscle?
    Answer: β_2 Receptors.
12. Identify the adrenergic receptor preference for phenylephrine, norepinephrine, epinephrine, and isoproterenol.
    Answer: Phenylephrine—α receptors (α_1 specifically).
    Norepinephrine—$\alpha > \beta$ receptors.
    Epinephrine—α and β receptors equally.
    Isoproterenol—β (β_1 and β_2 receptors).
13. What is the autoregulatory receptor on the sympathetic presynaptic neuron?
    Answer: α_2 Receptors.
14. Classify the following drugs by autonomic class and receptor preference: dopamine, ephedrine, albuterol, phentolamine, propranolol, and prazosin.
    Answer: Dopamine—sympathomimetic (dopamine receptors, α, β).
    Ephedrine—sympathomimetic (α and β).
    Albuterol—sympathomimetic (β_2 preferential).
    Phentolamine—α sympatholytic (α_1 and α_2).
    Propranolol—β sympatholytic (β_1 and β_2).
    Prazosin—α_1 sympatholytic.

15. What is the autoregulatory receptor on the parasympathetic presynaptic neuron at the terminal nerve site?
    Answer: The muscarinic receptor subtype M_2.

16. Contrast α_1 and α_2 receptor effects, in general.
    Answer: α_1 Effects are generally excitatory (e.g., vasoconstriction of peripheral blood vessels). α_2 Effects are generally inhibitory (e.g., inhibition of norepinephrine release from nerve terminals).

17. What substance may be the neurotransmitter in the NANC inhibitory nervous system in the lung?
    Answer: Vasoactive intestinal peptide (VIP) or possibly nitric oxide (NO).

18. What substance is the neurotransmitter in the NANC excitatory nervous system in the lung?
    Answer: Substance P.

Clinical Scenario

What may have led to the wheezing and dyspnea of the patient?
Answer: This is an example of altering the balance of autonomic control in the lung. Propranolol (Inderal) is a nonspecific β blocker (β_1 and β_2). As a β_1-blocking agent, the drug will slow the heart rate. However, the blockade of β_2 receptors in the airway prevents endogenous epinephrine and exogenous adrenergic agents from stimulating those receptors. The intravenous dose directly antagonizes the effect of the β receptor stimulation in the airways with the adrenergic bronchodilator albuterol, and it inhibits the degree of bronchodilation achieved in this asthmatic, whose airways tend to react to stimuli and constrict. The balance between adrenergic relaxation of the airway and cholinergic constriction is tipped in favor of an unbalanced cholinergic activity. She begins to exhibit symptoms of bronchoconstriction (wheezing, dyspnea).

What changes in the therapeutic approach would you suggest in a case such as this?
Answer: Prevention is the best approach. In a patient such as an asthmatic, β receptor stimulation is an important property to preserve. The use of a drug other than a β-blocking agent would be indicated for the SVT, to avoid the undesirable side effect of β blockade in the lung. Alternative drugs for tachycardia will be discussed in subsequent chapters; these would include a calcium channel blocking agent such as verapamil or an agent such as adenosine. Her use of the β-adrenergic bronchodilator (albuterol), which is a β_2 agonist, should be reviewed also, to ensure proper dosage and frequency of use. Although β_2 specific, an adrenergic agonist can stimulate the heart.

Chapter 6

Self-Assessment Questions

1. Identify three adrenergic bronchodilators used clinically that are catecholamines.
   Answer: Epinephrine, isoproterenol, isoetharine.

2. Which of the catecholamine bronchodilators given by aerosol is β_2 specific?
   Answer: Isoetharine.

3. What is the duration of action of the catecholamine bronchodilators?
   Answer: Approximately 1.5 hour; up to 3 hours at most.

4. Identify two advantages introduced with the modifications of the catecholamine structure in adrenergic bronchodilators.
   Answer: Increased β_2 specificity and longer duration of action.

5. Identify the usual dose by aerosol for an SVN for metaproterenol and albuterol.
   Answer: Metaproterenol—0.3 cc of a 5% concentration.
   Albuterol—0.5 cc of a 0.5% concentration.

6. What is an extremely common side effect with β_2-adrenergic bronchodilators?
   Answer: Muscle tremor.

7. Identify the approximate duration of action for isoetharine, pirbuterol and salmeterol.
   Answer: Isoetharine—1 to 3 hours.
   Pirbuterol—4 to 6 hours.
   Salmeterol—12 hours.

8. Identify the generic drug for each of the following brand names: Alupent, Tornalate, Maxair, Serevent, Brethaire, Ventolin.
   Answer: Alupent—metaproterenol.
   Tornalate—bitolterol.
   Maxair—pirbuterol.
   Serevent—salmeterol.
   Brethaire—terbutaline.
   Ventolin—albuterol.

9. Which route of administration is more likely to have greater severity of side effects with a β agonist, oral or inhaled aerosol?
   Answer: Oral (tremor is more severe).

10. You notice a pinkish tinge to aerosol rain-out in the large-bore tubing connecting a patient's mouthpiece to a nebulizer after a treatment with racemic epinephrine; what has caused this?

Answer: The catecholamine epinephrine will be broken down by light and air to the adrenochrome form, producing a pinkish, or pinkish-brown residue in tubing.

11. A patient exhibits paradoxical bronchoconstriction from the Freon propellant when using his albuterol by MDI. Suggest an alternative for the patient.

    Answer: Consider trying the HFA formulation or an alternative delivery form such as a DPI (the Rotahaler) or a nebulizer solution. If the albuterol is effective with the patient, this will allow him to continue use of the drug.

12. If you are working with an asthmatic with occasional symptoms of wheezing and chest tightness, which respond well to an inhaled β agonist, would you suggest using salmeterol?

    Answer: No; salmeterol is indicated for maintenance therapy of asthmatics needing regular use of a β agonist or Step 2 therapy (regular β agonist and inhaled corticosteroid or other agents).

13. Suggest a β agonist that would be appropriate for the patient in question 12.

    Answer: Any of the following: albuterol, pirbuterol, terbutaline, metaproterenol.

CLINICAL SCENARIO

How could you assess the presence of airflow obstruction in this patient?

Answer: A peak expiratory flow measure, which indicates approximately 80% of his predicted value. Alternatively, office spirometry would provide more complete information on his FEV_1 and mid-maximal flow rates. A "before and after" bronchodilator study would further determine if he has *reversible* obstruction; however, his history and symptoms suggest this.

Given his symptoms, your physical findings, and a reduced peak flow, would you recommend a β agonist?

Answer: Yes. He exhibits measures of airflow obstruction, and it is reasonable to treat him with a bronchodilator.

If you recommend a bronchodilator, suggest an appropriate agent.

Answer: A $β_2$-selective, short-acting inhaled drug would be appropriate for relief now. This could include levalbuterol, albuterol, pirbuterol, or terbutaline. A long-acting agent such as salmeterol is not appropriate because of its time course.

How could you assess his response to a β-agonist bronchodilator?

Answer: The simplest approach is to wait about 15 minutes after he inhales the β agonist and test his peak flow again or his FEV_1. Improvement in his flow rate indicates reversibility.

At this point, suggest a β agonist to prescribe for his use at home or work when he leaves the clinic.

Answer: At the least, he needs a rescue β-agonist bronchodilator. A short-acting agent such as albuterol, pirbuterol, or terbutaline in an MDI would be appropriate.

What type of instructions and follow-up would you suggest for this patient?

Answer: First, be sure to demonstrate correct use of the MDI, with a return demonstration using a placebo inhaler. If he has difficulty, a holding chamber should be prescribed. Second, he should be given a basic action plan to deal with reoccurrences of bronchospasm, which includes how much and often to use his β agonist inhaler and when to seek help. Third, follow-up testing for allergies and to establish a diagnosis of asthma requires an immediate referral to a pulmonologist or an allergist, for more complete assessment, ongoing monitoring, and management.

CHAPTER 7

SELF-ASSESSMENT QUESTIONS

1. What is the first FDA-approved anticholinergic bronchodilator for aerosol inhalation?

   Answer: Ipratropium (Atrovent).

2. What is the usual recommended dose of ipratropium by MDI and by SVN?

   Answer: MDI: 36 µg; 2 actuations, each 18 µg (from the mouthpiece). SVN: 500 µg; 2.5 ml of a 0.02% solution.

3. Identify a long-acting anticholinergic bronchodilator and give its duration of action.

   Answer: Tiotropium (Spiriva); duration of effect up to 24 hours.

4. What is the usual clinical indication for use of an anticholinergic bronchodilator such as ipratropium?

   Answer: Maintenance treatment of COPD.

5. Which disease state, asthma or COPD, may show greater response to an anticholinergic bronchodilator than to a β agonist?

Answer: COPD patients are likely to have a greater response to an anticholinergic agent rather than a β agonist in reversibility of airflow obstruction.

6. With which type of anticholinergic agent are you more likely to observe systemic side effects: the tertiary ammonium or quaternary ammonium compounds?

Answer: Tertiary; these are less ionized and are better absorbed and distributed through body tissues.

7. What are the most common side effects seen with inhaled ipratropium?

Answer: Dry mouth and cough.

8. Can ipratropium be used with subjects who have glaucoma?

Answer: Yes. However, use with caution, have patient notify the ophthalmologist, and monitor intraocular pressures.

9. Can ipratropium be alternated with or combined with a β agonist in the treatment of COPD and asthma?

Answer: Yes. The two types of agents may have additive effects in reversing airflow obstruction. In addition, they have complementary sites and mechanisms of action, and the time to peak effect is later for ipratropium compared with that of a β agonist, resulting in more sustained peak bronchodilation.

10. What precautions should you observe if administering ipratropium by SVN?

Answer: Protect the eyes from exposure to nebulized drug, using a mouthpiece instead of a mask whenever possible or covering the eyes if a facemask is used for administration. This is to avoid ocular effects of mydriasis and cycloplegia.

11. What is the clinical indication for the use of an anticholinergic intranasal spray?

Answer: Rhinorrhea associated with nonallergic perennial rhinitis, colds, and allergic rhinitis if unresponsive to intranasal corticosteroids.

CLINICAL SCENARIO

Would you recommend a bronchodilator for Mr. C.?
Answer: A bronchodilator should be considered after assessing the degree of reversibility of his airflow obstruction with spirometry after bronchodilator administration. In fact, Mr. C.'s FEV_1 and FEV_1/FVC improved by approximately 20% with a β agonist.

What type of bronchodilator would you think best to start for Mr. C.?
Answer: An anticholinergic bronchodilator, specifically ipratropium, is indicated for maintenance treatment of COPD with reversible airflow obstruction. The most convenient formulation is an MDI and a starting dose of 2 puffs (inhalations) qid could be prescribed.

If Mr. C. has trouble with MDI use, what actions could you take?
Answer: First, review instructions for correct use of the MDI with Mr. C. and have him practice using a placebo inhaler. Second, consider using a reservoir device with the MDI.

Third, if he is unable or unwilling to use the MDI, you could change to the nebulizer solution.

What lifestyle change(s) would you emphasize to Mr. C.?
Answer: First and foremost, quit smoking. Give smoking cessation material and program information to him. Secondly, consider a rehabilitation or disease management educational program, to incorporate knowledge of the disease, its treatment options, exercise, and nutrition.

CHAPTER 8

SELF-ASSESSMENT QUESTIONS

1. What drug in the xanthine group is used most often therapeutically?
Answer: Theophylline (aminophylline).

2. What is the difference between aminophylline and theophylline?
Answer: Aminophylline is a salt of theophylline to increase aqueous solubility for intravenous administration.

3. What is the recommended therapeutic plasma level for theophylline in asthma?
Answer: 5 to 15 μg/ml.

4. How do you know whether a given dose of theophylline will produce a satisfactory treatment effect in an asthmatic?
Answer: The most exact method is to monitor the plasma level of theophylline and adjust the dose to maintain a therapeutic plasma level. Alternatively, and less precisely, the dose can be adjusted to control of symptoms and side effects.

5. Identify at least three adverse side effects seen with theophylline.

Answer: Gastric irritation, insomnia, anxiety/shakiness, tachycardia, nausea, loss of appetite, headache.

6. What is meant by a "narrow therapeutic margin?"
Answer: The dose required to produce a therapeutic effect is close to the dose that begins to produce toxic side effects.

7. Although theophylline is a weak bronchodilator, what other effects make it useful in treating chronic airflow obstruction?
Answer: (1) Stimulation of ventilatory drive in the central nervous system and (2) strengthening of diaphragmatic contractile force.

8. True or False: Theophylline causes bronchodilation and improved airflow by inhibiting phosphodiesterase, which breaks down cAMP.
Answer: False. The mode of action of theophylline is unclear.

CLINICAL SCENARIO

What is the first drug that is indicated by this individual's blood sample values?
Answer: Oxygen. Although a PO_2 of 64 mm Hg on room air, with a saturation of 90%, appears to be satisfactory, this is achieved by a labored pattern of respiration, with tachypnea (RR, 22 breaths/min), and is accompanied by an increased blood pressure (170/112 mm Hg) and tachycardia (120 beats/min). In addition, he is mildly anemic. Relieving his hypoxemia, and thereby reducing his work of breathing and myocardial work, may prevent the need for ventilatory support.

Would you continue his use of ipratropium; if so, what dose would you suggest?
Answer: Yes; ipratropium is a drug of choice in COPD, including an acute exacerbation. However, a dose of 2 inhalations from the MDI may well be insufficient and the dose should be titrated to 6 or 8 actuations for inhalation, given immediately with a reservoir device, because he is tachypneic and may have trouble coordinating breathing and actuation. A larger dose of ipratropium can be administered if the SVN solution of 500 µg is administered instead.

What additional bronchodilator therapy could you recommend?
Answer: A β_2 agonist, such as albuterol, pirbuterol, terbutaline, or metaproterenol, should be administered by MDI with a reservoir preferably or, if available, as an SVN solution, by that mode. This should be adminis-

tered at the same time as the ipratropium. In addition, this patient may benefit from theophylline.

What is the rationale for use of theophylline in this patient?
Answer: Theophylline has a weak bronchodilating effect in the airways, which may help reverse his airflow obstruction. In addition, the drug can strengthen diaphragmatic contractile force, improving his ability to ventilate, and the drug is a ventilatory stimulant. Finally, theophylline has been shown to reduce dyspnea, even in the absence of improvement in objective measures of airflow.

What would you check before initiating therapy with theophylline?
Answer: Question the patient on use of theophylline before his admission to the hospital. Although he did not state use of theophylline in his initial assessment, this should be checked before administering the drug, because there is a narrow therapeutic margin. If he does recall regular use of the drug, or any use before admission, a theophylline blood level should be checked as soon as possible.

What serum theophylline level would you target, if the patient is started on theophylline?
Answer: Optimal results with minimal side effects will be obtained with a blood level of 10 to 12 µg/ml in most patients.

CHAPTER 9

SELF-ASSESSMENT QUESTIONS

1. Identify the two mucolytic agents approved for inhalation as an aerosol in the United States (give the generic and brand names).
Answer: Acetylcysteine (Mucomyst, others) and dornase alfa (Pulmozyme).

2. What is the mode of action for acetylcysteine?
Answer: Acetylcysteine reduces the viscosity of mucus by substituting a sulfhydril group for the disulfide (SS) bonds in mucus.

3. What is the mode of action for dornase alfa?
Answer: Dornase alfa acts as a peptide mucolytic by cleaving the DNA polymers from neutrophils in purulent secretions.

4. What is the clinical indication for use of dornase alfa?
Answer: Management of cystic fibrosis patients to decrease the frequency of respiratory infec-

tions requiring parenteral antibiotics and to improve pulmonary function.

5. What is the usual dose of acetylcysteine by nebulizer?
   Answer: 3 to 5 ml of a 10% solution, tid, qid, or as ordered; the 20% solution is more irritating to the airway and may provoke constriction or cough.

6. What is the recommended dose of dornase alfa?
   Answer: 2.5 mg daily, using a 1 mg/ml ampule solution, administered by suitable nebulizers such as the Hudson T Updraft II, the Marquest Acorn II (using the PulmoAide compressor), or the PARI LC jet nebulizer using the PARI PRONEB compressor.

7. How much active ingredient is contained in 4 cc of 10% acetylcysteine solution?
   Answer: 10% concentration is equal to 100 mg per cc; 4 cc would give 400 mg total dose.

   $$\text{Calculation: } 0.10 = xg/4 \text{ cc.}$$
   $$x\,g = 0.10 \times 4 \text{ cc} = 0.4 \text{ g, or } 400 \text{ mg.}$$

8. What is the percent strength of the 1 mg/ml solution of dornase alfa available for nebulization?
   Answer: $x = 0.001$ g/1 ml $= 0.001 = 0.1\%$ concentration.

9. What is a common side effect of acetylcysteine by nebulization? How is it detected?
   Answer: Airway irritation and bronchospasm are common with acetylcysteine and more likely with the 20% than the 10% strength. Check the concentration of the solution to be used. Airway reactivity predisposes to bronchoconstriction with use of acetylcysteine; check the diagnosis and history of the patient for asthma. The assessment for airway irritation and bronchoconstriction is recognition of wheezing through auscultation or, alternatively, patient complaints of chest tightness, difficulty in breathing, or similar statements.

10. What is a common side effect seen with administration of dornase alfa by aerosol?
    Answer: Voice alteration and pharyngitis.

Clinical Scenario

What aerosol medications would be indicated for her?

Answer: Her pulmonary function tests indicate mild to moderate airway obstruction, accompanied by the usual problematic secretions seen in cystic fibrosis. Her recent history also suggests recurrent pulmonary infec-

tions, with purulent sputum production and a need for intravenous antibiotic therapy and hospitalizations. She may benefit from dornase alfa (Pulmozyme), 2.5 mg daily by nebulizer. She may also find continued use of a β agonist such as albuterol helpful to improve or maintain lung function and secretion clearance. Finally, continued use of aerosolized antibiotic such as tobramycin should be considered to reduce the bacterial burden of her respiratory secretions.

What outcomes would you assess to determine the effectiveness of dornase alfa in her case?

Answer: (1) The use of parenteral antibiotics over the coming year; (2) the use of oral quinolones such as ciprofloxacin over the year; (3) the need for hospitalizations for acute exacerbations; and (4) maintenance or hopefully even improvement in her pulmonary function.

Chapter 10

Self-Assessment Questions

1. What is the definition of a surface-active substance?
   Answer: An agent that can change surface tension at liquid-air interfaces.

2. What clinical problem was ethyl alcohol used for in the past?
   Answer: Acute pulmonary edema, usually from congestive heart failure.

3. In general, what is the clinical indication for use of exogenous surfactants?
   Answer: Prevention (prophylaxis) of RDS in premature newborns with immature lungs or newborns with evidence of immature lung development, and treatment (rescue) of infants who have developed RDS.

4. What type (category) of exogenous surfactant is each of the following: colfosceril palmitate, beractant, calfactant, and poractant alfa?
   Answer: Colfosceril palmitate (Exosurf Neonatal)—artificial.
   Beractant (Survanta)—modified natural bovine extract.
   Calfactant (Infasurf)—natural bovine extract.
   Poractant alfa (Curosurf)—natural porcine extract.

5. What are the major ingredients of natural pulmonary surfactant?
   Answer: Lipids (about 90%), including DPPC; proteins, 10%.

6. Give the dosage schedule of each of the current exogenous surfactants:
   Answer: Exosurf—5 ml/kg.
   Survanta—100 mg/kg, or 4 ml/kg.
   Infasurf—3 ml/kg.
   Curosurf—2.5 ml/kg.

7. What is the difference between "rescue" and "prophylaxis" treatment with these agents?
   Answer: Rescue—drug given in presence of RDS. Prophylaxis—drug given *before* onset of RDS.

8. Identify at least three possible adverse effects with use of exogenous surfactant treatment.
   Answer: Apnea, overventilation, overoxygenation, airway occlusion, desaturation, and bradycardia.

9. Why does the improvement in lung compliance last, after only one or two administrations of exogenous surfactant?
   Answer: Apparently, exogenous surfactant enters the recycling pool in alveolar cells.

10. How does the artificial surfactant colfosceril palmitate compensate for lack of the natural surfactant-associated proteins, such as SP-B or SP-C?
    Answer: Cetyl alcohol and tyloxapol are substituted for the surfactant proteins to promote adsorption and spreading of the colfosceril palmitate which is synthetic DPPC.

11. Which exogenous surfactants contain the proteins found in natural surfactant, such as SP-B?
    Answer: The modified natural products beractant (Survanta), calfactant (Infasurf), and poractant alfa (Curosurf).

12. How would you assess the effectiveness of exogenous surfactant treatment in a premature newborn with respiratory distress?
    Answer: Monitor vital signs, including color and activity, for evidence of airway occlusion, desaturation, and bradycardia. Be prepared to manually ventilate and suction the airway. Assess changes in level of ventilation: chest rise, Sao_2 or $tcPo_2$, and exhaled volumes or peak inspiratory pressures. Modify ventilator settings and Fio_2 based on changes.

Clinical Scenario

Is there an indication for administration of an exogenous surfactant in this case? Support your decision with the available data.
Answer: Yes. The gestational age and low birth weight indicate prematurity, which is associated with lung immaturity and lack of endogenous surfactant. The chest radiograph confirms the presence of neonatal RDS. Beractant (Survanta) was chosen for administration, and ABG values after treatment were pH, 7.38; $Paco_2$, 48 mm Hg; and Pao_2, 62 mm Hg. There was good chest rise, and exhaled tidal volume averaged 5 to 6 ml/kg body weight. Pulse oximetry readings stabilized in the range of 93% to 96%. Over the next few hours, the Fio_2 was lowered to 0.60, and the PIP decreased to 17 cm H_2O.

Would this administration of surfactant be a rescue or prophylactic treatment, if given immediately after placement on ventilatory support?
Answer: Although RDS is present on the radiograph, immediate treatment with surfactant is considered prophylactic rather than rescue; the infant has not yet developed full-blown respiratory failure (note Apgar score at 5 minutes). However, this is likely to occur without treatment.

What pharmacological treatment is now indicated?
Answer: A second dose of surfactant should be administered in an attempt to reverse the subsequent decline in lung function indicated by the decrease in compliance, deteriorating vital signs, and oxygenation. Ventilation and oxygenation should be monitored after a repeat dose, and adjustments made to avoid overventilation and overoxygenation.

Chapter 11

Self-Assessment Questions

1. Identify five corticosteroids approved for clinical use by oral inhalation in the United States, using generic names.
   Answer: Beclomethasone dipropionate, triamcinolone acetonide, flunisolide, fluticasone, and budesonide.

2. What is the major therapeutic effect of corticosteroids?
   Answer: Their antiinflammatory effect.

3. Identify two common respiratory diseases in which inhaled corticosteroids are prescribed.
   Answer: Asthma, and (less frequently) chronic obstructive pulmonary disease (COPD).

4. What is the rationale for use of inhaled corticosteroids instead of oral routes in asthma?
   Answer: By targeting the lung directly with corticosteroids that have a high topical potency, systemic levels can be minimized and systemic side effects decreased or avoided.

5. Contrast the effects of β agonists with those of corticosteroids, in their effects on the early and late phase of asthma.

    Answer: β Agonists may relieve the early phase of bronchoconstriction, whereas corticosteroids can reduce airway inflammation, preventing both the early and late phases of asthma.

6. What is the effect of orally administered corticosteroids on growth, bone density, and adrenal function?

    Answer: Growth is decreased in children; bone density is decreased, causing osteoporosis; normal adrenal steroid secretion is suppressed, and in general the HPA axis activity is suppressed.

7. What is the purpose of alternate-day steroid therapy?

    Answer: To reduce exposure of the body to exogenous corticosteroids and thereby reduce systemic side effects, such as adrenal suppression.

8. Can you transfer an asthmatic patient from oral steroid use to inhaled steroid use? Explain the precautions or reasons, as appropriate.

    Answer: Transfer can be accomplished; however, the patient should be weaned from the oral dose using tapering doses while initiating inhaled steroids, to allow adequate recovery of adrenal function, because inhaled steroids will not maintain significant plasma levels using recommended doses.

9. Identify a common side effect with inhaled steroids.

    Answer: Oral thrush (candidiasis), dysphonia.

10. Identify two methods of minimizing the side effect identified in question 9.

    Answer: (1) Use of a reservoir device with MDI orally inhaled corticosteroids; (2) rinsing of the throat with gargling after inhaling a corticosteroid.

11. Have inhaled corticosteroids traditionally been used with an asthmatic during an acute episode?

    Answer: No; there is no acute bronchodilating effect, and the dose of inhaled steroids is too low for acute management of airway inflammation. However, inhaled corticosteroids have been investigated for emergency department treatment of acute severe asthma, along with aggressive bronchodilator therapy (see discussion in Chapter 11).

CLINICAL SCENARIO

What inhaled aerosol agents would you recommend as appropriate at this time for discharge?

Answer: A bronchodilator as a reliever and a corticosteroid as a controller would seem to benefit this individual, given her history. An inhaled steroid by either MDI or DPI, depending on drug choice, should be recommended. A shorter, more rapid-acting β agonist, such as albuterol by MDI, should also be prescribed for as-needed use in acute symptoms. Salmeterol by MDI twice daily can be added as an additional controller agent if symptoms persist and may prevent the need for increasing the inhaled corticosteroid dose. The combination product, fluticasone/salmeterol in a DPI formulation is available for convenient dosing.

What precautions and recommendations would you make with this patient?

Answer: Check to see if she has been on oral or intravenous steroids during her hospital stay; if so, taper the dose with oral prednisone while she begins using an inhaled steroid. This is intended to prevent adrenal suppression and exacerbation of symptoms. Instruct her to use a reservoir device with her inhaled steroid if an MDI formulation is prescribed, unless an integral spacing tube is supplied with the drug (e.g., triamcinolone acetonide, Azmacort). Instruct her to rinse her throat with water after inhalation to avoid oropharyngeal side effects such as dysphonia or oral thrush. Explain that poor compliance with the inhaled steroid will prevent a full therapeutic effect and that regular use is needed for control of airway inflammation, even though she may not "feel" an immediate effect. Clarify the use of the long-acting agent salmeterol versus the shorter-acting agent albuterol. Salmeterol is not helpful for acute symptoms, and overuse may lead to toxic accumulation. Albuterol has favorable pharmacokinetics for treating acute symptoms. Review correct use of an MDI and reservoir device, with a return demonstration from the individual. Finally, she should be instructed in self-assessment with a peak flow measuring device and told to contact her physician if her symptoms return and are not controlled by this regimen.

CHAPTER 12

SELF-ASSESSMENT QUESTIONS

1. Identify five nonsteroidal antiasthmatic drugs used in the management of chronic asthma (give both generic and brand names).

Answer: Cromolyn sodium (Intal), nedocromil sodium (Tilade), montelukast (Singulair), zafirlukast (Accolate), and zileuton (Zyflo).

2. Which immunoglobulin is implicated in allergy and is termed cytophilic?

Answer: Immunoglobulin E (IgE).

3. Which type of asthma involves allergic reaction to an antigenic stimulus?

Answer: Extrinsic, or atopic.

4. Which type of helper T cell, Th1 or Th2, is involved primarily in the atopic allergic response?

Answer: Th2 cells (helper type 2 lymphocytes).

5. A resident wishes to order nebulized cromolyn sodium for a young asthmatic patient in the emergency department who is wheezing and in moderate distress. Would you agree?

Answer: No. Cromolyn sodium, as a mediator antagonist, is a prophylactic agent to *prevent* mast cell degranulation and mediator release; the drug has no bronchodilating properties.

6. Which of the following could be recommended as possible choices for the asthmatic patient in question 5: inhaled albuterol, inhaled salmeterol, inhaled ipratropium, theophylline either orally or intravenously?

Answer: All of the agents listed could be used in an acute asthma episode, except for salmeterol, because its pharmacokinetics are not useful for an acute attack.

7. What is the usual dose of nedocromil sodium by inhalation in adults?

Answer: By MDI, 2 actuations with 1.75 mg per actuation, four times daily.

8. An asthmatic patient has been on 40 mg of oral prednisone for a week after an acute asthma attack and an emergency department visit. His physician now wants to switch him to inhaled nedocromil and discontinue the oral prednisone. What is the risk in doing this and what would you recommend?

Answer: There is risk of adrenal insufficiency caused by the steroid therapy and HPA suppression, and the fact that nedocromil is not a steroid. A tapered dose regimen of the oral prednisone while the nedocromil is started should be recommended.

9. Briefly compare and distinguish the mode of action of nedocromil sodium versus cromolyn sodium.

Answer: Nedocromil sodium has a broader effect, with inhibition of multiple inflammatory cells, including mast cell degranulation, eosinophil protein release, cytokine release from airway epithelial cells, suppression of adhesion molecules from epithelial cells (e.g., ICAM-1), and inhibition of sensory nerve activation; cromolyn sodium has a more specific action inhibiting IgE-mediated mast cell degranulation and mediator release.

10. How does the mode of action of zafirlukast and montelukast differ from that of zileuton?

Answer: Zafirlukast and montelukast act by competitive antagonism of leukotriene receptors ($CysLT_1$), whereas zileuton acts by inhibition of the 5-lipoxygenase enzyme.

11. What are the recommended dose and route of administration for zafirlukast, montelukast, and zileuton?

Answer: Zafirlukast—20 mg twice daily, by the oral route.
Montelukast—10 mg once daily, orally.
Zileuton—600 mg four times daily, orally.

12. Which of the three antileukotriene agents in question 11 offers the most convenient dosing and fewest drug interactions?

Answer: Montelukast (Singulair), with once daily dosing, and no significant drug interactions such as can occur with zileuton or zafirlukast.

CLINICAL SCENARIO

How would you treat her asthma attack at this point?

Answer: She was placed on oxygen at 2 L/min by nasal cannula and given albuterol, 4 actuations using an MDI with holding chamber, every 20 minutes. A plasma theophylline level showed 12.8 µg/ml. After approximately 1 hour (three albuterol treatments), her respiratory rate had decreased to 14 breaths/min, she appeared comfortable, and her wheezing had diminished, with breath sounds heard over both lung fields. She stated her chest felt "much more open." She was given a prescription for 1 week of oral prednisone, tapered dose, and asked to see her physician within a week.

What medications would you consider for maintenance of her asthma, given her recent history and prior medications?

Answer: Her increasing use of the inhaled β agonist on most days of the week indicates the need for an antiinflammatory agent. A trial of either cromolyn sodium or nedocromil sodium could be considered to target her inflammation. Given her recent cough symptoms, aspirin sensitivity, and history of nasal polyps, she may be a good candidate for use of an antileukotriene agent. Alternatively, the broad inhibitory effect of nedocromil sodium on the inflammatory process may prove beneficial. Either type of agent is an alternative to use of inhaled steroids. The inhaled β agonist should be continued. The theophylline could be discontinued in light of her headaches, gastrointestinal symptoms, and insomnia and replaced with either nedocromil or an antileukotriene while monitoring for any deterioration of her asthma symptoms. She was started on nedocromil sodium, 2 inhalations by MDI four times daily, together with pirbuterol, 2 to 4 inhalations as needed. She was also instructed in the use of a peak flow meter, to evaluate control of her symptoms. Because she had occasional mornings with chest tightness and a need for use of the pirbuterol, and because of more convenient dosing, she subsequently changed to oral montelukast, 10 mg each evening. She has done well on this combination of rescue β agonist and an antileukotriene.

CHAPTER 13

SELF-ASSESSMENT QUESTIONS

1. Identify the disease states each of these drugs are used for when inhaled as an aerosol: pentamidine, ribavirin, tobramycin, and zanamivir.
   Answer: Pentamidine—PCP prophylaxis in AIDS (second-line).
   Ribavirin—RSV treatment with risk of severe or complicated infection.
   Tobramycin—management of *P. aeruginosa* in cystic fibrosis.
   Zanamivir—treatment of acute influenza infection.
2. Briefly, what is the rationale for aerosolizing an antibiotic such as tobramycin, in cystic fibrosis?
   Answer: Oral route gives inadequate lung levels; inhaled and intravenous routes give higher lung tissue levels.
3. What is the brand name of aerosol pentamidine?
   Answer: NebuPent.
4. What is the dose and frequency for aerosol pentamidine?
   Answer: 300 mg q4wk.
5. What device is approved for aerosolization of pentamidine?
   Answer: Respirgard II.

6. Identify the common airway effects with aerosol pentamidine, and suggest a method for preventing or lessening these.
   Answer: Cough, bronchoconstriction; pretreat with a β agonist.
7. What is a major risk to the caregiver when aerosolizing pentamidine to a patient with AIDS?
   Answer: Contraction of TB infection.
8. What is the current Centers for Disease Control (CDC) recommended prophylactic treatment for PCP in AIDS patients?
   Answer: Use TMP-SMX orally as long as side effects are tolerated and acceptable. If side effects are too severe, switch to inhaled pentamidine (NebuPent).
9. What is the brand name and dose for aerosol ribavirin?
   Answer: Virazole 6 g/300 ml (2%) 12 to 18 hr/day for 3 to 7 days.
10. What is the mode of action of ribavirin?
    Answer: Virostatic. As a nucleoside analogue, ribavirin interferes with viral transcription and replication.
11. Identify two serious hazards when ribavirin is given to a patient on mechanical ventilation.
    Answer: (1) Occlusion of endotracheal tube. (2) Expiratory valve and sensor occlusion.
12. How, in general, can you prevent environmental contamination when delivering ribavirin to an oxyhood?
    Answer: A containment/scavenging system around hood.
13. What is the recommended dosage for inhaled tobramycin?
    Answer: 300 mg by PARI LC Plus SVN twice daily, alternating 28 days on/28 days off.
14. What common side effects have been observed with aerosolized tobramycin?
    Answer: Tinnitus and voice changes.
15. Identify two potential hazards to family members with aerosolized tobramycin at home.
    Answer: Exposure to aerosol drug in ambient air may lead to (1) allergic reactions in those sensitive to the drug and (2) fetal harm in a pregnant female.
16. Give the brand name and dosage for zanamivir.
    Answer: Relenza 2 inhalations (10 mg) twice daily 12 hours apart, for 5 days.
17. In one sentence describe the mode of action of zanamivir.

Answer: Zanamivir inhibits the viral enzyme neuraminidase, causing viral aggregation and clumping, preventing viral release and spreading.

18. What are common hazards in the use of inhaled zanamivir?

    Answer: Pulmonary function deterioration, including bronchospasm in those with reactive airways disease, and inappropriate treatment or undertreatment of nonviral bacterial infections.

19. What factors cause debate over use of zanamivir in treating influenza?

    Answer: Essentially cost versus efficacy—small reduction in symptoms, no inexpensive easily available test to confirm influenza infection, increased possible risk in airways disease.

CLINICAL SCENARIO

Identify key elements of his respiratory care plan that you would suggest.

Answer: Continue with his usual cystic fibrosis medications (vitamins, iron supplement, Pancrease enzymes). *Oxygen* is indicated by his SpO_2 value. *Antibiotic therapy* will be needed to reduce his bacterial burden, as indicated by his temperature and WBC count. An aggressive program of bronchial hygiene is usual to clear his secretions, and would include *chest physiotherapy* with postural drainage and percussion as tolerated for mobilization of secretions; β_2 *agonist* by aerosol to maintain airway patency; possible administration of the anticholinergic bronchodilator, *ipratropium* by either SVN or MDI; and, finally, adequate fluid intake and balanced nutrition.

What is the risk of using the ciprofloxacin as an antibiotic to treat his symptoms of infection?

Answer: Because he has completed a course of ciprofloxacin and symptoms are now recurring, there is the possibility of resistance to the ciprofloxacin. A different, or at the least an additional, antibiotic may be needed.

His physician decides to institute a course of tobramycin rather than repeating the ciprofloxacin. Can this antibiotic be given orally as an effective antibacterial agent for Mr. P's respiratory infection?

Answer: No. Oral administration of aminoglycosides, antibiotics that are very effective in treating the gram-negative infections typical in cystic fibrosis, do not give suitably high lung levels.

Identify two alternative routes of administration for tobramycin in this case.

Either intravenously or by aerosol. Aerosol administration would directly target the lung.

Mr. P's physician orders intravenous tobramycin, as well as by aerosol, 300 mg bid, and he asks you to make a detailed suggestion on administration by nebulizer. What would you suggest?

Answer: The nebulizer used in clinical trials of aerosolized tobramycin was the PARI LC Plus. Other nebulizers may give suitable drug output and particle size. The PARI should be operated either by a suitable powerful compressor, such as the Pulmo-Aide, or used with 6 to 8 L/min of air powered by 50 psi. Administer the β_2 agonist by MDI before the antibiotic treatment. A nebulizer system with one-way intake and expiratory valves and a scavenging filter on the expiratory side is strongly recommended, to reduce personnel exposure to ambient aerosol of the antibiotic.

How would you evaluate (1) the aerosolized antibiotic therapy and (2) the treatment plan for Mr. P?

Answer: (1). The aerosol antibiotic therapy can be evaluated during and after a treatment by monitoring respiratory rate and pattern, pulse, and breath sounds. (2). Over the course of his therapy, vital signs, including temperature, chest radiograph, WBC count, sputum production characteristics (color, amount, consistency), sputum cultures, and bedside spirometry (especially FEV_1) will provide information on his progress. The treatment plan described in the question above on key elements, including intravenous and aerosol tobramycin, was in fact successfully implemented, and Mr P. steadily improved. On his eighth day of admission, intravenous antibiotic therapy was discontinued, and on his eleventh day, Mr. P. was discharged, with no wheezing and some rales on auscultation of his lung fields.

CHAPTER 14

SELF-ASSESSMENT QUESTIONS

1. What is the difference between bacteriostatic and bactericidal antimicrobial agents?

   Answer: Bacteriostatic agents inhibit the growth of bacteria, whereas bactericidal agents kill bacteria.

2. Describe the difference between antimicrobial agents that act in a concentration-dependent manner and agents that act in a time-dependent manner.
   Answer: Concentration-dependent antimicrobials have a proportional increase in their rate of microbial kill when their concentrations are increased. Time-dependent (or concentration-independent) antimicrobials do not have proportional increases in microbial kill with increasing concentrations of the agent. Time-dependent agents require maintenance of drug concentration above the minimal inhibitory concentration (MIC) (or some factor of the MIC) for optimal activity.

3. Describe at least three parameters that may indicate antibiotic failure in a patient.
   Answer: Continued fever spikes, elevated WBC count, repeated positive cultures, and nonresolution or worsening of symptoms (such as hypotension or mental status change) may indicate antibiotic failure.

4. Why is it useful to use combination antimicrobial therapy (be specific)?
   Answer: Antimicrobial combinations can provide broad-spectrum activity as part of an empiric regimen. Certain infections are polymicrobial and so require a combination of antimicrobials to be therapeutically effective. Antimicrobial combinations can be used for their synergistic effect and reduce the emergence of resistance.

5. Describe the mechanism of action of penicillin antibiotics. Name at least two additional antibiotic classes with similar mechanisms of action.
   Answer: Penicillins bind to cell wall proteins to inhibit the cross-linkage of peptidoglycan, which reduces the structural integrity of the cell wall, resulting in lysis. Cephalosporins, carbepenems, and monobactams have a similar mechanism of action.

6. Which β-lactam antibiotic is least likely to cause an allergic reaction in a patient with a penicillin allergy?
   Answer: Aztreonam.

7. Name three antimicrobial agents that would be useful in the treatment of community-acquired pneumonia?
   Answer: Azithromycin, clarithromycin, levofloxacin, gatifloxacin, moxifloxacin, cefuroxime, or erythromycin.

8. What is the antimicrobial agent of choice for the treatment of *Pneumocystis carinii* pneumonia (PCP)?
   Answer: Trimethoprim-sulfamethoxazole.

9. What agents are considered first-line therapy for the treatment of pulmonary tuberculosis?
   Answer: Isoniazid, rifampin or rifabutin, pyrazinamide, and ethambutol.

10. Which antimicrobial agents are useful for the treatment of nosocomial pneumonia caused by *Pseudomonas aeruginosa?*
    Answer: Imipenem or meropenem or cefepime or ceftazidime or piperacillin/tazobactam + an aminoglycoside (gentamicin, tobramycin or amikacin) or ciprofloxacin.

CLINICAL SCENARIO

What signs and symptoms of infection in this patient are consistent with the diagnosis of community-acquired pneumonia?
Answer: The symptoms consistent with this diagnosis include productive cough, fever, chills, and shortness of breath. The signs of infection include his elevated temperature, heart and respiratory rates, decreased oxygen saturation, bilateral respiratory crackles, elevated WBC count, many WBCs in his sputum, and left lower lobe infiltrate on chest x-ray film.

What is the most likely pathogen responsible for community-acquired pneumonia in this patient?
Answer: The Gram stain reveals gram-positive cocci in pairs and chains, which is consistent with the most likely pathogen, *Streptococcus pneumoniae.*

Name two antibiotics that can be used to treat this patient's community-acquired pneumonia.
Answer: Numerous antibiotics may be used, including azithromycin, clarithromycin, levofloxacin, gatifloxacin, or moxifloxacin. A β-lactam (e.g., a penicillin or cephalosporin) must be avoided because of the patient's allergy history.

If the sputum stains are acid-fast positive, what precautions should be taken and what drug therapy should be initiated?
Answer: The patient must be placed in respiratory isolation using a negative-pressure room. Health care personnel should wear fitted respiratory masks when tending to this patient. The patient should

be initiated on isoniazid, rifampin, pyrazina-mide, ethambutol, and pyridoxine for treatment of tuberculosis.

CHAPTER 15

SELF-ASSESSMENT QUESTIONS

1. Identify the four classes of ingredients found in cold medications.
   Answer: Adrenergic decongestants, antihistamines (H_1 blockers), expectorants, antitussives; note: analgesic may be added.
2. For each of the following agents, identify the category (e.g., adrenergic, antitussive, etc.): codeine, chlorpheniramine, phenylpropanolamine, dextromethorphan, pseudoephedrine.
   Answer: Codeine—antitussive.
   Chlorpheniramine—antihistamine.
   Phenylpropanolamine—adrenergic.
   Dextromethorphan—antitussive.
   Pseudoephedrine—adrenergic.
3. What is the intended purpose of α-adrenergic agents in cold medications?
   Answer: Topical vasoconstriction, to open upper (nasal) airway.
4. What is the intended effect of antihistamines (H_1 blockers) in cold medications?
   Answer: To dry secretions (rhinitis) produced by histamine release and stimulation of H_1 receptors.
5. Are antihistamines in cold remedies H_1 or H_2 blockers?
   Answer: H_1 blockers. (H_2 blockers, e.g., ranitidine [Zantac], are antiulcer drugs.)
6. You drink several beers at a friend's house after taking a dose of Chlor-Trimeton. Should you drive home, and why or why not?
   Answer: No. Antihistamines cause drowsiness, and alcohol produces an additive effect on this—reflexes are decreased.
7. Identify the most common expectorant in OTC cold remedies.
   Answer: Guaifenesin (glyceryl guaiacolate).
8. Briefly explain how guaifenesin stimulates mucus production?
   Answer: Probably through stimulation of vagal receptors in the stomach.
9. List some specific fluids you would recommend to someone with a cold.
   Answer: Water, juices, milk.
10. Differentiate a "cold" from the "flu."
    Answer: Cold—nonbacterial upper respiratory infection with mild malaise and runny, stuffy nose (more localized than the flu).
    Flu—systemic viral infection with fever, chills, headache, muscle ache, extreme fatigue.

CLINICAL SCENARIO

What other symptoms would you ask about to differentiate his complaint as a cold versus the flu?
Answer: Temperature, headache, muscle ache, degree of malaise, and rapidity of onset. In response to questioning, he denies headache or muscle ache, describes the malaise as a very mild fatigue, and states that he noticed a gradually increasing rhinitis over a period of hours, with sneezing beginning during the first 6 hours of these symptoms. He has no fever. You could also ask if he has any ache in the area of his sinuses. A general question about history of any upper respiratory problems would be helpful.

What is your conclusion, at this point?
Answer: His symptoms indicate a cold rather than the flu.

Based on your information, what would you suggest to him for self-treatment?
Answer: Point out that there is no "cure" if this is a rhinovirus infection. He should treat his symptoms, however. An adrenergic *decongestant* may be helpful in opening his nasal passages and reducing some of the rhinitis. The use of a topical agent will give fewer systemic effects, such as a feeling of shakiness, and central nervous system stimulation than an oral agent. Caution him to use the decongestant sparingly to avoid rebound nasal congestion; treating the rebound congestion with additional sprays can produce a self-sustaining congestion. An antitussive agent, such as dextromethorphan, can be helpful if he has a nonproductive, dry, irritating cough, particularly if this prevents adequate rest at night. The use of an antihistamine should be avoided if possible, to prevent impaction of secretions and subsequent sinus problems. However, if an antihistamine is used, it should only be taken at night or when alert activity (including driving) is not needed. Rest and good nutrition, including juices, will assist his own immune response to recover from the infection.

What is your assessment now?

Answer: Based on his symptoms, there is a secondary infection, probably bacterial, causing an acute bronchitis. Identification of a causative organism would be desirable, but in its absence treatment with a broad-spectrum antibiotic should be considered. This could be with penicillin, tetracycline, or a third-generation cephalosporin to cover gram-negative bacteria.

CHAPTER 16

SELF-ASSESSMENT QUESTIONS

1. What is the disease state in which an α_1-proteinase inhibitor (API) is indicated?
   Answer: Congenital α_1-antitrypsin deficiency.
2. What is the route of administration for α_1-proteinase inhibitor?
   Answer: Intravenous.
3. What is the mode of action of α_1-proteinase inhibitor in treating emphysema associated with inadequate API levels?
   Answer: Intravenous administration of exogenous α_1-proteinase increases blood levels and diffuses into the lung tissue to increase epithelial fluid levels, where the API inactivates the enzyme neutrophil elastase (NE), which can destroy lung tissue.
4. Is treatment with API indicated for age-related emphysema or in general for those who smoke and have emphysema later in life?
   Answer: No. Use of API is recommended only for those who have congenital α_1-AT deficiency and severe COPD. Such individuals often are smokers, which is a risk factor for development of COPD in α_1-AT deficiency, usually at an early age (third or fourth decade).
5. Identify three pharmaceutical formulations of nicotine that are used as smoking cessation aids.
   Answer: The transdermal patch, chewing gum, nasal spray.
6. What is the usual effect of nicotine, whether in a smoking cessation aid or in cigarettes, on blood pressure?
   Answer: Nicotine acts at the ganglionic synapses to increase blood pressure, with peripheral vasoconstriction; epinephrine is released from the adrenal medulla, contributing to hypertension, tachycardia, and vasoconstriction.
7. What is the effect of inhaled nitric oxide?
   Answer: Relaxation of the pulmonary vascular endothelium and a reduction of pulmonary hypertension.
8. Identify two potentially toxic by-products of inhaled nitric oxide.
   Answer: Methemoglobin and nitrogen dioxide.
9. What is the usual dose of inhaled nitric oxide?
   Answer: The recommended dose is 20 ppm, maintained up to 14 days or until the underlying oxygen desaturation has resolved and weaning from inhaled nitric oxide can be accomplished.
10. Identify two disease states in which nitric oxide has been used to reverse pulmonary hypertension.
    Answer: Persistent pulmonary hypertension of the newborn and acute respiratory distress syndrome.

CLINICAL SCENARIO

Given this presenting scenario, what laboratory tests would you obtain to further evaluate her respiratory status?

Answer: Important laboratory tests to evaluate her respiratory status would be a CBC and differential, electrolytes, sputum sample, chest radiograph (anteroposterior and lateral), ABGs, and pulmonary function test. These tests were performed, and the results showed a mild elevation of her WBC count (13.1×10^3/mm³), normal hemoglobin and hematocrit, normal electrolytes, and *Pseudomonas* and normal flora in her sputum. Her chest radiograph showed some hyperlucency; hyperinflation with moderately lowered, somewhat flattened hemidiaphragms on full inspiration; and an infiltrate in the right lower lobe. ABG values on room air were pH, 7.35; Pa_{CO_2}, 54 mm Hg; Pa_{O_2}, 66 mm Hg; HCO_3^-, 30 mEq/L; and an Sa_{O_2}, 92%. Pulmonary function tests revealed an FEV_1 that was 60% of predicted, with an elevated residual volume and RV/TLC ratio, an increased TLC above predicted, and a decreased DL_{CO}.

Based on her clinical picture and the laboratory results, what further test would you want now?

Answer: Her clinical and laboratory findings support a diagnosis of chronic obstructive pulmonary disease (COPD). However, her smoking history is not sufficient to produce the degree of severity seen, and her age is incompatible with the usual presentation of COPD. You may want to obtain an α_1-proteinase inhibitor blood level. This was obtained, in fact, and her value was found to be approximately 5 μM, by the purified laboratory standard.

With these results, would the use of α_1-proteinase inhibitor therapy be indicated?

Answer: Yes. She was subsequently started on Prolastin, 60 mg/kg intravenously once a week, with a diagnosis of moderately severe emphysema secondary to α_1-proteinase inhibitor deficiency.

CHAPTER 17

SELF-ASSESSMENT QUESTIONS

1. Can an aerosol formulation for oral inhalation be administered to neonatal and pediatric patients?
   Answer: Yes. Using appropriate devices and techniques and with a duly licensed physician's order.
2. Can an adrenergic bronchodilator such as albuterol reduce airway resistance when used in infants and children?
   Answer: Yes. Multiple studies cited in Table 17-5 have found improved airway mechanics with aerosolized albuterol delivered by either MDI/reservoir system or nebulizer.
3. Based on the data reviewed in this chapter, does the adult dose of an aerosol drug need to be reduced with pediatric subjects based on weight?
   Answer: No. Because of multiple factors in neonatal and pediatric patients, the actual dose of an inhaled aerosol reaching the lungs is proportionately less than an adult lung dose and increases/decreases with increasing/decreasing age.
4. What aerosol delivery devices could be used with a 2-year-old child?
   Answer: A nebulizer (with mask if necessary) or an MDI with a reservoir and mask.

CLINICAL SCENARIO

What methods of aerosol delivery are *appropriate* and *available* for albuterol?

Answer: Either an MDI or an SVN could be used, based on the age and patient interface (ETT).

What would you recommend to the physician?

Answer: A dose of 2.5 mg of albuterol is the maximal recommended dose. Because the side effect of sinus tachycardia is noted with this dose, it would be appropriate to reduce the dose. The dose schedule of 0.05 mg/kg would result in an ineffectively low dose of only 0.04 mg, which is less than 0.01 ml of a 0.5% solution. The minimal recommended dose of 1.25 mg would be reasonable and, in fact, was then delivered after allowing the heart rate to return to baseline. The heart rate remained at 164 to 176 beats/min throughout the subsequent treatment, and improved volume exchange was noted.

CHAPTER 18

SELF-ASSESSMENT QUESTIONS

1. List four general uses of skeletal muscle relaxants.
   Answer: (1). To facilitate endotracheal intubation.
   (2). For muscle relaxation during surgery.
   (3). To enhance CO_2 removal in difficult-to-ventilate patients.
   (4). To reduce intracranial pressure in intubated patients with uncontrolled intracranial pressure.
2. What are the two types of neuromuscular blocking agents?
   Answer: Nondepolarizing and depolarizing.
3. Identify each of the following agents by type: tubocurarine, vecuronium, succinylcholine, and pancuronium.
   Answer: Tubocurarine—nondepolarizing.
   Vecuronium—nondepolarizing.
   Succinylcholine—depolarizing.
   Pancuronium—nondepolarizing.
4. Which type of neuromuscular blocker can be reversed?
   Answer: Nondepolarizing.
5. What type of drug would you use to reverse vecuronium?
   Answer: Cholinesterase inhibitor (e.g., neostigmine).
6. Identify another drug that you would want to give before you reverse the vecuronium.
   Answer: Atropine or glycopyrrolate (antimuscarinic agents).
7. Briefly explain why you might need to paralyze a patient receiving mechanical ventilation.
   Answer: To relax chest wall and prevent spontaneous breathing efforts that are out of phase with the ventilator, causing increased intrathoracic pressure and decreased alveolar ventilation.
8. Neuromuscular blocking agents do not block consciousness; what two types or classes of drugs would be indicated in a paralyzed patient on a mechanical ventilator?
   Answer: Analgesics and sedatives.
9. Identify at least two neuromuscular blocking agents that would be preferred for paralysis in a patient receiving mechanical ventilation (assume normal renal and hepatic function).

Answer: Doxacurium and vecuronium have minimal histamine release and cardiovascular effects; mivacurium, atracurium, and rocuronium are also alternatives.

10. You are called to the recovery room to set up a ventilator for a young woman who has just undergone a hysterectomy and has failed to breathe after a single dose of succinylcholine. What might the problem be?

    Answer: Atypical plasma cholinesterase.

11. What would you do first to assess a ventilated patient who is restless, and "fighting" the ventilator, before using a paralyzing agent?

    Answer: Assess ventilator function and patient status.

    Ventilator—possible malfunction; inappropriate settings (flow, FIO_2, volume, I:E, etc.)

    Patient—airway patency, SaO_2 or SpO_2, possible pain or anxiety requiring analgesia and sedation rather than paralysis.

CLINICAL SCENARIO

What additional drug is immediately indicated, given her laboratory results?

Answer: Oxygen, because she has an SpO_2 of only 80% on room air. She was started on a nasal cannula at 3 L/min and her SpO_2 improved to 95%.

What additional laboratory information would be most helpful in assessing this patient and determining further treatment?

Answser: An arterial blood gas. Her desaturation and poor FEV_1 indicate a severe attack, and pulse oximetry does not give her pH or carbon dioxide level. ABG values obtained immediately after placing her on a nasal cannula at 3 L/min revealed pH, 7.37; $PaCO_2$, 37 mm Hg; PaO_2, 104 mm Hg; and a base excess of -2.9. She was also given 4 actuations of albuterol by MDI using a reservoir device. She was admitted to the intensive care unit for aggressive treatment and close monitoring.

What other drugs would you consider at this point for treating her acute asthma?

Answer: An intravenous corticosteroid such as methylprednisolone or an oral formulation is reasonable, and the intravenous dose was given. In addition, inhalation of albuterol by MDI, 4 to 6 puffs with a reservoir, was ordered every 20 minutes for up to 1 hour, as limited by tachycardia or unac-

ceptable muscle tremor. She was also placed on cefuroxime.

What neuromuscular blocking agent would you consider for a rapid-sequence intubation?

Answer: Either a nondepolarizing or a depolarizing agent could be used. However, succinylcholine has the advantage of rapid onset and short duration. This will avoid the need to manually ventilate the patient for several minutes, because of the slower onset of action using a nondepolarizing agent. After sedation, succinylcholine was administered and the patient was nasally intubated.

What agent would you use?

Answer: A nondepolarizing agent is indicated in this situation, because a longer duration of action is needed. Fortunately the patient is young and has normal hepatic and renal function. Given that she has asthma and high intrathoracic pressures resulting from intrinsic positive end-expiratory pressure (PEEP), a nondepolarizing agent that combines low histamine release and minimal cardiovascular effects is desirable. Pancuronium has often been chosen for its low histamine release, but it can cause increases in heart rate or mean arterial blood pressure. Vecuronium has both a low histamine release, important in this asthmatic to avoid exacerbation of airway inflammation, and minimal cardiovascular effects. Paralysis was maintained with an infusion of vecuronium over the next 24 hours, with no adverse consequences. Ventilation and arterial blood gas values improved, and 2 days later the patient was extubated uneventfully.

How will you monitor the effectiveness of this therapy?

Answer: Using peripheral (ulnar) nerve stimulation, the neuromuscular blocking drug should be titrated to maintain at least one twitch during TOF evaluation. This will minimize the amount of blocking agent and prevent overdosage. TOF peripheral nerve stimulation should be monitored at 15- to 30-minute intervals while the neuromuscular blocking infusion continues. The goals of neuromuscular blockade in this patient should also be assessed. Ventilatory pressures with an adequate respiratory rate and I:E ratio should be seen. The improvement noted in arterial blood gases reflects improved gas exchange with the level of ventilatory support.

If the patient were in renal or hepatic failure, what neuromuscular blocking agent would you recommend?

Answer: This additional factor leads to consideration of atracurium or cisatracurium, neither of which is eliminated in the liver or kidneys. However, monitoring for cerebral toxicity and excitation caused by the metabolite, laudanosine, is needed. Alternatively, mivacurium provides a blocking agent not dependent on significant liver or kidney elimination. Mivacurium has a relatively short duration of action, which can be prolonged in end-stage liver or kidney disease. All three agents can cause more histamine release than vecuronium or pancuronium.

CHAPTER 19

SELF-ASSESSMENT QUESTIONS

1. Should pulmonary function testing be done at baseline for all patients who are started on chronic amiodarone therapy?

    Answer: No. Pulmonary function testing may be done at baseline when patients have preexisting lung disease, but it is typically done only if patients become symptomatic during amiodarone therapy.

2. Should patients with early-onset amiodarone hypersensitivity syndrome continue to receive amiodarone?

    Answer: No. Amiodarone should be discontinued and corticosteroid therapy initiated if amiodarone pulmonary hypersensitivity is suspected.

3. Is vasopressin an alternative to epinephrine therapy for ventricular fibrillation?

    Answer: Yes. Vasopressin is now an alternative to epinephrine for the treatment of persistent ventricular fibrillation.

4. What is a positive inotropic effect?

    Answer: A positive inotropic effect is an increase in the force of contraction of the heart. Decreased contractility would be a negative inotropic effect. Chronotropic changes refer to changes in heart rate.

5. What is the general effect on cardiac function of the cardiac glycosides such as digitalis?

    Answer: Increased contractility (positive inotropic effect). Improved contractility and cardiac output may in turn lead to a reduction in heart rate (a negative chronotropic effect).

6. What effect does milrinone have on cardiac contractility?

    Answer: Milrinone, and inamrinone are both phosphodiesterase inhibitors and are classified as positive inotropic agents, which increase cardiac contractility.

7. Which class of cardiac antiarrhythmics includes lidocaine?

    Answer: Lidocaine is a Class I antiarrhythmic and is more specifically categorized as a Class IB agent. Class I agents slow the fast inward sodium channel, to delay the myocardial action potential.

8. To which class of antiarrhythmic does esmolol (Brevibloc) belong?

    Answer: Esmolol is a Class II agent and a cardioselective β blocker, which can reduce heart rate.

9. What is the mechanism of action for Class IV agents such as diltiazem or verapamil?

    Answer: Class IV agents are calcium channel blockers and inhibit the influx of calcium to slow supraventricular tachyarrhythmias.

10. In which type of cardiac arrhythmia would atropine be used?

    Answer: Atropine is a parasympatholytic (anticholinergic) agent used in symptomatic bradycardia or asystole. Blocking the parasympathetic (vagal) slowing of the heart can increase the heart rate.

CLINICAL SCENARIO

Is oxygen therapy indicated for immediate support of the patient?

Answer: Yes. Her pulse oximetry reading (89%) indicates moderate hypoxemia, equivalent to a Pao_2 of 55 to 60 mm Hg. She is maintaining this oxygenation with a respiratory rate of 34 breaths/min and a pulse rate of 110 beats/min. Supplemental oxygen will protect her heart from the need to compensate for hypoxemia with an increased rate, which would increase myocardial oxygen consumption in an already failing heart.

At this point, would initiation of an intravenous inotrope to improve cardiac output be a good choice?

Answer: Yes. A patient with an acute onset of congestive heart failure needs therapy to improve cardiac output. An inotrope is usually initiated early in therapy. Other treatments may include the use of diuretics and vasodilators.

Would dopamine be a good choice as an intravenous inotrope in this patient?

Answer: No. The potential for dopamine to worsen the tachycardia makes it a less desirable inotrope for most patients.

What potential side effect of dopamine would be of greatest concern?

Answer: Although dopamine has several side effects, including the ability to raise blood pressure and act as a positive inotrope, it may cause an elevation of heart rate, which makes it less desirable. Dopamine may improve renal blood flow and urine output through its effect on the dopaminergic receptor, but that would be beneficial to this patient.

What inotrope may be a better alternative than her current therapy?

Answer: Dobutamine. Although less likely than dopamine to cause tachycardia, dobutamine also shares that risk. In patients with tachyarrhythmias on dobutamine, milrinone is considered an alternative therapy. Dopamine and isoproterenol would sustain or worsen the tachycardia. Amiodarone is a treatment option for atrial arrhythmias but is not an inotrope.

What electrolyte therapy would you recommend?

Answer: Magnesium. Patients with hypomagnesemia are prone to develop a variety of arrhythmias. Replacement of magnesium and potassium are often needed in a patient with a new-onset arrhythmia. Although patients with hypercalcemia can have arrhythmias, it is uncommon with hypocalcemia. Sodium and chloride are extracellular electrolytes and do not significantly influence the risk of arrhythmias.

If the tachycardia produces severe hypotension, what therapy would be recommended?

Answer: Cardioversion/defibrillation. In an emergent situation, the most rapid treatment of an arrhythmia is defibrillation. Drug therapies may be used in a less urgent situation. Once a cardiac resuscitation has been started, agents such as epinephrine, vasopressin, and lidocaine may all be part of the supportive care therapies, but only defibrillation is a rapid means to convert the arrhythmia.

What is the preferred initial drug therapy for control of her ventricular response rate?

Answer: A calcium channel blocker. The calcium channel blockers diltiazem and verapamil will slow atrioventricular conduction and reduce the ventricular response rate in atrial fibrillation. Dofetilide is used for chronic treatment of atrial arrhythmias and is not recommended for acute treatment. Procainamide can be used to convert the arrhythmia to sinus rhythm, after another agent is used to control the heart rate. Epinephrine would increase the heart rate.

CHAPTER 20

SELF-ASSESSMENT QUESTIONS

1. List the adverse effects associated with angiotensin-converting–enzyme inhibitors (ACEIs).
    Answer: The most common ACEI-induced adverse effect is a persistent nonproductive dry cough, with an incidence of 20% to 30%. ACEI-induced adverse effects include rash, dysgeusia, hyperkalemia, orthostatic hypotension, blood dyscrasias, angioedema, and proteinuria.

2. Which of the β blockers possess intrinsic sympathomimetic activity (ISA)?
    Answer: The β blockers with ISA are acebutolol, carteolol, penbutolol, and pindolol.

3. Which of the β blockers possess selective β_1 blocker activity?
    Answer: The β blockers with α_1 selectivity are acebutolol, atenolol, betaxolol, bisoprolol, and metoprolol

4. List the adverse effects associated with β_1-adrenergic antagonists?
    Answer: α_1-Adrenergic antagonists adverse effects include orthostatic hypotension, dizziness, syncope, reflex tachycardia, palpitations, and headaches. These adverse effects are generally a manifestation of the first-dose phenomenon.

5. What are the most common side effects of nitrates?
    Answer: The most common side effects of nitrates include tachycardia, palpitations, headaches, dizziness, and flushing.

6. List the metabolic effects associated with thiazide diuretics.
    Answer: The metabolic effects of thiazide diuretics include hypokalemia, hypomagnesemia, hypercalcemia, hyperuricemia, and hyperglycemia.

7. List five medications that may cause drug-induced increases in blood pressure.
    Answer: Five drugs that may cause drug-induced increases in blood pressure are venlafaxine,

cyclosporine, ma huang, ibuprofen, and rofecoxib.

8. Which calcium channel blocker is most likely to cause constipation?

    Answer: Verapamil is the calcium-channel blocker most likely to cause constipation.

9. What is the best parameter available to monitor the effects of coumarin?

    Answer: The International Normalization Ratio is the best parameter available to monitor the effects of coumarin.

10. What is the antidote for heparin?

    Answer: Protamine is the antidote for heparin.

11. What is the mechanism of action of coumarin?

    Answer: Coumarin exerts its effect by interfering with the hepatic synthesis of vitamin K–dependent clotting factors II, VII, IX, and X.

12. Name the pharmacological class responsible for inhibiting the final pathway in platelet aggregation.

    Answer: The glycoprotein IIbIIIa inhibitors are responsible for inhibiting the final pathway in platelet aggregation.

13. Which thrombolytic is recommended for patients greater than 75 years of age who present with ST-segment-elevation myocardial infarction?

    Answer: Streptokinase is the thrombolytic recommended for patients greater than 75 years of age who present with ST-segment-elevation myocardial infarction.

14. Name the only ACEI that is available in a parenteral dosage form.

    Answer: Enalaprilat is the only ACEI that is available in a parenteral dosage form.

15. What is the best parameter available to monitor the effects of heparin?

    Answer: Activated partial thromboplastin time (APTT) is the best parameter available to monitor the effects of heparin.

CLINICAL SCENARIO

Is this patient a candidate for immediate administration of a glycoprotein IIb/IIIa inhibitor?

Answer: Yes, considering the significant role of platelets in non–ST-segment elevated myocardial infarction, glycoprotein IIb/IIIa inhibitors would provide benefit by inhibiting platelet aggregation and thrombus formation after an atherosclerotic plaque rupture. The use of glycoprotein IIb/IIIa inhibitors reduce the risk of death or nonfatal myocardial infarction.

Is this patient a candidate for immediate administration of thrombolytic therapy?

Answer: No. This patient does not have ST-segment elevation myocardial infarction and therefore is not a candidate for thrombolytic therapy. Immediate reperfusion of the infarcted artery is indicated in patients with persistent ST-segment elevations. Whether thrombolytics are beneficial in non–ST-segment elevation myocardial infarction has not been well elucidated and studies are being conducted in this area.

CHAPTER 21

SELF-ASSESSMENT QUESTIONS

1. What is a diuretic?

    Answer: A diuretic is any substance that increases urine output.

2. Identify the five major groups of diuretics used clinically.

    Answer: Osmotic, carbonic anhydrase inhibitors, thiazide, loop, and potassium-sparing.

3. If an agent such as one of the loop diuretics causes a loss of potassium, how will this lead to a metabolic alkalosis?

    Answer: Sodium that is still reabsorbed will exchange for either potassium or hydrogen. Low potassium, resulting from excretion, forces reabsorbed sodium to exchange for hydrogen, depleting hydrogen ions and raising pH. Hydrogen is also excreted as a result of the diuretic, adding to the alkalosis. Potassium replacement is usually necessary to prevent hypokalemia.

4. Which diuretics would preserve potassium?

    Answer: The potassium-sparing agents, such as amiloride, triamterene, or spironolactone.

5. What is the potential effect of a carbonic anhydrase inhibitor on acid-base balance?

    Answer: A loss of bicarbonate leading to a metabolic acidosis.

6. Explain how a diuretic such as furosemide can be helpful in acute congestive (left ventricular) heart failure with pulmonary and vascular edema?

    Answer: A potent diuretic such as furosemide will cause excretion of volume from the circulatory system by limiting sodium and therefore water retention. This will decrease the amount of volume leaking from the vasculature both in the lung and in the periphery, as well as venous return to the heart. Reduced pulmonary edema will improve oxygenation, which will also improve oxygen available to the heart. Reduced preload also reduces the work of the myocardium. Reduced preload and improved oxygenation are beneficial to restoring the heart function.

Clinical Scenario

True or False: In addition to oxygen and morphine sulfate 2 mg intravenously, a thiazide-type diuretic should be administered immediately.

Answer: False. Thiazide diuretics are generally relatively weak in their effect and have a slow onset of action. They are typically used when mild diuresis is needed or as a treatment for chronic hypertension. In acute pulmonary edema, a more vigorous diuresis is needed. The patient should be given an intravenous diuretic that acts primarily in the loop of Henle (a loop diuretic). Any of the available loop diuretics would be acceptable. In general, because of its higher incidence of side effects, ethacrynic acid is reserved for patients who are allergic to the other loop diuretics or who fail to respond to them. This patient is currently taking furosemide 40 mg daily; thus an acceptable approach would be to double the oral dose and give it intravenously. Therefore furosemide 80 mg intravenously would be a reasonable choice.

If the patient fails to respond to furosemide 80 mg intravenously, should another loop diuretic be tried?

Answer: No. If within 30 to 45 minutes of receiving intravenous furosemide, the patient has not begun to diurese, another loop diuretic would be reasonable. However, typically the preceding dose of furosemide would be doubled, that is 160 mg, and administered. There are no substantial data supporting the superiority of one loop diuretic over another.

True or False: When the patient begins to diurese, close observation of the potassium level will be needed.

Answer: True. The patient does have mild renal insufficiency and is on a β blocker. Both of these probably attenuate the normal potassium wasting seen with diuretics; however, with vigorous diuresis, he would most certainly become hypokalemic without potassium replacement. This can lead to dangerous arrhythmias, particularly in patients with ischemic cardiomyopathy. The potassium should be followed closely and repleted to a level of 4.0 mEq/L or greater.

CHAPTER 22

Self-Assessment Questions

1. What is the difference between sedation and analgesia?
   Answer: Sedation—decreased response to stimuli, relaxes.
   Analgesia—relief of pain.
2. Identify the general class of each of the following agents (sedative-hypnotic, analgesic, tranquilizer, anesthetic, antipsychotic):
   Answer: Lorazepam—minor tranquilizer (antianxiety).
   Phenobarbital—sedative hypnotic.
   Doxapram—respiratory stimulant.
   Chloral hydrate—nonbarbiturate sedative-hypnotic.
   Thiopental—general (intravenous) anesthetic.
   Midazolam—general anesthetic.
   Nitrous oxide—general anesthetic (gas).
   Chlorpromazine—antipsychotic.
   Halothane—general anesthetic (gas).
   Morphine—narcotic analgesic.
   Ibuprofen—NSAID, analgesic.
3. You are planning to extubate and remove a patient from the ventilator. However, the nurse administers a large dose of lorazepam (Ativan) for anxiety. What problem may occur if you proceed?
   Answer: Hypoventilation, depressed ventilatory drive.
4. What is the most serious side effect of tranquilizers, sedatives, or analgesics (especially opioids)?
   Answer: Central nervous system depression resulting in respiratory depression—hypoventilation or respiratory arrest.
5. You have two patients, both of whom have overdosed on central nervous system depressants.
   Patient 1: Comatose, cyanotic, dilated pupils.
   Patient 2: Comatose, cyanotic, pinpoint pupils.
   Which patient may have taken a barbiturate and which a narcotic analgesic?
   Answer: Barbiturate—Patient 1.
   Narcotic—Patient 2.
6. Identify your initial priorities as a respiratory therapist in caring for a subject with an overdose of tranquilizers.
   Answer: (1). Maintenance or establishment of airway.

(2). Provide ventilation.

(3). Supplemental O_2 as needed to maintain Pao_2.

7. What is the mode of action of the benzodiazepines?

    Answer: Benzodiazepines bind to benzodiazepine receptors in the central nervous system, and facilitate the action of γ-aminobutyric acid in inhibiting neuronal transmission through increased chloride ion flow.

8. Identify an agent that can reverse the effects of benzodiazepines such as midazolam and triazolam.

    Answer: Flumazenil.

9. Will barbiturates be helpful in managing pain with a ventilator patient?

    Answer: No, unless a dose capable of producing unconsciousness is used. There is no direct effect on pain transmission.

10. Would meperidine be helpful to prevent or lessen perception of pain?

    Answer: Yes. Meperidine (Demerol) is a morphinelike narcotic and will occupy opiate receptors to block nerve transmission of pain.

11. For a patient with a bleeding disorder, such as hemophilia, or one who is on anticoagulants such as warfarin, suggest an analgesic for minor pain.

    Answer: Acetaminophen would be the drug of choice. Aspirin and NSAIDs can both inhibit platelet aggregation and prolong bleeding times, even in normal subjects, and should be avoided in those with bleeding disorders.

12. Are there any serious side effects to use of a ventilatory stimulant such as doxapram?

    Answer: Yes—central nervous system stimulation to the point of seizures.

CLINICAL SCENARIO

What are the toxic side effects of TCAs, and what class of drugs (and what drug in particular) do they mimic in this regard?

Answer: TCAs act to relieve depression by inhibiting the reuptake of norepinephrine or serotonin at the presynaptic junction in the central nervous system. However, these agents, including amitriptyline, have sedating, vasodilating, and anticholinergic effects. They can depress ventilatory drive and cause hypotension, particularly orthostatic hypotension. Their anticholinergic effects result in tachycardia, dry and warm or hot skin, blurred and unfocussed vision (paralysis of accommodation), mydriasis, increased intraocular pressure, constipation, and possible urinary retention. Confusion or other mental changes may occur. A "quinidine-like" effect can prolong the PR, QRS, and QT intervals. Their anticholinergic effects mimic the action of atropine sulfate, and this can help in understanding the effects of an overdose of TCAs. Note many of these effects in this patient: HR, 140 beats/min; BP, 110/60 mm Hg; pupillary mydriasis; very warm and dry skin; T, 39° C; absent bowel sounds; and prolonged PR and QRS intervals.

How is TCA overdose typically treated?

Answer: Instillation of activated charcoal slurry, in this case via the nasograstric tube, can reverse absorption of the drug from the gastrointestinal tract. Blood pressure is maintained with intravenous fluids. ECG monitoring is needed to detect changes in the P-QRS-T patterns and intervals. In the event of respiratory depression, the airway should be secured by endotracheal intubation to prevent aspiration pneumonitis and to provide for positive-pressure ventilation. Ventilatory support is maintained until the central nervous system depressant effects, particularly respiratory, have decreased, allowing a return to adequate spontaneous ventilation.

Why did the patient awaken and then fall back asleep in between doses of activated charcoal?

Answer: As the charcoal progresses through the gastrointestinal tract and is expelled, a favorable gradient for TCA diffusion from interstitial and adipose tissue to the bloodstream exists, causing a subsequent rise in blood levels of TCA, along with a renewed depressant effect. This continues until levels of TCA in the body are reduced to a sufficiently low level.

What implications does this phenomenon have for respiratory therapists in freeing TCA-overdosed patients from the ventilator? When would it have been deemed safe to extubate this patient?

Answer: Extubation and termination of ventilatory support levels should be delayed until the patient no longer falls asleep before the next dose of charcoal is due. If the patient is able to maintain his level of consciousness and adequate ventilation for over 6 hours, this would indicate a low level of remaining drug. Blood levels of TCA should be checked to determine the success of charcoal treatment, but this is only clinically helpful if the results are available within a few hours of taking the sample.

What did the ABG values on T-piece imply regarding the patient's ventilatory status? Could the patient have been extubated with these particular ABG values? Why or why not?

Answer: Compared with the previous ABG values (pH, 7.43; CO_2, 40 torr), the ABG values on T-piece indicates decreased ventilation (pH, 7.36; CO_2, 48 torr). This trend, coupled with the degree of drowsiness and sedation observed, implies that the levels of TCA have not been reduced sufficiently, and the depressant effects still prevail, jeopardizing adequate ventilation. Extubation at this point would have been premature, because the ABG values indicate a trend of hypoventilation and documents continuing depressant effects of the drug. Extubation with depressed ventilatory drive could then result in respiratory or cardiac arrest.

Was supplemental oxygen ever needed for this patient? Why or why not?

Answer: No. An estimate of his A-aDO_2 before placement on the T-piece shows a gradient of 35 torr on an FIO_2 of 0.35. There is no indication of impaired oxygenation, either by pulmonary history or by clinical signs. With adequate ventilation, gas exchange should be normal in this patient.

APPENDIX B

Units and Systems of Measurement

I. SCIENTIFIC NOTATION

Scientific notation is a method for expressing very large or very small numbers, using a single digit multiplied by a whole number power of 10.

USE OF SCIENTIFIC NOTATION

Place the decimal point of the number to the right of the first non-zero digit.

Multiply the number by 10 raised to a power equal to the number of places moved by the decimal point.

The exponent of 10 is positive for moves to the left and negative for moves to the right.

Large number, for example: 2292.0 is the same as 2.292×10^3

Small number, for example: 0.002292 is the same as 2.292×10^{-3}

II. METRIC SYSTEM

The metric system is based on multiples or fractions of 10.

Prefixes	Scale
Kilo	10^3
Hecto	10^2
Deca	10^1
Base unit	$10^0 = 1$
Deci	10^{-1}
Centi	10^{-2}
Milli	10^{-3}
Micro	10^{-6}
Nano	10^{-9}
Pico	10^{-12}

III. INTERNATIONAL SYSTEM OF UNITS (SI UNITS)

(Systeme International d'Unites)

SI BASE UNITS

Length:	meter, m
Mass:	kilogram, kg
Time:	second, s
Temperature:	kelvin, K
Amount of substance:	mole, mol

SI DERIVED UNITS

Area:	square meter, m^2
Volume:	cubic meter, m^3
Concentration:	mole per cubic meter, mol/m^3

IV. TEMPERATURE SCALES AND CONVERSIONS

Scale	Absolute Zero	Freezing, Water	Boiling, Water
Kelvin	0 degrees	273 degrees	373 degrees
Centigrade	−273 degrees	0 degrees	100 degrees
Fahrenheit	−460 degrees	32 degrees	212 degrees

CONVERSION: CENTIGRADE/KELVIN

To convert from Kelvin to centigrade:

$$\text{Centigrade (degrees)} = \text{Kelvin} - 273$$

To convert from centigrade to Kelvin:

$$\text{Kelvin (degrees)} = \text{Centigrade} + 273$$

CONVERSION: CENTIGRADE/FAHRENHEIT

To convert from Fahrenheit to Centigrade:

$$\text{Centigrade (degrees)} = 0.55 \times (\text{Fahrenheit} - 32)$$

To convert from Centigrade to Fahrenheit:

$$\text{Fahrenheit (degrees)} = (1.8 \times \text{Centigrade}) + 32$$

V. Household Units

Generally, the metric system of measure is used for drug amounts. However, household measures such as teaspoons or tablespoons are used for administering medications in the home environment. For example, a cough syrup may have a label giving a usual adult dose as "1 teaspoon every 6 hours." Household measures are not consistent; for example, a teaspoon may vary from 3 to 5 ml. Although the metric system, which is more exact and consistent with milligrams, micrograms, and milliliters, is recommended in place of household measures, the following equivalences may be helpful. Use of household measures such as teaspoons can be very helpful in discussing amounts of substance with a patient.

1 teaspoon = 5 ml = 60 drops
1 tablespoon = 15 ml (or 3 teaspoons)
1 cup = 240 ml (or 8 fluid ounces)

Recommendations on the Use of Aerosol Generators

I. Use of Traditional Small Volume Nebulizers

Brands of nebulizers can differ considerably in performance capability. The following recommendations are based on average performance capability of disposable *constant-output* small volume nebulizers (SVNs).[1] These specifications may not apply to newer or investigational nebulizers that have greater delivery efficiency.

- **Filling volume:** Minimum of 3 ml; optimum = 5 ml at 10 L/min.
- **Power gas flow rate:** 8 to 10 L/min.
- **Treatment time:** 10 minutes or less.
- **Pattern of inhalation:** Tidal breathing is effective; occasional slow, deep breaths with an inspiratory hold if possible.
- **Inspiratory nebulization:** Power on inspiration only will increase delivery but lengthen treatment time
- **Cleaning:** Rinse after each use to prevent drug concentration; rinse with detergent and distilled water daily, and dry thoroughly.

Cleaning Small Volume Nebulizers

- **After each use:** Rinse the mouthpiece, T-piece, and cup with distilled or sterile water. Tap water is discouraged.[2]
- **Once a day:** Wash the mouthpiece, T-piece, and cup with mild soap and warm water. Rinse with distilled or sterile water and air-dry.
- **Once or twice a week:** Wash with mild soap and warm water, rinse well. Soak in solution of 1 part distilled white vinegar to 2 parts distilled water; do not reuse vinegar solution for later disinfection. Rinse well with warm running distilled or sterile water and air-dry.[3]

II. Use of Metered Dose Inhalers

The following instructions for use of bronchodilator or corticosteroid aerosols with metered dose inhalers (MDIs) are written in terms that may be helpful for patient education. Package inserts on particular agents should always be checked, and these protocols should be modified as needed, especially for other drug classes.

Critical Steps in Metered Dose Inhaler Use[4]

1. Remove cap, inspect for foreign matter, and push the canister into the nozzle receptacle of the mouthpiece actuator.
2. Shake the inhaler, and if not used in 24 hours or more, discharge a priming dose.
3. Exhale to functional residual capacity (easier for subject) or to residual volume.
4. Hold MDI about an inch in front of open mouth or, alternatively, place in mouth with teeth apart and with tongue flat.
5. Begin to breathe in slowly through mouth while actuating inhaler by pressing down on canister. Inspiration should take about 3 to 4 seconds.
6. Continue inhaling to total lung capacity, and hold breath for up to 10 seconds. (Only 1 puff for inhalation.)
7. Exhale normally, shake canister, wait 20 to 30 seconds to allow valve refill, and repeat dose if prescribed.

*NOTE: If you have trouble aiming the MDI at your open mouth, you can place the mouthpiece directly in your mouth and rest it on the lower front teeth without sealing your lips around it. If you find it hard to coordinate breathing and activating the MDI, you may wish to ask your physician to prescribe a reservoir device.

TO INHALE A CORTICOSTEROID

Use the same procedure as above, except for the following:

1. If you use both a bronchodilator and corticosteroid, inhale the bronchodilator first and wait 1 to 2 minutes before inhaling the corticosteroid.
2. Always use an extension or spacer device when inhaling a corticosteroid. If you do not have such a device, try to hyperextend (straighten) your head and neck as much as possible when inhaling (in other words, look at the ceiling).
3. Rinse your mouth and throat with water after finishing.

COMMON ERRORS IN USE

The number of patients using MDIs incorrectly varies from 12% to 89% in studies available.[5]

PRINCIPAL TYPES OF ERRORS

* Failure to coordinate actuation of MDI with inhalation (27%)
* Too short a period of breath-hold after inhalation (26%)
* Too rapid an inspiratory flow rate (19%)
* Inadequate shaking and mixing of MDI contents before use (13%)
* Abrupt cessation of inspiration as aerosol strikes throat (cold Freon effect) (6%)
* Actuation of MDI at total lung capacity (4%)
* Firing of MDI into mouth but inhaling through nose (2%)
* Exhaling during MDI actuation
* Placing wrong end of inhaler in mouth, or holding in wrong (nonvertical) position
* Failure to take cap off before use
* Firing of MDI multiple times during a single inhalation

CLEANING INSTRUCTIONS: METERED DOSE INHALER

Once a day: Remove the canister, and clean the plastic actuator case in warm running water. Thoroughly dry the actuator before reinserting the canister.*

---

*Based on manufacturers' recommendations.

CHECK CANISTER FULLNESS

The best approach is to keep a patient log of use, showing date of initial use and subsequent numbers of actuations each day. If an MDI is used regularly (e.g., 2 actuations 4 times daily), the projected date of depletion can be calculated. For occasional use, tallies at the end of the day on a self-stick note kept in a convenient place, such as the bathroom, can be useful. The use of flotation in water is no longer recommended; it is imprecise, varies with different drugs, and can clog MDI nozzles.

III. USE OF RESERVOIR DEVICES

There is variation in design and use of reservoir devices. The following steps are generic and are intended to describe most reservoir devices for handheld use. Specific brand instructions should be reviewed before use or instruction of patients.

1. Remove protective cap from mouthpiece if found on reservoir; inspect for foreign matter.
2. Assemble if needed for brand being used.
3. Shake MDI well, discharge if not used for more than 24 hours, and insert into reservoir.
   * Some reservoirs (e.g., AeroChamber) accept entire mouthpiece/actuator; others accept only MDI canister nozzle.
4. Exhale normally to functional residual capacity.
5. Place mouth on mouthpiece and close lips.
6. Actuate MDI canister into reservoir. (NOTE: OptiHaler: Begin to inhale, and then actuate MDI into reservoir.)
7. Inhale through mouth (not nose) slowly and deeply to total lung capacity. If flow signal indicator sounds (usually approximately 30 L/min), slow inspiration.
8. Hold breath for 5 to 10 seconds, if possible, and exhale (many units have an exhalation port).
9. Shake canister, wait 20 to 30 seconds, and repeat dose as prescribed.

TIPS ON USE[6-8]

* Inhale simultaneously or right after actuating MDI, to maximize dose.
* Use single inhalation with each MDI actuation. Multiple MDI actuations followed by a single inhalation will reduce dose available.
* Have small children or infants inhale through device for 5 or 6 breaths to maximize emptying of chamber.

COMMON ERRORS IN USE

- Incorrect assembly
- Incorrect (nonvertical) position of MDI canister on reservoir
- Waiting too long to inhale after actuating MDI
- Inhaling too rapidly (may reduce dose?)
- Firing of multiple puffs into reservoir before inhaling
- Firing of puffs from two different MDIs before inhaling
- Failure to take mouthpiece cap off before use

IV. USE OF DRY POWDER INHALERS

Specific instructions for use of the various dry powder inhalers (DPIs) currently available should be reviewed in the package insert before use or patient education.

GENERIC RECOMMENDATIONS THAT APPLY TO ALL OF THE DEVICES

1. Be sure mouthpiece is clear of all foreign matter.
2. Load the powder dose as instructed for the particular inhaler.
3. Exhale normally, *away* from the inhaler (humidity reduces dose).
4. Inhale from mouthpiece forcefully, to total lung capacity.
5. Hold breath up to 10 seconds, if possible.
6. Remove from mouth and exhale away from device.

Manufacturers' recommended use is summarized for the Rotahaler, the Turbuhaler, and the Diskus. As new devices become available in the United States, package inserts can provide instructions on use.

USE OF THE ROTAHALER

1. Check the device for foreign objects in the mouthpiece before use.
2. Turn the Rotahaler vertically, with the darker mouthpiece end down, and turn the upper portion in one direction and then the other, as far as it will go.
3. Insert the clear end of a Ventolin Rotacaps capsule in the raised octagonal hole at the end opposite the mouthpiece, and push in the capsule until it is level with the top of the hole. (If a previously used capsule is in the hole, force the old capsule in with the new one.)

4. Hold the Rotahaler horizontally with the white dot up, and turn the upper portion as far as it will go. This will open the capsule.
5. With the Rotahaler horizontal, breathe out fully away from the mouthpiece, place the mouthpiece in your mouth with teeth apart, and breathe in through your mouth as quickly and deeply as you can.
6. Hold your breath for a few seconds, remove the Rotahaler from your mouth, and then exhale normally.
7. After use, open the device and discard previously used capsule fragments.

Care: Once or twice a week, wash the device with warm water and allow to dry thoroughly before reassembling.

USE OF THE TURBUHALER

1. Remove the cover.
2. Hold the inhaler *upright* and turn base of device completely to the right and then to the left until it clicks.
3. Exhale *away* from inhaler to functional residual capacity or residual volume.
4. Put mouthpiece between lips, holding upright or horizontally.
5. Breathe in forcefully and deeply.
6. Don't exhale; remove inhaler from mouth.
7. Hold breath according to comfort (5 to 10 seconds).
8. Exhale; wait a minimum of 20 to 30 seconds before second inhalation.
9. Rinse mouth with water (for Pulmicort, a steroid).

Before *first* use, prime the Turbuhaler using steps 1 to 3, and then *repeat these steps* for the first dose.

Do not shake the inhaler, nor wash it. When a red mark appears at the window next to the mouthpiece, 20 doses remain.

USE OF THE DISKUS INHALER

1. Push the thumbgrip away from you, to expose the mouthpiece.
2. Hold the Diskus in a level horizontal position, and slide the lever next to the mouthpiece away from you until it clicks.
3. Hold the Diskus level, and exhale *away* from the mouthpiece.

4. Put mouthpiece to lips, and inhale steadily and deeply through Diskus.
5. Remove Diskus from mouth, hold breath for about 10 seconds if possible, and breathe out slowly *away* from device.
6. Close the mouthpiece cover by sliding the thumb-grip back toward you.

Do not wash any part of the device; keep it dry.

REFERENCES

1. Hess D and others: Medication nebulizer performance, *Chest* 110:498, 1996.
2. Clinical Practice Guidelines, *Respir Care* 39:803, 1994; *Respir Care* 41:647, 1996.
3. Clinical Practice Guidelines, *Respir Care* 40:1325, 1995.
4. Kesten S and others: Pharmacist knowledge and ability to use inhaled medication delivery systems, *Chest* 104:1737, 1993.
5. McFadden Jr ER: Improper patient techniques with metered dose inhalers: clinical consequences and solutions to misuse, *J Allergy Clin Immunol* 96:278, 1995.
6. O'Callaghan C, Cant M, Robertson C: Delivery of beclomethasone dipropionate from a spacer device: what dose is available for inhalation? *Thorax* 49:961, 1994.
7. Rau JL, Restrepo RD, Deshpande V: Inhalation of single vs multiple metered-dose bronchodilator actuations from reservoir devices: an in vitro study, *Chest* 109:969, 1996.
8. Fink JB: Aerosol device selection: evidence to practice, *Respir Care* 45:874, 2000.

Pharmacological Management of Asthma and Chronic Obstructive Pulmonary Disease

PHARMACOLOGICAL MANAGEMENT OF ASTHMA

DEFINITION OF ASTHMA

Asthma is a chronic inflammatory disorder of the airways in which many cells and cellular elements play a role, in particular, mast cells, eosinophils, T lymphocytes, macrophages, neutrophils, and epithelial cells. In susceptible individuals, this inflammation causes recurrent episodes of wheezing, breathlessness, chest tightness, and coughing, particularly at night or in the early morning. These episodes are usually associated with widespread but variable airflow obstruction that is often reversible either spontaneously or with treatment. The inflammation also causes an associated increase in the existing bronchial hyperresponsiveness to a variety of stimuli.*

---

*(National Asthma Education and Prevention Program, Expert Panel Report II: *Guidelines for the diagnosis and management of asthma,* Bethesda, Md, 1997, National Institutes of Health, 1997.)

STEPWISE DRUG THERAPY OF ASTHMA FOR ADULTS AND CHILDREN OLDER THAN 5 YEARS

The following table summarizes levels of drug therapy for maintenance of chronic asthma. The complete NAEPP document should be consulted for details on managing asthma.

Goals of Therapy
- Minimal or no chronic symptoms day or night
- Minimal or no episodes
- No limitations on activities; no school/work missed
- PEF $\geq$80% of personal best
- Minimal use of inhaled short-acting β_2 agonist (<1 per day)
- No or minimal adverse effects from medications

SEVERITY	LONG-TERM CONTROL	QUICK-RELIEF
STEP 1: *Mild intermittent* Days with symptoms: ≤2/week Nocturnal symptoms: ≤2/month PEF or FEV_1 ≥80% PEF variability <20%	• None	• Short-acting* **inhaled β_2-agonist** as needed (Use of short-acting inhaled β_2-agonists >2 times/week may indicate the need to initiate long-term control therapy)
STEP 2: *Mild persistent* Days with symptoms: 3-6/week Nocturnal symptoms: 3-4/month PEF or FEV_1 ≥80% PEF variability <20%-30%	• **Inhaled corticosteroid** (low dose) or **cromolyn** or **nedocromil** (children usually begin with trial of cromolyn or nedocromil) • Sustained-release theophylline to serum levels 5-15 μg/ml is an alternative but not preferred therapy • Zafirlukast or zileuton, for ≥12 years; position not fully established in 1997 EPR II Guidelines (montelukast is approved for pediatric use ≥2 years of age, but was not available at time of 1997 Guidelines)	• Short-acting **inhaled β_2-agonists** as needed for symptoms
STEP 3: *Moderate persistent* Days with symptoms: daily Nocturnal symptoms: ≥5/month PEF or FEV_1 60%-80% PEF variability >30%	• **Inhaled corticosteroid** (medium dose) *or* • **Inhaled corticosteroid** (low-medium dose) and either **long-acting inhaled β_2-agonist,** sustained-release theophylline or oral long-acting β_2-agonist tablets • **If needed,** increase medications up to: **inhaled steroid** (medium-high dose) *and* • **Long-acting inhaled β_2-agonist,** sustained-release theophylline, or oral long-acting β_2-agonist tablets	• Short-acting **inhaled β_2-agonists** as needed for symptoms
STEP 4: *Severe persistent* Days with symptoms: continual Nocturnal symptoms: frequent PEF or FEV_1 ≤60% PEF variability >30%	• **Inhaled corticosteroid** (high dose) *and* • **Long-acting inhaled β_2-agonist,** sustained-release theophylline, or oral long-acting β_2-agonist tablets *and* • Corticosteroid tablets or syrup long term Make repeated attempts to reduce oral steroids	• Short-acting **inhaled β_2-agonists** as needed for symptoms

• Preferred treatments are given in **bold** print, based on NAEPP Guidelines.
• Evaluate control of asthma and step up or step down treatment as indicated.
• A rescue course of oral corticosteroid may be needed at times at any step.
EPR, National Asthma Education and Prevention Program, Expert Panel Report II; FEV_1, forced expiratory volume in 1 second; *PEF,* peak expiratory flow.
*Short-acting refers to β_2-agonists such as albuterol, with a duration of 4-6 hours.

STEPWISE THERAPY FOR INFANTS AND CHILDREN 5 YEARS OF AGE OR YOUNGER WITH ACUTE OR CHRONIC ASTHMA SYMPTOMS

The following table summarizes levels of drug therapy for maintenance of asthma. The complete NAEPP document should be consulted for details on managing asthma.

SEVERITY	LONG-TERM CONTROL	QUICK-RELIEF

STEP 1: *Mild intermittent*
 Days with symptoms:
 ≤2/week
 Nocturnal symptoms:
 ≤2/month
	• None	• **Inhaled short-acting β$_2$-agonists** by SVN or MDI/reservoir with face mask, as needed for symptoms <2 times/week
		 or
		 • Oral β$_2$ agonists
		 • With viral respiratory infection:
		  • Bronchodilator q4-6h, up to 24 hours (longer with physician consult), but generally move up to next step if repeated more than once q6wk
		  • Consider systemic corticosteroid if current exacerbation is severe or history of previous severe exacerbations

STEP 2: *Mild persistent* Days with symptoms: 3-6/week Nocturnal symptoms: 3-4/month	**Daily antiinflammatory medication:** • **Cromolyn** (SVN preferred or MDI) or **nedocromil** MDI (usually begin with one of the above two drugs) *or* • **Low-dose inhaled corticosteroid** with reservoir and face mask	• Bronchodilator as needed for symptoms (see Step 1)
STEP 3: *Moderate persistent* Days with symptoms: daily Nocturnal symptoms: ≥5/month	**Daily antiinflammatory medication:** • **Medium-dose inhaled corticosteroid** with reservoir/face mask *or* • Once control is established: medium-dose inhaled corticosteroid and nedocromil *or* • Medium-dose inhaled corticosteroid and long-acting bronchodilator (theophylline)	• Bronchodilator as needed for symptoms (see Step 1) up to 3 times/day
STEP 4: *Severe persistent* Days with symptoms: continual Nocturnal symptoms: frequent	**Daily antiinflammatory medication:** • **High-dose inhaled corticosteroid** with reservoir/mask; if needed, add **systemic corticosteroid** 2 mg/kg/day and reduce to lowest daily or alternate-day dose that stabilizes symptoms	• Bronchodilator as needed for symptoms (see Step 1) up to 3 times/day

In addition to the qualifications given for adult management, the following should be noted:
• There are very few studies on asthma therapy for infants.
• The Guidelines offer a general plan, and not specific prescriptions.
• Consultation with an asthma specialist is recommended for those with moderate or severe persistent asthma in this age-group.
• A course of oral steroids (prednisolone) may be needed at any time and step.
MDI, Metered dose inhaler; *SVN*, small volume nebulizer.

USUAL DOSAGES FOR QUICK-RELIEF MEDICATIONS

DRUG*	DOSAGE FORM	ADULT DOSE	CHILD DOSE
SHORT-ACTING INHALED β_2-AGONISTS			
Albuterol	MDI: 90 μg/puff	2 puffs, 5 min before exercise; 2 puffs tid-qid prn	1-2 puffs 5 min before exercise
Albuterol HFA	MDI: 90 μg/puff		
Albuterol Rotahaler	DPI: 200 μg/capsule	1-2 caps q4-6h as needed and before exercise	1 cap q4-6h as needed and before exercise
Albuterol	SVN: 5 mg/ml (0.5%)	1.25-5 mg (0.25-1 cc) in 2-3 cc of saline q4-8h	0.05 mg/kg (min 1.25 mg, max 2.5 mg) in 2-3 cc of saline q4-6h
Bitolterol	SVN: 2 mg/ml (0.2%)	0.5-3.5 mg (0.25-1 cc) in 2-3 cc of saline q4-8h	Not established
ANTICHOLINERGIC			
Ipratropium	MDI: 18 μg/puff SVN: 0.2 mg/ml (0.02%)	2-3 puffs, q6h 0.25-0.5 mg q6h	1-2 puffs, q6h 0.25 mg
SYSTEMIC CORTICOSTEROIDS			
Methylprednisolone	2, 4, 8, 16, 32 mg tabs	Short course "burst": 40-60 mg/day as single or 2 divided doses for 3-10 days	Short course "burst": 1-2 mg/kg/day, maximum 60 mg/day, for 3-10 days
Prednisolone	5 mg tabs, 5 mg/5cc, 15 mg/5 cc	Short course "burst": 40-60 mg/day as single or 2 divided doses for 3-10 days	Short course "burst": 1-2 mg/kg/day, maximum 60 mg/day, for 3-10 days
Prednisone	1, 2.5, 5, 10, 20, 25 mg tabs; 5 mg/cc, 5 mg/5 cc	Short course "burst": 40-60 mg/day as single or 2 divided doses for 3-10 days	Short course "burst": 1-2 mg/kg/day, maximum 60 mg/day, for 3-10 days

*See NAEPP EPR II Guidelines for complete details and comments on use of these agents in asthma.
DPI, Dry powder inhaler; *MDI,* metered dose inhaler; *SVN,* small volume nebulizer.

USUAL DOSAGES FOR LONG-TERM CONTROL MEDICATIONS

DRUG*	DOSAGE FORM	ADULT DOSE	CHILD DOSE
SYSTEMIC CORTICOSTEROIDS			
Methylprednisolone	2, 4, 8, 16, 32 mg tabs	7.5-60 mg daily in a single dose or qid as needed for control. Short-course "burst": 40-60 mg per day as single or 2 divided doses for 3-10 days	0.25-2 mg/kg daily in single dose or qid as needed for control
Prednisolone	5 mg tabs, 5 mg/cc, 15 mg/cc	7.5-60 mg daily in a single dose or qid as needed for control. Short-course "burst": 40-60 mg per day as single or 2 divided doses for 3-10 days	0.25-2 mg/kg daily in single dose or qid as needed for control
Prednisone	1, 2.5, 5, 10, 20, 25 mg tabs; 5 mg/cc solution	7.5-60 mg daily in a single dose or qid as needed for control. Short-course "burst": 40-60 mg per day as single or 2 divided doses for 3-10 days	Short-course "burst": 1-2 mg/kg/day, maximum 60 mg/day, for 3-10 days
CROMOLYN AND NEDOCROMIL			
Cromolyn	MDI: 1 mg/puff	2-4 puffs tid-qid	1-2 puffs tid-qid
	SVN: 20 mg/ampule	1 ampule tid-qid	1 ampule tid-qid
Nedocromil	MDI: 1.75 mg/puff	2-4 puffs bid-qid	1-2 puffs bid-qid
LONG-ACTING β_2-AGONISTS			
Salmeterol	MDI: 21 μg/puff	2 puffs q12h	1-2 puffs q12h
	DPI: 50 μg/blister	l blister q12h	1 blister q12h
Sustained-release albuterol	Tablet: 4 mg	4 mg q12h	0.3-0.6 mg/kg/day, not to exceed 8 mg/day
METHYLXANTHINES			
Theophylline	Liquids, sustained- release tabs, capsules	Starting dose: 10 mg/kg/day up to 300 mg max; usual max 800 mg/day	Starting dose 10 mg/kg/day; usual max: <1 year of age: 0.2 (age in weeks) + 5 = mg/kg/day ≥1 year of age: 16 mg/kg/day

*See NAEPP EPR II Guidelines for complete details and comments on use of these agents in asthma.
DPI, Dry powder inhaler; *MDI,* metered dose inhaler; *SVN,* small volume nebulizer.

Dosages of Drugs for Asthma Exacerbations in Emergency Medical Care or Hospital

DRUG*	ADULTS	CHILDREN
INHALED SHORT-ACTING β-AGONISTS		
Albuterol		
Nebulizer solution (5 mg/ml)	2.5-5 mg q20min for 3 doses, then 2.5-10 mg q1-4h as needed or 10-15 mg/hr continuously	0.15 mg/kg (min dose 2.5 mg) q20min for 3 doses, then 0.15-0.3 mg/kg up to 10 mg q1-4h as needed, or 0.5 mg/kg/hr by continuous nebulization
Metered dose inhaler (90 μg/puff)	4-8 puffs q20min up to 4 hours, then q1-4h as needed	4-8 puffs q20min for 3 doses, then q1-4h as needed
SYSTEMIC (INJECTED) β$_2$-AGONISTS		
Epinephrine 1:1000 (1 mg/ml)	0.3-0.5 mg q20min for 3 doses SC	0.01 mg/kg up to 0.3-0.5 mg q20min for 3 doses SC
Terbutaline (1 mg/mL)	0.25 mg q20min for 3 doses SC	0.01 mg/kg q20min for 3 doses, then q2-6h SC as needed
ANTICHOLINERGICS		
Ipratropium		
Nebulizer solution (0.2 mg/ml)	0.5 mg q30min for 3 doses, then q2-4h as needed	0.25 mg q20min for 3 doses, then q2-4h
Metered dose inhaler (18 μg/puff)	4-8 puffs as needed	4-8 puffs as needed

*See NAEPP EPR II Guidelines for complete details and comments on use of these agents in asthma.

Management of Asthma Exacerbations: Emergency Department and Hospital-Based Care

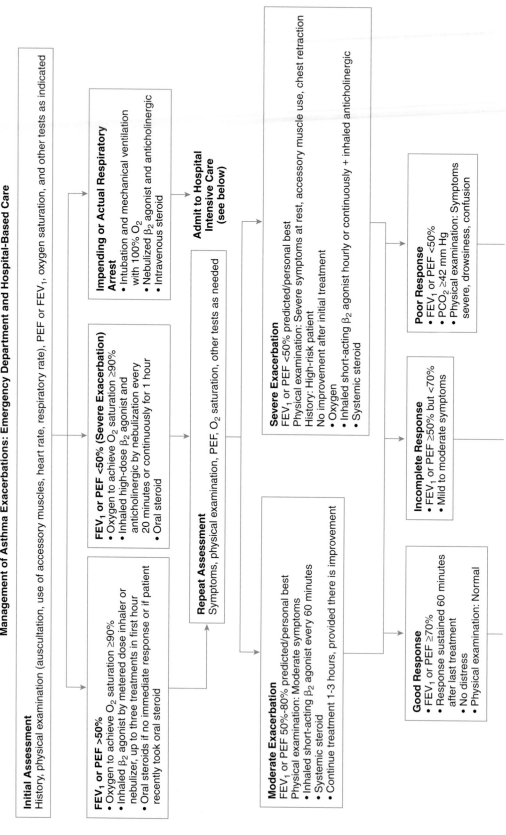

Initial Assessment
History, physical examination (auscultation, use of accessory muscles, heart rate, respiratory rate), PEF or FEV_1, oxygen saturation, and other tests as indicated

FEV_1 or PEF >50%
• Oxygen to achieve O_2 saturation ≥90%
• Inhaled β_2 agonist by metered dose inhaler or nebulizer, up to three treatments in first hour
• Oral steroids if no immediate response or if patient recently took oral steroid

FEV_1 or PEF <50% (Severe Exacerbation)
• Oxygen to achieve O_2 saturation ≥90%
• Inhaled high-dose β_2 agonist and anticholinergic by nebulization every 20 minutes or continuously for 1 hour
• Oral steroid

Impending or Actual Respiratory Arrest
• Intubation and mechanical ventilation with 100% O_2
• Nebulized β_2 agonist and anticholinergic
• Intravenous steroid

Admit to Hospital Intensive Care (see below)

Repeat Assessment
Symptoms, physical examination, PEF, O_2 saturation, other tests as needed

Moderate Exacerbation
FEV_1 or PEF 50%-80% predicted/personal best
Physical examination: Moderate symptoms
• Inhaled short-acting β_2 agonist every 60 minutes
• Systemic steroid
• Continue treatment 1-3 hours, provided there is improvement

Severe Exacerbation
FEV_1 or PEF <50% predicted/personal best
Physical examination: Severe symptoms at rest, accessory muscle use, chest retraction
History: High-risk patient
No improvement after initial treatment
• Oxygen
• Inhaled short-acting β_2 agonist hourly or continuously + inhaled anticholinergic
• Systemic steroid

Good Response
• FEV_1 or PEF ≥70%
• Response sustained 60 minutes after last treatment
• No distress
• Physical examination: Normal

Incomplete Response
• FEV_1 or PEF ≥50% but <70%
• Mild to moderate symptoms

Poor Response
• FEV_1 or PEF <50%
• PCO_2 ≥42 mm Hg
• Physical examination: Symptoms severe, drowsiness, confusion

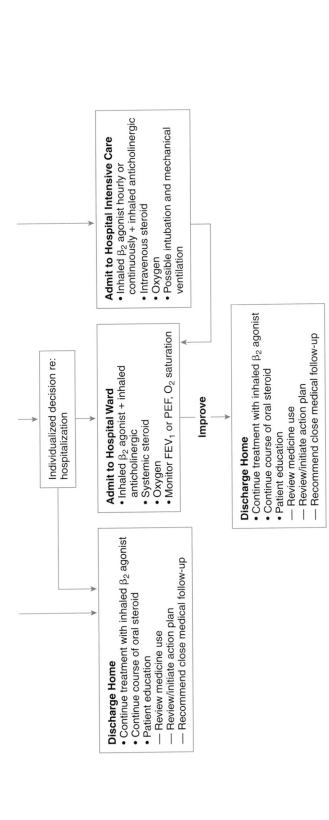

Figure D-1.   Algorithm for management of asthma exacerbations for emergency department and hospital-based care. (From National Asthma Education and Prevention Program, Expert Panel Report II: *Guidelines for the diagnosis and management of asthma*, Bethesda, Md, 1997, National Institutes of Health.)

PHARMACOLOGICAL MANAGEMENT OF CHRONIC OBSTRUCTIVE PULMONARY DISEASE*

DEFINITION OF CHRONIC OBSTRUCTIVE PULMONARY DISEASE

Chronic obstructive pulmonary disease (COPD) is a disease state characterized by airflow limitation that is not fully reversible. The airflow limitation is usually both progressive and associated with an abnormal inflammatory response of the lungs to noxious particles or gases.

CLASSIFICATION OF CHRONIC OBSTRUCTIVE PULMONARY DISEASE BY SEVERITY

STAGE	CHARACTERISTICS
0: At risk	Normal spirometry; chronic symptoms (cough, sputum production)
1: Mild COPD	FEV_1*/FVC <70% FEV_1 ≥80% predicted With or without chronic symptoms (cough, sputum production)
II: Moderate COPD	FEV_1/FVC <70% IIA: 50% ≤FEV_1 <80% predicted IIB: 30% ≤FEV_1<50% predicted With or without chronic symptoms (cough, sputum production, dyspnea)
III: Severe COPD	FEV_1/FVC <70% FEV_1 <30% predicted or FEV_1 <50% predicted plus respiratory failure† or clinical signs of right heart failure

COPD, Chronic obstructive pulmonary disease; *FEV_1,* forced expiratory volume in 1 second; *FVC,* forced vital capacity.
*All FEV_1 values in the GOLD Workshop Report refer to postbronchodilator FEV_1.
†Respiratory failure: PaO_2 less than 8.0 kPa (60 mm Hg) with or without $PaCO_2$ greater than 6.7 kPa (50 mm Hg) while breathing air at sea level.

*From Global Initiative for Chronic Obstructive Lung Disease (GOLD), Workshop Report: *Global strategy for the diagnosis, management, and prevention of COPD,* Bethesda, Md, 2000, National Heart, Lung, and Blood Institute and the World Health Organization.

GOALS OF LONG-TERM MANAGEMENT OF CHRONIC OBSTRUCTIVE PULMONARY DISEASE

- Prevent disease progression
- Relieve symptoms (dyspnea, cough, fatigue)
- Improve exercise tolerance
- Improve health status
- Prevent and treat complications
- Prevent and treat exacerbations
- Reduce mortality

GENERAL MANAGEMENT OF STABLE CHRONIC OBSTRUCTIVE PULMONARY DISEASE

The overall approach to management in stable COPD is a stepwise increase in treatment depending on the severity of the disease.

- Health eduction, including smoking cessation
- Pharmacological management
- Exercise training programs to improve exercise tolerance and reduce symptoms of dyspnea and fatigue
- Long-term oxygen (>15 hours per day) to patients with chronic respiratory failure

PHARMACOLOGICAL TREATMENT OF STABLE CHRONIC OBSTRUCTIVE PULMONARY DISEASE

None of the existing medications for COPD has been shown to modify the long-term decline in lung function. Pharmacological therapy is used to prevent and control symptoms, reduce the frequency and severity of exacerbations, and improve health status and exercise tolerance. The following table summarizes the GOLD guidelines for treatment at each stage of COPD. *The complete GOLD Guidelines should be consulted for more detail in drug management of COPD.*

THERAPY AT EACH STAGE OF CHRONIC OBSTRUCTIVE PULMONARY DISEASE

Patients must be taught how and when to use their treatments, and treatments being prescribed for other conditions should be reviewed. β-Blocking agents (including eye drop formulations) should be avoided.

STAGE	CHARACTERISTIC	RECOMMENDED TREATMENT
All		• Avoidance of risk factor(s) • Influenza vaccination
0: At risk	• Chronic symptoms (cough, sputum) • Exposure to risk factors • Normal spirometry	
I: Mild COPD	• FEV_1/FVC <70% • FEV_1 ≥80% predicted with or without symptoms	• Short-acting bronchodilator when needed
II: Moderate COPD	• FEV_1/FVC <70% • IIA: 50% ≤FEV_1 <80% predicted with or without symptoms • IIB: 30% ≤FEV_1<50% predicted with or without symptoms	• Regular treatment with one or more bronchodilators • Rehabilitation • Inhaled glucocorticoids if significant symptoms and lung function response* • Regular treatment with one or more bronchodilators • Rehabilitation • Inhaled glucocorticoids if significant symptoms and lung function response* or if repeated exacerbations
III: Severe COPD	• FEV_1/FVC <70% • FEV_1<30% predicted or respiratory failure† or clinical signs of right heart failure	• Regular treatment with one or more bronchodilators • Inhaled glucocorticoids if significant symptoms and lung function response* or if repeated exacerbations • Treatment of complications • Rehabilitation • Long-term oxygen therapy if respiratory failure • Consider surgical treatments

COPD, Chronic obstructive pulmonary disease; FEV_1, forced expiratory volume in 1 second; FVC, forced vital capacity.
*Criteria for response: trial of inhaled glucocorticosteroids for 6 weeks to 3 months, with an increase in FEV_1 of 200 ml and 15% of the postbronchodilator response baseline.
†Respiratory failure: PaO_2 less than 8.0 kPa (60 mm Hg) with or without $PaCO_2$ greater than kPa (50 mm Hg) while breathing air at sea level.

The GOLD Guidelines provide the following comments on each class of drug therapy in stable COPD.

Bronchodilators

- Bronchodilator medications are central to symptom management in COPD.
- Inhaled therapy is preferred (theophylline is effective in COPD, but because of potential toxicity, inhaled bronchodilators are preferred when available).
- The choice between β_2-agonist, anticholinergic, theophylline, or combination therapy depends on availability and individual response in terms of symptom relief and side effects.
- Bronchodilators are prescribed on an as-needed or a regular basis to prevent or reduce symptoms.
- Long-acting inhaled bronchodilators are more convenient.
- Combining bronchodilators may improve efficacy and decrease the risk of side effects compared with increasing the dose of a single bronchodilator.

Glucocorticoids

- Regular treatment with inhaled glucocorticosteroids is only appropriate for symptomatic COPD patients with a documented spirometric response to inhaled glucocorticosteroids, or in those with an FEV_1 less than 50% of predicted (Stage IIB: Moderate COPD and Stage III: Severe COPD) and repeated exacerbations requiring treatment with antibiotics or oral glucocorticosteroids.
- Long-term treatment with oral glucocorticosteroids is not recommended in management of stable COPD.

Other Pharmacological Treatments

- **Vaccines:** Influenza vaccines are recommended; pneumococcal vaccine lacks sufficient data to support general use in COPD.
- **α_1-Antitrypsin augmentation therapy:** This therapy is recommended in young patients with severe hereditary α_1-antitrypsin deficiency and established emphysema; not recommended for COPD unrelated to α_1-antitrypsin deficiency.
- **Antibiotics:** Use of antibiotics other than to treat infectious exacerbations and other bacterial infections is not recommended.
- **Mucolytic (mucokinetic and mucoregulator) agents:** A few patients with viscous sputum may

benefit from mucolytics, although overall benefits seem to be small; not recommended for widespread use. This group includes agents such as ambroxol, erdosteine, carbocysteine, iodinated glycerol.

- **Antioxidant agents:** Antioxidants, particularly N-acetylcysteine, have been shown to reduce the frequency of exacerbations and may be useful in patients with recurrent exacerbations. Additional studies needed for recommending in routine treatment.
- **Antitussives:** Regular use of antitussives is contraindicated in stable COPD.
- **Vasodilators:** In stable COPD, inhaled nitric oxide can worsen gas exchange and is contraindicated.
- **Respiratory stimulants:** Use of either intravenous doxapram or almitrine bismesylate is not recommended in stable COPD.
- **Narcotics:** These agents are contraindicated in COPD because of their respiratory depressant effects.
- **Others:** Nedocromil, leukotriene modifiers, or alternative healing methods (e.g., herbal medicine, acupuncture, homeopathy) have not been adequately tested in COPD patients and cannot be recommended at this time.

Management of Exacerbations

The complete GOLD Guidelines should be consulted for more detail in management of COPD exacerbations.

Home Management

The GOLD Guidelines note that when to treat an exacerbation at home and when to hospitalize a patient is a major outstanding issue.

Bronchodilator Therapy

- Increase dose and frequency of existing bronchodilator therapy.
- If not already used, add an anticholinergic agent until symptoms improve.
- High-dose nebulized therapy can be given on an as-needed basis for several days.

Glucocorticosteroids

- Consider if patient's baseline FEV_1 is less than 50% predicted. A dose of prednisolone 40 mg per day for 10 days is recommended.

ANTIBIOTICS

- Only effective when patients with worsening dyspnea and cough have increased sputum volume and purulence. Choice of agents should reflect local patterns of antibiotic sensitivity among *S. pneumoniae, H. inflenzae,* and *M. catarrhalis.*

HOSPITAL MANAGEMENT

- Assess severity of symptoms, blood gases, chest x-ray.
  - If life-threatening (development of respiratory acidosis, significant comorbidities, and the need for ventilatory support), admit directly to ICU.
- Administer controlled oxygen therapy; repeat arterial blood gas measurement after 30 minutes.
- Bronchodilators:
  - Increase doses or frequency.
  - Combine β_2-agonists and anticholinergics.
  - Use spacers or air-driven nebulizers.
  - Consider adding intravenous methylxanthine, if needed.
- Add oral or intravenous glucocorticosteroids.
- Consider antibiotics when signs of bacterial infection (worsening dyspnea, cough, increased sputum volume and purulence); oral or occasionally intravenous.
- Consider noninvasive mechanical ventilation.
- At all times:
  - Monitor fluid balance and nutrition.
  - Consider subcutaneous heparin.
  - Identify and treat associated conditions (e.g., heart failure, arrhythmias).
  - Closely monitor condition of the patient.

OUTCOME MEASURES FOR EVALUATING COPD THERAPY

- Spirometric measure of FEV_1 to evaluate airflow limitation and inhibition of long-term lung function decline seen in COPD.
- Number (decrease in) of exacerbations and hospitalizations.
- Relief of symptoms.
- Improvement in quality of life.
- Increase in performance status.
- Increase in life expectancy.

Modified from Pauwels RA: National and international guidelines for COPD: the need for evidence, *Chest* 117:2[Feb suppl]:20S, 2000.

Glossary of Selected Terms

An eclectic glossary of terms encountered in pharmacology, many from the basic sciences, is offered for convenience in using the text as a study source. This glossary is not intended to substitute for a comprehensive dictionary of medical terms. Selection of terms for inclusion is based on the author's experience in reading the literature of drug actions and effects. Terms that are frequently found or used in discussing drugs but may be less well known to the practicing clinician are included.

Acid A substance that contributes hydrogen ions (protons) in solution.

Strong acid An acid that completely dissociates in aqueous solution.

Weak acid An acid that incompletely dissociates in aqueous solution.

Afferent Toward; in neural control, toward the central nervous system, from the periphery; for example, the sensory neural signal is an afferent impulse.

Allele One of two genes, which contain inheritable characteristics, that are paired together.

Amine A group of compounds related to ammonia (NH_3) by having one or more alkyl groups (methyl, CH_3; ethyl, CH_3CH_2; etc.) attached directly to the nitrogen atom.

Amino acid A molecule with both an amine group and a carboxyl (COOH) group.

Anion An ion with a negative charge, attracted to the anode (positive) terminal.

Apoptosis A disintegration of cells into particles that can be phagocytosed by other cells. This type of cell death is not associated with signs of inflammation and is contrasted with necrosis. Also referred to as *programmed cell death*. See *phagocytosis, phagocyte*.

Autocrine Refers to secretory activity of the cell that influences only the cell itself. See *paracrine*.

Autosomal Refers to an autosome or one of the 22 non-sex chromosomes.

Capsid Protein covering around the central core of a virus particle. Capsid develops from protein units termed *protomers* and protect the nucleic acid in the core of the virus from enzymes in biological fluids; promotes attachment of virus to susceptible cells.

Capsomer Short ribbons of protein that make up a portion of the capsid viral particle. See *capsid*.

Cation An ion with a positive charge, attracted to the cathode (negative) terminal.

Chemokine Chemotactic cytokines that guide leukocytes from blood vessels into the tissues. Different types of leukocytes (e.g., neutrophils, eosinophils) have chemokine receptors that draw the leukocyte to chemokines in the tissues. See *Cytokine*.

Clone A group of genetically identical cells with a common ancestor.

Conjugate A compound resulting from the combination of drug or drug metabolite with a substrate such as glucuronic acid, by means of a catalyzing enzyme (a transferase), to form an inactive drug conjugate; this is usually a polar (water-soluble) molecule and is readily excreted.

Cycloplegia Flattening of the eye lens by paralysis of the ciliary muscle attached to the lens.

Cytokine A protein secreted by a variety of cells such as monocytes or lymphocytes, which regulate and control immune responses, including local and systemic inflammatory responses. Examples are interluekins, interferon, tumor necrosis factor (TNF).

Efferent Away from; in neural control, a nervous impulse from the central nervous system to the periphery; for example, the neuromuscular fiber is an efferent fiber.

Enzyme induction A process by which exposure to a drug induces or increases production of the enzyme responsible for metabolizing the drug.

G protein One of a family of guanine nucleotide binding proteins, on the cytoplasmic face of the cell membrane, that links to receptors and transduces drug or neurotransmitter signals to the cell; it has a trimeric structure, designated as alpha (α), beta (β), or gamma (γ). The α subunit binds guanine nucleotides.

Glycogenolysis Conversion of glycogen (a polysaccharide, starch formed from sugar) into glucose in tissues.

Heme An iron-containing nonprotein portion of the hemoglobin molecule in which the iron is in the ferrous (Fe^{++}) state.

Hemoprotein Any protein combined with heme, a blood pigment.

Heterozygous A combination of a dominant and recessive allele; two different parent genes.

Homozygous Having similar or identical alleles (one of each pair of genes from parents).

Hydrolysis Chemical decomposition in which a substance is split into simpler compounds by the addition of the elements of water; for example, H_2O + salt $\longleftrightarrow$ acid and base.

Hygroscopic A tendency to absorb water.

Ligand In immunology a small molecule bound to another chemical group or molecule.

Lipocyte A fat cell.

Lipolysis The breakdown or decomposition of fat.

Lipophilic Having an affinity for fat or lipids; lipid-soluble.

Lymphokine A cytokine produced by lymphocytes. See *cytokine.*

Miosis A term describing the constriction of the circular iris muscle, causing pupillary contraction.

Mydriasis Describes dilation of the pupil, by constriction of the radial iris muscle.

Neuroeffector site Refers to the terminal site of a nerve fiber; the target site or tissue of a nerve fiber.

Neurotransmitter A chemical, such as acetylcholine or norepinephrine, that is released when the presynaptic neuron of an axon is excited, diffuses across the synapse, and attaches to postsynaptic receptors to transmit the nerve impulse.

Nucleotide A compound of phosphoric acid, a sugar, and a base group, which constitutes the structural unit of nucleic acid, either deoxyribonucleic acid (DNA) or ribonucleic acid (RNA).

Paracrine Refers to the secretion of a hormone from a source other than an endocrine gland; *paracrine control* is a general term referring to a control mechanism by which one cell secretes a substance that acts on nearby cells in the area. See *autocrine.*

Peptide A compound of two or more amino acids; the carboxyl group of one amino acid is linked with the amino group of another, forming a peptide bond, —CO—NH—.

Phagocyte A cell such as the macrophage that can ingest and digest particles such as bacteria or cell debris.

Phagocytosis The process of ingestion and digestion of bacteria and particles by phagocytes.

Phenotype Physical appearance, partially or completely determined by heredity; for example, blood groups.

Polar Having positive and negatively charged sites.

Polypeptide A union of two or more amino acids.

Protein A nitrogenous compound formed by a series of amino acids.

Protonated Having a proton, the positively charged hydrogen ion.

Recessive Not dominant; a gene that is recessive does not express itself when paired with its dominant allele (one of two paired genes); when an individual has identical alleles, whether dominant or recessive, this is described as *homozygous* for the gene. A combination of a dominant and recessive allele is termed *heterozygous.*

Solution Physically homogeneous mixture of two or more substances (liquid).

Isotonic Solutions that have equal osmotic pressures.

Buffer Solution; an aqueous solution able to resist changes of pH with addition of acid/base.

Normal One gram–equivalent weight of solute per liter of solution.

Molar One mole of solute per liter of solution.

Molal One mole of solute per 1000 g of solvent.

Osmolar One osmole per liter of solution.

Osmolal One osmole per kilogram of solvent.

Substrate The substance acted upon by an enzyme.

Tachykinin A family of small peptide mediators that stimulate a variety of neurokinin receptors on target membranes. Examples are neurokinin A or substance P.

Index

A page number followed by b indicates a
box; a page number followed by f indicates an illustration, and a page number
followed by t indicates a table.